55,000+
Baby
Names

by Bruce Lansky

Meadowbrook Press

Distributed by Simon & Schuster
New York

Library of Congress Cataloging-in-Publication Data

Lansky, Bruce.
  55,000+ baby names / by Bruce Lansky.
    p. cm.
  ISBN 0-88166-504-5 (Meadowbrook Press) ISBN 0-684-03724-6 (Simon & Schuster)
  1. Names, Personal--Dictionaries. I. Title: Fifty-five thousand plus baby names. II. Title.
  CS2377.L3543 2005
  929.4'4'03--dc22   2005018344

Editorial Director: Christine Zuchora-Walske
Editors: Megan McGinnis, Angela Wiechmann
Editorial Assistants: Andrea Patch, Maureen Burns
Production Manager: Paul Woods
Graphic Design Manager: Tamara Peterson
Researcher and Translator: David Rochelero
Researcher: Kelsey Anderson
Data Programmer: Sean Beaton
Cover Art: © Corbis, © Getty Images, Inc.

© 2005 by Bruce Lansky

ISBN 13: 978-0-684-03724-X
ISBN 10: 0-684-03724-6

Published by:
Meadowbrook Press • 5451 Smetana Drive • Minnetonka, MN • 55343

www.meadowbrookpress.com

BOOK TRADE DISTRIBUTION by Simon and Schuster, a division of Simon and Schuster, Inc., 1230 Avenue of the Americas, New York, New York 10020

09 08 07 06   10 9 8 7 6 5 4 3 2

Printed in the United States of America

Contents

Introduction

Searching for just the right name for your baby can be a pleasure if you have just the right book. Let me tell you why I think *55,000+ Baby Names* is the right book.

It contains the most names—complete with origins, meanings, variations, fascinating facts, and famous namesakes—of any book in its price range. Here you'll find the most names from major ethnic origins, such as:

- Nearly 7,000 American names, many of which African-American families choose for their children

- Over 5,000 names Hispanic families commonly use

- Over 4,000 French names; 9,000 English names; 6,000 Latin names; 4,000 Irish names; and 6,000 Greek names

- Nearly 6,000 Hebrew names; 2,500 Arabic names; and 4,000 German names

- Thousands of Scottish, Welsh, Italian, Russian, Japanese, Chinese, Scandinavian, Polish, Native American, Hawaiian, African, and Hindi names.

But there's more in *55,000+ Baby Names* than just pages and pages of names. There are also over 150 fun, helpful lists that will get you brainstorming names without having to read the book cover to cover. You'll find the most recently available lists of the top 100 girls' and boys' names, and I've also included data to help you compare rankings from the previous year's list. This way, you can see which names are climbing, which are falling, and which are holding steady. To quickly see what's hot and what's not, check out the Big Gains and Big Losses lists. And to quickly find the most popular names in the Girls' Names and Boys' Names sections, look for the special ☆ icon. If you're expecting a double dose of joy, take a look at the lists of the most popular names for twins. Lastly, if you're interested in tracking names over the years or just looking for a timeless name, you'll love the lists of popular names over the last one hundred years.

Want to know what parents in Canada, Australia, Sweden, and Japan are naming their babies? Want to find that perfect name to reflect your heritage? *55,000+ Baby Names* features lists of popular names around the world as well as lists of common and interesting names from many different origins. Want to name your baby after your favorite movie star, religious figure, or locale? Check out the lists featuring names inspired by people, places, and things. These lists will get you thinking about names that have special meaning to you. In fact, don't miss "How to Pick a Name You and Your Baby Will Love." In three simple steps, complete with easy-to-use worksheets, you can select a name that has personal meaning but is also practical. It's the perfect approach for parents who find the idea of reading over 55,000 baby names a bit overwhelming.

55,000+ Baby Names also has an exclusive new feature to help parents make informed choices about names. Recently, naming trends have been heading in less traditional directions. One such trend is to use traditional boys' names for girls and vice versa. Throughout the Girls' Names and Boys' Names sections, you'll find special icons highlighting names that are shared by both genders. The icons will indicate whether a shared name is used mostly for boys BG, used mostly for girls GB, or used about evenly by both genders BG. Some parents want androgynous or gender-jumping names and other parents want names with clear gender identification. Either way, the icons will help you make an informed choice.

As you browse the names with these special icons, you may be surprised to learn that certain names are shared. It's important to keep several factors in mind:

1. The data may include errors. Amanda is listed in the boys' section because records show that 1 out of every 100,000 boys are named Amanda. It's reasonable to think that some boy "Amandas" are simply recording errors, but perhaps some aren't.

2. Names have different roles in different cultures. In the U.S., Andrea is primarily a girls' name, whereas in Italy, it's often used as a boys' name (for example, opera star Andrea Bocelli).

3. This book defines a name by its spelling, not by its pronunciation or meaning. This explains why a name like Julian is listed as a shared name. Julian (pronounced "JOO-lee-en") is a form of Julius, and therefore in the Boys' Names section. Julian (pronounced "Joo-lee-ANN") is a form of Julianne, and therefore in the Girls' Names section. You could argue that these are two different names, but because this book defines a name by its spelling, it treats them as one name.

4. The gender "assignment" of names change—often in surprising ways. For years, Ashley was used often for boys. (Remember Ashley Wilkes in *Gone with the Wind?*) Twenty-five years ago, it was in the top 300 of boys' names. Today it doesn't crack the top 1000, whereas it's the eighth-most-popular name for girls. In 2000, over twice as many boys than girls were named Reese. By 2004, actress Reese Witherspoon had helped those numbers switch places—now nearly twice as many girls than boys are named Reese.

I hope you find this book fun, helpful, and easy to use as you search for just the right name that will help your baby put his or her best foot forward in life.

Bruce Lansky

How to Pick a Name You and Your Baby Will Like

The first edition of *The Best Baby Name Book in the Whole Wide World,* which I wrote back in 1978, had about 10,000 names on 120 pages. So, you could read the introductory material about "15 Things to Consider When You Name Your Baby" and browse all the main listings (and even pause to read the origins, meanings, and variations for names that appealed to you) in a few hours. It's something a couple could even do together.

55,000+ Baby Names, my latest book, has more than 55,000 names on 736 pages. I don't know how long it would take you and your partner to browse all the main listings and pause to read more about your favorites, but it could be a daunting task. If you're up to the challenge, go for it. You'll certainly find your favorite names and discover some new names as well.

But if the idea of wading through a sea of 55,000 names sounds overwhelming, I'd like to propose another method. The method I suggest involves generating lists of names you and your partner love and then narrowing down the lists based on how well the names might work for your baby. It's a fun, easy way to come up with a name that has special meaning but is practical as well. Let's get started.

Step 1: Make a List of Names with Special Meaning

Make a list of names to consider by writing down your answers to the following questions. (You can each make your own list.) These questions are based on the lists starting on page 11. Browse those lists to help you answer the questions and to brainstorm other questions specific to your background, preferences, and experiences.

Popular Names (pages 11–23)

What are your favorite names from the most recent Top 100 lists?
What are your favorite names from the lists of most popular names over the past 100 years?
If any of your relatives' names appear in the popularity lists from previous generations, what are your favorites?

Names around the World (pages 24–36)

What country are your parents or grandparents from? What country are you and your partner from?

If any of your relatives' names appear in the international lists, what are your favorites?

What are your favorite names that are currently popular in other countries?

What language(s) do you speak?

Where did you go on your honeymoon?

Where do you like to vacation?

Where did you conceive?

Impressions Names Make (pages 37–47)

What might your baby's personality be like?

How might your baby look physically?

What impression would you like your baby's name to make about him/her?

Names Inspired by People, Places, and Things (pages 38–66)

Who are your favorite artists?

Who are your favorite athletes?

Who are your favorite musicians?

Who are your favorite movie stars?

Who are your favorite authors?

Who are your favorite fictional, biblical, and mythological characters?

Who are your favorite presidents and military figures?

What are your favorite flowers?

What are your favorite gems?

What are your favorite aspects of nature?

Once you answer these questions, turn to the Girls' Names and Boys' Names sections to find interesting spellings or variations based on the names from your list. (As you flip through the book, you might stumble across a few new names that capture your attention, too.) That will give you a long list of names to consider for the next step.

Step 2: Narrow the List Based on What Will Work Best for Your Baby

Now that you've each created a list based on personal considerations, it's time to narrow them down based on practical considerations. This way, you'll choose a name that works well for you and for your baby. You may love a particular name, but if it doesn't hold up to these basic criteria, your baby probably won't love it. It can be unpleasant going through life with a name that for whatever reason doesn't work for you.

Make enough copies of the table on the following page for each name on your list. Have your partner do the same. Rate each name on twelve factors. Example: Consider popularity for the name Jacob—if you think there might be too many Jacobs in his school, check "too popular." Consider nicknames—if you love Jake, check "appealing." Another example: Consider sound for the name Rafael—if it's music to your ears, check "pleasing." Consider its fit with your last name—if you don't think it goes so well with Abramovitz, check "doesn't fit."

When you've completed the table, add up the score by giving three points for every check in the Positive column, two points for every check in the Neutral column, and one point for every check in the Negative column. Scoring each name might help make the subjective process of selecting a name more objective to you.

(Note: If you're pinched for time, mentally complete the table for each name, keeping track of a rough score. The important part is to narrow the list to your top five boys' and girls' names.)

Name:_____

Factors	Positive	Neutral	Negative
1. Spelling	❏ easy	❏ medium	❏ hard
2. Pronunciation	❏ easy	❏ medium	❏ hard
3. Sound	❏ pleasing	❏ okay	❏ unpleasing
4. Last name	❏ fits well	❏ fits okay	❏ doesn't fit
5. Gender ID	❏ clear	❏ neutral	❏ confusing
6. Nicknames	❏ appealing	❏ okay	❏ unappealing
7. Popularity	❏ not too popular	❏ popular	❏ too popular
8. Uniqueness	❏ not too unique	❏ unique	❏ too unique
9. Impression	❏ positive	❏ okay	❏ negative
10. Namesakes	❏ positive	❏ okay	❏ negative
11. Initials	❏ pleasing	❏ okay	❏ unpleasing
12. Meaning	❏ positive	❏ okay	❏ negative

Final Score:_____

Step 3: Make the Final Choice

List your top five boys' and girls' names in the chart below, and have your partner do the same. It's now time to share the names. If you have names in common, compare your scores; perhaps average them. If you have different names on your lists, swap names and rate them using the same table as before. In the end, you'll have a handful of names that work well for you, your partner, and your baby. Now all you have to do is make the final decision. Good luck!

Mom's Top Five Names

1._____ Mom's Score: ____ Dad's Score: ____

2._____ Mom's Score: ____ Dad's Score: ____

3._____ Mom's Score: ____ Dad's Score: ____

4._____ Mom's Score: ____ Dad's Score: ____

5._____ Mom's Score: ____ Dad's Score: ____

Dad's Top Five Names

1._____ Dad's Score: ____ Mom's Score: ____

2._____ Dad's Score: ____ Mom's Score: ____

3._____ Dad's Score: ____ Mom's Score: ____

4._____ Dad's Score: ____ Mom's Score: ____

5._____ Dad's Score: ____ Mom's Score: ____

The Most Popular Names from 1900 to 2004

The popularity of names, like the length of hemlines and the width of ties, is subject to change every year. The changes become even more noticeable when you think about the changes in name "fashions" over long periods.

Think about the names of your grandparents' generation: Margaret, Shirley, George, Harold. Very few of those names are in the current list of top 100 names. Most names from your parents' generation—Susan, Cheryl, Gary, Ronald—don't make the current list of top 100 names either.

It seems that every decade a new group of names rises in popularity and an old group of names declines. So, when choosing a name for your baby, it's wise to consider whether a name's popularity is rising, declining, or holding steady.

To help you assess name popularity trends, we are presenting the latest top 100 names given to baby boys and girls in the United States. The rankings are derived from a survey of new births nationwide conducted by the Social Security Administration. (Alternate spellings of each name are treated as separate names. For example, Sarah and Sara are ranked separately.) You can see from the data how the names have risen or fallen since the previous year's survey. If you're expecting two bundles of joy, don't miss the lists of most popular names for twins in the U.S. In addition, you can track popularity trends over the years with the lists of top 25 names given to girls and boys in each decade since 1900.

Enjoy the following data, but remember that the popularity issue cuts two ways: 1) Psychologists say a child with a common or popular name seems to have better odds of success in life than a child with an uncommon name. 2) A child whose name is at the top of the popularity poll may not feel as unique and special as a child whose name is less common.

Top 100 Girls' Names
in 2004

2004 Rank	Name	2003 Rank	Rank Change	2004 Rank	Name	2003 Rank	Rank Change
1	Emily	1	-	26	Jasmine	27	+1
2	Emma	2	-	27	Sydney	25	−2
3	Madison	3	-	28	Victoria	22	−6
4	Olivia	5	+1	29	Ella	44	+15
5	Hannah	4	−1	30	Mia	36	+6
6	Abigail	6	-	31	Morgan	29	−2
7	Isabella	11	+4	32	Julia	33	+1
8	Ashley	8	-	33	Kaitlyn	32	−1
9	Samantha	10	+1	34	Rachel	28	−6
10	Elizabeth	9	−1	35	Katherine	35	-
11	Alexis	7	−4	36	Megan	30	−6
12	Sarah	12	-	37	Alexandra	38	+1
13	Grace	13	-	38	Jennifer	31	−7
14	Alyssa	14	-	39	Destiny	37	−2
15	Sophia	20	+5	40	Allison	46	+6
16	Lauren	15	−1	41	Savannah	41	-
17	Brianna	17	-	42	Haley	34	−8
18	Kayla	16	−2	43	Mackenzie	45	+2
19	Natalie	23	+4	44	Brooke	43	−1
20	Anna	21	+1	45	Maria	42	−3
21	Jessica	18	−3	46	Nicole	40	−6
22	Taylor	19	−3	47	Makayla	51	+4
23	Chloe	24	+1	48	Trinity	56	+8
24	Hailey	26	+2	49	Kylie	52	+3
25	Ava	39	+14	50	Kaylee	53	+3

2004 Rank	Name	2003 Rank	Rank Change	2004 Rank	Name	2003 Rank	Rank Change
51	Paige	47	−4	76	Gabriella	77	+1
52	Lily	69	+17	77	Avery	89	+12
53	Faith	50	−3	78	Marissa	95	+17
54	Zoe	57	+3	79	Ariana	85	+6
55	Stephanie	49	−6	80	Audrey	78	−2
56	Jenna	54	−2	81	Jada	79	−2
57	Andrea	61	+4	82	Autumn	75	−7
58	Riley	72	+14	83	Evelyn	88	+5
59	Katelyn	58	−1	84	Jocelyn	87	+3
60	Angelina	71	+11	85	Maya	84	−1
61	Kimberly	64	+3	86	Arianna	86	-
62	Madeline	60	−2	87	Isabel	83	−4
63	Mary	59	−4	88	Amber	74	−14
64	Leah	81	+17	89	Melanie	93	+4
65	Lillian	76	+11	90	Diana	108	+18
66	Michelle	62	−4	91	Danielle	82	−9
67	Amanda	55	−12	92	Sierra	73	−19
68	Sara	65	−3	93	Leslie	91	−2
69	Sofia	97	+28	94	Aaliyah	90	−4
70	Jordan	48	−22	95	Erin	80	−15
71	Alexa	66	−5	96	Amelia	110	+14
72	Rebecca	63	−9	97	Molly	100	+3
73	Gabrielle	67	−6	98	Claire	92	−6
74	Caroline	68	−6	99	Bailey	98	−1
75	Vanessa	70	−5	100	Melissa	96	−4

Top 100 Boys' Names
in 2004

2004 Rank	Name	2003 Rank	Rank Change	2004 Rank	Name	2003 Rank	Rank Change
1	Jacob	1	-	26	Zachary	20	–6
2	Michael	2	-	27	Logan	28	+1
3	Joshua	3	-	28	Jose	30	+2
4	Matthew	4	-	29	Noah	31	+2
5	Ethan	6	+1	30	Justin	26	–4
6	Andrew	5	–1	31	Elijah	37	+6
7	Daniel	8	+1	32	Gabriel	29	–3
8	William	11	+3	33	Caleb	34	+1
9	Joseph	7	–2	34	Kevin	32	–2
10	Christopher	9	–1	35	Austin	33	–2
11	Anthony	10	–1	36	Robert	35	–1
12	Ryan	13	+1	37	Thomas	36	–1
13	Nicholas	12	–1	38	Connor	43	+5
14	David	14	-	39	Evan	44	+5
15	Alexander	16	+1	40	Aidan	39	–1
16	Tyler	15	–1	41	Jack	45	+4
17	James	18	+1	42	Luke	46	+4
18	John	17	–1	43	Jordan	38	–5
19	Dylan	19	-	44	Angel	47	+3
20	Nathan	27	+7	45	Isaiah	50	+5
21	Jonathan	22	+1	46	Isaac	48	+2
22	Brandon	21	–1	47	Jason	42	–5
23	Samuel	23	-	48	Jackson	52	+4
24	Christian	25	+1	49	Hunter	41	–8
25	Benjamin	24	–1	50	Cameron	40	–10

2004 Rank	Name	2003 Rank	Rank Change	2004 Rank	Name	2003 Rank	Rank Change
51	Gavin	51	-	76	Ashton	101	+25
52	Mason	54	+2	77	Steven	70	−7
53	Aaron	49	−4	78	Jeremiah	90	+12
54	Juan	55	+1	79	Timothy	76	−3
55	Kyle	53	−2	80	Chase	87	+7
56	Charles	57	+1	81	Devin	74	−7
57	Luis	60	+3	82	Seth	80	−2
58	Adam	59	+1	83	Jaden	82	−1
59	Brian	58	−1	84	Colin	88	+4
60	Aiden	73	+13	85	Cody	78	−7
61	Eric	56	−5	86	Landon	97	+11
62	Jayden	75	+13	87	Carter	102	+15
63	Alex	62	−1	88	Hayden	84	−4
64	Bryan	64	-	89	Xavier	85	−4
65	Sean	61	−4	90	Wyatt	109	+19
66	Owen	72	+6	91	Dominic	81	−10
67	Lucas	71	+4	92	Richard	86	−6
68	Nathaniel	63	−5	93	Antonio	92	−1
69	Ian	65	−4	94	Jesse	95	+1
70	Jesus	67	−3	95	Blake	79	−16
71	Carlos	66	−5	96	Sebastian	93	−3
72	Adrian	68	−4	97	Miguel	94	−3
73	Diego	83	+10	98	Jake	98	-
74	Julian	77	+3	99	Alejandro	100	+1
75	Cole	69	−6	100	Patrick	91	−9

Big Gains from 2003 to 2004

Big Losses from 2003 to 2004

Girls		Boys		Girls		Boys	
Sofia	+28	Ashton	+25	Jordan	−22	Blake	−16
Diana	+18	Wyatt	+19	Sierra	−19	Cameron	−10
Lily	+17	Carter	+15	Erin	−15	Dominic	−10
Leah	+17	Aiden	+13	Amber	−14	Patrick	−9
Marissa	+17	Jayden	+13	Amanda	−12	Hunter	−8
Ella	+15	Jeremiah	+12	Rebecca	−9	Steven	−7
Ava	+14	Landon	+11	Danielle	−9	Devin	−7
Riley	+14	Diego	+10	Haley	−8	Cody	−7
Amelia	+14	Nathan	+7	Jennifer	−7	Zachary	−6
Avery	+12	Chase	+7	Autumn	−7	Cole	−6

The Most Popular Names for Twins in 2004

Twin Girls	Twin Boys	Twin Girl & Boy
Faith, Hope	Jacob, Joshua	Taylor, Tyler
Madison, Morgan	Matthew, Michael	Emma, Ethan
Mackenzie, Madison	Daniel, David	Natalie, Nathan
Hailey, Hannah	Ethan, Evan	Madison, Matthew
Anna, Emma	Alexander, Andrew	Madison, Mason
Ella, Emma	Nathan, Nicholas	Jada, Jaden
Ashley, Emily	Christian, Christopher	Brianna, Brian
Elizabeth, Katherine	Joseph, Joshua	Alexis, Alexander
Jennifer, Jessica	Andrew, Matthew	Brianna, Brandon
Abigail, Emma	Alexander, Nicholas	Emily, Matthew
Gabriella, Isabella	Isaac, Isaiah	Emma, Jacob
Hannah, Sarah	Jacob, Joseph	Zoe, Zachary
Olivia, Sophia	Jonathan, Joshua	Emily, Ethan
Haley, Hannah	Elijah, Isaiah	
Abigail, Emily	Alexander, Zachary	
Emily, Sarah	James, John	
Faith, Grace	Benjamin, Samuel	
Megan, Morgan	John, William	
Elizabeth, Emily	Joshua, Justin	
Isabella, Sophia	Joshua, Matthew	
Emma, Grace	Alexander, Benjamin	
Grace, Hannah	Hayden, Hunter	
Elizabeth, Emma	Jacob, Matthew	
Isabella, Emma	Jason, Justin	
Isabella, Olivia	Jordan, Justin	

The Most Popular Names through the Decades

Most Popular Names 2000–2004		Most Popular Names 1990–1999	
Girls	**Boys**	**Girls**	**Boys**
Emily	Jacob	Ashley	Michael
Madison	Michael	Jessica	Christopher
Hannah	Joshua	Emily	Matthew
Emma	Matthew	Sarah	Joshua
Ashley	Andrew	Samantha	Jacob
Alexis	Christopher	Brittany	Andrew
Samantha	Joseph	Amanda	Daniel
Sarah	Nicholas	Elizabeth	Nicholas
Abigail	Daniel	Taylor	Tyler
Olivia	William	Megan	Joseph
Elizabeth	Ethan	Stephanie	David
Alyssa	Anthony	Kayla	Brandon
Jessica	Ryan	Lauren	James
Grace	Tyler	Jennifer	John
Lauren	David	Rachel	Ryan
Taylor	John	Hannah	Zachary
Kayla	Alexander	Nicole	Justin
Brianna	James	Amber	Anthony
Isabella	Zachary	Alexis	William
Anna	Brandon	Courtney	Robert
Victoria	Jonathan	Victoria	Jonathan
Sydney	Dylan	Danielle	Kyle
Megan	Justin	Alyssa	Austin
Rachel	Christian	Rebecca	Alexander
Jasmine	Samuel	Jasmine	Kevin

Most Popular Names 1980–1989

Girls	Boys
Jessica	Michael
Jennifer	Christopher
Amanda	Matthew
Ashley	Joshua
Sarah	David
Stephanie	Daniel
Melissa	James
Nicole	Robert
Elizabeth	John
Heather	Joseph
Tiffany	Jason
Michelle	Justin
Amber	Andrew
Megan	Ryan
Rachel	William
Amy	Brian
Lauren	Jonathan
Kimberly	Brandon
Christina	Nicholas
Brittany	Anthony
Crystal	Eric
Rebecca	Adam
Laura	Kevin
Emily	Steven
Danielle	Thomas

Most Popular Names 1970–1979

Girls	Boys
Jennifer	Michael
Amy	Christopher
Melissa	Jason
Michelle	David
Kimberly	James
Lisa	John
Angela	Robert
Heather	Brian
Stephanie	William
Jessica	Matthew
Elizabeth	Daniel
Nicole	Joseph
Rebecca	Kevin
Kelly	Eric
Mary	Jeffrey
Christina	Richard
Amanda	Scott
Sarah	Mark
Laura	Steven
Julie	Timothy
Shannon	Thomas
Christine	Anthony
Tammy	Charles
Karen	Jeremy
Tracy	Joshua

Most Popular Names 1960–1969

Girls	Boys
Lisa	Michael
Mary	David
Karen	John
Susan	James
Kimberly	Robert
Patricia	Mark
Linda	William
Donna	Richard
Michelle	Thomas
Cynthia	Jeffrey
Sandra	Steven
Deborah	Joseph
Pamela	Timothy
Tammy	Kevin
Laura	Scott
Lori	Brian
Elizabeth	Charles
Julie	Daniel
Jennifer	Paul
Brenda	Christopher
Angela	Kenneth
Barbara	Anthony
Debra	Gregory
Sharon	Ronald
Teresa	Donald

Most Popular Names 1950–1959

Girls	Boys
Mary	Michael
Linda	James
Patricia	Robert
Susan	John
Deborah	David
Barbara	William
Debra	Richard
Karen	Thomas
Nancy	Mark
Donna	Charles
Cynthia	Steven
Sandra	Gary
Pamela	Joseph
Sharon	Donald
Kathleen	Ronald
Carol	Kenneth
Diane	Paul
Brenda	Larry
Cheryl	Daniel
Elizabeth	Stephen
Janet	Dennis
Kathy	Timothy
Margaret	Edward
Janice	Jeffrey
Carolyn	George

Most Popular Names
1940–1949

Girls	Boys
Mary	James
Linda	Robert
Barbara	John
Patricia	William
Carol	Richard
Sandra	David
Nancy	Charles
Judith	Thomas
Sharon	Michael
Susan	Ronald
Betty	Larry
Carolyn	Donald
Shirley	Joseph
Margaret	Gary
Karen	George
Donna	Kenneth
Judy	Paul
Kathleen	Edward
Joyce	Jerry
Dorothy	Dennis
Janet	Frank
Diane	Daniel
Elizabeth	Raymond
Janice	Stephen
Joan	Roger

Most Popular Names
1930–1939

Girls	Boys
Mary	Robert
Betty	James
Barbara	John
Shirley	William
Patricia	Richard
Dorothy	Charles
Joan	Donald
Margaret	George
Nancy	Thomas
Helen	Joseph
Carol	David
Joyce	Edward
Doris	Ronald
Ruth	Paul
Virginia	Kenneth
Marilyn	Frank
Elizabeth	Raymond
Jean	Jack
Frances	Harold
Dolores	Billy
Beverly	Gerald
Donna	Walter
Alice	Jerry
Lois	Eugene
Janet	Henry

Most Popular Names
1920–1929

Girls	Boys
Mary	Robert
Dorothy	John
Helen	James
Betty	William
Margaret	Charles
Ruth	George
Virginia	Joseph
Doris	Richard
Mildred	Edward
Elizabeth	Donald
Frances	Thomas
Anna	Frank
Evelyn	Paul
Alice	Harold
Marie	Walter
Jean	Raymond
Shirley	Jack
Barbara	Henry
Irene	Arthur
Marjorie	Kenneth
Lois	Albert
Florence	David
Rose	Harry
Martha	Ralph
Louise	Eugene

Most Popular Names
1910–1919

Girls	Boys
Mary	John
Helen	William
Dorothy	James
Margaret	Robert
Ruth	Joseph
Mildred	George
Anna	Charles
Elizabeth	Edward
Frances	Frank
Marie	Walter
Evelyn	Thomas
Virginia	Henry
Alice	Harold
Florence	Paul
Rose	Raymond
Lillian	Arthur
Irene	Richard
Louise	Albert
Edna	Harry
Gladys	Donald
Catherine	Ralph
Ethel	Louis
Josephine	Clarence
Ruby	Carl
Martha	Fred

Most Popular Names
1900–1909

Girls	Boys
Mary	John
Helen	William
Margaret	James
Anna	George
Ruth	Joseph
Elizabeth	Charles
Dorothy	Robert
Marie	Frank
Mildred	Edward
Alice	Henry
Florence	Walter
Ethel	Thomas
Lillian	Harry
Rose	Arthur
Gladys	Harold
Frances	Albert
Edna	Paul
Grace	Clarence
Catherine	Fred
Hazel	Carl
Irene	Louis
Gertrude	Raymond
Clara	Ralph
Louise	Roy
Edith	Richard

Names around the World

Want to track popularity trends across the globe? Want to give your baby a name that reflects your heritage, language, or favorite travel destination? The following lists feature names with international flair. You'll learn the latest popular names given to baby girls and boys in several countries. Just as the U.S. popularity lists come from data compiled by the Social Security Administration, these international lists come from records kept by similar organizations across the globe. You'll also discover a sampling of interesting names from particular cultural origins. Use those lists to get you thinking, but don't forget that there are thousands more names in the Girls' Names and Boys' Names sections with the origins you're looking for.

The Most Popular Names around the World

Most Popular Names in Austria in 2003

Girls	Boys
Sarah	Lukas
Anna	Florian
Julia	Tobias
Laura	David
Lena	Alexander
Hannah	Fabian
Lisa	Michael
Katharina	Julian
Leonie	Daniel
Vanessa	Simon

Most Popular Names in Belgium in 2003

Girls	Boys
Emma	Thomas
Laura	Lucas
Marie	Noah
Julie	Nathan
Sarah	Maxime
Manon	Hugo
Léa	Louis
Luna	Arthur
Lisa	Robbe
Charlotte	Nicolas
Camille	Simon
Louise	Alexandre
Amber	Romain
Clara	Tom
Lotte	Mohamed

Emilie	Théo
Elise	Robin
Chloé	Antoine
Océane	Milan
Eva	Wout
Jana	Senne
Pauline	Luca
Britt	Victor
Lara	Jonas
Femke	Jelle

Most Popular Names in British Columbia, Canada in 2004

Girls	Boys
Emma	Ethan
Emily	Jacob
Hannah	Matthew
Olivia	Ryan
Madison	Joshua
Sarah	Nathan
Jessica	Benjamin
Ella	Alexander
Grace	Nicholas
Sophia	Owen
Hailey	Daniel
Isabella	Liam
Abigail	Dylan
Megan	Logan
Samantha	Tyler
Lauren	Andrew
Paige	Evan
Ava	Noah
Rachel	William
Ashley	Samuel
Chloe	James
Anna	Connor
Taylor	Lucas
Julia	Adam
Mackenzie	Michael

Most Popular Names in Denmark in 2003

Girls	Boys
Emma	Mikkel
Julie	Frederik
Mathilde	Mathias
Sofia	Mads
Laura	Rasmus
Caroline	Emil
Cecilie	Oliver
Ida	Christian
Sarah	Magnus
Freja	Lucas

Most Popular Names in England/Wales in 2004

Girls	Boys
Emily	Jack
Ellie	Joshua
Jessica	Thomas
Sophie	James
Chloe	Daniel
Lucy	Samuel
Olivia	Oliver
Charlotte	William
Katie	Benjamin
Megan	Joseph
Grace	Harry
Hannah	Matthew
Amy	Lewis
Ella	Ethan
Mia	Luke
Lily	Charlie
Abigail	George
Emma	Callum
Amelia	Alexander
Molly	Mohammed
Lauren	Ryan
Millie	Dylan
Holly	Jacob

Girls	Boys
Leah	Adam
Caitlin	Ben

Most Popular Names in France in 2003

Girls	Boys
Lea	Lucas
Manon	Theo
Emma	Thomas
Chloe	Hugo
Camille	Enzo
Clara	Maxime
Oceane	Clement
Ines	Leo
Sarah	Antoine
Marie	Alexandre
Lucie	Mathis
Anais	Louis
Jade	Quentin
Lisa	Alexis
Mathilde	Romain
Julie	Tom
Laura	Nicolas
Pauline	Nathan
Eva	Baptiste
Maeva	Paul
Marine	Arthur
Lola	Matteo
Justine	Noah
Juliette	Matheo
Celia	Valentin

Most Popular Names in Germany in 2004

Girls	Boys
Marie	Maximilian
Sophie	Alexander
Maria	Paul
Anna, Anne	Leon
Leonie	Lukas/Lucas

Lea(h)	Luca
Laura	Felix
Lena	Jonas
Katharina	Tim
Johanna	David

Most Popular Names in Ireland in 2003

Girls	Boys
Emma	Sean
Sarah	Jack
Aoife	Adam
Ciara	Conor
Katie	James
Sophie	Daniel
Rachel	Michael
Chloe	Cian
Amy	David
Leah	Dylan
Niamh	Luke
Caoimhe	Ryan
Hannah	Aaron
Ella	Thomas
Lauren	Darragh
Megan	Eoin
Kate	Joshua
Rebecca	Ben
Jessica	Patrick
Emily	Oisin
Laura	Shane
Anna	John
Grace	Jamie
Ava	Liam
Ellen	Matthew

Most Popular Names in Japan in 2002

Girls	Boys
Misaki	Shun
Aoi	Takumi
Nanami	Shou

Miu	Ren
Riko	Shouta
Miyu	Souta
Moe	Kaito
Mitsuki	Kenta
Yuuka	Daiki
Rin	Yuu

Most Popular Names in New South Wales, Australia in 2004

Girls	Boys
Emily	Jack
Chloe	Joshua
Olivia	Lachlan
Sophie	Thomas
Jessica	William
Charlotte	James
Ella	Ethan
Isabella	Samuel
Sarah	Daniel
Emma	Ryan
Grace	Benjamin
Mia	Nicholas
Hannah	Matthew
Georgia	Luke
Jasmine	Liam
Lily	Jacob
Amelia	Alexander
Zoe	Riley
Hayley	Dylan
Ruby	Jayden
Madison	Jake
Jade	Harrison
Holly	Oliver
Maddison	Cooper
Alyssa	Max

Most Popular Names in Norway in 2004

Girls	Boys
Emma	Mathias
Julie	Markus
Thea	Martin
Ida	Kristian
Nora	Andreas
Emilie	Jonas
Maria	Tobias
Sara	Daniel
Hanna	Sander
Ingrid	Alexander
Malin	Kristoffer
Tuva	Magnus
Sofie	Adrian
Amalie	Henrik
Anna	Emil
Frida	Elias
Vilde	Fredrik
Andrea	Sebastian
Mia	Sondre
Marte	Thomas
Marie	Oliver
Karoline	Nikolai
Hedda	Jakob
Martine	Mats
Silje	Marius

Most Popular Names in Quebec, Canada in 2004

Girls	Boys
Lea	Samuel
Rosalie	William
Noemie	Alexis
Laurence	Gabriel
Jade	Jeremy
Megane	Xavier
Sarah	Felix
Audrey	Thomas

Girls	Boys
Camille	Antoine
Coralie	Olivier
Megan	Mathis
Ariane	Anthony
Florence	Nathan
Gabrielle	Zachary
Laurie	Nicolas
Oceane	Alexandre
Emilie	Justin
Juliette	Jacob
Chloe	Raphael
Amelie	Vincent
Emy	Benjamin
Maude	Emile
Justine	Mathieu
Alicia	Maxime
Catherine	Simon

Most Popular Names in Scotland in 2004

Girls	Boys
Emma	Lewis
Sophie	Jack
Ellie	James
Amy	Cameron
Chloe	Ryan
Katie	Liam
Erin	Jamie
Emily	Ben
Lucy	Kyle
Hannah	Callum
Rebecca	Matthew
Rachel	Daniel
Abbie	Connor
Lauren	Adam
Megan	Dylan
Aimee	Andrew
Olivia	Aidan
Caitlin	Ross
Leah	Scott
Niamh	Nathan
Sarah	Thomas
Jessica	Kieran
Holly	Alexander
Anna	Aaron
Eilidh	Joshua

Most Popular Names in Spain in 2003

Girls	Boys
Lucia	Alejandro
Maria	Daniel
Paula	Pablo
Laura	David
Marta	Javier
Andrea	Adrian
Alba	Alvaro
Sara	Sergio
Claudia	Carlos
Ana	Hugo
Nerea	Mario
Carla	Jorge
Elena	Diego
Cristina	Ivan
Ainhoa	Raul
Natalia	Manuel
Marina	Miguel
Irene	Antonio
Carmen	Ruben
Nuria	Juan
Julia	Victor
Angela	Marcos
Sofia	Alberto
Rocio	Marc
Sandra	Jesus

Most Popular Names in
Sweden in 2004

Girls	Boys
Emma	William
Maja	Filip
Ida	Oscar
Elin	Lucas
Julia	Erik
Linnéa	Emil
Hanna	Isak
Alva	Alexander
Wilma	Viktor
Klara	Anton
Ebba	Elias
Ella	Simon
Alice	Hugo
Matilda	Gustav
Moa	Albin
Amanda	Axel
Elsa	Jonathan
Sara	Linus
Emilia	Oliver
Tilda	Ludvig
Ellen	Rasmus
Saga	Max
Felicia	Adam
Tindra	Jacob
Emelie	David

Names from around the World

African

Girls	Boys
Afi	Afram
Adia	Axi
Adanna	Bello
Ama	Ekon
Ashanti	Enzi
Batini	Idi
Eshe	Jabari
Fayola	Kayin
Femi	Kitwana
Goma	Kosey
Halla	Kwasi
Imena	Liu
Kameke	Mansa
Kamilah	Moswen
Kia	Mzuzi
Mosi	Nwa
Pita	Nwake
Poni	Ogun
Reta	Ohin
Sharik	Okapi
Siko	Ottah
Tawia	Senwe
Thema	Ulan
Winna	Uzoma
Zina	Zareb

American

Girls	Boys
Abelina	Adarius
Akayla	Buster
Amberlyn	Caden
Betsy	Daevon
Blinda	Dantrell
Coralee	Demarius
Darilynn	Dionte
Doneshia	Jadrien
Emmylou	Jailen
Jaycee	Jamar
Jessalyn	Jareth
Johnessa	Jayce
Karolane	Lashawn
Krystalynn	Lavon
Lakiesha	Montel
Lashana	Mychal
Liza	Reno
Roshawna	Reshawn
Shaniqua	Ryker
Shantel	Tevin
Takayla	Tiger
Tenesha	Treshawn
Teralyn	Tyrees
Trixia	Woody
Tyesha	Ziggy

Arabic

Girls	Boys
Abia	Abdul
Aleah	Ahmad
Cantara	Asad
Emani	Bilal
Fatima	Fadi
Ghada	Fahaad
Habiba	Ferran
Halimah	Ghazi
Imani	Gilad
Jalila	Habib
Kalila	Hadi
Laela	Hakim
Lilith	Hassan
Maja	Imad

Marya	Ismael
Nalia	Jabir
Omaira	Jamaal
Qadira	Mohamed
Rabi	Nadim
Rasha	Omar
Rayya	Rafiq
Samira	Rahul
Shahar	Rashad
Tabina	Samír
Vega	Sayyid

Chinese

Girls	Boys
An	Chen
Bo	Cheung
Chultua	Chi
Hua	Chung
Jun	De
Lee	Dewei
Lian	Fai
Lien	Gan
Lin	Guotin
Ling	Ho
Mani	Hu
Marrim	Jin
Meiying	Keung
Nuwa	Kong
Ping	Lei
Shu	Li
Syá	Liang
Sying	On
Tao	Park
Tu	Po Sin
Ushi	Quon
Xiang	Shing
Xiu Mei	Tung
Yáng	Wing
Yen	Yu

English

Girls	Boys
Addison	Alfie
Ashley	Ashton
Beverly	Baxter
Britany	Blake
Cady	Chip
Chelsea	Cody
Ellen	Dawson
Evelyn	Edward
Hailey	Franklin
Holly	Gordon
Hope	Harry
Janet	Jamison
Jill	Jeffrey
Julie	Jeremy
Leigh	Lane
Maddie	Maxwell
Millicent	Ned
Paige	Parker
Piper	Rodney
Robin	Scott
Sally	Slade
Scarlet	Ted
Shelby	Tucker
Sigourney	Wallace
Twyla	William

French

Girls	Boys
Angelique	Adrien
Annette	Alexandre
Aubrey	Andre
Belle	Antoine
Camille	Christophe
Charlotte	Donatien
Christelle	Edouard
Cosette	François
Desiree	Gage

Estelle	Guillaume
Gabrielle	Henri
Genevieve	Jacques
Juliette	Jean
Jolie	Leroy
Lourdes	Luc
Margaux	Marc
Maribel	Marquis
Michelle	Philippe
Monique	Pierre
Nicole	Quincy
Paris	Remy
Raquel	Russel
Salina	Sebastien
Sydney	Stéphane
Yvonne	Sylvian

German

Girls	Boys
Adelaide	Adler
Amelia	Adolf
Christa	Arnold
Edda	Bernard
Elke	Claus
Elsbeth	Conrad
Emma	Derek
Frederica	Dieter
Giselle	Dustin
Gretchen	Frederick
Heidi	Fritz
Hetta	Gerald
Hilda	Harvey
Ida	Johan
Johana	Karl
Katrina	Lance
Klarise	Louis
Lisele	Milo
Lorelei	Philipp
Margret	Roger
Milia	Roland

Monika	Sigmund
Reynalda	Terrell
Velma	Ulrich
Wanda	Walter

Greek

Girls	Boys
Alexandra	Achilles
Amaryllis	Adonis
Anastasia	Alexis
Athena	Christos
Callista	Cristobal
Daphne	Damian
Delia	Darius
Delphine	Demetris
Eleanora	Elias
Eudora	Feoras
Evangelina	Gaylen
Gaea	Georgios
Helena	Julius
Hermione	Krisopher
Ianthe	Leander
Kalliope	Nicholas
Kassandra	Panos
Maia	Paris
Medea	Petros
Oceana	Rhodes
Odelia	Sebastian
Ophelia	Stefanos
Phoebe	Thanos
Rhea	Urian
Selena	Xander

Hebrew

Girls	Boys
Alia	Aaron
Anais	Abel
Becca	Ahab
Beth	Azriel

Cayla	Benjamin
Deborah	Boaz
Dinah	Caleb
Eliane	Coby
Eliza	Daniel
Hannah	Elijah
Ilisha	Emmanuel
Jana	Ira
Judith	Isaak
Kaela	Jacob
Leeza	Jeremiah
Lena	Michael
Mariam	Nathaniel
Mikala	Noah
Naomi	Oren
Rachael	Raphael
Rebecca	Reuben
Ruth	Seth
Sarah	Tobin
Tirza	Zachariah
Yael	Zachary

Irish

Girls	**Boys**
Aileen	Aidan
Alanna	Brenden
Blaine	Clancy
Breanna	Desmond
Brigit	Donovan
Carlin	Eagan
Colleen	Flynn
Dacia	Garret
Dierdre	Grady
Erin	Keegan
Fallon	Keenan
Ilene	Kevin
Kaitlin	Liam
Keara	Logan
Kelly	Mahon
Kyleigh	Makenzie

Maura	Nevin
Maureen	Nolan
Moira	Owen
Quincy	Phinean
Raleigh	Quinn
Reagan	Reilly
Sinead	Ryan
Sloane	Seamus
Taryn	Sedric

Latin

Girls	**Boys**
Allegra	Amadeus
Aurora	Antony
Beatrice	Austin
Bella	Benedict
Cecily	Bennett
Celeste	Camilo
Deana	Cecil
Felicia	Delfino
Imogene	Dominic
Josalyn	Favian
Karmen	Felix
Laurel	Griffin
Luna	Horacio
Mabel	Hugo
Madonna	Ignatius
Maren	Jerome
Maxine	Jude
Nova	Loren
Olivia	Marius
Paxton	Octavio
Persis	Oliver
Pomona	Quentin
Regina	Roman
Rose	Silas
Sabina	Valentin

Japanese

Girls	Boys
Aiko	Akemi
Aneko	Akira
Dai	Botan
Hachi	Goro
Hoshi	Hiroshi
Ishi	Isas
Jin	Joben
Keiko	Joji
Kioko	Jum
Kumiko	Kaemon
Leiko	Kentaro
Maeko	Masao
Mai	Michio
Mariko	Minoru
Masago	Naoko
Nari	Raiden
Oki	Rei
Raku	Saburo
Ran	Sen
Ruri	Takeo
Seki	Toru
Tazu	Udo
Yasu	Yasuo
Yei	Yóshi
Yoko	Yuki

Native American

Girls	Boys
Aiyana	Ahanu
Cherokee	Anoki
Dakota	Bly
Dena	Delsin
Halona	Demothi
Heta	Elan
Imala	Elsu
Izusa	Etu
Kachina	Hakan
Kanda	Huslu
Kiona	Inteus
Leotie	Istu
Magena	Iye
Netis	Jolon
Nuna	Knoton
Olathe	Lenno
Oneida	Mingan
Sakuna	Motega
Sora	Muraco
Taima	Neka
Tala	Nodin
Utina	Patwin
Wyanet	Sahale
Wyoming	Songan
Yenene	Wingi

Russian

Girls	Boys
Alena	Alexi
Annika	Christoff
Breasha	Dimitri
Duscha	Egor
Galina	Feliks
Irina	Fyodor
Karina	Gena
Katia	Gyorgy
Lelya	Igor
Liolya	Ilya
Marisha	Iosif
Masha	Ivan
Natasha	Kolya
Natalia	Leonid
Nikita	Maxim
Olena	Michail
Orlenda	Panas
Raisa	Pasha
Sasha	Pavel
Shura	Pyotr
Svetlana	Sacha

Tanya	Sergei
Valera	Valerii
Yekaterina	Viktor
Yelena	Vladimir

Scandinavian

Girls	Boys
Anneka	Anders
Birgitte	Burr
Britta	Frans
Carina	Gustaf
Elga	Hadrian
Freja	Halen
Freya	Hilmar
Gala	Kjell
Gerda	Krister
Gunda	Kristofer
Haldana	Lauris
Ingrid	Lennart
Kalle	Lunt
Karena	Mats
Karin	Mikael
Kolina	Nansen
Lena	Niklas
Lusa	Nils
Maija	Per
Malena	Reinhold
Rika	Rikard
Runa	Rolle
Ulla	Steffan
Unn	Torkel
Valma	Valter

Scottish

Girls	Boys
Aili	Adair
Ailsa	Alastair
Ainsley	Angus
Berkley	Boyd

Blair	Bret
Camden	Caelan
Connor	Cameron
Christal	Dougal
Davonna	Duncan
Elspeth	Geordan
Greer	Gregor
Isela	Henderson
Jeana	Ian
Jinny	Kennan
Keita	Kenzie
Kelsea	Lennox
Leslie	Leslie
Maisie	Macaulay
Marjie	Malcolm
Mckenzie	Morgan
Mhairie	Perth
Paisley	Ronald
Rhona	Seumas
Roslyn	Stratton
Tavie	Tavish

Spanish

Girls	Boys
Alejandra	Armando
Benita	Carlos
Clarita	Eduardo
Esmeralda	Enrique
Esperanza	Estéban
Felicia	Felipe
Gracia	Fernando
Isabel	Garcia
Jacinthe	Gerardo
Juana	Heraldo
Lola	Jose
Lucia	Jorge
Madrona	Juan
Marisol	Luis
Marquita	Marcos
Nelia	Mateo

Girls	Boys
Oleda	Pablo
Pilar	Pedro
Reina	Rafael
Rosalinda	Ramón
Rosita	Renaldo
Salvadora	Salvador
Soledad	Santiago
Toya	Tobal
Ynez	Vincinte

Vietnamese

Girls	Boys
Am	Anh
Bian	Antoan
Cai	Binh
Cam	Cadao
Hoa	Cham
Hoai	Duc
Hong	Dinh
Huong	Gia
Kim	Hai
Kima	Hieu
Lan	Hoang
Le	Huy
Mai	Lap
Nu	Minh
Nue	Nam
Ping	Ngai
Tam	Nguyen
Tao	Nien
Thanh	Phuok
Thao	Pin
Thi	Tai
Thuy	Thanh
Tuyen	Thian
Tuyet	Tuan
Xuan	Tuyen

Welsh

Girls	Boys
Bevanne	Bevan
Bronwyn	Bowen
Carys	Broderick
Deryn	Bryce
Enid	Caddock
Glynnis	Cairn
Guinevere	Davis
Gwyneth	Dylan
Idelle	Eoin
Isolde	Gareth
Linette	Gavin
Mab	Griffith
Meghan	Howell
Meredith	Jestin
Olwen	Kynan
Owena	Lewis
Rhiannon	Llewellyn
Rhonda	Lloyd
Ronelle	Maddock
Rowena	Price
Sulwen	Rhett
Teagan	Rhys
Vanora	Tristan
Wenda	Vaughn
Wynne	Wren

The Impressions Names Make

Consciously or unconsciously, we all have private pictures associated with certain names. Jackie could be sophisticated and beautiful, like Jackie Kennedy, or fat and funny, like Jackie Gleason. These pictures come from personal experience as well as from images we absorb from the mass media, and thus they may conflict in interesting ways. The name Charlton strikes many people as a sissified, passive, whiny brat—until they think of Charlton Heston. Marilyn may personify voluptuous femininity—until you think of Marilyn, your neighbor with the ratty bathrobe, curlers, and a cigarette dangling out of her mouth.

Over the years, researchers have been fascinated by this question of the "real" meanings of names and their effects. When asked to stereotype names by age, trustworthiness, attractiveness, sociability, kindness, aggressiveness, popularity, masculinity/femininity, degree of activity or passivity, etc., people actually do tend to agree on each name's characteristics.

So if people think of Mallory as cute and likeable, does that influence a girl named Mallory to become cute and likeable? Experts agree that names don't guarantee instant success or condemn people to certain failure, but they do affect self-images, influence relationships with others, and help (or hinder) success in work and school.

Robert Rosenthal's classic experiment identified what he named the Pygmalion effect: randomly selected children who'd been labeled "intellectual bloomers" actually did bloom. Here's how the Pygmalion effect works with names: Researcher S. Gray Garwood conducted a study on sixth graders in New Orleans. He found that students given names popular with teachers scored higher in skills tests, were better adjusted and more consistent in their self-perceptions, were more realistic in their evaluations of themselves, and more frequently expected that they would attain their goals—even though their goals were more ambitious than ones set by their peers. A research study in San Diego suggested that average essays by Davids, Michaels, Karens, and Lisas got better grades than average essays written by Elmers, Huberts, Adelles, and Berthas. The reason? Teachers expected kids with popular names to do better, and thus they assigned those kids higher grades in a self-fulfilling prophecy.

The Sinrod Marketing Group's International Opinion panel surveyed over 100,000 parents to discover their opinions about names. Results of this poll are presented in *The Baby Name Survey Book* by Bruce Lansky and Barry Sinrod. Their book contains the names people most often associate with hundreds of personal attributes such as intelligent, athletic, attractive, and nice (as well as dumb, klutzy, ugly, and nasty). It also contains personality profiles of over 1,700 common and unusual boys' and girls' names and includes real or fictional famous namesakes who may have influenced people's perception of each name.

What the authors found was that most names have very clear images; some even have multiple images. The following are lists of boys' and girls' names that were found to have particular image associations.

Athletic

Girls	Boys
Bailey	Alex
Billie	Ali
Bobbie	Alonso
Casey	Bart
Chris	Brian
Colleen	Buck
Dena	Chuck
Gabriella	Connor
Jackie	Cooper
Jessie	Daniel
Jill	Derek
Jody	Emmitt
Josie	Hakeem
Katie	Houston
Kelsey	Jake
Lindsay	Jock
Lola	Kareem
Martina	Kevin
Mia	Kirby
Morgan	Lynn
Natalia	Marcus
Nora	Riley
Steffi	Rod
Sue	Terry
Tammy	Trey

Beautiful/Handsome

Girls	Boys
Adrienne	Adam
Ariel	Ahmad
Aurora	Alejandro
Bella	Alonzo
Bonita	Austin
Carmen	Beau
Cassandra	Blake
Catherine	Bo
Danielle	Bryant
Ebony	Chaz
Farrah	Christopher
Genevieve	Clint
Jasmine	Damian
Jewel	David
Kendra	Demetrius
Kiera	Denzel
Lydia	Douglas
Marisa	Grant
Maya	Humphrey
Sarah	Joe
Scarlett	Jude
Simone	Kiefer
Tanya	Mitchell
Tessa	Tevin
Whitney	Vance

Blonde

Girls	Boys
Bambie	Aubrey
Barbie	Austin
Bianca	Bjorn
Blanche	Brett
Brigitte	Bud
Bunny	Chance
Candy	Chick
Daisy	Colin
Dolly	Corbin
Heidi	Dalton
Inga	Dane
Jillian	Dennis
Krystal	Dwayne
Lara	Eric
Lorna	Josh
Madonna	Keith
Marcia	Kerry
Marnie	Kipp
Olivia	Kyle
Randi	Lars
Sally	Leif
Shannon	Louis
Sheila	Martin
Tracy	Olaf
Vanna	Sven

Cute

Girls	Boys
Annie	Andrew
Becca	Antoine
Bobbie	Antonio
Cheryl	Barry
Christy	Benjamin
Deanna	Chick
Debbie	Cory
Dee Dee	Danny
Emily	Eric
Jennifer	Francisco
Jody	Franky
Kari	Jon
Lacie	Kipp
Mallory	Linus
Mandy	Louis
Megan	Matthew
Peggy	Mike
Porsha	Nicholas
Randi	Rene
Serena	Robbie
Shannon	Rory
Shirley	Sonny
Stacy	Stevie
Tammy	Timothy
Trudy	Wade

Friendly		Funny	
Girls	**Boys**	**Girls**	**Boys**
Bernadette	Allen	Dionne	Abbott
Bobbie	Aubrey	Ellen	Ace
Bonnie	Barrett	Erma	Allen
Carol	Bennie	Fanny	Archie
Christy	Bing	Gilda	Artie
Dorothy	Cal	Gillian	Bennie
Elaine	Casper	Jenny	Bobby
Gwen	Cole	Julie	Carson
Joy	Dan	Lucille	Chase
Kathy	Denny	Lucy	Diego
Kenya	Donovan	Maggie	Dudley
Kim	Ed	Marge	Eddie
Lila	Fred	Marsha	Edsel
Marcie	Gary	Maud	Eduardo
Millie	Hakeem	Melinda	Fletcher
Nancy	Jeff	Mickey	Fraser
Nikki	Jerry	Patty	Grady
Opal	Jim	Paula	Jerome
Patricia	Khalil	Rosie	Keenan
Rhoda	Rob	Roxanne	Rochester
Rose	Russ	Sally	Rollie
Ruby	Sandy	Stevie	Roscoe
Sandy	Tony	Sunny	Sid
Vivian	Vinny	Sydney	Tim
Wendy	Wally	Vivian	Vinny

Hippie

Girls and Boys

Angel
Autumn
Baby
Breezy
Crystal
Dawn
Happy
Harmony
Honey
Indigo
Kharma
Love
Lucky
Meadow
Misty
Moon
Passion
Rainbow
River
Serenity
Skye
Sparkle
Sprout
Star
Sunshine

Intelligent

Girls	Boys
Abigail	Adlai
Agatha	Alexander
Alexis	Barton
Barbara	Brock
Dana	Clifford
Daria	Colin
Diana	Dalton
Eleanor	David
Grace	Donovan
Helen	Edward
Jade	Esteban
Jillian	Fraser
Kate	Jefferson
Kaylyn	Jerome
Laura	John
Leah	Kelsey
Lillian	Kenneth
Mackenzie	Merlin
Marcella	Ned
Meredith	Nelson
Meryl	Roderick
Michaela	Samuel
Shauna	Sebastian
Shelley	Tim
Vanessa	Virgil

Nerdy

Boys

Arnie
Barrett
Bernie
Clarence
Clifford
Creighton
Dexter
Egbert
Khalil
Marvin
Mortimer
Myron
Newt
Norman
Sanford
Seymour
Sheldon
Sinclair
Tracy
Truman
Ulysses
Vern
Vladimir
Waldo
Xavier

Old-Fashioned

Girls	Boys
Abigail	Abe
Adelaide	Amos
Adelle	Arthur
Bea	Bertrand
Charlotte	Clarence
Clementine	Cy
Cora	Cyril
Dinah	Dennis
Edith	Erasmus
Elsie	Erskine
Esther	Ezekiel
Eugenia	Giuseppe
Hattie	Grover
Ida	Herbert
Mamie	Herschel
Martha	Jerome
Maureen	Kermit
Meryl	Lloyd
Mildred	Sanford
Nellie	Silas
Prudence	Spencer
Rosalie	Stanley
Thelma	Sven
Verna	Vic
Wilma	Wilfred

Quiet

Girls	Boys
Bernice	Aaron
Beth	Adrian
Cathleen	Angel
Chloe	Benedict
Diana	Bryce
Donna	Carlo
Faith	Curtis
Fawn	Cy
Fay	Douglas
Grace	Gerald
Jocelyn	Gideon
Leona	Jeremiah
Lisa	Jermaine
Lori	Kiefer
Lydia	Kyle
Moira	Riley
Natalia	Robert
Nina	Robin
Rena	Samson
Sheryl	Spencer
Tessa	Toby
Theresa	Tommy
Ursula	Tucker
Violet	Vaughn
Yoko	Virgil

Rich/Wealthy

Girls	Boys
Alexis	Bartholomew
Amanda	Bradley
Ariel	Brock
Blair	Bryce
Chanel	Burke
Chantal	Cameron
Chastity	Carlos
Chelsea	Chet
Christina	Claybourne
Clara	Clinton
Crystal	Colby
Darlene	Colin
Deandra	Corbin
Jewel	Dane
Larissa	Dante
Madison	Dillon
Marina	Frederick
Meredith	Geoffrey
Moira	Hamilton
Porsha	Harper
Rachel	Montgomery
Taryn	Roosevelt
Tiffany	Sterling
Trisha	Winslow
Zsa Zsa	Winthrop

Sexy	Southern	
Girls	**Girls**	**Boys**
Alana	Ada	Ashley
Angie	Alma	Beau
Bambi	Annabel	Bobby
Brooke	Belle	Cletus
Caresse	Carolina	Clint
Cari	Charlotte	Dale
Carmen	Clementine	Earl
Dani	Dixie	Jackson
Desiree	Dolly	Jeb
Donna	Dottie	Jed
Honey	Ellie	Jefferson
Jillian	Georgeanne	Jesse
Kirstie	Georgia	Jethro
Kitty	Jolene	Jimmy
Kyra	LeeAnn	Johnny
Latoya	Luella	Lee
Leah	Mirabel	Luke
Lola	Ophelia	Luther
Marilyn	Patsy	Moses
Marlo	Polly	Otis
Raquel	Priscilla	Peyton
Sabrina	Rosalind	Rhett
Sandra	Scarlet	Robert
Simone	Tara	Roscoe
Zsa Zsa	Winona	Wade

Strong/Tough

Sweet

Boys

Amos
Ben
Brandon
Brock
Bronson
Bruce
Bruno
Cain
Christopher
Clint
Cody
Coleman
Colin
Delbert
Demetrius
Duke
Jed
Judd
Kurt
Nick
Sampson
Stefan
Thor
Vince
Zeb

Girls

Abby
Alyssa
Angela
Betsy
Candy
Cheryl
Cindy
Dana
Desiree
Elise
Ellie
Esther
Heather
Heidi
Kara
Kristi
Laura
Linda
Marjorie
Melinda
Melissa
Olivia
Rose
Shauna
Sue

Trendy

Girls	Boys
Alexia	Adrian
Alia	Alec
Britney	Angelo
Chanel	Bradley
Char	Carson
Delia	Connor
Destiny	Davis
Gwyneth	Dominic
Hannah	Ellery
India	Garrett
Isabella	Harley
Jen	Harper
Julianna	Jefferson
Keely	Kellan
Lane	Levi
Macy	Liam
Madeleine	Neil
Madison	Olaf
Morgan	Omar
Nadia	Orlando
Natalia	Parker
Olivia	Pierce
Paris	Remington
Ricki	Simon
Taylor	Warren

Weird

Girls	Boys
Abra	Abner
Aida	Barton
Annelise	Boris
Athalie	Cosmo
Belicia	Earl
Calla	Edward
Devonna	Ferris
Dianthe	Gaylord
Elvira	Ira
Garland	Jules
Giselle	Maynard
Happy	Mervin
Hestia	Neville
Keiko	Newt
Kyrene	Nolan
Mahalia	Rod
Modesty	Roscoe
Novia	Seth
Opal	Siegfried
Poppy	Sylvester
Rani	Thaddeus
Sapphire	Tristan
Tierney	Vernon
Twyla	Victor
Velvet	Ward

Wimpy

Boys

Antoine
Archibald
Barton
Bernard
Bradford
Burke
Cecil
Cyril
Dalton
Darren
Duane
Edwin
Gaylord
Homer
Horton
Napoleon
Percival
Prescott
Roosevelt
Rupert
Ulysses
Wesley
Winslow
Winthrop
Yale

Names Inspired by People, Places, and Things

What's in a name? Some parents choose names that carry special meaning. They're sports buffs who name their children after legendary athletes, bookworms who name their children after beloved characters, and nature lovers who name their children after the things they see in their favorite vistas. Then again, some people choose names not because they carry personal significance but simply because they fall in love with them. They may not be sports buffs, bookworms, or nature lovers, but they still choose names like Jordan, Bridget, and Willow.

However you approach it, here are several lists of girls' and boys' names inspired by people, places, and things. (To learn more about choosing names with special meaning, check out the "How to Pick a Name You and Your Baby Will Like" feature on page 5.)

Art and Literature

Artists

Male and Female

Andy (Warhol)
Ansel (Adams)
Claude (Monet)
Edgar (Degas)
Edward (Hopper)
Frida (Kahlo)
Henri (Matisse)
Diego (Rivera)
Georgia (O'Keeffe)
Gustav (Klimt)
Jackson (Pollock)
Jasper (Johns)
Leonardo (da Vinci)

Marc (Chagall)
Mary (Cassatt)
Michelangelo (Buonarroti)
Norman (Rockwell)
Pablo (Picasso)
Paul (Cézanne)
Rembrandt (van Rijn)
Robert (Mapplethorpe)
Roy (Lichtenstein)
Salvador (Dali)
Sandro (Botticelli)
Vincent (van Gogh)

Authors

Female	Male
Anne (Tyler)	Ambrose (Bierce)
Barbara (Kingsolver)	Bram (Stoker)
Carolyn (Keene)	Cormac (McCarthy)
Charlotte (Brontë)	Dan (Brown)
Doris (Lessing)	Ernest (Hemingway)
Elizabeth (Barrett Browning)	George (Orwell)
Emily (Dickinson)	Henry David (Thoreau)
Harper (Lee)	Homer
Harriet (Beecher Stowe)	J. D. (Salinger)
Jane (Austen)	Jules (Verne)
Joanne Kathleen (J. K. Rowling)	Leo (Tolstoy)
Judy (Blume)	Lewis (Carroll)
Katherine (Mansfield)	Mario (Puzo)
Louisa (May Alcott)	Nicholas (Sparks)
Lucy Maud (Montgomery)	Oscar (Wilde)
Madeleine (L'Engle)	Ray (Bradbury)
Margaret (Atwood)	Samuel (Clemens)
Marge (Piercy)	Scott (Fitzgerald)
Mary (Shelley)	Stephen (King)
Maya (Angelou)	Tennessee (Williams)
Paula (Danziger)	Tom (Clancy)
Rebecca (Wells)	Truman (Capote)
Sylvia (Plath)	Virgil
Virginia (Woolf)	Walt (Whitman)
Willa (Cather)	William (Faulkner)

Fictional Characters

Female	Male
Anna (Karenina)	Atticus (Finch)
Anne (Shirley)	Billy (Coleman)
Antonia (Shimerda)	Boo (Radley)
Bridget (Jones)	Cyrus (Trask)
Cosette (Valjean)	Edmond (Dantés)
Daisy (Buchanan)	Ethan (Frome)
Dorothea (Brooke)	Frodo (Baggins)
Edna (Pontellier)	Guy (Montag)
Elizabeth (Bennet)	Harry (Potter)
Emma (Woodhouse)	Heathcliff
Hermione (Granger)	Henry (Fleming)
Hester (Prynne)	Holden (Caulfield)
Isabel (Archer)	Huck (Finn)
Jane (Eyre)	Jake (Barnes)
Josephine (March)	Jay (Gatsby)
Juliet (Capulet)	Jean (Valjean)
Junie (B. Jones)	John (Proctor)
Mary (Lennox)	Odysseus
Meg (Murry)	Owen (Meany)
Ophelia	Pip (Philip Pirrip)
Phoebe (Caulfield)	Rhett (Butler)
Pippi (Longstocking)	Robinson (Crusoe)
Scarlett (O'Hara)	Romeo (Montague)
Scout (Finch)	Santiago
Serena (Joy)	Victor (Frankenstein)

History

Presidents	Military Figures
Male	**Female and Male**
Abraham (Lincoln)	Alexander (the Great)
Andrew (Jackson)	Andrew (Johnson)
Bill (Clinton)	Anna (Warner Bailey)
Calvin (Coolidge)	Attila (the Hun)
Chester (Arthur)	Charles (de Gaulle)
Dwight (D. Eisenhower)	Douglas (MacArthur)
Franklin (D. Roosevelt)	Dwight (D. Eisenhower)
George (Washington)	Genghis (Khan)
Gerald (Ford)	George (S. Patton)
Grover (Cleveland)	Ivan (Stepanovich Konev)
Harry (S. Truman)	Jennie (Hodgers)
Herbert (Hoover)	Joan (of Arc)
James (Madison)	Julius (Caesar)
Jimmy (Carter)	Lucy (Brewer)
John (F. Kennedy)	Moshe (Dayan)
Lyndon (B. Johnson)	Napoleon (Bonaparte)
Martin (Van Buren)	Oliver (Cromwell)
Millard (Fillmore)	Omar (Bradley)
Richard (Nixon)	Peter (the Great)
Ronald (Reagan)	Robert (E. Lee)
Rutherford (B. Hayes)	Tecumseh
Thomas (Jefferson)	Ulysses (S. Grant)
Ulysses (S. Grant)	William (Wallace)
Warren (G. Harding)	Winfield (Scott)
Woodrow (Wilson)	Winston (Churchill)

Movies and Music

Country Stars

Female	Male
Alison (Krauss)	Alan (Jackson)
Carolyn Dawn (Johnson)	Billy Ray (Cyrus)
Chely (Wright)	Brad (Paisley)
Crystal (Gayle)	Charley (Pride)
Cyndi (Thomson)	Chet (Atkins)
Dolly (Parton)	Clint (Black)
Faith (Hill)	Darryl (Worley)
Gretchen (Wilson)	Don (Everly)
Jamie (O'Neal)	Garth (Brooks)
Jo Dee (Messina)	Gene (Autry)
Julie (Roberts)	George (Strait)
LeAnn (Rimes)	Hank (Williams)
Loretta (Lynn)	Joe (Nichols)
Martie (Maguire)	Johnny (Cash)
Martina (McBride)	Keith (Urban)
Mary (Chapin Carpenter)	Kenny (Chesney)
Mindy (McCready)	Kix (Brooks)
Natalie (Maines)	Randy (Travis)
Patsy (Cline)	Ronnie (Dunn)
Patty (Loveless)	Tim (McGraw)
Reba (McEntire)	Toby (Keith)
Sara (Evans)	Trace (Adkins)
Shania (Twain)	Vince (Gill)
Tammy (Wynette)	Waylon (Jennings)
Terri (Clark)	Willie (Nelson)

Movie Stars

Female	Male
Angelina (Jolie)	Benicio (Del Toro)
Anjelica (Huston)	Bing (Crosby)
Audrey (Hepburn)	Bruce (Willis)
Betty (Grable)	Cary (Grant)
Cameron (Diaz)	Chevy (Chase)
Catherine (Zeta-Jones)	Clark (Gable)
Cher	Clint (Eastwood)
Drew (Barrymore)	Dustin (Hoffman)
Elizabeth (Taylor)	Harrison (Ford)
Emma (Thompson)	Jack (Nicholson)
Gwyneth (Paltrow)	John (Wayne)
Halle (Berry)	Leonardo (DiCaprio)
Jodie (Foster)	Martin (Sheen)
Julia (Roberts)	Mel (Gibson)
Katharine (Hepburn)	Mickey (Rooney)
Liv (Tyler)	Orlando (Bloom)
Meg (Ryan)	Patrick (Swayze)
Meryl (Streep)	Robert (De Niro)
Michelle (Pfeiffer)	Robin (Williams)
Nicole (Kidman)	Rock (Hudson)
Penelope (Cruz)	Russell (Crowe)
Salma (Hayek)	Sean (Connery)
Sandra (Bullock)	Spencer (Tracy)
Shirley (Temple)	Sylvester (Stallone)
Sissy (Spacek)	Tom (Cruise)

Notorious Celebrity Baby Names

Female and Male

Ahmet Emuukha Rodan (son of Frank and Gail Zappa)
Apple Blythe Alison (daughter of Gwyneth Paltrow and Chris Martin)
Audio Science (son of Shannyn Sossamon and Dallas Clayton)
Coco Riley (daughter of Courteney Cox Arquette and David Arquette)
Daisy Boo (daughter of Jamie and Jools Oliver)
Dweezil (son of Frank and Gail Zappa)
Elijah Bob Patricus Guggi Q (son of Bono and Alison Stewart)
Fifi Trixiebelle (daughter of Paula Yates and Bob Geldof)
Hazel Patricia (daughter of Julia Roberts and Danny Moder)
Heavenly Hirani Tiger Lily (daughter of Paula Yates and Michael Hutchence)
Lourdes Maria Ciccone (daughter of Madonna and Carlos Leon)
Moon Unit (daughter of Frank and Gail Zappa)
Moxie CrimeFighter (daughter of Penn and Emily Jillette)
Peaches Honeyblossom (daughter of Paula Yates and Bob Geldof)
Phinnaeus Walter (son of Julia Roberts and Danny Moder)
Pilot Inspektor (son of Jason Lee and Beth Riesgraf)
Pirate Howsmon (son of Jonathan and Deven Davis)
Poppy Honey (daughter of Jamie and Jools Oliver)
Prince Michael (son of Michael Jackson and Debbie Rowe)
Prince Michael II (son of Michael Jackson)
Rocco (son of Madonna and Guy Ritchie)
Rumer Glenn (daughter of Demi Moore and Bruce Willis)
Scout LaRue (daughter of Demi Moore and Bruce Willis)
Seven Sirius (son of Andre 3000 and Erykah Badu)
Tallulah Belle (daughter of Demi Moore and Bruce Willis)

Opera Composers and Stars

Female and Male

Andrea (Bocelli)
Anne (Sofie von Otter)
Camille (Saint-Saëns)
Danielle (Millet)
Elisabeth (Schwarzkopf)
Floriana (Cavalli)
Georges (Bizet)
Giacomo (Puccini)
Gioacchino (Rossini)
Giuseppe (Campora)
Helga (Dernesch)
Jane (Berbié)
Jeannine (Collard)
José (Carreras)
Kiri (Te Kanawa)
Lucia (Popp)
Luciano (Pavarotti)
Mady (Mesplé)
Margaret (Marshall)
Maria (Callas)
Montserrat (Caballe)
Placido (Domingo)
Renata (Scotto)
Renée (Fleming)
Richard (Wagner)

Pop/Rock Stars

Female	Male
Aaliyah	Alice (Cooper)
Alanis (Morissette)	Axl (Rose)
Alicia (Keys)	B. B. King
Annie (Lennox)	Billy (Joel)
Aretha (Franklin)	Carlos (Santana)
Beyonce (Knowles)	Cat (Stevens)
Britney (Spears)	Don (Henley)
Christina (Aguilera)	Elton (John)
Courtney (Love)	Jack (Johnson)
Dido	Jerry (Garcia)
Fiona (Apple)	Jimi (Hendrix)
Gwen (Stefani)	John (Lennon)
Janet (Jackson)	Justin (Timberlake)
Jennifer (Lopez)	Kurt (Cobain)
Jessica (Simpson)	Marshall ("Eminem" Mathers)
Jewel	Michael (Jackson)
Lauryn (Hill)	Paul (McCartney)
Madonna	Prince
Mariah (Carey)	Ray (Charles)
Melissa (Etheridge)	Ricky (Martin)
Missy (Elliott)	Ringo (Starr)
Natalie (Imbruglia)	Sean ("P. Diddy" Combs)
Norah (Jones)	Steven (Tyler)
Shania (Twain)	Stevie (Wonder)
Whitney (Houston)	Van (Morrison)

Nature and Places

Flowers

Female

Angelica
Calla
Dahlia
Daisy
Fern
Flora
Flower
Holly
Hyacinth
Iris
Jasmine
Laurel
Lavender
Lilac
Lily
Marigold
Pansy
Poppy
Posy
Rose
Sage
Tulip
Verbena
Vine
Violet

Rocks, Gems, Minerals

Female and Male

Beryl
Clay
Coal
Coral
Crystal
Diamond
Esmerelda
Flint
Garnet
Gemma
Goldie
Jade
Jasper
Jewel
Mercury
Mica
Opal
Pearl
Rock
Ruby
Sandy
Sapphire
Steele
Stone
Topaz

Natural Elements

Female	Male
Amber	Ash
Autumn	Branch
Breezy	Bud
Blossom	Burr
Briar	Canyon
Brook	Cliff
Delta	Crag
Gale	Dale
Hailey	Eddy
Heather	Field
Ivy	Ford
Marina	Forest
Rain	Heath
Rainbow	Lake
Savannah	Marsh
Sequoia	Moss
Sierra	Oakes
Skye	Thorne
Star	Ridge
Summer	River
Sunny	Rye
Terra	Rock
Tempest	Stone
Willow	Storm
Windy	Woody

Places

Female	Male
Africa	Afton
Asia	Austin
Augusta	Boston
Brooklyn	Chad
Cheyenne	Cleveland
China	Cuba
Dakota	Dakota
Florence	Dallas
Georgia	Denver
Holland	Diego
India	Indiana
Italia	Israel
Jamaica	Kent
Kenya	Laramie
Lourdes	London
Madison	Montreal
Montana	Nevada
Olympia	Orlando
Paris	Phoenix
Regina	Reno
Savannah	Rhodes
Sydney	Rio
Tijuana	Sydney
Victoria	Tennessee
Vienna	Washington

Religion and Mythology

Biblical Figures	Old Testament Figures
Female	**Male**
Abigail	Abel
Bathsheba	Abraham
Deborah	Adam
Delilah	Cain
Dinah	Caleb
Eden	Daniel
Elizabeth	David
Esther	Eli
Eve	Esau
Hagar	Ezekiel
Hannah	Ezra
Jezebel	Isaac
Joy	Isaiah
Julia	Jacob
Leah	Jeremiah
Maria	Job
Martha	Joel
Mary	Joshua
Miriam	Moses
Naomi	Nemiah
Phoebe	Noah
Rachel	Samson
Rebekah	Samuel
Ruth	Solomon
Sarah	

New Testament Figures	Mythology Figures	
Male	**Female**	**Male**
Agrippa	Aphrodite	Achilles
Andrew	Artemis	Aeolus
Annas	Athena	Ajax
Aquila	Chloe	Apollo
Gabriel	Concordia	Aries
Herod	Daphne	Atlas
James	Diana	Eros
Jesus	Eros	Hector
John	Gaia	Helios
Joseph	Grace	Hercules
Judas	Hebe	Hermes
Jude	Helen	Hyrem
Luke	Hera	Jason
Mark	Hestia	Loki
Matthew	Iris	Mars
Nicolas	Lorelei	Midas
Paul	Luna	Neptune
Peter	Lyssa	Odysseus
Philip	Maia	Orion
Simon	Minerva	Pan
Stephen	Nike	Paris
Thomas	Penelope	Perseus
Timothy	Persephone	Pollux
Titus	Rhea	Thor
Zechariah	Venus	Zeus

Sports

Athletes

Female	Male
Anna (Kournikova)	Andre (Agassi)
Annika (Sorenstam)	Andy (Roddick)
Diana (Taurasi)	Babe (Ruth)
Jackie (Joyner-Kersee)	Bernie (Williams)
Jennie (Finch)	Dale (Earnhardt)
Kerri (Strug)	David (Beckham)
Kristi (Yamaguchi)	Elvis (Stojko)
Florence (Griffith Joyner)	Hulk (Hogan)
Laila (Ali)	Kasey (Kahne)
Lisa (Leslie)	Kobe (Bryant)
Marion (Jones)	Lance (Armstrong)
Martina (Hingis)	Mark (Spitz)
Mary Lou (Retton)	Michael (Jordan)
Mia (Hamm)	Mike (Tyson)
Monica (Seles)	Muhammad (Ali)
Nadia (Comaneci)	Orenthal James ("O. J." Simpson)
Babe (Didrikson Zaharias)	Oscar (De La Hoya)
Oksana (Baiul)	Red (Grange)
Picabo (Street)	Riddick (Bowe)
Rebecca (Lobo)	Rocky (Balboa)
Sarah (Hughes)	Scott (Hamilton)
Serena (Williams)	Tiger (Woods)
Sheryl (Swoopes)	Tony (Hawk)
Steffi (Graf)	Wayne (Gretzky)
Venus (Williams)	Yao (Ming)

Baseball Players

Male

Alex (Rodriguez)
Babe (Ruth)
Barry (Bonds)
Catfish (Hunter)
Cy (Young)
Derek (Jeter)
Dizzy (Dean)
Cal (Ripken, Jr.)
Hank (Aaron)
Ichiro (Suzuki)
Jackie (Robinson)
Ken (Griffey, Jr.)
Kirby (Puckett)
Mark (McGwire)
Mickey (Mantle)
Nolan (Ryan)
Pete (Rose)
Randy (Johnson)
Roger (Clemens)
Rollie (Fingers)
Sammy (Sosa)
Ted (Williams)
Torii (Hunter)
Wade (Boggs)
Willie (Mays)

Basketball Players

Female	Male
Alana (Beard)	Alonzo (Mourning)
Alicia (Thompson)	Anfernee ("Penny" Hardaway)
Chantelle (Anderson)	Bill (Russell)
Coco (Miller)	Carmelo (Anthony)
Dominique (Canty)	Clyde (Drexler)
Ebony (Hoffman)	Dennis (Rodman)
Felicia (Ragland)	Earvin ("Magic" Johnson)
Giuliana (Mendiola)	Isiah (Thomas)
Gwen (Jackson)	Jerry (West)
Jessie (Hicks)	Julius (Erving)
Kaayla (Chones)	Kareem (Abdul-Jabbar)
Katie (Douglas)	Karl (Malone)
Kiesha (Brown)	Kevin (Garnett)
Lisa (Leslie)	Kobe (Bryant)
Lucienne (Berthieu)	Larry (Bird)
Michele (Van Gorp)	Latrell (Sprewell)
Natalie (Williams)	LeBron (James)
Nykesha (Sales)	Michael (Jordan)
Olympia (Scott-Richardson)	Moses (Malone)
Sheryl (Swoopes)	Patrick (Ewing)
Simone (Edwards)	Scottie (Pippen)
Tai (Dillard)	Shaquille (O'Neal)
Tamicha (Jackson)	Spud (Webb)
Tangela (Smith)	Wilt (Chamberlain)
Tari (Phillips)	Yao (Ming)

Football Players

Male
Barry (Sanders)
Bo (Jackson)
Brett (Favre)
Donovan (McNabb)
Carl (Eller)
Dan (Marino)
Deion (Sanders)
Johnny (Unitas)
Eli (Manning)
Emmitt (Smith)
Frank (Gifford)
Jeremy (Shockey)
Jerry (Rice)
Jim (Kelly)
Joe (Montana)
John (Elway)
Ahman (Green)
Peyton (Manning)
Randy (Moss)
Steve (Young)
Tiki (Barber)
Troy (Aikman)
Vince (Lombardi)
William ("The Refrigerator" Perry)
Woody (Hayes)

Golfers

Female	Male
Amy (Alcott)	Arnold (Palmer)
Annika (Sorenstam)	Chi Chi (Rodriguez)
Babe (Didrikson Zaharias)	Claude (Harmon)
Beth (Daniel)	Craig (Stadler)
Betsy (King)	Eldrick ("Tiger" Woods)
Betty (Jameson)	Ernie (Els)
Carol (Mann)	Gene (Littler)
Dinah (Shore)	Greg (Norman)
Donna (Caponi)	Hale (Irwin)
Dottie (Pepper)	Happy (Gilmore)
Hollis (Stacy)	Harvey (Penick)
JoAnne (Carner)	Jack (Nicklaus)
Judy (Rankin)	Jeff (Maggert)
Juli (Inkster)	Jesper (Parnevik)
Karrie (Webb)	Ken (Venturi)
Kathy (Whitworth)	Nick (Price)
Laura (Davies)	Payne (Stewart)
Louise (Suggs)	Phil (Mickelson)
Marlene (Hagge)	Raymond (Floyd)
Michelle (Wie)	Retief (Goosen)
Nancy (Lopez)	Sam (Snead)
Pat (Bradley)	Sergio (Garcia)
Patty (Berg)	Tommy (Bolt)
Sandra (Haynie)	Vijay (Singh)
Se (Ri Pak)	Walter (Hagen)

Race Car Drivers

A. J. (Foyt)
Al (Unser, Jr.)
Ashton (Lewis)
Bill (Elliott)
Bobby (Labonte)
Cole (Trickle)
Dale (Earnhardt)
Danica (Patrick)
Darrell (Waltrip)
Jeff (Gordon)
Jimmie (Johnson)
Jimmy (Spencer)
John (Andretti)
Justin (Ashburn)
Kenny (Irwin)
Kevin (Harvick)
Kyle (Petty)
Mario (Andretti)
Matt (Kenseth)
Richard (Petty)
Ricky (Rudd)
Rusty (Wallace)
Sterling (Marlin)
Terry (Labonte)
Tony (Stewart)

Girls

'Aolani (Hawaiian) heavenly cloud.

'Aulani (Hawaiian) royal messenger.
Lani, Lanie

A GB (American) an initial used as a first name.

Aaleyah (Hebrew) a form of Aliya.
Aalayah, Aalayaha, Aalea, Aaleah, Aaleaha, Aaleeyah, Aaleyiah, Aaleyyah

Aaliah (Hebrew) a form of Aliya.
Aaliaya, Aaliayah

Aalisha (Greek) a form of Alisha.
Aaleasha, Aaliesha

Aaliyah ☆ GB (Hebrew) a form of Aliya.
Aahliyah, Aailiyah, Aailyah, Aalaiya, Aaleah, Aalia, Aalieyha, Aaliya, Aaliyaha, Aaliyha, Aalliah, Aalliyah, Aalyah, Aalyiah

Aaron BG (Hebrew) enlightened. (Arabic) messenger.

Abagail (Hebrew) a form of Abigale.
Abagael, Abagaile, Abagale, Abagayle, Abageal, Abagil, Abaigael, Abaigeal

Abbagail (Hebrew) a form of Abigale.
Abbagale, Abbagayle, Abbegail, Abbegale, Abbegayle

Abbey, Abbie, Abby GB (Hebrew) familiar forms of Abigail.
Aabbee, Abbe, Abbea, Abbeigh, Abbi, Abbye, Abeey, Abey, Abi, Abia, Abie, Aby

Abbigail GB (Hebrew) a form of Abigail.

Abbygail (Hebrew) a form of Abigail.
Abbeygale, Abbygale, Abbygayl, Abbygayle

Abegail (Hebrew) a form of Abigail.
Abegale, Abegaile, Abegayle

Abel BG (Hebrew) breath. (Assyrian) meadow. (German) a short form of Abelard (see Boys' Names).

Abelina (American) a combination of Abbey + Lina.
Abilana, Abilene

Abia (Arabic) great.
Abbia, Abbiah, Abiah, Abya

Abianne (American) a combination of Abbey + Ann.
Abena, Abeni, Abian, Abinaya

Abida (Arabic) worshiper.
Abedah, Abidah

Abigail ★ (Hebrew) father's joy.
Bible: one of the wives of King
David. See also Gail.
*Abagail, Abbagail, Abbey,
Abbiegail, Abbiegayle, Abbigael,
Abbigal, Abbigale, Abbigayl,
Abbigayle, Abbygail, Abegail,
Abgail, Abgale, Abgayle, Abigael,
Abigaile, Abigaill, Abigal,
Abigale, Abigayil, Abigayl,
Abigayle, Abigel, Abigial,
Abugail, Abygail, Avigail*

Abigaíl (Spanish) a form of
Abigail.

Abinaya (American) a form of
Abiann.
*Abenaa, Abenaya, Abinaa,
Abinaiya, Abinayan*

Abira (Hebrew) my strength.
*Abbira, Abeer, Abeerah, Abeir,
Abera, Aberah, Abhira, Abiir, Abir*

Abra (Hebrew) mother of many
nations.
Abree, Abri, Abria

Abria (Hebrew) a form of Abra.
*Abréa, Abrea, Abreia, Abriah,
Abriéa, Abrya*

Abrial (French) open; secure,
protected.
*Abrail, Abreal, Abreale, Abriale,
Abrielle*

Abriana (Italian) a form of Abra.
*Abbrienna, Abbryana, Abreana,
Abreanna, Abreanne, Abreeana,
Abreona, Abreonia, Abriann,
Abrianna, Abriannah, Abrieana,*

*Abrien, Abrienna, Abrienne,
Abrietta, Abrion, Abrionée,
Abrionne, Abriunna, Abryann,
Abryanna, Abryona*

Abrielle (French) a form of
Abrial.
Aabriella, Abriel, Abriell, Abryell

Abrienda (Spanish) opening.

Abril (French) a form of Abrial.
Abrilla, Abrille

Abygail (Hebrew) a form of
Abigail.
Abygael, Abygale, Abygayle

Acacia (Greek) thorny.
Mythology: the acacia tree
symbolizes immortality and
resurrection. See also Casey.
*Acasha, Acatia, Accassia, Acey,
Acie, Akacia, Cacia, Casia, Kasia*

Acalia (Latin) adoptive mother of
Romulus and Remus.

Ada (German) a short form of
Adelaide. (English) prosperous;
happy.
*Adabelle, Adah, Adan, Adaya,
Adda, Auda*

Adabella (Spanish) a
combination of Ada and Bella.

Adah (Hebrew) ornament.
Ada, Addah

Adair **GB** (Greek) a form of
Adara.
Adaire

Adalene (Spanish) a form of Adalia.
Adalane, Adalena, Adalin, Adalina, Adaline, Adalinn, Adalyn, Adalynn, Adalynne, Addalyn, Addalynn

Adalgisa (German) noble hostage.

Adalia (German, Spanish) noble.
Adal, Adala, Adalea, Adaleah, Adalee, Adalene, Adali, Adalie, Adaly, Addal, Addala, Addaly

Adaluz (Spanish) a combination of Ada and Luz.

Adam BG (Phoenician) man; mankind. (Hebrew) earth; of the red earth.

Adama (Phoenician, Hebrew) a form of Adam.

Adamma (Ibo) child of beauty.

Adana (Spanish) a form of Adama.

Adanna (Nigerian) her father's daughter.
Adanya

Adara (Greek) beauty. (Arabic) virgin.
Adair, Adaira, Adaora, Adar, Adarah, Adare, Adaria, Adarra, Adasha, Adauré, Adra

Adaya (American) a form of Ada.
Adaija, Adaijah, Adaja, Adajah, Adayja, Adayjah, Adejah

Addie (Greek, German) a familiar form of Adelaide, Adrienne.
Aday, Adde, Addee, Addey, Addi, Addia, Addy, Ade, Adee, Adei, Adey, Adeye, Adi, Adie, Ady, Atti, Attie, Atty

Addison BG (English) child of Adam.
Addis, Addisen, Addisson, Adison

Addyson (English) a form of Addison.

Adela (English) a short form of Adelaide.
Adelae, Adelia, Adelista, Adella

Adelaide (German) noble and serene. See also Ada, Adela, Adeline, Adelle, Ailis, Delia, Della, Ela, Elke, Heidi.
Adelade, Adelaid, Adelaida, Adelei, Adelheid, Adeliade, Adelka, Aley, Laidey, Laidy

Adele (English) a form of Adelle.
Adel, Adelie, Adile

Adelfa (Spanish) adelfa flower.

Adelina (English) a form of Adeline.
Adalina, Adeleana, Adelena, Adellyna, Adeliana, Adellena, Adileena, Adlena

Adeline (English) a form of Adelaide.
Adaline, Adelaine, Adelin, Adelina, Adelind, Adelita, Adeliya, Adelle, Adelyn, Adelynn, Adelynne, Adilene, Adlin, Adline, Adlyn, Adlynn, Aline

Adelle (German, English) a short form of Adelaide, Adeline.
Adele, Adell

Adelma (Teutonic) protector of the needy.

Adena (Hebrew) noble; adorned.
Adeana, Adeen, Adeena, Aden, Adene, Adenia, Adenna, Adina

Adhara (Arabic) name of a star in the Canis constellation.

Adia (Swahili) gift.
Addia, Adéa, Adea, Adiah

Adila (Arabic) equal.
Adeala, Adeela, Adela, Adelah, Adeola, Adilah, Adileh, Adilia, Adyla

Adilene (English) a form of Adeline.
Adilen, Adileni, Adilenne, Adlen, Adlene

Adina (Hebrew) a form of Adena. See also Dina.
Adeana, Adiana, Adiena, Adinah, Adine, Adinna, Adyna

Adira (Hebrew) strong.
Ader, Adera, Aderah, Aderra, Adhira, Adirah, Adirana

Adison, Adyson (English) forms of Addison, Addyson.
Adis, Adisa, Adisen, Adisynne, Adysen

Aditi (Hindi) unbound. Religion: the mother of the Hindu sun gods.
Adithi, Aditti

Adleigh (Hebrew) my ornament.
Adla, Adleni

Adoncia (Spanish) sweet.

Adonia (Spanish) beautiful.
Adonica, Adonis, Adonna, Adonnica, Adonya

Adora (Latin) beloved. See also Dora.
Adore, Adoree, Adoria

Adoración (Latin) action of venerating the magical gods.

Adra (Arabic) virgin.
Adara

Adreana, Adreanna (Latin) forms of Adrienne.
Adrean, Adreanne, Adreauna, Adreeanna, Adreen, Adreena, Adreeyana, Adrena, Adrene, Adrenea, Adréona, Adreonia, Adreonna

Adria (English) a short form of Adriana, Adriene.
Adrea, Adriani, Adrya

Adriadna (Greek) she who is very holy, who doesn't yield.

Adrian BG (English) a form of Adriane.

Adriana GB (Italian) a form of Adrienne.
Adreiana, Adreinna, Adria

Adriane, Adrianne (English) forms of Adrienne.
Addrian, Adranne, Adria, Adrian, Adreinne, Adriann, Adriayon, Adrion

Adrianna (Italian) a form of Adriana.
Addrianna, Addriyanna, Adriannea, Adriannia, Adrionna

Adrielle (Hebrew) member of God's flock.
Adriel, Adrielli, Adryelle

Adrien, Adriene BG (English) forms of Adrienne.

Adrienna (Italian) a form of Adrienne. See also Edrianna.
Adreana, Adrieanna, Adrieaunna, Adriena, Adrienia, Adriennah, Adrieunna

Adrienne GB (Greek) rich. (Latin) dark. See also Hadriane.
Addie, Adrien, Adriana, Adriane, Adrianna, Adrianne, Adrie, Adrieanne, Adrien, Adrienna, Adriyanna

Adrina (English) a short form of Adriana.
Adrinah, Adrinne

Adriyanna (American) a form of Adrienne.
Adrieyana, Adriyana, Adryan, Adryana, Adryane, Adryanna, Adryanne

Adya (Hindi) Sunday.
Adia

Aerial, Aeriel (Hebrew) forms of Ariel.
Aeriale, Aeriela, Aerielle, Aeril, Aerile, Aeryal

Afi (African) born on Friday.
Affi, Afia, Efi, Efia

Afra (Hebrew) young doe. (Arabic) earth color. See also Aphra.
Affery, Affrey, Affrie, Afraa

Africa (Latin, Greek) sunny; not cold. Geography: one of the seven continents.
Affrica, Afric, Africah, Africaya, Africia, Africiana, Afrika, Aifric

Afrika (Irish) a form of Africa.
Afrikah

Afrodite, Aphrodite (Greek) Mythology: the goddess of love and beauty.
Afrodita

Afton GB (English) from Afton, England.
Aftan, Aftine, Aftinn, Aftyn

Agacia (Greek) kind.

Agalia (Spanish) bright, joy.

Agapita (Greek) she who is beloved and wanted.

Agar (Hebrew) she who fled.

Agate (English) a semiprecious stone.
Aggie

Agatha (Greek) good, kind. Literature: Agatha Christie was a British writer of more than seventy detective novels. See also Gasha.
Agace, Agaisha, Agasha, Agata, Agatah, Agathe, Agathi, Agatka,

Agetha, Aggie, Ágota, Ágotha, Agueda, Atka

Agathe (Greek) a form of Agatha.

Aggie (Greek) a short form of Agatha, Agnes.
Ag, Aggy, Agi

Aglaia (Greek) splendorous one; beautiful; resplendent.

Agnes (Greek) pure. See also Aneesa, Anessa, Anice, Anisha, Ina, Inez, Necha, Nessa, Nessie, Neza, Nyusha, Una, Ynez.
Aganetha, Aggie, Agna, Agne, Agneis, Agnelia, Agnella, Agnés, Agnesa, Agnesca, Agnese, Agnesina, Agness, Agnessa, Agnesse, Agneta, Agneti, Agnetta, Agnies, Agnieszka, Agniya, Agnola, Agnus, Aignéis, Aneska, Anka

Agostina (Spanish) a form of Agustina.
Agostiña

Agripina (Greek) from the Agripa family.

Agüeda (Greek) having many virtues.

Águeda (Spanish) a form of Agatha.

Agustina (Latin) a form of Augustine.

Ahava (Hebrew) beloved.
Ahivia

Ahliya (Hebrew) a form of Aliya.
Ahlai, Ahlaia, Ahlaya, Ahleah, Ahleeyah, Ahley, Ahleya, Ahlia, Ahliah, Ahliyah

Ahmed BG (Swahili) praiseworthy.

Aida (Latin) helpful. (English) a form of Ada.
Aída, Aidah, Aidan, Aide, Aidee

Aidan, Aiden BG (Latin) forms of Aida.

Aidia (Spanish) help.

Aiesha (Swahili, Arabic) a form of Aisha.
Aeisha, Aeshia, Aieshia, Aieysha, Aiiesha

Aiko (Japanese) beloved.

Ailani (Hawaiian) chief.
Aelani, Ailana

Aileen (Scottish) light bearer. (Irish) a form of Helen. See also Eileen.
Ailean, Aileena, Ailen, Ailene, Aili, Ailina, Ailinn, Aillen

Ailén (Mapuche) ember.

Aili (Scottish) a form of Alice. (Finnish) a form of Helen.
Aila, Ailee, Ailey, Ailie, Aily

Ailín (Mapuche) transparent, very clear.

Ailis (Irish) a form of Adelaide.
Ailesh, Ailish, Ailyse, Eilis

Ailsa (Scottish) island dweller. Geography: Ailsa Craig is an island in Scotland.
Ailsha

Ailya (Hebrew) a form of Aliya.
Ailiyah

Aimee (Latin) a form of Amy. (French) loved.
Aime, Aimée, Aimey, Aimi, Aimia, Aimie, Aimy

Ainara (Basque) swallow.

Ainhoa (Basque) allusion to the Virgin Mary.

Ainoa (Basque) she who has fertile soil.

Ainsley 🆎 (Scottish) my own meadow.
Ainslee, Ainsleigh, Ainslie, Ainsly, Ansley, Aynslee, Aynsley, Aynslie

Airiana (English) a form of Ariana, Arianna.
Airana, Airanna, Aireana, Aireanah, Aireanna, Aireona, Aireonna, Aireyonna, Airianna, Airianne, Airiona, Airriana, Airrion, Airryon, Airyana, Airyanna

Airiél (Hebrew) a form of Ariel.
Aieral, Aierel, Aiiryel, Aire, Aireal, Aireale, Aireel, Airel, Airele, Airelle, Airi, Airial, Airiale, Airrel

Aisha (Swahili) life. (Arabic) woman. See also Asha, Asia, Iesha, Isha, Keisha, Yiesha.
Aaisha, Aaishah, Aesha, Aeshah, Aheesha, Aiasha, Aiesha,

Aieshah, Aisa, Aischa, Aish, Aishah, Aisheh, Aishia, Aishiah, Aiysha, Aiyesha, Ayesha, Aysa, Ayse, Aytza

Aislinn, Aislynn (Irish) forms of Ashlyn.
Aishellyn, Aishlinn, Aislee, Aisley, Aislin, Aisling, Aislyn, Aislynne

Aiyana (Native American) forever flowering.
Aiyhana, Aiyona, Aiyonia, Ayana

Aiyanna (Hindi) a form of Ayanna.
Aianna, Aiyannah, Aiyonna, Aiyunna

Aja 🆎 (Hindi) goat.
Ahjah, Aija, Aijah, Ajá, Ajada, Ajah, Ajara, Ajaran, Ajare, Ajaree, Ajha, Ajia

Ajanae (American) a combination of the letter A + Janae.
Ajahnae, Ajahne, Ajana, Ajanaé, Ajane, Ajané, Ajanee, Ajanique, Ajena, Ajenae, Ajené

Ajia (Hindi) a form of Aja.
Aijia, Ajhia, Aji, Ajjia

Akayla (American) a combination of the letter A + Kayla.
Akaela, Akaelia, Akaila, Akailah, Akala, Akaylah, Akaylia

Akeisha (American) a combination of the letter A + Keisha.
Akaesha, Akaisha, Akasha, Akasia, Akeecia, Akeesha, Akeishia, Akeshia, Akisha

Akela (Hawaiian) noble.
Ahkayla, Ahkeelah, Akelah, Akelia, Akeliah, Akeya, Akeyla, Akeylah

Akeria (American) a form of Akira.
Akera, Akerah, Akeri, Akerra, Akerra

Aki (Japanese) born in autumn.
Akeeye

Akia (American) a combination of the letter A + Kia.
Akaja, Akeia, Akeya, Akiá, Akiah, Akiane, Akiaya, Akiea, Akiya, Akiyah, Akya, Akyan, Akyia, Akyiah

Akiko (Japanese) bright light.

Akilah (Arabic) intelligent.
Aikiela, Aikilah, Akeela, Akeelah, Akeila, Akeilah, Akeiyla, Akiela, Akielah, Akila, Akilaih, Akilia, Akilka, Akillah, Akkila, Akyla, Akylah

Akili (Tanzanian) wisdom.

Akina (Japanese) spring flower.

Akira GB (American) a combination of the letter A + Kira.
Akeria, Akiera, Akierra, Akirah, Akire, Akiria, Akirrah, Akyra

Alaina, Alayna (Irish) forms of Alana.
Aalaina, Alainah, Alaine, Alainna, Alainnah, Alane, Alaynah, Alayne, Alaynna, Aleine, Alleyna, Alleynah, Alleyne

Alair (French) a form of Hilary.
Alaira, Ali, Allaire

Alamea (Hawaiian) ripe; precious.

Alameda (Spanish) poplar tree.

Alan BG (Irish) beautiful; peaceful.

Alana (Irish) a form of Alan. (Hawaiian) offering. See also Lana.
Alaana, Alaina, Alanae, Alanah, Alane, Alanea, Alani, Alania, Alanis, Alanna, Alawna, Alayna, Allana, Allanah, Allyn, Alonna

Alandra, Alandria (Spanish) forms of Alexandra, Alexandria.
Alandrea, Alantra, Aleandra, Aleandrea

Alani (Hawaiian) orange tree. (Irish) a form of Alana.
Alaini, Alainie, Alania, Alanie, Alaney, Alannie

Alanna (Irish) a form of Alana.
Alannah

Alanza (Spanish) noble and eager.

Alaysha, Alaysia (American) forms of Alicia.
Alaysh, Alayshia

Alba (Latin) from Alba Longa, an ancient city near Rome, Italy.
Albana, Albani, Albanie, Albany, Albeni, Albina, Albine, Albinia, Albinka

Albert BG (German, French)
noble and bright.

Alberta (German, French) a form
of Albert. See also Auberte,
Bertha, Elberta.
*Albertina, Albertine, Albertyna,
Albertyne, Alverta*

Albreanna (American) a
combination of Alberta +
Breanna (see Breana).
*Albré, Albrea, Albreona,
Albreonna, Albreyon*

Alcina (Greek) strong-minded.
*Alceena, Alcine, Alcinia, Alseena,
Alsinia, Alsyna, Alzina*

Alcira (German) adornment of
nobility.

Alda (German) old; elder.
Aldina, Aldine

Aldana (Spanish) a combination
of Alda and Ana.

Alden BG (English) old; wise
protector.
Aldan, Aldon, Aldyn

Aldina, Aldine (Hebrew) forms
of Alda.
*Aldeana, Aldene, Aldona, Aldyna,
Aldyne*

Aldonsa, Aldonza (Spanish)
nice.

Alea, Aleah (Arabic) high,
exalted. (Persian) God's being.
*Aileah, Aleea, Aleeah, Aleia,
Aleiah, Allea, Alleah, Alleea,
Alleeah*

Aleasha, Aleesha (Greek)
forms of Alisha.
*Aleashae, Aleashea, Aleashia,
Aleassa, Aleeshia*

Alec, Alek BG (Greek) short
forms of Alexander.

Alecia (Greek) a form of Alicia.
*Aalecia, Ahlasia, Aleacia, Aleacya,
Aleasia, Alecea, Aleceea, Aleceia,
Aleciya, Aleciyah, Alecy, Alecya,
Aleeceia, Aleecia, Aleesia,
Aleesiya, Aleicia, Alesha, Alesia,
Allecia, Alleecia*

Aleela (Swahili) she cries.
Aleelah, Alila, Alile

Aleena (Dutch) a form of Aleene.
Ahleena, Aleana, Aleeanna

Aleene (Dutch) alone.
Aleen, Aleena, Alene, Alleen

Aleeya (Hebrew) a form of Aliya.
*Alee, Aleea, Aleeyah, Aleiya,
Aleiyah*

Aleeza (Hebrew) a form of Aliza.
See also Leeza.
Aleiza

Alegria (Spanish) cheerful.
*Aleggra, Alegra, Alegría, Allegra,
Allegria*

Aleisha, Alesha (Greek) forms
of Alecia, Alisha.
*Aleasha, Aleashea, Aleasia,
Aleesha, Aleeshah, Aleeshia,
Aleeshya, Aleisa, Alesa, Alesah,
Aleisha, Aleshia, Aleshya, Alesia,
Alessia*

Alejandra GB (Spanish) a form of Alexandra.
Aleiandra, Alejanda, Alejandr, Alejandrea, Alejandria, Alejandrina, Alejandro

Alejandro BG (Spanish) a form of Alejandra.

Aleka (Hawaiian) a form of Alice.
Aleeka, Alekah

Aleksandra (Greek) a form of Alexandra.
Alecsandra, Aleksasha, Aleksandrija, Aleksandriya

Alena (Russian) a form of Helen.
Alenah, Alene, Alenea, Aleni, Alenia, Alenka, Alenna, Alennah, Alenya, Alyna

Alesia, Alessia (Greek) forms of Alice, Alicia, Alisha.
Alessea, Alesya, Allesia

Alessa (Greek) a form of Alice.
Alessi, Allessa

Alessandra (Italian) a form of Alexandra.
Alesandra, Alesandrea, Alissandra, Alissondra, Allesand, Allessandra

Alessandro BG (Italian) a form of Alexander.

Aleta (Greek) a form of Alida. See also Leta.
Aletta, Alletta

Alethea (Greek) truth.
Alathea, Alathia, Aletea, Aletha, Aletheia, Alethia, Aletia, Alithea, Alithia

Alette (Latin) wing.

Alex BG (Greek) a short form of Alexander, Alexandra.
Aleix, Aleks, Alexe, Alexx, Allex, Allexx

Alexa ☆ GB (Greek) a short form of Alexandra.
Aleixa, Alekia, Aleksa, Aleksha, Aleksi, Alexah, Alexsa, Alexssa, Alexxa, Allexa, Alyxa

Alexander BG (Greek) defender of humankind.

Alexandra ☆ GB (Greek) a form of Alexander. History: the last czarina of Russia. See also Lexia, Lexie, Olesia, Ritsa, Sandra, Sandrine, Sasha, Shura, Sondra, Xandra, Zandra.
Alandra, Alaxandra, Aleczandra, Alejandra, Aleksandra, Alessandra, Alex, Alexa, Alexande, Alexandera, Alexandre, Alexas, Alexi, Alexina, Alexine, Alexis, Alexsandra, Alexius, Alexsis, Alexus, Alexxandra, Alexys, Alexzandra, Alix, Alixandra, Aljexi, Alla, Alyx, Alyxandra, Lexandra

Alexandre BG (Greek) a form of Alexandra.

Alexandrea (Greek) a form of Alexandria.
Alexandreana, Alexandreia, Alexandriea, Alexandrieah, Alexanndrea

Alexandria 🇬🇧 (Greek) a form of Alexandra. See also Drinka, Xandra, Zandra.
Alaxandria, Alecsandria, Aleczandria, Alexanderia, Alexanderine, Alexandrea, Alexandrena, Alexandrie, Alexandrina, Alexandrine, Alexanndria, Alexandrya, Alexendria, Alexendrine, Alexia, Alixandrea, Alyxandria

Alexandrine (Greek) a form of Alexandra.
Alexandrina

Alexanne (American) a combination of Alex + Anne.
Alexan, Alexanna, Alexane, Alexann, Alexanna, Alexian, Alexiana

Alexas, Alexes (Greek) short forms of Alexandra.
Alexess

Alexe 🇬🇧 (Greek) a form of Alex.

Alexi, Alexie 🇬🇧 (Greek) short forms of Alexandra.
Aleksey, Aleksi, Alexey, Alexy

Alexia (Greek) a short form of Alexandria. See also Lexia.
Aleksia, Aleska, Alexcia, Alexea, Alexsia, Alexsiya, Allexia, Alyxia

Alexis ☀ 🇬🇧 (Greek) a short form of Alexandra.
Aalexis, Ahlexis, Alaxis, Alecsis, Alecxis, Aleexis, Aleksis, Alexcis, Alexias, Alexiou, Alexiss, Alexiz, Alexxis, Alixis, Allexis, Elexis, Lexis

Alexius (Greek) a short form of Alexandra.
Allexius

Alexsandra (Greek) a form of Alexandra.
Alexsandria, Alexsandro, Alixsandra

Alexsis, Alexxis (Greek) short forms of Alexandra.
Alexxiz

Alexus 🇬🇧 (Greek) a short form of Alexandra.
Aalexus, Aalexxus, Aelexus, Ahlexus, Alecsus, Alexsus, Alexuss, Alexxus, Alixus, Allexus, Elexus, Lexus

Alexys (Greek) a short form of Alexandra.
Alexsys, Alexyes, Alexyis, Alexyss, Allexys

Alexzandra, Alexzandra (Greek) forms of Alexandra.
Alexzand, Alexzandrea, Alexzandriah, Alexzandrya, Alixzandria

Aleya, Aleyah (Hebrew) forms of Aliya.
Alayah, Aleayah, Aleeya, Aléyah, Aleyia, Aleyiah

Alfa (Greek) symbolizes the beginning of all.

Alfie 🇧🇬 (English) a familiar form of Alfreda.
Alfi, Alfy

Alfonsa (Spanish) noble.

Alfonsina (German) noble and ready for battle.

Alfreda (English) elf counselor; wise counselor. See also Effie, Elfrida, Freda, Frederica.
Alfie, Alfredda, Alfredia, Alfreeda, Alfreida, Alfrieda

Alhertina (Spanish) noble.

Ali, Aly BG (Greek) familiar forms of Alice, Alicia, Alisha, Alison.
Allea, Alli, Allie, Ally

Alia, Aliah (Hebrew) forms of Aliya. See also Aaliyah, Alea.
Aelia, Allia, Alya

Alice GB (Greek) truthful. (German) noble. See also Aili, Aleka, Alie, Alisa, Alison, Alli, Alysa, Alyssa, Alysse, Elke.
Adelice, Alecia, Aleece, Alesia, Alicie, Aliece, Alise, Alix, Alize, Alla, Alleece, Allice, Allis, Allise, Allix

Alicia GB (English) a form of Alice. See also Elicia, Licia.
Aelicia, Alaysha, Alecea, Alecia, Aleecia, Ali, Alicea, Alicha, Alichia, Aliciah, Alician, Alicja, Alicya, Aliecia, Alisha, Allicea, Allicia, Alycia, Ilysa

Alida (Latin) small and winged. (Spanish) noble. See also Aleta, Lida, Oleda.
Aleda, Aleida, Alidia, Alita, Alleda, Allida, Allidah, Alyda, Alydia, Elida, Elidia

Alie (Greek) a familiar form of Alice.

Aliesha (Greek) a form of Alisha.
Alieshai, Alieshia, Alliesha

Alika (Hawaiian) truthful. (Swahili) most beautiful.
Aleka, Alica, Alikah, Alike, Alikee, Aliki

Alima (Arabic) sea maiden; musical.

Alina, Alyna (Slavic) bright. (Scottish) fair. (English) short forms of Adeline. See also Alena.
Aliana, Alianna, Alinah, Aline, Alinna, Allyna, Alynna, Alyona

Aline (Scottish) a form of Alina.
Alianne, Allene, Alline, Allyn, Allyne, Alyne, Alynne

Alisa (Greek) a form of Alice. See also Elisa, Ilisa.
Aalissah, Aaliysah, Aleessa, Alisah, Alisea, Alisia, Alisza, Alisza, Aliysa, Allissa, Alyssa

Alise, Allise (Greek) forms of Alice.
Alics, Aliese, Alis, Aliss, Alisse, Alisse, Alles, Allesse, Allis, Allisse

Alisha GB (Greek) truthful. (German) noble. (English) a form of Alicia. See also Elisha, Ilisha, Lisha.
Aalisha, Aleasha, Aleesha, Aleisha, Alesha, Ali, Aliesha, Aliscia, Alishah, Alishay, Alishaye, Alishia, Alishya, Alitsha, Allisha, Allysha, Alysha

Alishia, Alisia, Alissia
(English) forms of Alisha.
*Alishea, Alisheia, Alishiana,
Alyssaya, Alisea, Alissya, Alisyia,
Allissia*

Alison 🇬🇧 (English) a form of
Alice.
*Ali, Alicen, Alicyn, Alisan,
Alisann, Alisanne, Alisen,
Alisenne, Alisin, Alision, Alisonn,
Alisson, Alisun*

Alissa 🇬🇧 (Greek) a form of
Alice. See also Elisa, Ilisa.
*Aelicia, Alaysha, Alecea, Alecia,
Aleecia, Ali, Alicea, Alicha,
Alichia, Aliciah, Alician, Alicja,
Alicya, Aliecia, Alisha, Allicea,
Allicia, Alycia, Ilysa*

Alita (Spanish) a form of Alida.
Allita

Alivia (Latin) a form of Olivia.
Alivah

Alix 🇬🇧 (Greek) a short form of
Alexandra, Alice.
Alixe, Alixia, Allix, Alyx

Alixandra, Alixandria (Greek)
forms of Alexandria.
*Alixandriya, Allixandra,
Allixandria, Allixandrya*

Aliya (Hebrew) ascender.
*Aaleyah, Aaliyah, Aeliyah, Ahliya,
Ailya, Alea, Aleya, Alia, Alieya,
Alieyah, Aliyah, Aliyiah, Aliyyah,
Allia, Alliyah, Aly, Alyah*

Aliye (Arabic) noble.
Aliyeh

Aliza (Hebrew) joyful. See also
Aleeza, Eliza.
*Alieza, Aliezah, Alitza, Aliz,
Alizah, Alize, Alizee*

Alizabeth (Hebrew) a form of
Elizabeth.
Alyzabeth

Allan 🇧🇬 (Irish) a form of Alan.

Allana, Allanah (Irish) forms of
Alana.
Allanie, Allanna, Allauna

Allegra (Latin) cheerful.
Legra

Allen 🇧🇬 (Irish) a form of Alan.

Allena (Irish) a form of Alana.
Alleen, Alleyna, Alleynah

Alli, Ally (Greek) familiar forms
of Alice.
Ali, Alley

Allia, Alliah (Hebrew) forms of
Aliya.

Allie 🇬🇧 (Greek) familiar forms
of Alice.

Allison ☀ 🇬🇧 (English) a form
of Alice. See also Lissie.
*Alles, Allesse, Alleyson, Allie,
Allisson, Allisyn, Allix, Allsun*

Allissa (Greek) a form of Alyssa.
Allisa

Alliyah (Hebrew) a form of Aliya.
*Alliya, Alliyha, Alliyia, Alliyyah,
Allya, Allyah*

Allysa, Allyssa (Greek) a form
of Alyssa.
*Allissa, Allyisa, Allysa, Allysah,
Allyssah*

Allysha (English) a form of
Alisha.
Alishia, Allysia

Allyson, Alyson (English) forms
of Alison.
*Allysen, Allyson, Allysonn,
Allysson, Allysun, Alyson*

Alma 🄶🄱 (Arabic) learned.
(Latin) soul.
Almah

Almeda (Arabic) ambitious.
*Allmeda, Allmedah, Allmeta,
Allmita, Almea, Almedah,
Almeta, Almida, Almita*

Almira (Arabic) aristocratic,
princess; exalted. (Spanish) from
Almeíra, Spain. See also Elmira,
Mira.
*Allmeera, Allmeria, Allmira,
Almeera, Almeeria, Almeira,
Almeria, Almire*

Almudena (Spanish) city.

Almunda (Spanish) refers to the
Virgin Mary.

Almundena, Almundina
(Spanish) forms of Almunda.

Aloha (Hawaiian) loving,
kindhearted, charitable.
Alohi

Aloisa (German) famous warrior.
Aloisia, Aloysia

Aloma (Latin) a short form of
Paloma.

Alondra 🄶🄱 (Spanish) a form of
Alexandra.
Allandra, Alonda

Alonna (Irish) a form of Alana.
Alona, Alonnah, Alonya, Alonyah

Alonsa (English) eager for battle.

Alonza (English) noble and eager.

Alora (American) a combination
of the letter A + Lora.
*Alorah, Alorha, Alorie, Aloura,
Alouria*

Alpha (Greek) first-born.
Linguistics: the first letter of the
Greek alphabet.
Alphia

Alta (Latin) high; tall.
*Allta, Altah, Altana, Altanna,
Altea, Alto*

Altagracia (Spanish) refers to
the high grace of the Virgin Mary.

Althea (Greek) wholesome;
healer. History: Althea Gibson was
the first African American to win
a major tennis title. See also
Thea.
*Altha, Altheda, Altheya, Althia,
Elthea, Eltheya, Elthia*

Aluminé (Mapuche) she who
shines.

Alva 🄱🄶 (Latin, Spanish) white;
light skinned. See also Elva.
Alvana, Alvanna, Alvannah

Alvarita, Alvera (Spanish) speaker of truth.

Alvina (English) friend to all; noble friend; friend to elves. See also Elva, Vina.
Alveanea, Alveen, Alveena, Alveenia, Alvenea, Alvie, Alvinae, Alvincia, Alvine, Alvinea, Alvinesha, Alvinia, Alvinna, Alvita, Alvona, Alvyna, Alwin, Alwina, Alwyn

Alyah, Alyiah (Hebrew) forms of Aliya.
Aly, Alya, Aleah, Alyia

Alycia, Alyssia (English) forms of Alicia.
Allyce, Alycea, Alyciah, Alyse, Lycia

Alysa, Alyse, Alysse (Greek) forms of Alice.
Allys, Allyse, Allyss, Alys, Alyss

Alysha, Alysia (Greek) forms of Alisha.
Allysea, Allyscia, Alysea, Alyshia, Alysssha, Alyssia

Alyssa ☀ GB (Greek) rational. Botany: alyssum is a flowering herb. See also Alice, Elissa.
Ahlyssa, Alissa, Allissa, Allyssa, Alyesa, Alyessa, Alyissa, Alysah, Ilyssa, Lyssa, Lyssah

Alysse (Greek) a form of Alice.
Allyce, Allys, Allyse, Allyss, Alys, Alyss

Alyx, Alyxis (Greek) short forms of Alexandra.

Alyxandra, Alyxandria (Greek) forms of Alexandria.
Alyxandrea, Alyxzandrya

Am (Vietnamese) lunar; female.

Ama (African) born on Saturday.

Amabel (Latin) lovable. See also Bel, Mabel.

Amada (Spanish) beloved.
Amadea, Amadi, Amadia, Amadita

Amadis (Latin) great love, the most beloved.

Amairani (Greek) a form of Amara.
Amairaine, Amairane, Amairanie, Amairany

Amal GB (Hebrew) worker. (Arabic) hopeful.
Amala

Amalia (German) a form of Amelia.
Ahmalia, Amalea, Amaleah, Amaleta, Amalija, Amalina, Amalisa, Amalita, Amaliya, Amalya, Amalyn

Amalie (German) a form of Amelia.
Amalee, Amali, Amaly

Amalsinda (German) one that God points to.

Aman, Amani (Arabic) forms of Imani.
Aamani, Ahmani, Amane, Amanee, Amaney, Amanie, Ammanu

Amanada (Latin) a form of Amanda.

Amancái, Amancay (Quechua) voice that gives a name to a beautiful yellow flower streaked with red.

Amanda ☆ GB (Latin) lovable. See also Manda.
Amada, Amanada, Amandah, Amandalee, Amandalyn, Amandi, Amandie, Amandine, Amandy

Amandeep BG (Punjabi) peaceful light.

Amapola (Arabic) poppy.

Amara (Greek) eternally beautiful. See also Mara.
Amar, Amaira, Amairani, Amarah, Amari, Amaria, Amariah

Amaranta (Spanish) a flower that never fades.

Amari (Greek) a form of Amara.
Amaree, Amarie, Amarii, Amarri

Amarilia, Amarilla (Greek) she who shines.

Amarinda (Greek) she who shines.

Amaris (Hebrew) promised by God.
Amarissa, Amarys, Maris

Amarú (Quechua) snake, boa.

Amaryllis (Greek) fresh; flower.
Amarillis, Amarylis

Amaui (Hawaiian) thrush.

Amaya (Japanese) night rain.

Ambar GB (French) a form of Amber.

Amber ☆ GB (French) amber.
Aamber, Ahmber, Amberia, Amberise, Amberly, Ambria, Ambur, Ambyr, Ambyre, Ammber, Ember

Amberly (American) a familiar form of Amber.
Amberle, Amberlea, Amberlee, Amberleigh, Amberley, Amberli, Amberlie, Amberlly, Amberlye

Amberlyn, Amberlynn (American) combinations of Amber + Lynn.
Amberlin, Amberlina, Amberlyne, Amberlynne

Ambria (American) a form of Amber.
Ambrea, Ambra, Ambriah

Ambrosia (Greek) she who is immortal.

Amedia (Spanish) beloved.

Amelia ☆ (German) hard working. (Latin) a form of Emily. History: Amelia Earhart, an American aviator, was the first woman to fly solo across the Atlantic Ocean. See also Ima, Melia, Millie, Nuela, Yamelia.
Aemilia, Aimilia, Amalia, Amalie, Amaliya, Ameila, Ameilia, Amelie, Amelina, Ameline, Amelisa, Amelita, Amella, Amilia, Amilina, Amilisa, Amilita, Amilyn, Amylia

Amélia (Portuguese) a form of
Amelia.

Amelie (German) a familiar form
of Amelia.
*Amaley, Amalie, Amelee,
Ameleigh, Ameley, Amélie,
Amely, Amilie*

America (Teutonic) industrious.
América, Americana, Amerika

Ami, Amie (French) forms of
Amy.
*Aami, Amiee, Amii, Amiiee,
Ammee, Ammie, Ammiee*

Amilia, Amilie (Latin, German)
forms of Amelia.
*Amilee, Amili, Amillia, Amily,
Amilya*

Amina (Arabic) trustworthy,
faithful. History: the mother of the
prophet Muhammad.
*Aamena, Aamina, Aaminah,
Ameena, Ameenah, Aminah,
Aminda, Amindah, Aminta,
Amintah*

Amir GB (Hebrew) proclaimed.
(Punjabi) wealthy; king's
minister. (Arabic) prince.

Amira (Hebrew) speech;
utterance. (Arabic) princess. See
also Mira.
Ameera, Ameerah, Amirah

Amissa (Hebrew) truth.
Amissah

Amita (Hebrew) truth.
Amitha

Amity (Latin) friendship.
Amitie

Amlika (Hindi) mother.
Amlikah

Amma (Hindi) god, godlike.
Religion: another name for the
Hindu goddess Shakti.

Amor (German) a form of Amorie.

Amora (Spanish) a form of Amor.

Amorie (German) industrious
leader.

Amorina (Spanish) she who falls
in love easily.

Amparo (Spanish) protected.

Amrit BG (Sanskrit) nectar.
Amrita

Amuillan (Mapuche) useful,
helpful; enthusiastic woman who
does all that she can to serve
those around her.

Amy GB (Latin) beloved. See also
Aimee, Emma, Esmé.
*Amata, Ame, Amey, Ami, Amia,
Amie, Amio, Ammy, Amye,
Amylyn*

An BG (Chinese) peaceful.

Ana (Hawaiian, Spanish) a form
of Hannah.
Anai, Anaia

Anaba (Native American) she
returns from battle.

Anabel, Anabelle (English)
forms of Annabel.
Anabela, Anabele, Anabell,
Anabella

Anaclara (Spanish) a
combination of Ana and Clara.

Anacleta (Greek) she who has
been called on; the required one.

Anahí, Anahid (Guarani)
alluding to the flower of the
Ceibo plant.

Anahita (Persian) a river and
water goddess.
Anahai, Anahi, Anahit, Anahy

Anais (Hebrew) gracious.
Anaise, Anaïse

Anala (Hindi) fine.

Analena (Spanish) a form of Ana.

Analía (Spanish) a combination
of Ana and Lía.

Analisa, Analise (English)
combinations of Ana + Lisa.
Analice, Analicia, Analis,
Analisha, Analisia, Analissa

Anamaria (English) a
combination of Ana + Maria.
Anamarie, Anamary

Ananda (Hindi) blissful.

Anarosa (English) a form of Ana.

Anastacia (Greek) a form of
Anastasia.
Anastace, Anastacie

Anastasia (Greek) resurrection.
See also Nastasia, Stacey, Stacia,
Stasya.
Anastacia, Anastase, Anastascia,
Anastasha, Anastashia, Anastasie,
Anastasija, Anastassia, Anastassya,
Anastasya, Anastatia, Anastaysia,
Anastazia, Anastice, Annastasia,
Annastasija, Annastaysia,
Annastazia, Annstás

Anatilde (Spanish) a combination
of Ana and Matilde.

Anatola (Greek) from the east.

Anatolia (Greek) east.

Ancarla (Spanish) a combination
of Ana and Carla.

Ancelín (Latin) single woman.

Anci (Hungarian) a form of
Hannah.
Annus, Annushka

Andeana (Spanish) leaving.

Andee, Andi, Andie (American)
short forms of Andrea, Fernanda.
Ande, Andea, Andy

Andere (Greek) valiant,
courageous.

Anderson BG (Swedish) child of
Andrew.

Andre, André BG (French)
forms of Andrew.

Andrea ☀ 🏳 (Greek) strong;
courageous. See also Ondrea.
*Aindrea, Andee, Andera,
Anderea, Andra, Andrah, Andraia,
Andraya, Andreah, Andreaka,
Andreana, Andreane, Andree,
Andrée, Andreea, Andreia,
Andreja, Andreka, Andrel,
Andrell, Andrelle, Andreo,
Andressa, Andrette, Andreya,
Andria, Andriana, Andrieka,
Andrietta, Andris, Aundrea*

Andréa, Andréia (Portuguese)
valiant, courageous.

Andreana, Andreanna (Greek)
forms of Andrea.
*Ahndrianna, Andreina, Andrena,
Andreyana, Andreyonna, Andrina,
Andriona, Andrionna*

Andreane, Andreanne (Greek)
forms of Andrea.
*Andrean, Andreeanne, Andree
Anne, Andrene, Andrian,
Andrienne*

Andreas 🏳 (Greek) a form of
Andrew.

Andreína (Spanish) a form of
Andrea.

Andres 🏳 (Spanish) a form of
Andrew.

Andresa (Spanish) a form of
Andrea.

Andrew 🏳 (Greek) strong;
courageous.

Andria (Greek) a form of Andrea.
Andri, Andriea

Andriana, Andrianna (Greek)
forms of Andrea.

Andromaca (Greek) she who
battles with a man.

Andromeda (Greek) in Greek
mythology, the daughter of
Cassiopeia and Cepheus.

Andy 🏳 (American) a form of
Andee.

Aneesa, Aneesha (Greek)
forms of Agnes.
*Ahnesha, Ahnesia, Ahnesshia,
Anee, Aneesah, Aneese,
Aneeshah, Aneesia, Aneisa,
Aneisha, Anessa, Anessia*

Aneko (Japanese) older sister.

Anela (Hawaiian) angel.
Anel, Anelle

Anelida, Anelina (Spanish)
combinations of Ana and Elida.

Anessa (Greek) a form of Agnes.
*Anesha, Aneshia, Anesia,
Anessia, Annessa*

Anetra (American) a form of
Annette.
Anitra

Anezka (Czech) a form of
Hannah.

Angel 🏳 (Greek) a short form of
Angela.
*Angele, Angéle, Angell, Angelle,
Angil, Anjel*

Angela GB (Greek) angel;
messenger.
*Angala, Anganita, Angel,
Angelanell, Angelanette,
Angelee, Angeleigh, Angeles,
Angeli, Angelia, Angelica,
Angelina, Angelique, Angelita,
Angella, Angellita, Angie, Anglea,
Anjela, Anjelica*

Ángela (Spanish) a form of Angela.

Ángeles (Catalonian) angels.

Angelia (Greek) a form of
Angela.
Angelea, Angeleah, Angelie

Angelica, Angelika (Greek)
forms of Angela.
*Angalic, Angelic, Angelici,
Angelicia, Angelike, Angeliki,
Angellica, Angilica*

Angélica (Spanish) a form of
Angela.

Angelina ✲ GB (Russian) a
form of Angela.
*Angalena, Angalina, Angelena,
Angeliana, Angeleana, Angellina,
Angelyna, Anhelina, Anjelina*

Angeline (Russian) a form of
Angela.
*Angeleen, Angelene, Angelyn,
Angelyna, Angelyne, Angelynn,
Angelynne*

Angelique (French) a form of
Angela.
*Angeliqua, Angélique, Angilique,
Anjelique*

Angeni (Native American) spirit.

Angie (Greek) a familiar form of
Angela.
Ange, Angee, Angey, Angi, Angy

Angustias (Latin) she who suffers
from grief or sorrow.

Ani (Hawaiian) beautiful.
Aany, Aanye

Ania (Polish) a form of Hannah.
Ahnia, Anaya, Aniah

Anica, Anika (Czech) familiar
forms of Anna.
*Aanika, Anaka, Aneeky, Aneka,
Anekah, Anicka, Anik, Anikah,
Anike, Anikka, Anikke, Aniko,
Anneka, Annik, Annika, Anouska,
Anuska*

Anice (English) a form of Agnes.
*Anesse, Anis, Anise, Annes,
Annice, Annis, Annus*

Aniceta (Spanish) she who is
invincible because of her great
strength.

Anik GB (Czech) a form of Anica.

Anila (Hindi) Religion: an
attendant of the Hindu god
Vishnu.
Anilla

Anillang (Mapuche) stable altar;
decisive and courageously noble
woman.

Anisa, Anisah (Arabic) friendly.
Annissah

Anisha GB (English) a form of
Agnes, Ann.
Aanisha, Aeniesha, Annisha

Anissa (English) a form of Agnes,
Ann.
*Anis, Anisa, Anissah, Anise,
Annisa, Annissa, Anyssa*

Anita GB (Spanish) a form of
Ann, Anna. See also Nita.
*Aneeta, Aneetah, Aneethah,
Anetha, Anitha, Anithah, Anitia,
Anitra, Anitte*

Anjelica (Greek) a form of
Angela.
Anjelika

Anjelita (Spanish) heavenly
messenger.

Anka GB (Polish) a familiar form
of Hannah.
Anke

Ann (English) gracious. See also
Anne.
*Anissa, Anita, Annchen, Annette,
Annie, Annik, Annika, Annze,
Anouche*

Anna ☆ GB (German, Italian,
Czech, Swedish) gracious.
Culture: Anna Pavlova was a
famous Russian ballerina. See
also Anica, Anissa, Nina.
*Ahnna, Ana, Anah, Anica, Anita,
Annah, Annina, Annora, Anona,
Anya, Anyu, Aska*

Annabel (English) a combination
of Anna + Bel.
*Amabel, Anabel, Annabal,
Annabelle*

Annabelle (English) a form of
Annabel.
Anabelle, Annabell, Annabella

Annalie (Finnish) a form of
Hannah.
*Analee, Annalea, Annaleah,
Annalee, Annaleigh, Annaleigha,
Annali, Anneli, Annelie*

Annalisa, Annalise (English)
combinations of Anna + Lisa.
*Analisa, Analise, Annaliesa,
Annaliese, Annalissa, Annalisse*

**Annamarie, Annemarie,
Annmarie, Anne-Marie**
(English) combinations of Anne
+ Marie.
*Annamaria, Anna-Maria, Anna-
Marie, Annmaria*

Anneka (Swedish) a form of
Hannah.
*Annaka, Anneke, Annika, Anniki,
Annikki*

Annelisa (English) a combination
of Ann + Lisa.
*Analiese, Anelisa, Anelise,
Anneliese, Annelise*

Anne GB (English) gracious.

Annette (French) a form of Ann.
See also Anetra, Nettie.
*Anet, Aneta, Anetra, Anett,
Anetta, Anette, Anneth, Annett,
Annetta*

Annie (English) a familiar form of
Ann.
Anni, Anny

Annik, Annika (Russian) forms
of Ann.
*Aneka, Anekah, Annick, Annicka,
Annike, Annikka, Anninka, Anouk*

Annjanette (American) a
combination of Ann + Janette.
*Angen, Angenett, Angenette,
Anjane, Anjanetta, Anjani*

Anona (English) pineapple.

Anouhea (Hawaiian) cool, soft
fragrance.

Anselma (German, Dutch, Italian,
Spanish) helmet; protection.

Ansley GB (Scottish) forms of
Ainsley.
Anslea, Anslee, Ansleigh, Anslie

Anthea (Greek) flower.
Antha, Anthe, Anthia, Thia

Anthony BG (Latin) praiseworthy.
(Greek) flourishing.

Antía (Galician) priceless;
flourishing; flower.

Antígona (Greek) distinguished
by her brothers.

Antione BG (French) a form of
Anthony.

Antionette (French) a form of
Antonia.
Antionet, Antionett, Anntionett

Antoinette (French) a form of
Antonia. See also Netti, Toinette,
Toni.
*Anta, Antanette, Antoinella,
Antoinet, Antonella, Antonetta,
Antonette, Antonice, Antonieta,
Antonietta, Antonique*

Antolina (Spanish) flourishing,
beautiful as a flower.

Antonia GB (Greek) flourishing.
(Latin) praiseworthy. See also
Toni, Tonya, Tosha.
*Ansonia, Ansonya, Antania,
Antinia, Antionette, Antoinette,
Antona, Antoñía, Antonice,
Antonie, Antonina, Antonine,
Antoniya, Antonnea, Antonnia,
Antonya*

Antónia (Portuguese) a form of
Antonia.

Antonice (Latin) a form of
Antonia.
*Antanise, Antanisha, Antonesha,
Antoneshia, Antonise, Antonisha*

Antoniña (Latin) she who
confronts or is the adversary.

Antonio BG (Italian) a form of
Anthony.

Anuncia (Latin) announcer,
messenger.

Anunciación (Spanish)
annunciation.

Anunciada (Spanish) a form of
Anunciación.

Anunciata (Italian) a form of
Anunciación.

Anya (Russian) a form of Anna.
Aaniyah, Aniya, Aniyah, Anja

Anyssa (English) a form of
Anissa.
Anysa, Anysha

Aphra (Hebrew) young doe. See
also Afra.

Apia (Latin) devout woman.

Apolinaria (Spanish) sun
goddess.

Apolinia (Latin) sun goddess.

Apolonia (Greek) devoted to the
god, Apollo.

April ☑ (Latin) opening. See also
Avril.
*Aprele, Aprelle, Apriell, Aprielle,
Aprila, Aprile, Aprilette, Aprili,
Aprill, Apryl*

Apryl (Latin) a form of April.
Apryle

Aquene (Native American)
peaceful.

Aquilina (Latin) eagle.

Aquilinia (Spanish) eagle.

Ara (Arabic) opinionated.
*Ahraya, Aira, Arae, Arah, Araya,
Arayah*

Arabel (Latin) beautiful altar.

Arabella (Latin) beautiful altar.
See also Belle, Orabella.
Arabela, Arabele, Arabelle

Araceli, Aracely (Latin)
heavenly altar.
*Aracele, Aracelia, Aracelli,
Araseli, Arasely, Arcelia, Arceli*

Aracelis (Spanish) altar of
heaven.

Arama (Spanish) reference to the
Virgin Mary.

Arán (Catalonian) she is a
conflicted virgin.

Aránzazu (Basque) you in the
thorn.

Aranzuru (Spanish) a form of
Aránzazu.

Arcadia (Latin) adventurous.

Arcángela (Greek) archangel.

Arcilla (Latin) altar of heaven.

Ardelle (Latin) warm;
enthusiastic.
Ardelia, Ardelis, Ardella

Arden ☑ (English) valley of the
eagle. Literature: in Shakespeare,
a romantic place of refuge.
*Ardeen, Ardeena, Ardena,
Ardene, Ardenia, Ardi, Ardin,
Ardina, Ardine*

Ardi (Hebrew) a short form of
Arden, Ardice, Ardith.
Ardie, Arti, Artie

Ardice (Hebrew) a form of
Ardith.
Ardis, Artis, Ardiss, Ardyce, Ardys

Ardith (Hebrew) flowering field.
Ardath, Ardi, Ardice, Ardyth

Arebela (Latin) beautiful altar.

Areli GB (American) a form of
Oralee.
*Areil, Areile, Arelee, Arelis,
Arelli, Arellia*

Arella (Hebrew) angel;
messenger.
Arela, Arelle, Orella, Orelle

Arely (American) a form of
Oralee.
Arelly

Ares (Catalonian) virgin of the
Pyrenees mountains.

Aretha (Greek) virtuous. See also
Oretha.
*Areatha, Areetha, Areta, Aretina,
Aretta, Arette, Arita, Aritha,
Retha, Ritha*

Aretusa (Greek) Mythology: one
of Artemis's companions.

Argelia (Latin) jewelry boxes full
of treasures.

Argentina (Latin) she who shines
like gold.

Ari GB (Hebrew) a short form of
Ariel.

Arie (Hebrew) a short form of
Ariel.

Aria (Hebrew) a short form of
Ariel.
Ariah, Ariea, Aryia

Ariadna (Spanish) most holy.

Ariadne (Greek) holy. Mythology:
the daughter of King Minos of
Crete.

Ariana ☆ GB (Greek) holy.
*Aeriana, Ahriana, Airiana,
Arieana, Ariona*

Ariane, Arianne GB (French,
English) forms of Ariana,
Arianna.
*Aerian, Aeriann, Aerion,
Aerionne, Airiann, Ari, Arianie,
Ariann, Ariannie, Arieann, Arien,
Ariene, Arienne, Arieon, Arionne,
Aryane, Aryann, Aryanne*

Arianna ☆ (Greek) a form of
Ariana.
*Aerianna, Aerionna, Ahreanna,
Ahrianna, Arionna, Aryonna*

Arica (Scandinavian) a form of
Erica.
*Aerica, Aericka, Aeryka, Aricca,
Aricka, Arika, Arike, Arikka*

Aricela (Latin) altar of heaven.

Ariel GB (Hebrew) lion of God.
*Aerial, Aeriale, Aeriel, Aeriela,
Aeryal, Ahriel, Aire, Aireal, Airial,
Ari, Aria, Arial, Ariale, Arieal,
Ariela, Arielle, Arrieal, Arriel,
Aryel, Auriel*

Arielle (French) a form of Ariel.
*Aeriell, Ariella, Arriele, Arriell,
Arrielle, Aryelle, Aurielle*

Arin (Hebrew) enlightened.
(Arabic) messenger. See also
Erin.
*Aaren, Aerin, Aieron, Aieren,
Arinn, Aryn*

Arista (Greek) best.
Aris, Arissa, Aristana, Aristen

Arla (German) a form of Carla.

Arleigh (English) a form of
Harley.
Arlea, Arlee, Arley, Arlie, Arly

Arlene (Irish) pledge. See also
Lena, Lina.
*Airlen, Arlana, Arleen, Arleene,
Arlen, Arlena, Arlenis, Arlette,
Arleyne, Arliene, Arlina, Arlinda,
Arline, Arlis*

Arlette (English) a form of
Arlene.
Arleta, Arletta, Arletty

Arlynn (American) a combination
of Arlene + Lynn.
Arlyn, Arlyne, Arlynne

Armanda (Latin) noble.

Armani 🅱🅶 (Persian) desire, goal.
*Armahni, Arman, Armanee,
Armanii*

Armentaria (Latin) pastor of
older livestock.

Armida (Spanish) a form of
Arminda.

Arminda (German) warrior.

Armine (Latin) noble. (German)
soldier. (French) a form of
Herman (see Boys' Names).
Armina

Armonía (Spanish) balance,
harmony.

Arnalda (Spanish) strong as an
eagle.

Arnelle (German) eagle.
Arnell, Arnella

Aroa (German) good person.

Aron, Arron 🅱🅶 (Hebrew) forms
of Aaron.

Artemia (Greek) Greek goddess
of the moon and hunt.

Artemisa (Spanish) Greek
goddess of the hunt.

Artemisia (Greek) perfection.

Artha (Hindi) wealthy,
prosperous.
Arthi, Arti, Artie

Arthur 🅱🅶 (Irish) noble; lofty hill.
(Scottish) bear. (English) rock.
(Icelandic) follower of Thor.

Artis (Irish, Scottish, English,
Icelandic) a form of Arthur.
*Arthea, Arthelia, Arthene,
Arthette, Arthurette, Arthurina,
Arthurine, Artina, Artice*

Artura (Celtic) noble, follower of
Thor.

Aryana, Aryanna (Italian) forms of Ariana.
Aryan, Aryanah, Aryannah

Aryn (Hebrew) a form of Arin.
Aerryn, Aeryn, Airyn, Aryne, Arynn, Arynne

Asa BG (Japanese) born in the morning.

Ascención (Spanish) ascension.

Asha (Arabic, Swahili) a form of Aisha, Ashia.

Ashanti GB (Swahili) from a tribe in West Africa.
Achante, Achanti, Asante, Ashanta, Ashantae, Ashante, Ashanté, Ashantee, Ashantie, Ashaunta, Ashauntae, Ashauntee, Ashaunti, Ashonti, Ashuntae, Ashunti

Ashely (English) form of Ashley.
Ashelee, Ashelei, Asheley, Ashelie, Ashelley, Ashelly

Ashia (Arabic) life.
Asha, Ashya, Ashyah, Ashyia, Ayshia

Ashlee GB (English) a form of Ashley.
Ashle, Ashlea, Ashleah, Ashleeh

Ashleigh GB (English) a form of Ashley.
Ahsleigh, Asheleigh, Ashlei, Ashliegh

Ashley ☆ GB (English) ash-tree meadow. See also Lee.
Ahslee, Aishlee, Ashala, Ashalee,
Ashalei, Ashaley, Ashely, Ashla, Ashlay, Ashleay, Ashlee, Ashleigh, Ashleye, Ashli, Ashlie, Ashly, Ashlye

Ashli, Ashlie, Ashly (English) forms of Ashley.
Ashliee

Ashlin (English) a form of Ashlyn.
Ashlean, Ashliann, Ashlianne, Ashline

Ashlyn, Ashlynn GB (English) ash-tree pool. (Irish) vision, dream.
Ashlan, Ashleann, Ashleen, Ashleene, Ashlen, Ashlene, Ashlin, Ashling, Ashlyne, Ashlynne

Ashten, Ashtin (English) forms of Ashton.
Ashtine

Ashton BG (English) ash-tree settlement.
Ashten, Ashtyn

Ashtyn GB (English) a form of Ashton.
Ashtynne

Asia (Greek) resurrection. (English) eastern sunrise. (Swahili) a form of Aisha.
Ahsia, Aisia, Aisian, Asiah, Asian, Asianae, Asya, Aysia, Aysiah, Aysian, Ayzia

Aspasia (Greek) follower of the philosopher Aristotle.

Aspen GB (English) aspen tree.
Aspin, Aspyn

Assunção (Portuguese)
Assumption.

Aster (English) a form of Astra.
Astera, Asteria, Astyr

Astra (Greek) star.
Asta, Astara, Aster, Astraea,
Astrea

Astrid (Scandinavian) divine
strength.
Astri, Astrida, Astrik, Astrud, Atti,
Estrid

Astriz (German) of the stars.

Astryd (German) beloved one of
the gods.

Asunción (Spanish) Assumption.

Asunta (Spanish) to go up, to
ascend.

Atala (Greek) youthful one.

Atalanta (Greek) mighty
huntress. Mythology: an athletic
young woman who refused to
marry any man who could not
outrun her in a footrace. See also
Lani.
Atalaya, Atlanta, Atlante, Atlee

Atalía (Spanish) guard tower.

Atanasia (Spanish) one who will
be reborn; immortal.

Atara (Hebrew) crown.
Atarah, Ataree

Atenea (Greek) evokes the figure
of Palas Atenea, goddess
protectorate of the Athenians.

Athena (Greek) wise. Mythology:
the goddess of wisdom.
Athenea, Athene, Athina, Atina

Ática (Greek) city of Athens.

Atira (Hebrew) prayer.

Auberte (French) a form of
Alberta.
Auberta, Aubertha, Auberthe,
Aubine

Aubree, Aubrie GB (French)
forms of Aubrey.
Auberi, Aubre, Aubrei, Aubreigh,
Aubri, Aubrielle

Aubrey GB (German) noble;
bearlike. (French) blond ruler;
elf ruler.
Aubary, Aubery, Aubray, Aubrea,
Aubreah, Aubree, Aubrette,
Aubria, Aubrie, Aubry, Aubury,
Avery

Aubriana, Aubrianna (English)
combinations of Aubrey + Anna.
Aubreyana, Aubreyanna,
Aubreyanne, Aubreyena,
Aubrianne

Audelina (German) nobility,
strength.

Audey (English) a familiar form
of Audrey.
Aude, Audi, Audie

Audra GB (French) a form of
Audrey.
Audria, Audriea

Audreanne (English) a
combination of Audrey + Anne.
*Audrea, Audreen, Audrianne,
Audrienne*

Audree, Audrie (English) forms
of Audrey.
Audre, Audri

Audrey ☆ GB (English) noble
strength.
*Adrey, Audey, Audra, Audray,
Audree, Audrie, Audrin, Audriya,
Audry, Audrye*

Audriana, Audrianna (English)
combinations of Audrey + Anna.
Audreanna, Audrienna, Audrina

Audris (German) fortunate,
wealthy.
Audrys

August BG (Latin) a form of
Augusta.

Augusta (Latin) a short form of
Augustine. See also Gusta.
*Agusta, August, Auguste,
Augustia, Augustus, Austina*

Augustine BG (Latin) majestic.
Religion: Saint Augustine was the
first archbishop of Canterbury.
See also Tina.
*Augusta, Augustina, Augustyna,
Augustyne, Austin*

Aundrea (Greek) a form of
Andrea.
Aundreah

Aura (Greek) soft breeze. (Latin)
golden. See also Ora.

Aurelia (Latin) golden. See also
Oralia.
*Auralea, Auralia, Aurea, Aureal,
Aurel, Aurele, Aurelea, Aureliana,
Aurelie, Auria, Aurie, Aurilia,
Aurita*

Aurelie (Latin) a form of Aurelia.
*Auralee, Auralei, Aurelee,
Aurelei, Aurelle*

Auristela (Latin) golden star.

Aurora (Latin) dawn. Mythology:
Aurora was the goddess of dawn.
Aurore, Ora, Ori, Orie, Rora

Austen BG (Latin) a form of
Austin.

Austin (Latin) a short form of
Augustine.

Austyn (Latin) a form of Austin.
Austynn

Autumn ☆ GB (Latin) autumn.
Autum

Ava ☆ (Greek) a form of Eva.
Avada, Avae, Ave, Aveen

Avalon (Latin) island.
Avallon

Avelina (Latin) she who was born
in Avella.

Avery ☆ BG (English) a form of
Aubrey.
Aivree, Averi, Averie, Avry

Avis (Latin) bird.
*Avais, Avi, Avia, Aviana, Avianca,
Aviance, Avianna*

Aviva (Hebrew) springtime. See
also Viva.
*Aviv, Avivah, Avivi, Avivice, Avni,
Avnit, Avri, Avrit, Avy*

Avneet GB (Hebrew) a form of
Avner (see Boys' Names).

Avril (French) a form of April.
*Averil, Averyl, Avra, Avri, Avrilia,
Avrill, Avrille, Avrillia, Avy*

Axelle (Latin) axe. (German)
small oak tree; source of life.
Aixa

Aya (Hebrew) bird; fly swiftly.
Aia, Aiah, Aiya, Aiyah

Ayalga (Asturian) treasure.

Ayanna (Hindi) innocent.
*Ahyana, Aiyanna, Ayan, Ayana,
Ayania, Ayannica, Ayna*

Ayelen (Mapuche) she who
represents joy; smiling.

Ayelén (Araucanian) joy.

Ayesha (Persian) a form of Aisha.
*Ayasha, Ayeshah, Ayessa,
Ayisha, Ayishah, Aysha, Ayshah,
Ayshe, Ayshea, Aysia*

Ayinhual (Mapuche) beloved,
darling, generous and preferred
huala (Great Grebe).

Ayinleo (Mapuche) deep,
inextinguishable love.

Ayiqueo (Mapuche) soft-spoken;
pleasant.

Ayita (Cherokee) first in the
dance.

Ayla (Hebrew) oak tree.
*Aylana, Aylee, Ayleen, Aylene,
Aylie, Aylin*

Aymara (Spanish) people and
language of the south Andes.

Ayme (Mapuche) significant.

Aza (Arabic) comfort.
Aiza, Aizha, Aizia, Azia

Azalea (Latin) desert flower.

Aziza (Swahili) precious.
Azize

Azucena (Arabic) admirable
mother.

Azura (Spanish) sky blue.

Baba (African) born on Thursday.
Aba

B

B BG (American) an initial used as
a first name.

Babe (Latin) a familiar form of
Barbara. (American) a form of
Baby.
Babby

Babette (French, German) a
familiar form of Barbara.
Babita, Barbette

Babs (American) a familiar form
of Barbara.
Bab

Baby (American) baby.
Babby, Babe, Bebe

Bailee GB (English) a form of
Bailey.
Baelee, Bailea, Bailei, Baillee

Baileigh, Baleigh (English)
forms of Bailey.
Baeleigh

Bailey ☆ GB (English) bailiff.
*Baeley, Bailee, Baileigh, Bailley,
Bailly, Baily, Bali, Balley, Baylee,
Bayley*

Bailie (English) a form of Bailey.
Baeli, Baillie, Bailli

Baka (Hindi) crane.

Bakula (Hindi) flower.

Balbina (Latin) she who mutters.

Baldomera (Spanish) bold,
brave; famous.

Bambi (Italian) child.
Bambee, Bambie, Bamby

Bandi BG (Punjabi) prisoner.
Banda, Bandy

Baptista (Latin) baptizer.
*Baptiste, Batista, Battista,
Bautista*

Bara, Barra (Hebrew) chosen.
Bára, Bari

Barb (Latin) a short form of
Barbara.
Barba, Barbe

Barbara (Latin) stranger,
foreigner. See also Bebe, Varvara,
Wava.
*Babara, Babb, Babbie, Babe,
Babette, Babina, Babs, Barb,
Barbara-Ann, Barbarit, Barbarita,
Barbary, Barbeeleen, Barbera,
Barbie, Barbora, Barborah,
Barborka, Barbra, Barbraann,
Barbro, Barùska, Basha, Bebe,
Bobbi, Bobbie*

Bárbara (Greek) a form of
Barbara.

Barbie (American) a familiar
form of Barbara.
*Barbee, Barbey, Barbi, Barby,
Baubie*

Barbra (American) a form of
Barbara.
Barbro

Barrett BG (German) strong as a
bear.

Barrie (Irish) spear;
markswoman.
Bari, Barri, Berri, Berrie, Berry

Barry BG (Welsh) child of Harry.
(Irish) spear, marksman.
(French) gate, fence.

Bartolomea (Spanish) daughter
of Talmai.

Basia (Hebrew) daughter of God.
*Basya, Bathia, Batia, Batya, Bitya,
Bithia*

Basiana (Spanish) having acute
judgment.

Basilia (Greek) queen, princess;
governor.

Bathsheba (Hebrew) daughter of
the oath; seventh daughter. Bible:
a wife of King David. See also
Sheba.
*Bathshua, Batsheva, Bersaba,
Bethsabee, Bethsheba*

Batilde (German) she who
battles.

Batini (Swahili) inner thoughts.

Baudilia (Teutonic) audacious
and brave.

Baylee GB (English) a form of
Bailey.
*Bayla, Bayle, Baylea, Bayleah,
Baylei, Bayli, Bayliee*

Bayleigh, Baylie (English)
forms of Bailey.
Bayliegh

Bayley GB (English) a form of
Bailey.
Bayly

Bayo (Yoruba) joy is found.

Bea, Bee (American) short forms
of Beatrice.

Beata (Latin) a short form of
Beatrice.
Beatta

Beatrice (Latin) blessed; happy;
bringer of joy. See also Trish,
Trixie.
*Bea, Beata, Beatrica, Béatrice,
Beatricia, Beatriks, Beatrisa,
Beatrise, Beatrissa, Beatriz,
Beattie, Beatty, Bebe, Bee, Trice*

Beatriz GB (Latin) a form of
Beatrice.
Beatris, Beatriss, Beatrix, Beitris

Beau BG (French) beautiful.

Bebe BG (Spanish) a form of
Barbara, Beatrice.
BB, Beebee, Bibi

Becca (Hebrew) a short form of
Rebecca.
Beca, Becka, Bekah, Bekka

Becky (American) a familiar form
of Rebecca.
Beckey, Becki, Beckie

Bedelia (Irish) a form of Bridget.
Bedeelia, Biddy, Bidelia

Begoña (Basque) place of the
dominant hill.

Begonia (Spanish) begonia
flower.

Bel (Hindi) sacred wood of apple
trees. A short form of Amabel,
Belinda, Isabel.

Bela BG (Czech) white.
(Hungarian) bright.
Belah, Biela

Belarmina (Spanish) having
beautiful armor.

Belen GB (Greek) arrow.
(Spanish) Bethlehem.
Belina

Belicia (Spanish) dedicated to
God.
Beli, Belia, Belica

Belinda (Spanish) beautiful.
Literature: a name coined by
English poet Alexander Pope in
The Rape of the Lock. See also
Blinda, Linda.
Bel, Belindra, Belle, Belynda

Belisa (Latin) most slender.

Belisaria (Greek) right-handed
archer; she who shoots arrows
skillfully.

Bella (Latin) beautiful.
Bellah

Belle (French) beautiful. A short
form of Arabella, Belinda, Isabel.
See also Billie.
Belita, Bell, Belli, Bellina

Belva (Latin) beautiful view.
Belvia

Bena (Native American) pheasant.
See also Bina.
Benea

Benecia (Latin) a short form of
Benedicta.
*Beneisha, Benicia, Benish,
Benisha, Benishia, Bennicia*

Benedicta (Latin) blessed.
*Bendite, Benecia, Benedetta,
Benedicte, Benedikta, Bengta,*

*Benita, Benna, Benni, Bennicia,
Benoîte, Binney*

Benedicte (Latin) a form of
Benedicta.

Benedita (Portuguese) blessed.

Benicio (Spanish) benevolent
one.

Benigna (Spanish) kind.

Benilda (German) she who fights
with the bears.

Benilde (Spanish) a form of
Benilda.

Benita (Spanish) a form of
Benedicta.
*Beneta, Benetta, Benitta,
Bennita, Neeta*

Benjamin BG (Hebrew) child of
my right hand.

Benjamina (Spanish) preferred
daughter.

Bennett BG (Latin) little blessed
one.
Bennet, Bennetta

Benni (Latin) a familiar form of
Benedicta.
Bennie, Binni, Binnie, Binny

Bente (Latin) blessed.

Berenice (Greek) a form of
Bernice.
*Berenise, Berenisse, Bereniz,
Berenize*

Berget (Irish) a form of Bridget.
Bergette, Bergit

Berit (German) glorious.
Beret, Berette

Berkley (Scottish, English) birch-tree meadow.
Berkeley, Berkly

Berlynn (English) a combination of Bertha + Lynn.
Berla, Berlin, Berlinda, Berline, Berling, Berlyn, Berlyne, Berlynne

Bernabela (Hebrew) child of prophecy.

Bernabella (Spanish) a form of Bernabela.

Bernadette 🆖🅱 (French) a form of Bernadine. See also Nadette.
Bera, Beradette, Berna, Bernadet, Bernadete, Bernadett, Bernadetta, Bernarda, Bernardette, Bernedet, Bernedette, Bernessa, Berneta

Bernadine (English, German) brave as a bear.
Bernadene, Bernadette, Bernadin, Bernadina, Bernardina, Bernardine, Berni

Berneta (French) a short form of Bernadette.
Bernatta, Bernetta, Bernette, Bernita

Berni (English) a familiar form of Bernadine, Bernice.
Bernie, Berny

Bernice (Greek) bringer of victory. See also Bunny, Vernice.
Berenice, Berenike, Bernessa, Berni, Bernicia, Bernise, Nixie

Berta (German) a form of Berit.

Bertha (German) bright; illustrious; brilliant ruler. A short form of Alberta. See also Birdie, Peke.
Barta, Bartha, Berta, Berthe, Bertille, Bertita, Bertrona, Bertus, Birtha

Berti (German, English) a familiar form of Gilberte, Bertina.
Berte, Bertie, Berty

Bertilda (German) she who fights; the distinguished one.

Bertilia (German, Latin) a form of Berta.

Bertille (French) a form of Bertha.

Bertina (English) bright, shining.
Bertine

Beryl (Greek) sea green jewel.
Beryle

Bess, Bessie (Hebrew) familiar forms of Elizabeth.
Bessi, Bessy

Betania (Hebrew) name of a village in ancient Palestine.

Beth (Hebrew, Aramaic) house of God. A short form of Bethany, Elizabeth.
Betha, Bethe, Bethia

Bethani, Bethanie (Aramaic) forms of Bethany.
Bethanee, Bethania, Bethannie, Bethni, Bethnie

Bethann (English) a combination of Beth + Ann.
Beth-Ann, Bethan, Bethane, Bethanne, Beth-Anne

Bethany (Aramaic) house of figs. Bible: the site of Lazarus's resurrection.
Beth, Bethaney, Bethani, Bethanney, Bethanny, Bethena, Betheny, Bethia, Bethina, Bethney, Bethny, Betthany

Betsabe (Hebrew) daughter of an oath or pact.
Betsabé

Betsy (American) a familiar form of Elizabeth.
Betsey, Betsi, Betsie

Bette (French) a form of Betty.
Beta, Beti, Betka, Bett, Betta

Bettina (American) a combination of Beth + Tina.
Betina, Betine, Betti, Bettine

Betty (Hebrew) consecrated to God. (English) a familiar form of Elizabeth.
Bette, Bettey, Betti, Bettie, Bettye, Bettyjean, Betty-Jean, Bettyjo, Betty-Jo, Bettylou, Betty-Lou, Bety, Boski, Bözsi

Betula (Hebrew) girl, maiden.

Beulah (Hebrew) married. Bible: Beulah is a name for Israel.
Beula, Beulla, Beullah

Bev (English) a short form of Beverly.

Bevanne (Welsh) child of Evan.
Bevan, Bevann, Bevany

Beverly GB (English) beaver field. See also Buffy.
Bev, Bevalee, Beverle, Beverlee, Beverley, Beverlie, Beverlly, Bevlyn, Bevlynn, Bevlynne, Bevvy, Verly

Beverlyann (American) a combination of Beverly + Ann.
Beverliann, Beverlianne, Beverlyanne

Bian (Vietnamese) hidden; secretive.

Bianca GB (Italian) white. See also Blanca, Vianca.
Biancca, Biancha, Biancia, Bianco, Bianey, Bianica, Bianka, Biannca, Binney, Bionca, Blanca, Blanche, Byanca

Bianka (Italian) a form of Bianca.
Beyanka, Biannka

Bibi (Latin) a short form of Bibiana. (Arabic) lady. (Spanish) a form of Bebe.

Bibiana (Latin) lively.
Bibi

Biblis (Latin) swallow.

Biddy (Irish) a familiar form of Bedelia.
Biddie

Bienvenida (Spanish) welcome.

Billi (English) a form of Billie.

Billy 🅱🅖 (English) a form of Billie.
Billye

Billie 🅖🅑 (English) strong willed. (German, French) a familiar form of Belle, Wilhelmina.
Bilee, Bileigh, Bili, Bilie, Billee, Billi, Billy, Billye

Billie-Jean (American) a combination of Billie + Jean.
Billiejean, Billyjean, Billy-Jean

Billie-Jo (American) a combination of Billie + Jo.
Billiejo, Billyjo, Billy-Jo

Bina (Hebrew) wise; understanding. (Swahili) dancer. (Latin) a short form of Sabina. See also Bena.
Binah, Binney, Binta, Bintah

Binney (English) a familiar form of Benedicta, Bianca, Bina.
Binnee, Binni, Binnie, Binny

Bionca (Italian) a form of Bianca.
Beonca, Beyonca, Beyonka, Bioncha, Bionica, Bionka, Bionnca

Birdie (English) bird. (German) a familiar form of Bertha.
Bird, Birdee, Birdella, Birdena, Birdey, Birdi, Birdy, Byrd, Byrdey, Byrdie, Byrdy

Birgitte (Swedish) a form of Bridget.
Birgit, Birgita, Birgitta

Blaine 🅱🅖 (Irish) thin.
Blane, Blayne

Blair 🅱🅖 (Scottish) plains dweller.
Blaire

Blaire (Scottish) a form of Blair.
Blare, Blayre

Blaise 🅱🅖 (French) one who stammers.
Blaize, Blasha, Blasia, Blaza, Blaze, Blazena

Blake 🅱🅖 (English) dark.
Blaque, Blayke

Blakely 🅱🅖 (English) dark meadow.
Blakelea, Blakelee, Blakeleigh, Blakeley, Blakeli, Blakelyn, Blakelynn, Blakesley, Blakley, Blakli

Blanca 🅖🅑 (Italian) a form of Bianca.
Bellanca, Blancka, Blanka

Blanche (French) a form of Bianca.
Blanch, Blancha, Blinney

Blandina (Latin) flattering.

Blasa (French) stammerer.

Blinda (American) a short form of Belinda.
Blynda

Bliss 🅖🅑 (English) blissful, joyful.
Blisse, Blyss, Blysse

Blodwyn (Welsh) flower. See also Wynne.
Blodwen, Blodwynne, Blodyn

Blondelle (French) blond, fair haired.
Blondell, Blondie

Blondie (American) a familiar form of Blondell.
Blondee, Blondey, Blondy

Blossom (English) flower.

Blum (Yiddish) flower.
Bluma

Blythe GB (English) happy, cheerful.
Blithe, Blyss, Blyth

Bo BG (Chinese) precious.

Boacha (Hebrew) blessed.

Bobbette (American) a familiar form of Roberta.
Bobbet, Bobbetta

Bobbi, Bobbie GB (American) familiar forms of Barbara, Roberta.
Baubie, Bobbe, Bobbey, Bobbisue, Bobby, Bobbye, Bobi, Bobie, Bobina, Bobbie-Jean, Bobbie-Lynn, Bobbie-Sue

Bobbi-Ann, Bobbie-Ann (American) combinations of Bobbi + Ann.
Bobbiann, Bobbi-Anne, Bobbianne, Bobbie-Anne, Bobby-Ann, Bobbyann, Bobby-Anne, Bobbyanne

Bobbi-Jo (American) a combination of Bobbi + Jo.
Bobbiejo, Bobbie-Jo, Bobbijo, Bobby-Jo, Bobijo

Bobbi-Lee (American) a combination of Bobbi + Lee.
Bobbie-Lee, Bobbilee, Bobbylee, Bobby-Leigh, Bobile

Bobby BG (American) a form of Bobbi.

Bonfila, Bonfilia (Italian) good daughter.

Bonifacia (Italian) benefactor.

Bonita (Spanish) pretty.
Bonesha, Bonetta, Bonnetta, Bonnie, Bonny

Bonnie, Bonny (English, Scottish) beautiful, pretty. (Spanish) familiar forms of Bonita.
Boni, Bonie, Bonne, Bonnee, Bonnell, Bonney, Bonni, Bonnin

Bonnie-Bell (American) a combination of Bonnie + Belle.
Bonnebell, Bonnebelle, Bonnibell, Bonnibelle, Bonniebell, Bonniebelle, Bonnybell, Bonnybelle

Brad BG (English) a short form of Bradley.

Braden BG (English) broad valley.

Bradley BG (English) broad meadow.
Bradlee, Bradleigh, Bradlie

Brady BG (Irish) spirited.
Bradee, Bradey, Bradi, Bradie, Braedi, Braidee, Braidi, Braidie, Braidey, Braidy, Braydee

Braeden BG (English) broad hill.
*Bradyn, Bradynn, Braedan,
Braedean, Braedyn, Braidan
Braidyn, Braydn*

Braelyn (American) a
combination of Braeden + Lynn.
*Braelee, Braeleigh, Braelin, Braelle,
Braelon, Braelynn, Braelynne,
Brailee, Brailenn, Brailey, Braili,
Brailyn, Braylee, Brayley, Braylin,
Braylon, Braylyn, Braylynn*

Braiden BG (English) a form of
Braeden.

Branca (Portuguese) white.

Branda (Hebrew) blessing.

Brandan BG (English) a form of
Branden.

Brandee (Dutch) a form of
Brandy.
Brande, Brandea, Brendee

Branden BG (English) beacon
valley.
Brendan, Brandyn, Brennan

Brandi, Brandie GB (Dutch)
forms of Brandy.
*Brandei, Brandice, Brandiee,
Brandii, Brandily, Brandin,
Brandis, Brandise, Brani,
Branndie, Brendi*

Brandon BG (English) a form of
Branden.

Brandy GB (Dutch) an after-
dinner drink made from distilled
wine.
Brand, Brandace, Brandaise,

*Brandala, Brandee, Brandeli,
Brandell, Brandi, Brandye,
Brandylee, Brandy-Lee, Brandy-
Leigh, Brann, Branyell, Brendy*

Brandy-Lynn (American) a
combination of Brandy + Lynn.
*Brandalyn, Brandalynn,
Brandelyn, Brandelynn,
Brandelynne, Brandilyn,
Brandilynn, Brandilynne, Brandlin,
Brandlyn, Brandlynn, Brandlynne,
Brandolyn, Brandolynn,
Brandolynne, Brandylyn, Brandy-
Lyn, Brandylynne, Brandy-Lynne*

Brantley BG (Dutch) a form of
Brandy.

Braulia (Teutonic) gleaming.

Braxton BG (English) Brock's
town.
Braxten, Braxtyn

Brayden BG (English) a form of
Braeden.

Braydon (English) a form of
Braeden.

Brea, Bria (Irish) short forms of
Breana, Briana.
Breah, Breea, Briah, Brya

Breana (Irish) a form of Briana.
*Brea, Breanah, Breanda, Bre-
Anna, Breasha, Breawna, Breila*

Breann (Irish) a short form of
Briana.
*Breane, Bree, Breean, Breelyn,
Breeon, Brieon*

Breanna GB (Irish) a form of
Briana.
*Bre-Anna, Breannah, Breannea,
Breannia, Breeanna*

Breanne GB (Irish) a short form
of Brianna.
*Bre-Anne, Breaunne, Breeann,
Breeanne, Breiann, Breighann,
Breyenne, Brieann*

Breasha (Russian) a familiar
form of Breana.

Breauna, Breunna, Briauna
(Irish) forms of Briana.
*Breaunna, Breeauna, Breuna,
Breuna, Briaunna*

Breck BG (Irish) freckled.
Brecken

Bree (English) broth. (Irish) a
short form of Breann. See also
Brie.
Breay, Brei, Breigh

Breeana, Breeanna (Irish)
forms of Briana.
Breeanah, Breeannah

Breena (Irish) fairy palace. A
form of Brina.
Breenea, Breene, Breina, Brina

Breiana, Breianna (Irish) forms
of Briana.
Breiane, Breiann, Breianne

Brenda GB (Irish) little raven.
(English) sword.
*Brendell, Brendelle, Brendette,
Brendie, Brendyl, Brenna*

Brenda-Lee (American) a
combination of Brenda + Lee.
*Brendalee, Brendaleigh, Brendali,
Brendaly, Brendalys, Brenlee,
Brenley*

Brendan BG (Irish) little raven.
(English) sword.

Brenden BG (Irish) a form of
Brendan.

Brenna GB (Irish) a form of
Brenda.
*Bren, Brenie, Brenin, Brenn,
Brennah, Brennaugh, Brenne*

Brennan BG (English) a form of
Brendan.
Brennea, Brennon, Brennyn

Brennen BG (English) a form of
Brennan.

Brenton BG (English) steep hill.

Breon BG (Irish, Scottish) a form
of Brian.

Breona, Breonna (Irish) forms
of Briana.
*Breeona, Breiona, Breionna,
Breonah, Breonia, Breonie,
Breonne*

Bret BG (Irish) a form of Brett.

Brett BG (Irish) a short form of
Britany. See also Brita.
Bret, Brette, Brettin, Bretton

Breyana, Breyann, Breyanna
(Irish) forms of Briana.
*Breyan, Breyane, Breyannah,
Breyanne*

Breyona, Breyonna (Irish)
forms of Briana.
Breyonia

Brian BG (Irish, Scottish) strong;
virtuous; honorable.

Briana GB (Irish) a form of Brian.
*Brana, Brea, Breana, Breauna,
Breeana, Breiana, Breona,
Breyana, Breyona, Bria, Briahna,
Brianah, Briand, Brianda, Brina,
Briona, Briyana, Bryona*

Brianna ☀ GB (Irish) a form of
Brian.
*Bhrianna, Breann, Briannah,
Brianne, Brianni, Briannon,
Brienna, Bryanna*

Brianne GB (Irish) a form of
Briana.
Briane, Briann, Brienne, Bryanne

Briar (French) heather.
Brear, Brier, Bryar

Brice BG (Welsh) alert; ambitious.
(English) child of Rice.

Bricia (Spanish) represents
strength.

Bridey (Irish) a familiar form of
Bridget.
Bridi, Bridie, Brydie

Bridget GB (Irish) strong. See
also Bedelia, Bryga, Gitta.
*Berget, Birgitte, Bride, Bridey,
Bridger, Bridgete, Bridgett,
Bridgette, Bridgid, Bridgot,
Brietta, Brigada, Briget, Brigid,
Brigida, Brigitte, Brita*

Bridgett, Bridgette (Irish)
forms of Bridget.
*Bridgitte, Brigette, Bridggett,
Briggitte, Bridgitt, Brigitta*

Brie (French) a type of cheese.
Geography: a region in France
known for its cheese. See also
Bree.
*Briea, Brielle, Briena, Brieon,
Brietta, Briette*

Brieana, Brieanna (American)
combinations of Brie + Anna.
Brieannah

Brieann, Brieanne (American)
combinations of Brie + Ann. See
also Briana.
Brie-Ann, Brie-Anne

Brielle GB (French) a form of
Brie.
Briel, Briele, Briell, Briella

Brienna, Brienne (Irish) forms
of Briana.
Briene, Brieon, Brieona, Brieonna

Brienne (French) a form of
Briana.
Brienn

Brigette (French) a form of
Bridget.
*Briget, Brigett, Brigetta,
Brigettee, Brigget*

Brígida (Celtic) strong,
victorious.

Brigidia (Celtic) strong.

Brigitte (French) a form of Bridget.
Briggitte, Brigit, Brigita

Brina (Latin) a short form of Sabrina. (Irish) a familiar form of Briana.
Brin, Brinan, Brinda, Brindi, Brindy, Briney, Brinia, Brinlee, Brinly, Brinn, Brinna, Brinnan, Briona, Bryn, Bryna

Briona (Irish) a form of Briana.
Brione, Brionna, Brionne, Briony, Briunna, Bryony

Brisa (Spanish) beloved. Mythology: Briseis was the Greek name of Achilles's beloved.
Breezy, Breza, Brisha, Brishia, Brissa, Bryssa

Briselda (Spanish) a form of Briselda.

Brisia, Briza (Greek) beloved.

Brita (Irish) a form of Bridget. (English) a short form of Britany.
Bretta, Brieta, Brietta, Brit, Britta

Britaney, Brittaney (English) forms of Britany, Brittany.
Britanee, Britanny, Britenee, Briteny, Britianey, British, Britkney, Britley, Britlyn, Britney, Briton

Britani, Brittani, Brittanie (English) forms of Britany.
Brit, Britania, Britanica, Britanie, Britanii, Britanni, Britannia, Britatani, Britia, Britini, Brittane, Brittanee, Brittanni, Brittannia, Brittannie, Brittenie, Brittiani, Brittianni

Britany, Brittany **GB** (English) from Britain. See also Brett.
Brita, Britana, Britaney, Britani, Britanna, Britlyn, Britney, Britt, Brittainny, Brittainy, Brittamy, Brittana, Brittaney, Brittani, Brittania, Brittanica, Brittanny, Brittany-Ann, Brittanyne, Brittell, Britteny, Brittiany, Brittini, Brittlin, Brittlynn, Brittnee, Brittony, Bryttany

Britin, Brittin (English) from Britain.
Britann, Brittan, Brittin, Brittina, Brittine, Brittini, Brittiny

Britney, Brittny (English) forms of Britany.
Bittney, Bridnee, Bridney, Britnay, Britne, Britnee, Britnei, Britni, Britny, Britnye, Brittnay, Brittnaye, Brytnea, Brytni

Britni, Brittni, Brittnie (English) forms of Britney, Brittny.
Britnie

Briton, Brittin (English) forms of Britin, Brittin.
Britton

Britt, Britta (Latin) short forms of Britany, Brittany. (Swedish) strong.
Brett, Briet, Brit, Brita, Britte

Britteny (English) a form of Britany, Brittany.
Britten, Brittenay, Brittenee, Britteney, Brittenie

Brittini, Brittiny (English) forms of Britany, Brittany.
Brittinee, Brittiney, Brittinie, Brittiny

Brittnee (English) a form of Britany, Brittany.
Brittne, Brittnea, Brittnei, Brittneigh

Brittney 🇬🇧 (English) a form of Britany.

Briyana, Briyanna (Irish) forms of Briana.

Brock 🇧🇬 (English) badger.

Brodie 🇧🇬 (Irish) ditch; canal builder.
Brodee, Brodi

Brody 🇧🇬 (Irish) a form of Brodie.

Bronnie (Welsh) a familiar form of Bronwyn.
Bron, Bronia, Bronney, Bronny, Bronya

Bronwyn 🇬🇧 (Welsh) white breasted.
Bronnie, Bronwen, Bronwin, Bronwynn, Bronwynne

Brook 🇬🇧 (English) brook, stream.
Bhrooke, Brookelle, Brookie, Brooky

Brooke ✵ 🇬🇧 (English) brook, stream.

Brooklyn, Brooklynn 🇬🇧 (American) combinations of Brook + Lynn.
Brookellen, Brookelyn, Brookelyne, Brookelynn, Brooklen, Brooklin, Brooklyne, Brooklynne

Brooks 🇧🇬 (English) a form of Brook.

Bruce 🇧🇬 (French) brushwood thicket; woods.

Bruna (German) a short form of Brunhilda.
Brona

Brunela (Italian) a form of Bruna.

Brunhilda (German) armored warrior.
Brinhilda, Brinhilde, Bruna, Brunhilde, Brünnhilde, Brynhild, Brynhilda, Brynhilde, Hilda

Brunilda (German) line of defense in battle.

Bryan 🇧🇬 (Irish) a form of Brian.

Bryana 🇬🇧 (Irish) a form of Bryan.

Bryanna, Bryanne (Irish) short forms of Bryana.
Bryann, Bryanni

Bryce 🇧🇬 (Welsh) alert; ambitious.

Bryden 🇧🇬 (English) a form of Braden.

Bryga (Polish) a form of Bridget.
Brygid, Brygida, Brygitka

Brylee 🇬🇧 (American) a form of Brylie.

Brylie (American) a combination
of the letter B + Riley.
Brylei, Bryley, Bryli

Bryn, Brynn GB (Latin) from the
boundary line. (Welsh) mound.
Brinn, Brynee, Brynne

Bryna (Latin, Irish) a form of
Brina.
Brynan, Brynna, Brynnan

Bryona, Bryonna (Irish) forms
of Briana.
Bryonia, Bryony

Bryson BG (Welsh) child of Brice.
Brysan, Brysen, Brysun, Brysyn

Bryton BG (English) a form of
Bryttani.

Bryttani, Bryttany (English)
forms of Britany.
*Brytani, Brytanie, Brytanny,
Brytany, Brytnee, Brytnie,
Bryttanee, Bryttanie, Bryttine,
Bryttney, Bryttnie, Brytton*

Buena (Spanish) good.

Buenaventura (Castilian) she
who wishes good fortune and joy
to those around her.

Buffy (American) buffalo; from
the plains.
Buffee, Buffey, Buffie, Buffye

Bunny (Greek) a familiar form of
Bernice. (English) little rabbit.
See also Bonnie.
Bunni, Bunnie

Burgundy (French) Geography: a
region of France known for its
Burgundy wine.
*Burgandi, Burgandie, Burgandy,
Burgunde*

C

C BG (American) an initial used as
a first name.

Cachet (French) prestigious;
desirous.
*Cachae, Cache, Cachea, Cachee,
Cachée*

Cade BG (English) a form of
Cady.

Caden BG (American) a form of
Kadin (see Boys' Names).

Cadence (Latin) rhythm.
Cadena, Cadenza, Kadena

Cady (English) a form of Kady.
*Cade, Cadee, Cadey, Cadi, Cadie,
Cadine, Cadye*

Caeley, Cailey, Cayley
(American) forms of Kaylee,
Kelly.
*Caela, Caelee, Caeleigh, Caeley,
Caeli, Caelie, Caelly, Caely,
Cailee, Caileigh, Caili, Cailie,
Cailley, Caillie, Caily, Caylee*

Caelin, Caelyn (American)
forms of Kaelyn.
*Caelan, Caelinn, Caelynn, Cailan,
Caylan*

Cai (Vietnamese) feminine.
Cae, Cay, Caye

Cailida (Spanish) adoring.
Kailida

Cailin, Cailyn (American) forms of Caitlin.
Caileen, Cailene, Cailine, Cailynn, Cailynne, Calen, Cayleen, Caylen, Caylene, Caylin, Cayline, Caylyn, Caylyne, Caylynne

Caitlan (Irish) a form of Caitlin.
Caitland, Caitlandt

Caitlin GB (Irish) pure. See also Kaitlin, Katalina, Katelin, Katelyn, Kaytlyn.
Caetlin, Cailin, Caitlan, Caitleen, Caitlen, Caitlene, Caitlenn, Caitline, Caitlinn, Caitlon, Caitlyn, Catlee, Catleen, Catleene, Catlin

Caitlyn, Caitlynn (Irish) forms of Caitlin. See also Kaitlyn.
Caitlyne, Caitlynne, Catelyn, Catlyn, Catlynn, Catlynne

Cala (Arabic) castle, fortress. See also Callie, Kala.
Calah, Calan, Calla, Callah

Calandra (Greek) lark.
Calan, Calandrea, Calandria, Caleida, Calendra, Calendre, Kalandra, Kalandria

Caleb BG (Hebrew) dog; faithful. (Arabic) bold, brave.

Caledonia (Spanish) native of Caledonia.

Caleigh GB (American) a form of Caeley.
Caileigh, Caleah

Caley (American) a form of Caeley.

Calfuray (Mapuche) blue or violet flower.

Cali, Calli (Greek) forms of Callie. See also Kali.
Calee

Calida (Spanish) warm; ardent.
Calina, Calinda, Callida, Callinda, Kalida

Calíope (Greek) a form of Calliope.

Calisto (Spanish, Portuguese) most beautiful.

Callie (Greek, Arabic) a familiar form of Cala, Callista. See also Kalli.
Cal, Cali, Calie, Callee, Calley, Calli, Cally, Caly

Calliope (Greek) beautiful voice. Mythology: the Muse of epic poetry.

Callista (Greek) most beautiful. See also Kallista.
Calesta, Calista, Callie, Calysta

Callum BG (Irish) dove.

Caltha (Latin) yellow flower.

Calvina (Latin) bald.
Calvine, Calvinetta, Calvinette

Calypso (Greek) concealer.
Botany: a pink orchid native to
northern regions. Mythology: the
sea nymph who held Odysseus
captive for seven years.
Caly, Lypsie, Lypsy

Cam BG (Vietnamese) sweet
citrus.
Kam

Camara (American) a form of
Cameron.
*Camera, Cameri, Cameria,
Camira, Camry*

Camberly (American) a form of
Kimberly.
Camber, Camberlee, Camberleigh

Cambria (Latin) from Wales. See
also Kambria.
*Camberry, Cambreia, Cambie,
Cambrea, Cambree, Cambrie,
Cambrina, Cambry, Cambrya,
Cami*

Camden BG (Scottish) winding
valley.
Camdyn

Camellia (Italian) Botany: a
camellia is an evergreen tree or
shrub with fragrant roselike
flowers.
*Camala, Camalia, Camallia,
Camela, Camelia, Camelita,
Camella, Camellita, Cami,
Kamelia, Kamellia*

Cameo (Latin) gem or shell on
which a portrait is carved.
Cami, Kameo

Cameron BG (Scottish) crooked
nose. See also Kameron, Kamryn.
*Camara, Cameran, Cameren,
Camira, Camiran, Camiron,
Camryn*

Cami (French) a short form of
Camille. See also Kami.
*Camey, Camie, Cammi, Cammie,
Cammy, Cammye, Camy*

Camila, Camilla (Italian) forms
of Camille. See also Kamila, Mila.
*Camia, Camilia, Camillia, Camilya,
Cammilla, Chamelea, Chamelia,
Chamika, Chamila, Chamilia*

Camille GB (French) young
ceremonial attendant. See also
Millie.
*Cam, Cami, Camiel, Camielle,
Camil, Camila, Camile, Camill,
Cammille, Cammillie, Cammilyn,
Cammyl, Cammyll, Camylle,
Chamelle, Chamille, Kamille*

Camisha (American) a
combination of Cami + Aisha.
*Cameasha, Cameesha, Cameisha,
Camesa, Camesha, Cameshaa,
Cameshia, Camiesha, Camyeshia*

Camri, Camrie (American) short
forms of Camryn. See also Kamri.
Camrea, Camree, Camrey, Camry

Camron BG (American) a form of
Camryn.

Camryn (American) a form of
Cameron. See also Kamryn.
Camri, Camrin, Camron, Camrynn

Camylle (French) a form of
Camille.
Camyle, Camyll

Cancia (Spanish) native of the
city of Anzio.

Canciana, Cancianila
(Spanish) forms of Cancia.

Candace (Greek) glittering white;
glowing. History: the title of the
queens of ancient Ethiopia. See
also Dacey, Kandace.
*Cace, Canace, Canda, Candas,
Candece, Candelle, Candi,
Candiace, Candice, Candyce*

Candela (Spanish) candle; fire.

Candelaria (Latin) Candlemas;
she who shines brightly.

Candelas (Spanish) a form of
Candela.

Candi, Candy (American)
familiar forms of Candace,
Candice, Candida. See also Kandi.
Candee, Candie

Candice 🄶🄱 (Greek) a form of
Candace.
Candise, Candiss

Candida (Latin) bright white.
*Candeea, Candi, Candia, Candide,
Candita*

Cándida (Latin) a form of
Candida.

Candis (Greek) a form of Candace.
*Candes, Candi, Candias, Candies,
Candus*

Candra (Latin) glowing. See also
Kandra.
Candrea, Candria

Candyce (Greek) a form of
Candace.
Candys, Candyse, Cyndyss

Canela (Latin) name of an
aromatic plant and the color of
its dry bark.

Cantara (Arabic) small crossing.
Cantarah

Cantrelle (French) song.
Cantrella

Capitolina (Latin) she who lives
with the gods.

Capri (Italian) a short form of
Caprice. Geography: an island off
the west coast of Italy. See also
Kapri.
Capria, Caprie, Capry

Caprice (Italian) fanciful.
*Cappi, Caprece, Caprecia,
Capresha, Capricia, Capriese,
Caprina, Capris, Caprise,
Caprisha, Capritta*

Cara (Latin) dear. (Irish) friend.
See also Karah.
*Caira, Caragh, Carah, Caralee,
Caranda, Carey, Carra*

Caralee (Irish) a form of Cara.
*Caralea, Caraleigh, Caralia,
Caralie, Carely*

Caralyn (English) a form of Caroline.
Caralin, Caraline, Caralynn, Caralynna, Caralynne

Carem (Spanish) a form of Karen.

Caressa (French) a form of Carissa.
Caresa, Carese, Caresse, Carissa, Charessa, Charesse, Karessa

Carey BG (Welsh) a familiar form of Cara, Caroline, Karen, Katherine. See also Carrie, Kari.
Caree, Cari, Carrey, Cary

Cari, Carie (Welsh) forms of Carey, Kari.

Caridad (Latin) she who gives love, affection, and tenderness to those around her.

Carina GB (Italian) dear little one. (Swedish) a form of Karen. (Greek) a familiar form of Cora.
Carena, Carinah, Carine, Carinna

Carine (Italian) a form of Carina.
Carin, Carinn, Carinne

Carisa, Carrisa (Greek) forms of Carissa.
Carise, Carisha, Carisia, Charisa

Carissa (Greek) beloved. See also Karissa.
Caressa, Carisa, Carrissa, Charissa

Carita (Latin) charitable.
Caritta, Karita, Karitta

Caritina (Latin) grace, graceful.

Carl BG (German, English) a short form of Carlton. A form of Charles. See also Carroll, Kale, Kalle, Karl.

Carla (German) farmer. (English) strong. (Latin) a form of Carol, Caroline.
Carila, Carilla, Carleta, Carlia, Carliqua, Carliyle, Carlonda, Carlyjo, Carlyle, Carlysle

Carlee, Carley GB (English) forms of Carly. See also Karlee.
Carle, Carlea, Carleah, Carleh

Carleen, Carlene (English) forms of Caroline. See also Karlene.
Carlaen, Carlaena, Carleena, Carlen, Carlena, Carlenna, Carline, Carlyn, Carlyne

Carleigh (English) a form of Carly.
Carli, Carlie GB (English) forms of Carly. See also Karli.

Carlin BG (Irish) little champion. (Latin) a short form of Caroline.
Carlan, Carlana, Carlandra, Carlina, Carlinda, Carline, Carling, Carllan, Carlyn, Carllen, Carrlin

Carlisa (American) a form of Carlissa.
Carilis, Carilise, Carilyse, Carleesia, Carlesia, Carletha, Carlethe, Carlicia, Carlis, Carlise, Carlisha, Carlisia, Carlyse

Carlissa (American) a combination of Carla + Lissa.
Carleeza, Carlisa, Carliss, Carlissah, Carlisse, Carlissia, Carlista

Carlos ☆☆ (Spanish) a form of Carl, Charles.

Carlotta (Italian) a form of Charlotte.
Carletta, Carlita, Carlota

Carlton ☆☆ (English) Carl's town.

Carly ☆☆ (English) a familiar form of Caroline, Charlotte. See also Karli.
Carlye

Carlyn, Carlynn (Irish) forms of Carlin.
Carlyna, Carlynne

Carme (Galician) garden.

Carmela, Carmella (Hebrew) garden; vineyard. Bible: Mount Carmel in Israel is often thought of as paradise. See also Karmel.
Carma, Carmalla, Carmarit, Carmel, Carmeli, Carmelia, Carmelina, Carmelit, Carmelle, Carmellia, Carmellina, Carmesa, Carmesha, Carmi, Carmie, Carmiel, Carmil, Carmila, Carmile, Carmilla, Carmille, Carmisha, Leeta, Lita

Carmelit (Hebrew) a form of Carmela.
Carmaletta, Carmalit, Carmalita, Carmelita, Carmelitha, Carmelitia, Carmellit, Carmellita, Carmellitha, Carmellitia

Carmen ☆☆ (Latin) song. Religion: Nuestra Señora del Carmen-Our Lady of Mount Carmel-is one of the titles of the Virgin Mary. See also Karmen.
Carma, Carmaine, Carman, Carmelina, Carmencita, Carmene, Carmi, Carmia, Carmin, Carmina, Carmine, Carmita, Carmon, Carmynn, Charmaine

Carmiña (Spanish) a form of Carmen.

Carminda (Spanish) beautiful song.

Carmo (Portuguese) garden.

Carnelian (Latin) precious, red rock.

Carol ☆☆ (German) farmer. (French) song of joy. (English) strong. See also Charlene, Kalle, Karoll.
Carel, Cariel, Caro, Carola, Carole, Carolenia, Carolinda, Caroline, Caroll, Carrie, Carrol, Carroll, Caryl

Carolane, Carolann, Carolanne (American) combinations of Carol + Ann. Forms of Caroline.
Carolan, Carol Ann, Carole-Anne

Carole (English) a form of Carol.
Carolee, Karole, Karrole

Carolina ☆☆ (Italian) a form of Caroline. See also Karolina.
Carilena, Carlena, Carlina, Caroleena, Caroleina, Carolena, Carrolena

Caroline ☀ GB (French) little
and strong. See also Carla,
Carleen, Carlin, Karolina.
*Caralin, Caraline, Carileen,
Carilene, Carilin, Cariline, Carling,
Carly, Caro, Carolann, Caroleen,
Carolin, Carolina, Carolyn, Carrie,
Carroleen, Carrolene, Carrolin,
Carroline, Cary, Charlene*

Carolyn GB (English) a form of
Caroline. See also Karolyn.
*Carilyn, Carilynn, Carilynne,
Carlyn, Carlynn, Carlynne,
Carolyne, Carolynn, Carolynne,
Carrolyn, Carrolynn, Carrolynne*

Caron (Welsh) loving,
kindhearted, charitable.
Caronne, Carron, Carrone

Carona (Spanish) crown.

Carra (Irish) a form of Cara.
Carrah

Carrie GB (English) a familiar
form of Carol, Caroline. See also
Carey, Kari, Karri.
*Carree, Carrey, Carri, Carria,
Carry, Cary*

Carrola (French) song of joy.

Carson BG (English) child of
Carr.
Carsen, Carsyn

Carter BG (English) cart driver.

Caryl (Latin) a form of Carol.
Caryle, Caryll, Carylle

Caryn (Danish) a form of Karen.
*Caren, Carren, Carrin, Carryn,
Caryna, Caryne, Carynn*

Carys (Welsh) love.
Caris, Caryse, Ceris, Cerys

Casandra (Greek) a form of
Cassandra.
*Casandera, Casandre, Casandrea,
Casandrey, Casandri, Casandria,
Casanndra, Casaundra,
Casaundre, Casaundri,
Casaundria, Casondra, Casondre,
Casondri, Casondria*

Casey BG (Irish) brave. (Greek)
a familiar form of Acacia. See
also Kasey.
*Cacy, Cascy, Casie, Casse,
Cassee, Cassey, Cassye, Casy,
Cayce, Cayse, Caysee, Caysy*

Casiana (Latin) empty, vain.

Casidy (Irish) a form of Cassidy.
Casidee, Casidi

Casie (Irish) a form of Casey.
*Caci, Caesi, Caisie, Casci, Cascie,
Casi, Cayci, Caysi, Caysie, Cazzi*

Casiel (Latin) mother of the
earth.

Casilda (Arabic) virgin carrier of
the lance.

Casimira (Polish) predicts peace.

Cass BG (Greek) a short form of
Cassandra.

Cassady (Irish) a form of Cassidy.
*Casadee, Casadi, Casadie,
Cassaday, Cassadee, Cassadey,
Cassadi, Cassadie, Cassadina*

Cassandra 🇬🇧 (Greek) helper of
men. Mythology: a prophetess of
ancient Greece whose prophesies
were not believed. See also
Kassandra, Sandra, Sandy, Zandra.
*Casandra, Cass, Cassandre,
Cassandri, Cassandry,
Cassaundra, Cassie, Cassondra*

Cassaundra (Greek) a form of
Cassandra.
*Cassaundre, Cassaundri,
Cassundra, Cassundre, Cassundri,
Cassundria*

Cassey, Cassi (Greek) familiar
forms of Cassandra, Catherine.
Cassee, Cassii, Cassy, Casy

Cassia (Greek) a cinnamon-like
spice. See also Kasia.
Casia, Cass, Casya

Cassidy 🇬🇧 (Irish) clever. See
also Kassidy.
*Casidy, Cassady, Casseday,
Cassiddy, Cassidee, Cassidi,
Cassidie, Cassity*

Cassie 🇬🇧 (Greek) a familiar
form of Cassandra, Catherine. See
also Kassie.

Cassiopeia (Greek) clever.
Mythology: the wife of the
Ethiopian king Cepheus; the
mother of Andromeda.
Cassio

Cassondra (Greek) a form of
Cassandra.
Cassondre, Cassondri, Cassondria

Casta (Greek) pure.

Castalia (Greek) fountain of
purity.

Castel (Spanish) to the castle.

Castora (Spanish) brilliant.

Catalina (Spanish) a form of
Catherine. See also Katalina.
*Cataleen, Catalena, Catalene,
Catalin, Catalyn, Catalyna,
Cateline*

Catarina (German) a form of
Catherine.
*Catarena, Catarin, Catarine,
Caterin, Caterina, Caterine*

Catelyn (Irish) a form of Caitlin.
*Catelin, Cateline, Catelyne,
Catelynn*

Catharine (Greek) a form of
Catherine.
*Catharen, Catharin, Catharina,
Catharyn*

Catherine 🇬🇧 (Greek) pure.
(English) a form of Katherine.
*Cat, Catalina, Catarina, Cate,
Cathann, Cathanne, Catharine,
Cathenne, Catheren, Catherene,
Catheria, Catherin, Catherina,
Catheryn, Catheryne, Cathi,
Cathleen, Cathrine, Cathryn,
Cathy, Catlaina, Catreeka,
Catrelle, Catrice, Catricia, Catrika,
Catrina*

Cathi, Cathy (Greek) familiar forms of Catherine, Cathleen. See also Kathy.
Catha, Cathe, Cathee, Cathey, Cathie

Cathleen (Irish) a form of Catherine. See also Caitlin, Kathleen.
Caithlyn, Cathaleen, Cathelin, Cathelina, Cathelyn, Cathi, Cathleana, Cathleene, Cathlene, Cathleyn, Cathlin, Cathline, Cathlyn, Cathlyne, Cathlynn, Cathy

Cathrine (Greek) a form of Catherine.

Cathryn (Greek) a form of Catherine.
Cathryne, Cathrynn, Catryn

Catrina (Slavic) a form of Catherine, Katrina.
Caitriana, Caitriona, Catina, Catreen, Catreena, Catrene, Catrenia, Catrin, Catrine, Catrinia, Catriona, Catroina

Cayetana (Spanish) native of the city of Gaeta.

Cayfutray (Mapuche) noise from the bluish sky; blue thread; crystalline, celestial waterfall from heaven.

Cayla (Hebrew) a form of Kayla.
Caylea, Caylia

Caylee, Caylie (American) forms of Caeley, Cailey, Cayley.
Cayle, Cayleigh, Cayli, Cayly

Ceara (Irish) a form of Ciara.
Ceaira, Ceairah, Ceairra, Cearaa, Cearie, Cearah, Cearra, Cera

Cecelia (Latin) a form of Cecilia. See also Sheila.
Caceli, Cacelia, Cece, Ceceilia, Ceceli, Cecelia, Cecelie, Cecely, Cecelyn, Cecette, Cescelia, Cescelie

Cecil BG (Latin) a short form of Cecilia.

Cecilia (Latin) blind. See also Cicely, Cissy, Secilia, Selia, Sissy.
Cacilia, Caecilia, Cecelia, Cecil, Cecila, Cecile, Cecilea, Cecilija, Cecilla, Cecille, Cecillia, Cecily, Cecilya, Ceclia, Cecylia, Cee, Ceil, Ceila, Ceilagh, Ceileh, Ceileigh, Ceilena, Celia, Cesilia, Cicelia

Cecília (Portuguese) a form of Cecilia.

Cecily (Latin) a form of Cecilia.
Cacilie, Cecilee, Ceciley, Cecilie, Cescily, Cicely, Cilley

Ceferina (German) caresses like a soft wind.

Ceil (Latin) a short form of Cecilia.
Ceel, Ciel

Ceira, Ceirra (Irish) forms of Ciara.
Ceire

Celedonia (German) like the celedonia flower.

Celena (Greek) a form of Selena.
*Celeena, Celene, Celenia, Celine,
Cena*

Celene (Greek) a form of Celena.
Celeen

Celerina (Spanish) quick.

Celeste (Latin) celestial, heavenly.
*Cele, Celeeste, Celense, Celes,
Celesia, Celesley, Celest, Celesta,
Celestia, Celestial, Celestin,
Celestina, Celestine, Celestinia,
Celestyn, Celestyna, Cellest,
Celleste, Selestina*

Celia (Latin) a short form of
Cecilia.
Ceilia, Celie

Célia (Portuguese) a form of Celia.

Celidonia (Greek) a certain type
of herbal medicine.

Celina (Greek) a form of Celena.
See also Selina.
*Caleena, Calena, Calina, Celena,
Celinda, Celinka, Celinna, Celka,
Cellina*

Celine 🇬🇧 (Greek) a form of
Celena.
*Caline, Celeen, Celene, Céline,
Cellinn*

Celmira (Arabic) brilliant one.

Celsa (Latin) very spiritual.

Cemelia (Punic) she has God
present.

Cenobia (Greek) stranger.

Centola (Arabic) light of
knowledge.

Cera (French) a short form of
Cerise.
Cerea, Ceri, Ceria, Cerra

Cercira (Greek) she who is from
the island of Circe.

Cerella (Latin) springtime.
Cerelisa, Ceres

Cerise (French) cherry; cherry
red.
*Cera, Cerese, Cerice, Cericia,
Cerissa, Cerria, Cerrice, Cerrina,
Cerrita, Cerryce, Ceryce, Cherise*

Cesar 🇧🇬 (Spanish) a form of
Caesar (see Boys' Names).

Cesara (Latin) longhaired.

**Cesare, Cesaria, Cesarina,
Cesira** (Latin) she who was
forcibly separated from her
mother.

Cesilia (Latin) a form of Cecilia.
Cesia, Cesya

Chabela (Hebrew) a form of
Isabel.

Chablis (French) a dry, white wine.
Geography: a region in France
where wine grapes are grown.
*Chabeli, Chabelly, Chabely,
Chablee, Chabley, Chabli*

Chad 🇧🇬 (English) warrior. A
short form of Chadwick (see
Boys' Names). Geography: a
country in north-central Africa.

Chadee (French) from Chad, a
country in north-central Africa.
See also Sade.
*Chaday, Chadday, Chade, Chadea,
Chadi*

Chai (Hebrew) life.
*Chae, Chaela, Chaeli, Chaella,
Chaena, Chaia*

Chaka (Sanskrit) a form of
Chakra. See also Shaka.
Chakai, Chakia, Chakka, Chakkah

Chakra (Sanskrit) circle of energy.
*Chaka, Chakara, Chakaria, Chakena,
Chakina, Chakira, Chakrah, Chakria,
Chakriya, Chakyra*

Chalice (French) goblet.
*Chalace, Chalcie, Chalece,
Chalicea, Chalie, Chaliese, Chalis,
Chalisa, Chalise, Chalisk, Chalissa,
Chalisse, Challa, Challaine,
Challis, Challisse, Challysse,
Chalsey, Chalyce, Chalyn, Chalyse,
Chalyssa, Chalysse*

Chalina (Spanish) a form of
Rose.
Chaline, Chalini

Chalonna (American) a combi-
nation of the prefix Cha + Lona.
*Chalon, Chalona, Chalonda,
Chalonn, Chalonne, Chalonte,
Shalon*

Chambray (French) a lightweight
fabric.
*Chambrae, Chambre, Chambree,
Chambrée, Chambrey, Chambria,
Chambrie*

Chan BG (Cambodian) sweet-
smelling tree.

Chana (Hebrew) a form of
Hannah.
*Chanae, Chanai, Chanay, Chanea,
Chanie*

Chance BG (English) a short
form of Chancey.

Chancey (English) chancellor;
church official.
*Chance, Chancee, Chancie,
Chancy*

Chanda (Sanskrit) short
tempered. Religion: the demon
defeated by the Hindu goddess
Chamunda. See also Shanda.
*Chandee, Chandey, Chandi,
Chandie, Chandin*

Chandelle (French) candle.
*Chandal, Chandel, Shandal,
Shandel*

Chandler BG (Hindi) moon. (Old
English) candlemaker.
*Chandlar, Chandlier, Chandlor,
Chandlyr*

Chandra (Sanskrit) moon.
Religion: the Hindu god of the
moon. See also Shandra.
*Chandrae, Chandray, Chandre,
Chandrea, Chandrelle, Chandria*

Chanel (English) channel. See
also Shanel.
*Chanal, Chaneel, Chaneil,
Chanele, Chanell, Channal,
Channel, Chenelle*

Chanell, Chanelle (English)
forms of Chanel.
Channell, Shanell

Chanise (American) a form of
Shanice.
Chanisse, Chenice, Chenise

Channa (Hindi) chickpea.
Channah

Chantal GB (French) song.
*Chandal, Chantaal, Chantael,
Chantala, Chantale, Chantall,
Chantalle, Chantara, Chantarai,
Chantasia, Chante, Chanteau,
Chantel, Chantle, Chantoya,
Chantrill, Chauntel*

Chante BG (French) a short form
of Chantal.
*Chanta, Chantae, Chantai,
Chantay, Chantaye, Chanté,
Chantéa, Chantee, Chanti,
Chantia, Chaunte, Chauntea,
Chauntéa, Chauntee*

Chantel, GB (French) a form of
Chantal. See also Shantel.

Chantell, Chantelle (French)
forms of Chantel.
*Chanteese, Chantela, Chantele,
Chantella, Chanter, Chantey,
Chantez, Chantrel, Chantrell,
Chantrelle, Chatell*

Chantilly (French) fine lace. See
also Shantille.
*Chantiel, Chantielle, Chantil,
Chantila, Chantilée, Chantill,
Chantille*

Chantrea (Cambodian) moon;
moonbeam.
*Chantra, Chantrey, Chantri,
Chantria*

Chantrice (French) singer. See
also Shantrice.
Chantreese, Chantress

Chardae, Charde (Punjabi)
charitable. (French) short forms
of Chardonnay. See also Shardae.
*Charda, Chardai, Charday,
Chardea, Chardee, Chardée,
Chardese, Chardey, Chardie*

Chardonnay (French) a dry white
wine.
*Char, Chardae, Chardnay,
Chardney, Chardon, Chardonae,
Chardonai, Chardonay,
Chardonaye, Chardonee,
Chardonna, Chardonnae,
Chardonnai, Chardonnee,
Chardonnée, Chardonney,
Shardonay, Shardonnay*

Charis (Greek) grace; kindness.
*Charece, Chareece, Chareeze,
Charese, Chari, Charice, Charie,
Charish, Charisse*

Charissa, Charisse (Greek)
forms of Charity.
*Charesa, Charese, Charessa,
Charesse, Charis, Charisa,
Charise, Charisha, Charissee,
Charista, Charyssa*

Charity GB (Latin) charity,
kindness.
Chariety, Charis, Charissa,

Charisse, Charista, Charita,
Chariti, Charitie, Sharity

Charla (French, English) a short
form of Charlene, Charlotte.
Char, Charlea

Charlaine (English) a form of
Charlene.
Charlaina, Charlane, Charlanna,
Charlayna, Charlayne

Charlee, Charley (German,
English) forms of Charlie.
Charle, Charleigh

Charlene (English) a form of
Caroline. See also Carol, Karla,
Sharlene.
Charla, Charlaine, Charlean,
Charleen, Charleene, Charleesa,
Charlena, Charlenae, Charlesena,
Charline, Charlyn, Charlyne,
Charlynn, Charlynne, Charlzina,
Charoline

Charles BG (German) farmer.
(English) strong.

Charlie BG (German, English) a
familiar form of Charles.
Charlee, Charley, Charli, Charyl,
Chatty, Sharli, Sharlie

Charlotte (French) a form of
Caroline. Literature: Charlotte
Brontë was a British novelist and
poet best known for her novel
Jane Eyre. See also Karlotte,
Lotte, Sharlotte, Tottie.
Carlotta, Carly, Chara, Charil,
Charl, Charla, Charlet, Charlett,
Charletta, Charlette, Charlisa,

Charlita, Charlott, Charlotta,
Charlottie, Charlotty, Charolet,
Charolette, Charolot, Charolotte

Charmaine (French) a form of
Carmen. See also Sharmaine.
Charamy, Charma, Charmae,
Charmagne, Charmaigne,
Charmain, Chamaine, Charmalique,
Charman, Charmane, Charmar,
Charmara, Charmayane,
Charmayne, Charmeen, Charmeine,
Charmene, Charmese, Charmian,
Charmin, Charmine, Charmion,
Charmisa, Charmon, Charmyn,
Charmyne, Charmynne

Charnette (American) a
combination of Charo + Annette.
Charnetta, Charnita

Charnika (American) a
combination of Charo + Nika.
Charneka, Charniqua, Charnique

Charo (Spanish) a familiar form
of Rosa.

Charyanna (American) a
combination of Charo + Anna.
Charian, Charyian, Cheryn

Chase BG (French) hunter.

Chasidy, Chassidy (Latin) forms
of Chastity.
Chasa Dee, Chasadie, Chasady,
Chasidee, Chasidey, Chasidie,
Chassedi, Chassidi, Chasydi

Chasity (Latin) a form of Chastity.
Chasiti, Chasitie, Chasitty,
Chassey, Chassie, Chassiti,
Chassity, Chassy

Chastity (Latin) pure.
*Chasidy, Chasity, Chasta,
Chastady, Chastidy, Chastin,
Chastitie, Chastney, Chasty*

Chauncey BG (English)
chancellor; church official.

Chauntel (French) a form of
Chantal.
*Chaunta, Chauntae, Chauntay,
Chaunte, Chauntell, Chauntelle,
Chawntel, Chawntell,
Chawntelle, Chontelle*

Chava (Hebrew) life. (Yiddish)
bird. Religion: the original name
of Eve.
*Chabah, Chavae, Chavah,
Chavalah, Chavarra, Chavarria,
Chave, Chavé, Chavette, Chaviva,
Chavvis, Hava, Kaÿa*

Chavela (Spanish) consecrated to
God.

Chavella (Spanish) a form of
Isabel.
*Chavel, Chaveli, Chavell, Chavelle,
Chevelle, Chavely, Chevie*

Chavi (Gypsy) girl.
Chavali

Chavon (Hebrew) a form of Jane.
*Chavona, Chavonda, Chavonn,
Chavonne, Shavon*

Chavonne (Hebrew) a form of
Chavon. (American) a
combination of the prefix Cha +
Yvonne.
*Chavondria, Chavonna, Chevon,
Chevonn, Chevonna*

Chaya (Hebrew) life; living.
*Chaike, Chaye, Chayka, Chayla,
Chaylah, Chaylea, Chaylee,
Chaylene, Chayra*

Chaz BG (English) a familiar form
of Charles.

Chela (Spanish) consolation.

Chelci, Chelcie (English) forms
of Chelsea.
Chelce, Chelcee, Chelcey, Chelcy

Chelo (Spanish) a form of
Consuelo.

Chelsea GB (English) seaport.
See also Kelsi, Shelsea.
*Chelci, Chelese, Chelesia, Chelsa,
Chelsae, Chelsah, Chelse,
Chelseah, Chelsee, Chelsey,
Chelsia, Chelsie, Chesea,
Cheslee, Chessea*

Chelsee (English) a form of
Chelsea.
Chelsei, Chelseigh

Chelsey GB (English) a form of
Chelsea. See also Kelsey.
Chelsay, Chelssey, Chesley

Chelsie (English) a form of
Chelsea.
*Chelli, Chellie, Chellise, Chellsie,
Chelsi, Chelssie, Cheslie, Chessie*

Chelsy (English) a form of
Chelsea.
Chelcy, Chelssy, Chelsye

Chenelle (English) a form of
Chanel.
Chenel, Chenell

Chenoa (Native American) white dove.
Chenee, Chenika, Chenita, Chenna, Chenoah

Cher (French) beloved, dearest. (English) a short form of Cherilyn.
Chere, Cheri, Cherie, Sher

Cherelle, Cherrelle (French) forms of Cheryl. See also Sherelle.
Charell, Charelle, Cherell, Cherrel, Cherrell

Cherese (Greek) a form of Cherish.
Chereese, Cheresa, Cheresse, Cherice

Cheri, Cherie (French) familiar forms of Cher.
Cheree, Chérie, Cheriee, Cherri, Cherrie

Cherilyn (English) a combination of Cheryl + Lynn.
Cher, Cheralyn, Chereen, Chereena, Cherilynn, Cherlyn, Cherlynn, Cherralyn, Cherrilyn, Cherrylyn, Cherylene, Cherylin, Cheryline, Cheryl-Lyn, Cheryl-Lynn, Cheryl-Lynne, Cherylyn, Cherylynn, Cherylynne, Sherilyn

Cherise (French) a form of Cherish. See also Sharice, Sherice.
Charisa, Charise, Cherece, Chereese, Cheresa, Cherice, Cheriss, Cherissa, Cherisse, Cherrise

Cherish (English) dearly held, precious.
Charish, Charisha, Cheerish, Cherise, Cherishe, Cherrish, Sherish

Cherokee GB (Native American) a tribal name.
Cherika, Cherkita, Cherrokee, Sherokee

Cherry (Latin) a familiar form of Charity. (French) cherry; cherry red.
Chere, Cheree, Cherey, Cherida, Cherita, Cherrey, Cherrita, Cherry-Ann, Cherry-Anne, Cherrye, Chery, Cherye

Cheryl (French) beloved. See also Sheryl.
Charel, Charil, Charyl, Cherelle, Cherrelle, Cheryl-Ann, Cheryl-Anne, Cheryle, Cherylee, Cheryll, Cherylle, Cheryl-Lee

Chesarey (American) a form of Desiree.
Chesarae, Chessa

Chesna (Slavic) peaceful.
Chesnee, Chesney, Chesnie, Chesny

Chessa (American) a short form of Chesarey.
Chessi, Chessie, Chessy

Cheyanne (Cheyenne) a form of Cheyenne.
Cheyan, Cheyana, Cheyane, Cheyann, Cheyanna, Cheyeana, Cheyeannna, Cheyeannne

Cheyenne GB (Cheyenne) a tribal name. See also Shaianne, Sheyenne, Shianne, Shyann.
Cheyanne, Cheyeene, Cheyena, Cheyene, Cheyenna, Cheyna, Chi, Chi-Anna, Chie, Chyanne

Cheyla (American) a form of Sheila.
Cheylan, Cheyleigh, Cheylo

Cheyna (American) a short form of Cheyenne.
Chey, Cheye, Cheyne, Cheynee, Cheyney, Cheynna

Chi BG (Chinese) younger generation. (Nigerian) personal guardian angel.

Chiara (Italian) a form of Clara.
Cheara, Chiarra

Chika (Japanese) near and dear.
Chikaka, Chikako, Chikara, Chikona

Chiku (Swahili) chatterer.

China GB (Chinese) fine porcelain. Geography: a country in eastern Asia. See also Ciana, Shina.
Chinaetta, Chinah, Chinasa, Chinda, Chinea, Chinesia, Chinita, Chinna, Chinwa, Chyna, Chynna

Chinira (Swahili) God receives.
Chinara, Chinarah, Chinirah

Chinue (Ibo) God's own blessing.

Chiquita (Spanish) little one. See also Shiquita.
Chaqueta, Chaquita, Chica, Chickie, Chicky, Chikata, Chikita, Chiqueta, Chiquila, Chiquite, Chiquitha, Chiquithe, Chiquitia, Chiquitta

Chiyo (Japanese) eternal.
Chiya

Chloe ☀ GB (Greek) blooming, verdant. Mythology: another name for Demeter, the goddess of agriculture.
Chloé, Chlöe, Chloee, Chloie, Cloe, Kloe

Chloris (Greek) pale. Mythology: the only daughter of Niobe to escape the vengeful arrows of Apollo and Artemis. See also Loris.
Cloris, Clorissa

Cho (Korean) beautiful.
Choe

Cholena (Native American) bird.

Chriki (Swahili) blessing.

Chris BG (Greek) a short form of Christina. See also Kris.
Chrys, Cris

Chrissa (Greek) a short form of Christina. See also Khrissa.
Chrysa, Chryssa, Crissa, Cryssa

Chrissy (English) a familiar form of Christina.
Chrisie, Chrissee, Chrissie, Crissie, Khrissy

Christa GB (German) a short form of Christina. History: Christa McAuliffe, an American school teacher, was the first civilian on a

U.S. space flight. See also Krista.
Chrysta, Crista, Crysta

Christabel (Latin, French)
beautiful Christian.
*Christabell, Christabella,
Christabelle, Christable, Cristabel,
Kristabel*

Christain **BG** (Greek) a form of
Christina.
Christana, Christann, Christanna

Christal (Latin) a form of Crystal.
(Scottish) a form of Christina.
*Christalene, Christalin, Christaline,
Christall, Christalle, Christalyn,
Christelle, Christle, Chrystal*

Christelle (French) a form of
Christal.
*Christel, Christele, Christell,
Chrystel, Chrystelle*

Christen **GB** (Greek) a form of
Christin. See also Kristen.
*Christan, Christyn, Chrystan,
Chrysten, Chrystyn, Crestienne*

Christena, Christen (Greek)
forms of Christina.

Christi (Greek) a short form of
Christina, Christine. See also
Kristi.
Christy, Chrysti, Chrysty

Christian **BG** (Greek) a form of
Christina.

Christiana, Christianna
(Greek) forms of Christina. See
also Kristian, Krystian.
Christiane, Christiann, Christi-

*Ann, Christianne, Christi-Anne,
Christianni, Christiaun, Christiean,
Christien, Christiena, Christienne,
Christinan, Christy-Ann, Christy-
Anne, Crystian, Chrystyann,
Chrystyanne, Crystiann,
Crystianne*

Christie **GB** (Greek) a short form
of Christina, Christine.
Christy, Chrysti, Chrysty

Christin **GB** (Greek) a short form
of Christina.
Chrystin

Christina **GB** (Greek) Christian;
anointed. See also Khristina,
Kristina, Stina, Tina.
*Chris, Chrissa, Chrissy, Christa,
Christain, Christal, Christeena,
Christella, Christen, Christena,
Christi, Christian, Christie,
Christin, Christinaa, Christine,
Christinea, Christinia, Christinna,
Christinnah, Christna, Christy,
Christyn, Christyna, Christynna,
Chrystina, Chrystyna, Cristeena,
Cristena, Cristina, Crystina,
Chrystena, Cristena*

Christine **GB** (French, English) a
form of Christina. See also
Kirsten, Kristen, Kristine.
*Chrisa, Christeen, Christen,
Christene, Christi, Christie,
Christy, Chrystine, Cristeen,
Cristene, Cristine, Crystine*

Christophe **BG** (Greek) a form of
Christopher.

Christopher BG (Greek) Christ-bearer.

Christy GB (English) a short form of Christina, Christine.
Cristy

Christyn (Greek) a form of Christina.
Christyne

Chrys (English) a form of Chris.
Krys

Chrystal (Latin) a form of Christal.
Chrystale, Chrystalla, Chrystallina, Chrystallynn

Chu Hua (Chinese) chrysanthemum.

Chumani (Lakota) dewdrops.
Chumany

Chun BG (Burmese) nature's renewal.

Chyanne, Chyenne (Cheyenne) forms of Cheyenne.
Chyan, Chyana, Chyane, Chyann, Chyanna, Chyeana, Chyenn, Chyenna, Chyennee

Chyna, Chynna (Chinese) forms of China.

Ciana (Chinese) a form of China. (Italian) a form of Jane.
Cian, Ciandra, Ciann, Cianna

Ciara, Ciarra GB (Irish) black. See also Sierra.
Ceara, Chiairah, Ciaara, Ciaera, Ciaira, Ciarah, Ciaria, Ciarrah, Cieara, Ciearra, Ciearria, Ciera, Cierra, Cioria, Cyarra

Cibeles (Greek) mythological goddess.

Cicely (English) a form of Cecilia. See also Sissy.
Cicelia, Cicelie, Ciciley, Cicilia, Cicilie, Cicily, Cile, Cilka, Cilla, Cilli, Cillie, Cilly

Cidney (French) a form of Sydney.
Cidnee, Cidni, Cidnie

Cielo (Latin) she who is celestial.

Ciera, Cierra (Irish) forms of Ciara.
Ceira, Cierah, Ciere, Cieria, Cierrah, Cierre, Cierria, Cierro

Cinderella (French, English) little cinder girl. Literature: a fairy tale heroine.
Cindella

Cindy GB (Greek) moon. (Latin) a familiar form of Cynthia. See also Sindy.
Cindee, Cindi, Cindie, Cyndi

Cinthia, Cinthya (Greek) forms of Cynthia.
Cinthiya, Cintia

Cíntia (Portuguese) a form of Cynthia.

Cipriana (Greek) from Cyprus.

Ciprina (Spanish) blessed by the goddess of love.

Cira (Spanish) a form of Cyrilla.

Circe (Greek) from Greek mythology.

Cirenia, Cirinea (Greek) native of Cyrene, Libya.

Ciri (Greek) lady-like.

Ciríaca (Spanish) she who is the property of the Lord; belonging to God.

Cirila (Greek) great king or Almighty One.

Cissy (American) a familiar form of Cecelia, Cicely.
Cissey, Cissi, Cissie

Citlali (Nahuatl) star.

Claire ☀ **GB** (French) a form of Clara.
Clair, Klaire, Klarye

Clairissa (Greek) a form of Clarissa.
Clairisa, Clairisse, Claraissa

Clara **GB** (Latin) clear; bright. Music: Clara Shumann was a famous nineteenth-century German composer. See also Chiara, Klara.
Claira, Claire, Clarabelle, Clare, Claresta, Clarice, Clarie, Clarina, Clarinda, Clarine, Clarissa, Clarita

Clarabelle (Latin) bright and beautiful.
Clarabella, Claribel, Claribell

Clare **GB** (English) a form of Clara.

Clarence **BG** (Latin) clear; victorious.

Clarice (Italian) a form of Clara.
Claris, Clarise, Clarisse, Claryce, Cleriese, Klarice, Klarise

Clarie (Latin) a familiar form of Clara.
Clarey, Clari, Clary

Clarisa (Greek) a form of Clarissa.
Claresa, Clarise, Clarisia

Clarissa **GB** (Greek) brilliant. (Italian) a form of Clara. See also Klarissa.
Clairissa, Clarecia, Claressa, Claresta, Clarisa, Clarissia, Claritza, Clarizza, Clarrisa, Clarrissa, Clerissa

Clarita (Spanish) a form of Clara.
Clairette, Clareta, Claretta, Clarette, Claritza

Clark **BG** (French) cleric; scholar.

Claude **BG** (Latin, French) lame.

Claudette (French) a form of Claudia.
Clauddetta

Claudia (Latin) lame. See also Gladys, Klaudia.
Claudeen, Claudel, Claudelle, Claudette, Claudex, Claudiana, Claudiane, Claudie, Claudie-Anne, Claudina, Claudine

Claudie **GB** (Latin) a form of Claudia.
Claudee

Claudio BG (Italian) a form of Claude.

Clayton BG (English) town built on clay.

Clea (Greek) a form of Cleo, Clio.

Clementine (Latin) merciful.
Clemence, Clemencia, Clemencie, Clemency, Clementia, Clementina, Clemenza, Clemette

Clemira (Arabic) illuminated, brilliant princess.

Cleo (Greek) a short form of Cleopatra.
Chleo, Clea

Cleodora (Greek) she who represents the gift of God.

Cleofe (Greek) she who shows signs of glory.

Cleone (Greek) famous.
Cleonie, Cleonna, Cliona

Cleopatra (Greek) her father's fame. History: a great Egyptian queen.
Cleo

Cleta (Greek) illustrious.

Clidia (Greek) agitated in the sea.

Clifton BG (English) cliff town.

Clio (Greek) proclaimer; glorifier. Mythology: the Muse of history.
Clea

Clío (Greek) a form of Clio.

Clitemestra (Greek) Mythology: a form of Clytemnestra, the daughter of Tyndareus and Leda.

Cloe (Greek) a form of Chloe.
Clo, Cloei, Cloey, Cloie

Clorinda (Greek) fresh, healthy-looking, and vital.

Clotilda (German) heroine.

Clotilde (Teutonic) illustrious warrior full of wisdom.

Clovis (Teutonic) illustrious warrior full of wisdom.

Coco GB (Spanish) coconut. See also Koko.

Codey BG (English) a form of Codi, Cody.

Codi BG (English) cushion. See also Kodi.
Coady, Codee, Codey, Codia, Codie

Codie BG (English) a form of Codi, Cody.

Cody BG (English) cushion.

Colby BG (English) coal town. Geography: a region in England known for cheese-making.
Cobi, Cobie, Colbi, Colbie

Cole BG (Irish) a short form of Colleen.

Coleman BG (Latin) cabbage farmer. (English) coal miner.

Coleta (French) victory of the people.

Colette (Greek, French) a familiar form of Nicole.
Coe, Coetta, Coletta, Collet, Collete, Collett, Colletta, Collette, Kolette, Kollette

Colin B**G** (Irish) young cub. (Greek) a short form of Nicholas (see Boys' Names).

Colleen (Irish) girl. See also Kolina.
Coe, Coel, Cole, Coleen, Colene, Coley, Coline, Colleene, Collen, Collene, Collie, Collina, Colline, Colly

Collin B**G** (Scottish) a form of Colin.

Collina (Irish) a form of Colleen.
Colena, Colina, Colinda

Collipal (Mapuche) colored star.

Coloma, Columbia (Spanish) forms of Colomba.

Colomba (Latin) dove.

Colt B**G** (English) young horse; frisky. A short form of Colton.

Colton B**G** (English) coal town.

Concepción (Latin) she who conceives; related to the virginal miracle of Jesus' mother.

Concetta (Italian) pure.
Concettina, Conchetta

Conchita (Spanish) conception.
Chita, Conceptia, Concha, Conciana

Concordia (Latin) harmonious. Mythology: the goddess governing the peace after war.
Con, Cordae, Cordaye

Conner B**G** (Scottish, Irish) a form of Connor.

Connie G**B** (Latin) a familiar form of Constance.
Con, Connee, Conni, Conny, Konnie, Konny

Connor B**G** (Scottish) wise. (Irish) praised; exalted.
Connar, Conner, Connery, Conor

Conor B**G** (Scottish, Irish) a form of Connor.

Consolación (Latin) consolation.

Constance (Latin) constant; firm. History: Constance Motley was the first African-American woman to be appointed to a U.S. federal judge. See also Konstance, Kosta.
Connie, Constancia, Constancy, Constanta, Constantia, Constantina, Constantine, Constanza, Constynse

Constanza (Spanish) a form of Constance.
Constanz, Constanze

Consuelo (Spanish) consolation. Religion: Nuestra Señora del Consuelo—Our Lady of Consolation—is a name for the Virgin Mary.
Consolata, Consuela, Consuella, Consula, Conzuelo, Konsuela, Konsuelo

Cooper B G (English) barrel maker.

Cora (Greek) maiden. Mythology: Kore is another name for Persephone, the goddess of the underworld. See also Kora.
Corah, Coralee, Coretta, Corissa, Corey, Corra

Corabelle (American) a combination of Cora + Belle.
Corabel, Corabella

Coral (Latin) coral. See also Koral.
Coraal, Corral

Coralee (American) a combination of Cora + Lee.
Coralea, Cora-Lee, Coralena, Coralene, Coraley, Coralie, Coraline, Coraly, Coralyn, Corella, Corilee, Koralie

Coralie (American) a form of Coralee.
Corali, Coralia, Coralina, Coralynn, Coralynne

Corazon (Spanish) heart.

Corbin B G (Latin) raven.
Corbe, Corbi, Corby, Corbyn, Corbynn

Cordasha (American) a combination of Cora + Dasha.

Cordelia (Latin) warm-hearted. (Welsh) sea jewel. See also Delia, Della.
Cordae, Cordelie, Cordett, Cordette, Cordi, Cordilia, Cordilla, Cordula, Kordelia, Kordula

Cordi (Welsh) a short form of Cordelia.
Cordey, Cordia, Cordie, Cordy

Coretta (Greek) a familiar form of Cora.
Coreta, Corette, Correta, Corretta, Corrette, Koretta, Korretta

Corey, Cory B G (Irish) from the hollow. (Greek) familiar forms of Cora. See also Kori.
Coree, Cori, Correy, Correye, Corry

Cori G B (Irish) a form of Corey.

Coriann, Corianne (American) combinations of Cori + Ann, Cori + Anne.
Corian, Coriane, Cori-Ann, Corri, Corrie-Ann, Corrianne, Corrie-Anne

Corie, Corrie (Irish) forms of Corey.

Corina, Corinna (Greek) familiar forms of Corinne. See also Korina.
Coreena, Coriana, Corianna, Corinda, Correna, Corrinna, Coryna

Corinne (Greek) maiden.
Coreen, Coren, Corin, Corina, Corine, Corinee, Corinn, Corinna, Corrina, Coryn, Corynn, Corynne

Corissa (Greek) a familiar form of Cora.
Coresa, Coressa, Corisa, Coryssa, Korissa

Corliss (English) cheerful; goodhearted.
Corlisa, Corlise, Corlissa, Corly, Korliss

Cornelia (Latin) horn colored. See also Kornelia, Nelia, Nellie.
Carna, Carniella, Corneilla, Cornela, Cornelie, Cornella, Cornelle, Cornie, Cornilear, Cornisha, Corny

Cornelius BG (Greek) cornel tree. (Latin) horn colored.

Corrina, Corrine (Greek) forms of Corinne.
Correen, Corren, Corrin, Corrinn, Corrinna, Corrinne, Corrinne, Corryn

Cortney GB (English) a form of Courtney.
Cortne, Cortnea, Cortnee, Cortneia, Cortni, Cortnie, Cortny, Cortnye, Corttney

Cosette (French) a familiar form of Nicole.
Cosetta, Cossetta, Cossette, Cozette

Coty BG (French) slope, hillside.

Courtenay (English) a form of Courtney.
Courtaney, Courtany, Courteney, Courteny

Courtnee, Courtnie (English) forms of Courtney.
Courtne, Courtnée, Courtnei, Courtneigh, Courtni, Courtnii

Courtney GB (English) from the court. See also Kortney, Kourtney.
Cortney, Courtena, Courtenay, Courtene, Courtnae, Courtnay, Courtnee, Courtny, Courtonie

Covadonga (Spanish) large cave that is close to Asturias, which is the scene of the Spanish avocation of the Virgin Mary.

Craig BG (Irish, Scottish) crag; steep rock.

Crescencia (Spanish) growth.

Crimilda (German) she fights wearing a helmet.

Crisanta (Spanish) golden flower.

Crisbell (American) a combination of Crista + Belle.
Crisbel, Cristabel

Crispina (Latin) having curly locks of hair.

Crista, Crysta (Italian) forms of Christa.
Cristah

Cristal GB (Latin) a form of Crystal.
Cristalie, Cristalina, Cristalle, Cristel, Cristela, Cristelia, Cristella, Cristelle, Cristhie, Cristle

Cristen, Cristin (Irish) forms of Christen, Christin. See also Kristin.
Cristan, Cristyn, Crystan, Crysten, Crystin, Crystyn

Cristian 🅱🅖 (Greek) a form of Christian.

Cristiana (Spanish) Christian, follower of Christ.

Cristina, Cristine (Greek) forms of Christina. See also Kristina.
Cristiona, Cristy

Cristy (English) a familiar form of Cristina. A form of Christy. See also Kristy.
Cristey, Cristi, Cristie, Crysti, Crystie, Crysty

Cruz 🅱🅖 (Portuguese, Spanish) cross.

Cruzita (Spanish) a form of Cruz.

Crystal 🅖🅑 (Latin) clear, brilliant glass. See also Kristal, Krystal.
Christal, Chrystal, Chrystal-Lynn, Chrystel, Cristal, Crystala, Crystale, Crystalee, Crystalin, Crystall, Crystalle, Crystaly, Crystel, Crystela, Crystelia, Crystelle, Crysthelle, Crystl, Crystle, Crystol, Crystole, Crystyl

Crystalin (Latin) crystal pool.
Crystal-Ann, Cristalanna, Crystal-Anne, Cristalina, Cristallina, Cristalyn, Crystallynn, Crystallynne, Cristilyn, Crystalina, Crystal-Lee, Crystal-Lynn, Crystalyn, Crystalynn

Crystina (Greek) a form of Christina.
Crystin, Crystine, Crystyn, Crystyna, Crystyne

Cullen 🅱🅖 (Irish) beautiful.

Curipán (Mapuche) brave lioness; black mountain; valorous soul.

Curran 🅱🅖 (Irish) heroine.
Cura, Curin, Curina, Curinna

Curtis 🅱🅖 (Latin) enclosure. (French) courteous.

Custodia (Latin) guardian angel.

Cuyen (Mapuche) moon.

Cybele (Greek) a form of Sybil.
Cybel, Cybil, Cybill, Cybille

Cydney (French) a form of Sydney.
Cydne, Cydnee, Cydnei, Cydni, Cydnie

Cyerra (Irish) a form of Ciara.
Cyera, Cyerria

Cyndi (Greek) a form of Cindy.
Cynda, Cyndal, Cyndale, Cyndall, Cyndee, Cyndel, Cyndia, Cyndie, Cyndle, Cyndy

Cynthia 🅖🅑 (Greek) moon. Mythology: another name for Artemis, the moon goddess. See also Hyacinth, Kynthia.
Cindy, Cinthia, Cyneria, Cynethia, Cynithia, Cynthea, Cynthiana, Cynthiann, Cynthie, Cynthria, Cynthy, Cynthya, Cyntia, Cyntreia, Cythia, Synthia

Cyrilla (Greek) noble.
Cerelia, Cerella, Cira, Cirilla, Cyrella, Cyrille

Cyteria (Greek) goddess of love.

D

D BG (American) an initial used as a first name.

D'andre BG (French) a form of Deandre.

Dabria (Latin) name of an angel.

Dacey GB (Irish) southerner. (Greek) a familiar form of Candace.
Dacee, Dacei, Daci, Dacia, Dacie, Dacy, Daicee, Daici, Daicie, Daicy, Daycee, Daycie, Daycy

Dacia (Irish) a form of Dacey.
Daciah

Dae (English) day. See also Dai.

Daeja (French) a form of Déja.
Daejah, Daejia

Daelynn (American) a combination of Dae + Lynn.
Daeleen, Daelena, Daelin, Daelyn, Daelynne

Daeshandra (American) a combination of Dae + Shandra.
Daeshandria, Daeshaundra, Daeshaundria, Daeshawndra, Daeshawndria, Daeshondra, Daeshondria

Daeshawna (American) a combination of Dae + Shawna.
Daeshan, Daeshaun, Daeshauna, Daeshavon, Daeshawn, Daeshawntia, Daeshon, Daeshona

Daeshonda (American) a combination of Dae + Shonda.
Daeshanda, Daeshawnda

Dafny (American) a form of Daphne.
Dafany, Daffany, Daffie, Daffy, Dafna, Dafne, Dafney, Dafnie

Dagmar (German) glorious.
Dagmara

Dagny (Scandinavian) day.
Dagna, Dagnanna, Dagne, Dagney, Dagnie

Dahlia (Scandinavian) valley. Botany: a perennial flower. See also Daliah.
Dahliah, Dahlya, Dahlye

Dai GB (Japanese) great. See also Dae.
Day, Daye

Daija, Daijah (French) forms of Déja.
Daijaah, Daijea, Daijha, Daijhah, Dayja

Daila (Latin) beautiful like a flower.

Daisha (American) a form of Dasha.
Daesha, Daishae, Daishia, Daishya, Daisia

Daisy (English) day's eye. Botany: a white and yellow flower.
Daisee, Daisey, Daisi, Daisia, Daisie, Dasey, Dasi, Dasie, Dasy, Daysi, Deisy

Daja, Dajah (French) forms of Déja.
Dajae, Dajai, Daje, Dajha, Dajia

Dakayla (American) a combination of the prefix Da + Kayla.
Dakala, Dakila

Dakira (American) a combination of the prefix Da + Kira.
Dakara, Dakaria, Dakarra, Dakirah, Dakyra

Dakota BG (Native American) a tribal name.
Dakkota, Dakoda, Dakotah, Dakotha, Dakotta, Dekoda, Dekota, Dekotah, Dekotha

Dakotah BG (Native American) a form of Dakota.

Dale BG (English) valley.
Dael, Dahl, Daile, Daleleana, Dalena, Dalina, Dayle

Dalia, Daliah (Hebrew) branch. See also Dahlia.
Daelia, Dailia, Daleah, Daleia, Dalialah, Daliyah

Dalila (Swahili) gentle.
Dalela, Dalida, Dalilah, Dalilia

Dalisha (American) a form of Dallas.
Dalisa, Dalishea, Dalishia, Dalishya, Dalisia, Dalissia

Dallas BG (Irish) wise.
Dalis, Dalise, Dalisha, Dalisse, Dallace, Dallis, Dallise, Dallus, Dallys, Dalyce, Dalys

Dallen BG (English) a form of Dallan (see Boys' Names).

Dallyn BG (English) pride's people.

Dalma (Spanish) a form of Dalmacia.

Dalmacia (Latin) native of Dalmacia.

Dalmira (Teutonic) illustrious; respected for her noble ancestry.

Dalton BG (English) town in the valley.

Damaris GB (Greek) gentle girl. See also Maris.
Dama, Damar, Damara, Damarius, Damary, Damarylis, Damarys, Dameress, Dameris, Damiris, Dammaris, Dammeris, Damris, Demaras, Demaris

Damasia (Spanish) a form of Dalmacia.

Damian BG (Greek) tamer; soother.

Damiana (Greek) a form of Damian.
Daimenia, Daimiona, Damia, Damiann, Damianna, Damianne, Damien, Damienne, Damiona, Damon, Demion

Damica (French) friendly.
Damee, Dameeka, Dameka, Damekah, Damicah, Damicia, Damicka, Damie, Damieka, Damika, Damikah, Damyka,

Demeeka, Demeka, Demekah,
Demica, Demicah

Damien BG (Greek) a form of
Damian.

Damita (Spanish) small
noblewoman.
Damee, Damesha, Dameshia,
Damesia, Dametia, Dametra,
Dametrah

Damon BG (Greek) a form of
Damian.

Damonica (American) a
combination of the prefix Da +
Monica.
Damonec, Damoneke, Damonik,
Damonika, Damonique,
Diamoniqua, Diamonique

Dan BG (Vietnamese) yes.
(Hebrew) a short form of Daniel.

Dana GB (English) from
Denmark; bright as day.
Daina, Dainna, Danah, Danaia,
Danan, Danarra, Dane, Danean,
Danna, Dayna

Danae (Greek) Mythology: the
mother of Perseus.
Danaë, Danay, Danayla, Danays,
Danai, Danea, Danee, Dannae,
Denae, Denee

Dánae (Greek) a form of Danae.

Danalyn (American) a
combination of Dana + Lynn.
Danalee, Donaleen

Danas (Spanish) a form of Dana.

Dane BG (English) a form of Dana.

Daneil (Hebrew) a form of
Danielle.
Daneal, Daneala, Daneale,
Daneel, Daneela, Daneila

Danella (American) a form of
Danielle.
Danayla, Danela, Danelia,
Danelle, Danna, Donella, Donnella

Danelle (Hebrew) a form of
Danielle.
Danael, Danalle, Danel, Danele,
Danell, Danella, Donelle, Donnelle

Danesha, Danisha (American)
forms of Danessa.
Daneisha, Daneshia, Daniesha,
Danishia

Danessa (American) a
combination of Danielle +
Vanessa. See also Doneshia.
Danasia, Danesa, Danesha,
Danessia, Daniesa, Danisa,
Danissa

Danessia (American) a form of
Danessa.
Danesia, Danieshia, Danisia,
Danissia

Danette (American) a form of
Danielle.
Danetra, Danett, Danetta,
Donnita

Dani (Hebrew) a familiar form of
Danielle.
Danee, Danie, Danne, Dannee,
Danni, Dannie, Danny, Dannye,
Dany

Dania, Danya (Hebrew) short forms of Danielle.
Daniah, Danja, Dannia, Danyae

Danica, Danika GB (Slavic) morning star. (Hebrew) forms of Danielle.
Daneca, Daneeka, Daneekah, Danicah, Danicka, Danieka, Danikah, Danikla, Danneeka, Dannica, Dannika, Dannikah, Danyka, Denica, Donica, Donika, Donnaica, Donnica, Donnika

Danice (American) a combination of Danielle + Janice.
Donice

Daniel BG (Hebrew, French) God is my judge.

Daniela (Italian) a form of Danielle.
Daniellah, Dannilla, Danijela

Danielan (Spanish) a form of Danielle.

Daniella (English) a form of Dana.
Danka, Danniella, Danyella

Danielle ☆ GB (Hebrew, French) a form of Daniel.
Daneen, Daneil, Daneille, Danelle, Dani, Danial, Danialle, Danica, Daniel, Daniela, Danielan, Daniele, Danielka, Daniell, Daniella, Danilka, Danille, Danit, Dannielle, Danyel, Donniella

Danille (American) a form of Danielle.
Danila, Danile, Danilla, Dannille

Danit (Hebrew) a form of Danielle.
Danett, Danis, Danisha, Daniss, Danita, Danitra, Danitrea, Danitria, Danitza, Daniz

Danna (Hebrew) a short form of Danella.
Dannah

Dannielle (Hebrew, French) a form of Danielle.
Danniel, Danniele, Danniell

Danny BG (Hebrew) a form of Dani.

Dante, Danté BG (Latin) lasting, enduring.

Dany BG (Hebrew) a form of Dani.

Danyel GB (American) a form of Danielle.
Daniyel, Danyae, Danyail, Danyaile, Danyal, Danyale, Danyea, Danyele, Danyiel, Danyle, Donnyale, Donyale

Danyell, Danyelle (American) forms of Danyel.
Danyielle, Donnyell, Donyell

Daphne (Greek) laurel tree.
Dafny, Daphane, Daphany, Dapheney, Daphna, Daphnee, Daphnique, Daphnit, Daphny

Daphnee (Greek) a form of
Daphne.
*Daphaney, Daphanie, Daphney,
Daphni, Daphnie*

Dara GB (Hebrew)
compassionate.
*Dahra, Daira, Dairah, Darah,
Daraka, Daralea, Daralee,
Daraleigh, Daralie, Daravie,
Darda, Darice, Darisa, Darissa,
Darja, Darra, Darrah*

Darby GB (Irish) free.
(Scandinavian) deer estate.
*Darb, Darbe, Darbee, Darbi,
Darbie, Darbra, Darbye*

Darcelle (French) a form of
Darci.
Darcel, Darcell, Darcella, Darselle

Darci, Darcy GB (Irish) dark.
(French) fortress.
*Darcee, Darcelle, Darcey, Darcie,
Darsey, Darsi, Darsie*

Daria (Greek) wealthy.
*Dari, Daría, Dariya, Darria, Darya,
Daryia*

Darian, Darrian BG (Greek)
forms of Daron.
*Dariana, Dariane, Dariann,
Darianna, Darianne, Dariyan,
Dariyanne, Darriana, Darriane,
Darriann, Darrianna, Darrianne,
Derrian, Driana*

Darielle (French) a form of
Daryl.
*Dariel, Dariela, Dariell, Darriel,
Darrielle*

Darien, Darrien BG (Greek)
forms of Daron.
Dariene, Darienne, Darriene

Darilynn (American) a form of
Darlene.
*Daralin, Daralyn, Daralynn,
Daralynne, Darilin, Darilyn,
Darilynne, Darlin, Darlyn, Darlynn,
Darlynne, Darylin, Darylyn,
Darylynn, Darylynne*

Darin BG (Irish) a form of
Darren.

Darion, Darrion BG (Irish)
forms of Daron.
*Dariona, Darione, Darionna,
Darionne, Darriona, Darrionna*

Darius BG (Greek) wealthy.

Darla (English) a short form of
Darlene.
*Darlecia, Darli, Darlice, Darlie,
Darlis, Darly, Darlys*

Darlene (French) little darling.
See also Daryl.
*Darilynn, Darla, Darlean, Darlee,
Darleen, Darleene, Darlena,
Darlenia, Darlenne, Darletha,
Darlin, Darline, Darling, Darlyn,
Darlynn, Darlynne*

Darnee (Irish) a familiar form of
Darnelle.

Darnell BG (English) a form of Darnelle.

Darnelle (English) hidden place.
Darnee, Darnel, Darnell, Darnella, Darnesha, Darnetta, Darnette, Darnice, Darniece, Darnita, Darnyell

Darnesha, Darnisha (American) forms of Darnelle.
Darneisha, Darneishia, Darneshea, Darneshia, Darnesia, Darniesha, Darnishia, Darnisia, Darrenisha

Daron (Irish) great.
Darian, Darien, Darion, Daronica, Daronice, Darron, Daryn

Darrell (English, French) a form of Daryl.

Darren BG (Irish) great. (English) small; rocky hill.

Darryl BG (English, French) a form of Daryl.

Darselle (French) a form of Darcelle.
Darsel, Darsell, Darsella

Daru (Hindi) pine tree.

Daryl BG (English) beloved. (French) a short form of Darlene.
Darelle, Darielle, Daril, Darilynn, Darrel, Darrell, Darrelle, Darreshia, Darryl, Darryll, Daryll, Darylle

Daryn (Greek) gifts. (Irish) great.
Daron, Daryan, Daryne, Darynn, Darynne

Dasha, Dasia (Russian) forms of Dorothy.
Daisha, Dashae, Dashenka, Dashia, Dashiah, Dasiah, Daysha

Dashawn BG (American) a form of Dashawna.

Dashawna (American) a combination of the prefix Da + Shawna.
Dashawnna, Dashay, Dashell, Dayshana, Dayshawnna, Dayshona, Deshawna

Dashiki (Swahili) loose-fitting shirt worn in Africa.
Dashi, Dashika, Dashka, Desheka, Deshiki

Dashonda (American) a combination of the prefix Da + Shonda.
Dashawnda, Dishante

Davalinda (American) a combination of Davida + Linda.
Davalynda, Davelinda, Davilinda, Davylinda

Davalynda (American) a form of Davalinda.
Davelynda, Davilynda, Davylynda

Davalynn (American) a combination of Davida + Lynn.
Davalin, Davalyn, Davalynne, Davelin, Davelyn, Davelynn, Davelynne, Davilin, Davilyn, Davilynn, Davilynne, Dayleen, Devlyn

Dave BG (Hebrew) a short form of David, Davis.

David BG (Hebrew) beloved.

Davida (Hebrew) a form of David. See also Vida.
Daveta, Davetta, Davette, Davika, Davita

Davin BG (Scottish) a form of Davina.

Davina (Scottish) a form of Davida. See also Vina.
Dava, Davannah, Davean, Davee, Daveen, Daveena, Davene, Daveon, Davey, Davi, Daviana, Davie, Davin, Davinder, Davine, Davineen, Davinia, Davinna, Davonna, Davria, Devean, Deveen, Devene, Devina

Davion BG (Scottish, English) a form of Davonna.

Davis BG (American) a form of Davisha.

Davisha (American) a combination of the prefix Da + Aisha.
Daveisha, Davesia, Davis, Davisa

Davon BG (Scottish, English) a short form of Davonna.

Davonna (Scottish, English) a form of Davina, Devonna.
Davion, Daviona, Davionna, Davon, Davona, Davonda, Davone, Davonia, Davonne, Davonnia

Davonte BG (American) a combination of Davon + the suffix Te.

Dawn GB (English) sunrise, dawn.
Dawana, Dawandrea, Dawanna, Dawin, Dawna, Dawne, Dawnee, Dawnetta, Dawnisha, Dawnlynn, Dawnn, Dawnrae

Dawna (English) a form of Dawn.
Dawnna, Dawnya

Dawnisha (American) a form of Dawn.
Dawnesha, Dawni, Dawniell, Dawnielle, Dawnisia, Dawniss, Dawnita, Dawnnisha, Dawnysha, Dawnysia

Dawnyelle (American) a combination of Dawn + Danielle.
Dawnele, Dawnell, Dawnelle, Dawnyel, Dawnyella

Dawson BG (English) child of David.

Dayana (Latin) a form of Diana.
Dayanara, Dayani, Dayanna, Dayanne, Dayanni, Deyanaira, Dyani, Dyanna, Dyia

Dayanira (Greek) she stirs up great passions.

Dayle (English) a form of Dale.
Dayla, Daylan, Daylea, Daylee

Dayna (Scandinavian) a form of Dana.
Daynah, Dayne, Daynna, Deyna

Daysha (American) a form of
Dasha.
Daysa, Dayshalie, Daysia, Deisha

Daysi, Deysi (English) forms of
Daisy.
*Daysee, Daysia, Daysie, Daysy,
Deysia, Deysy*

Dayton BG (English) day town;
bright, sunny town.

Daytona (English) a form of
Dayton.
Daytonia

De BG (Chinese) virtuous.

Dean BG (French) leader.
(English) valley.

Deana GB (Latin) divine.
(English) a form of Dean.
*Deanah, Deane, Deanielle,
Deanisha, Deanna, Deeana,
Deeann, Deeanna, Deena*

Deandra (American) a combi-
nation of Dee + Andrea.
*Dandrea, Deandre, Deandré,
Deandrea, Deandree, Deandreia,
Deandria, Deanndra, Deaundra,
Deaundria, Deeandra, Deyaneira,
Deondra, Diandra, Diandre,
Diandrea, Diondria, Dyandra*

Deandre BG (American) a form
of Deandra, Deanna.

Deangela (Italian) a combination
of the prefix De + Angela.
Deangala, Deangalique, Deangle

Deanna GB (Latin) a form of
Deana, Diana.
*Deaana, Deahana, Deandra,
Deandre, Déanna, Deannia,
Deeanna, Deena*

Deanne (Latin) a form of Diane.
*Deahanne, Deane, Deann,
Déanne, Deeann, Dee-Ann,
Deeanne*

Debbie (Hebrew) a short form of
Deborah.
*Debbee, Debbey, Debbi, Debby,
Debee, Debi, Debie*

Débora, Déborah (Hebrew)
forms of Deborah.

Deborah GB (Hebrew) bee.
Bible: a great Hebrew prophetess.
*Deb, Debbie, Debbora, Debborah,
Deberah, Debor, Debora,
Deboran, Deborha, Deborrah,
Debra, Debrena, Debrina,
Debroah, Devora, Dobra*

Debra (American) a form of
Deborah.
*Debbra, Debbrah, Debrah,
Debrea, Debria*

Dedra (American) a form of
Deirdre.
*Deeddra, Deedra, Deedrea,
Deedrie*

Dedriana (American) a
combination of Dedra + Adriana.
Dedranae

Dee (Welsh) black, dark.
*De, Dea, Deah, Dede, Dedie,
Deea, Deedee, Dee Dee, Didi*

Deena (American) a form of
Deana, Dena, Dinah.

Deidamia (Greek) she who is
patient in battle.

Deidra, Deidre (Irish) forms of
Deirdre.
Deidrah, Deidrea, Deidrie, Diedra,
Diedre, Dierdra

Deina (Spanish) religious holiday.

Deion BG (Greek) a form of Dion.

Deirdre (Irish) sorrowful;
wanderer.
Dedra, Deerdra, Deerdre, Deidra,
Deidre, Deirdree, Didi, Diedra,
Dierdre, Diérdre, Dierdrie

Deisy (English) a form of Daisy.
Deisi, Deissy

Deitra (Greek) a short form of
Demetria.
Deetra, Detria

Deja GB (French) a form of Déja.

Déja (French) before.
Daeja, Daija, Deejay, Dejae, Déjah,
Dejai, Dejanae, Dejanelle, Dejon

Dejanae (French) a form of Déja.
Dajahnae, Dajona, Dejana,
Dejanah, Dejanae, Dejanai,
Dejanay, Dejane, Dejanea,
Dejanee, Dejanna, Dejannaye,
Dejena, Dejonae

Dejanira (Greek) destroyer of men.

Dejon (French) a form of Déja.
Daijon, Dajan, Dejone, Dejonee,
Dejonelle, Dejonna

Deka (Somali) pleasing.
Dekah

Delacy (American) a combination
of the prefix De + Lacy.
Delaceya

Delainey (Irish) a form of Delaney.
Delaine, Delainee, Delaini,
Delainie, Delainy

Delana (German) noble
protector.
Dalanna, Dalayna, Daleena,
Dalena, Dalenna, Dalina, Dalinda,
Dalinna, Delaina, Delania,
Delanya, Delayna, Deleena,
Delena, Delenya, Delina, Dellaina

Delaney GB (Irish) descendant
of the challenger. (English) a
form of Adeline.
Dalaney, Dalania, Dalene,
Daleney, Daline, Del, Delainey,
Delane, Delanee, Delanie, Delany,
Delayne, Delayney, Delaynie,
Deleani, Déline, Della, Dellaney

Delanie (Irish) a form of Delaney.
Delani

Delfina (Greek) a form of
Delphine. (Spanish) dolphin.
Delfeena, Delfine

Delia (Greek) visible; from Delos,
Greece. (German, Welsh) a short
form of Adelaide, Cordelia.
Mythology: a festival of Apollo
held in ancient Greece.
Dehlia, Delea, Deli, Deliah,
Deliana, Delianne, Delinda,
Dellia, Dellya, Delya

Delicia (English) delightful.
Delecia, Delesha, Delice, Delisa, Delise, Delisha, Delishia, Delisiah, Delya, Delys, Delyse, Delysia, Doleesha

Delilah (Hebrew) brooder. Bible: the companion of Samson. See also Lila.
Dalialah, Dalila, Daliliah, Delila, Delilia

Della (English) a short form of Adelaide, Cordelia, Delaney.
Del, Dela, Dell, Delle, Delli, Dellie, Dells

Delma (German) noble protector.

Delmara (Latin) of the sea.

Delmira (Spanish) a form of Dalmira.

Delores (Spanish) a form of Dolores.
Delora, Delore, Deloria, Delories, Deloris, Delorise, Delorita, Delsie

Delphine GB (Greek) from Delphi, Greece. See also Delfina.
Delpha, Delphe, Delphi, Delphia, Delphina, Delphinia, Delvina

Delsie (English) a familiar form of Delores.
Delsa, Delsey, Delza

Delta (Greek) door. Linguistics: the fourth letter in the Greek alphabet. Geography: a triangular land mass at the mouth of a river.
Delte, Deltora, Deltoria, Deltra

Demetria GB (Greek) cover of the earth. Mythology: Demeter was the Greek goddess of the harvest.
Deitra, Demeta, Demeteria, Demetra, Demetriana, Demetrianna, Demetrias, Demetrice, Demetriona, Demetris, Demetrish, Demetrius, Demi, Demita, Demitra, Demitria, Dymitra

Demetrius BG (Greek) a form of Demetria.

Demi (French) half. (Greek) a short form of Demetria.
Demia, Demiah, Demii, Demmi, Demmie, Demy

Demofila (Greek) friend of the village.

Dena (English, Native American) valley. (Hebrew) a form of Dinah. See also Deana.
Deane, Deena, Deeyn, Denae, Denah, Dene, Denea, Deney, Denna, Deonna

Denae (Hebrew) a form of Dena.
Denaé, Denay, Denee, Deneé

Deni (French) a short form of Denise.
Deney, Denie, Denni, Dennie, Denny, Dinnie, Dinny

Denica, Denika (Slavic) forms of Danica.
Denikah, Denikia

Denis BG (Greek) a form of Dennis.

Denisa (Spanish) god of wine.

Denise GB (French) Mythology: follower of Dionysus, the god of wine.
Danice, Danise, Denese, Deni, Denice, Denicy, Deniece, Denisha, Denisse, Denize, Dennise, Dennys, Denyce, Denys, Denyse

Denisha (American) a form of Denise.
Deneesha, Deneichia, Deneisha, Deneishea, Denesha, Deneshia, Deniesha, Denishia

Denisse (French) a form of Denise.
Denesse, Denissa

Dennis BG (Greek) Mythology: a follower of Dionysus, the god of wine.

Denver BG (English) green valley. Geography: the capital of Colorado.

Denzel BG (Cornish) a form of Denzell (see Boys' Names).

Deon BG (English) a short form of Deonna.

Deonilde (German) she who fights.

Deonna (English) a form of Dena.
Deona, Deonah, Deondra, Deonne

Deonte BG (American) a form of Deontae (see Boys' Names).

Derek BG (German) a short form of Theodoric (see Boys' Names).

Derika (German) ruler of the people.
Dereka, Derekia, Derica, Dericka, Derrica, Derricka, Derrika

Derrick BG (German) ruler of the people. A form of Derek.

Derry BG (Irish) redhead.
Deri, Derie

Deryn (Welsh) bird.
Derien, Derienne, Derion, Derin, Deron, Derren, Derrin, Derrine, Derrion, Derriona, Deryne

Desarae (French) a form of Desiree.
Desara, Desarai, Desaraie, Desaray, Desare, Desaré, Desarea, Desaree, Desarie, Dezarae

Desdemona (Greek) she who is very unfortunate; unhappy one.

Deserae, Desirae (French) forms of Desiree.
Desera, Deserai, Deseray, Desere, Deseree, Deseret, Deseri, Deserie, Deserrae, Deserray, Deserré, Dessirae, Dezeray, Dezere, Dezerea, Dezrae, Dezyrae

Deshawn BG (American) a form of Deshawna.

Deshawna (American) a combination of the prefix De + Shawna.
Dashawna, Deshan, Deshane, Deshaun, Deshawn, Desheania, Deshona, Deshonna

Deshawnda (American) a combination of the prefix De + Shawnda.
Deshanda, Deshandra, Deshaundra, Deshawndra, Deshonda

Desi (French) a short form of Desiree.
Désir, Desira, Dezi, Dezia, Dezzia, Dezzie

Desideria (French) desired or longed for.

Desiree (French) desired, longed for. See also Dessa.
Chesarey, Desarae, Deserae, Desi, Desirae, Desirah, Desirai, Desiray, Desire, Desirea, Desireah, Desirée, Désirée, Desirey, Desiri, Desray, Desree, Dessie, Dessire, Dezarae, Dezirae, Deziree

Dessa (Greek) wanderer. (French) a form of Desiree.

Desta (Ethiopian) happy. (French) a short form of Destiny.
Desti, Destie, Desty

Destany (French) a form of Destiny.
Destanee, Destaney, Destani, Destanie, Destannee, Destannie

Destin BG (French) a form of Destiny.

Destina (Spanish) fate.

Destinee, Destini, Destinie (French) forms of Destiny.
Desteni, Destiana, Destine, Destinée, Destnie

Destiney (French) a form of Destiny.

Destiny ☆ GB (French) fate.
Desnine, Desta, Destany, Destenee, Destenie, Desteny, Destin, Destinee, Destiney, Destini, Destinie, Destonie, Destynee, Dezstany

Destynee, Destyni (French) forms of Destiny.
Desty, Destyn, Destyne, Destyne, Destynie

Deva (Hindi) divine.
Deeva

Devan BG (Irish) a form of Devin.
Devana, Devane, Devanee, Devaney, Devani, Devanie, Devann, Devanna, Devannae, Devanne, Devany

Deven BG (Irish) a form of Devin.

Devera (Spanish) task.

Devi (Hindi) goddess. Religion: the Hindu goddess of power and destruction.

Devin BG (Irish) poet.
Devan, Deven, Devena, Devenje, Deveny, Devine, Devinn, Devinne, Devyn

Devon BG (English) a short form of Devonna. (Irish) a form of Devin.
Deaven, Devion, Devione, Devionne, Devone, Devoni, Devonne

Devonna (English) from
Devonshire.
Davonna, Devon, Devona,
Devonda, Devondra, Devonia

Devonta **BG** (American) a
combination of Devon + the
suffix Ta.

Devonte **BG** (American) a combination of Devon + the suffix Te.

Devora (Hebrew) a form of
Deborah.
Deva, Devorah, Devra, Devrah

Devota (Latin) faithful to God.

Devyn **BG** (Irish) a form of Devin.
Deveyn, Devyne, Devynn,
Devynne

Dextra (Latin) adroit, skillful.
Dekstra, Dextria

Deyanira (Latin) destroyer of men.

Dezarae, Dezirae, Deziree
(French) forms of Desiree.
Dezaraee, Dezarai, Dezaray,
Dezare, Dezaree, Dezarey,
Dezerie, Deziray, Dezirea,
Dezirée, Dezorae, Dezra

Di (Latin) a short form of Diana,
Diane.
Dy

Dia (Latin) a short form of Diana,
Diane.

Diamond **GB** (Latin) precious
gem.
Diamantina, Diamon, Diamonda,
Diamonde, Diamonia,
Diamonique, Diamonte,
Diamontina, Dyamond

Diana ⭐ **GB** (Latin) divine.
Mythology: the goddess of the
hunt, the moon, and fertility. See
also Deanna, Deanne, Dyan.
Daiana, Daianna, Dayana,
Dayanna, Di, Dia, Dianah,
Dianalyn, Dianarose, Dianatris,
Dianca, Diandra, Diane, Dianelis,
Diania, Dianielle, Dianita, Dianna,
Dianys, Didi

Diane, Dianne (Latin) short
forms of Diana.
Deane, Deanne, Deeane,
Deeanne, Di, Dia, Diahann, Dian,
Diani, Dianie, Diann

Dianna (Latin) a form of Diana.
Diahanna, Diannah

Diantha (Greek) divine flower.
Diandre, Dianthe

Diedra (Irish) a form of Deirdre.
Didra, Diedre

Diega (Spanish) supplanter.

Diella (Latin) she who adores
God.

Digna (Latin) worthy.

Dillan **BG** (Irish) loyal, faithful.
Dillon, Dillyn

Dillon **BG** (Irish) a form of
Dillan.

Dilys (Welsh) perfect; true.

Dimitri **BG** (Russian) a form of
Demetrius.

Dina (Hebrew) a form of Dinah.
Dinna, Dyna

Dinah (Hebrew) vindicated. Bible:
a daughter of Jacob and Leah.
Dina, Dinnah, Dynah

Dinka (Swahili) people.

Dinora (Hebrew) avenged or
vindicated.

Dinorah (Aramic) she who
personifies light.

Diomira (Spanish) a form of
Teodomira.

Dion 🅱🅶 (Greek) a form of
Dionne.

Dionisa (Greek) divine.

Dionisia (Greek) lover of wine;
blessed by God in face of
adversity.

Dionna (Greek) a form of
Dionne.
*Deona, Deondra, Deonia,
Deonna, Deonyia, Diona, Diondra,
Diondrea*

Dionne (Greek) divine queen.
Mythology: Dione was the mother
of Aphrodite, the goddess of love.
*Deonne, Dion, Dione, Dionee,
Dionis, Dionna, Dionte*

Dior (French) golden.
Diora, Diore, Diorra, Diorre

Dita (Spanish) a form of Edith.
Ditka, Ditta

Diva (Latin) divine.

Divinia (Latin) divine.
*Devina, Devinae, Devinia,
Devinie, Devinna, Diveena,
Divina, Divine, Diviniea, Divya*

Dixie (French) tenth. (English)
wall; dike. Geography: a
nickname for the American
South.
Dix, Dixee, Dixi, Dixy

Diza (Hebrew) joyful.
Ditza, Ditzah, Dizah

Dodie (Hebrew) beloved. (Greek)
a familiar form of Dorothy.
Doda, Dode, Dodee, Dodi, Dody

Dolly (American) a short form of
Dolores, Dorothy.
*Dol, Doll, Dollee, Dolley, Dolli,
Dollie, Dollina*

Dolores 🅶🅱 (Spanish) sorrowful.
Religion: Nuestra Señora de los
Dolores—Our Lady of Sorrows—
is a name for the Virgin Mary. See
also Lola.
*Delores, Deloria, Dolly,
Dolorcitas, Dolorita, Doloritas*

Domenic 🅱🅶 (Latin) an alternate
form of Dominic.

Domicia (Greek) she who loves
her house.

Domiciana (Spanish) a form of
Domicia.

Dominga (Latin) a form of
Dominica.

Dominic 🅱🅶 (Latin) belonging to
the Lord.

Dominica, Dominika (Latin) a form of Dominic. See also Mika.
Domenica, Domenika, Domineca, Domineka, Domini, Dominick, Dominicka, Dominique, Dominixe, Domino, Dominyika, Domka, Domnicka, Domonica, Domonice, Domonika

Domínica (Latin) a form of Dominica.

Dominick BG (Latin) a form of Dominica.

Dominique, Domonique GB (French) forms of Dominica, Dominika.
Domanique, Domeneque, Domenique, Domineque, Dominiqua, Domino, Dominoque, Dominque, Dominuque, Domique, Domminique, Domoniqua

Domino (English) a short form of Dominica, Dominique.

Dominque BG (French) a form of Dominique.

Domítica (Spanish) a form of Dominga.

Domitila (Latin) she who loves her house.

Don BG (Scottish) a short form of Donald (see Boys' Names).

Dona (English) world leader; proud ruler. (Italian) a form of Donna.
Donae, Donah, Donalda, Donaldina, Donelda, Donellia, Doni

Doña (Italian) a form of Donna.
Donail, Donalea, Donalisa, Donay, Doni, Donia, Donie, Donise, Donitrae

Donata (Latin) gift.
Donatha, Donato, Donatta, Donetta, Donette, Donita, Donnette, Donnita, Donte

Dondi (American) a familiar form of Donna.
Dondra, Dondrea, Dondria

Doneshia, Donisha (American) forms of Danessa.
Donasha, Donashay, Doneisha, Doneishia, Donesha, Donisa, Donisha, Donishia, Donneshia, Donnisha

Donina (Latin) gift of God.

Donna (Italian) lady.
Doña, Dondi, Donnae, Donnalee, Donnalen, Donnay, Donne, Donnell, Donni, Donnie, Donnise, Donny, Dontia, Donya

Donnell BG (Italian) a form of Donna.

Donnie BG (Italian) a familiar form of Donna.

Donniella (American) a form of Danielle.
Donella, Doniele, Doniell, Doniella, Donielle, Donnella, Donnielle, Donnyella, Donyelle

Donosa (Latin) she who has grace and charm.

Donte B☿ (Latin) a form of Donata.

Dontrell B☿ (American) a form of Dantrell (see Boys' Names).

Dora (Greek) gift. A short form of Adora, Eudora, Pandora, Theodora.
Dorah, Doralia, Doralie, Doralisa, Doraly, Doralynn, Doran, Dorchen, Dore, Dorece, Doree, Doreece, Doreen, Dorelia, Dorella, Dorelle, Doresha, Doressa, Doretta, Dori, Dorielle, Dorika, Doriley, Dorilis, Dorinda, Dorion, Dorita, Doro, Dory

Doralynn (English) a combination of Dora + Lynn.
Doralin, Doralyn, Doralynne, Dorlin

Dorana (Spanish) a form of Dorotea.

Dorbeta (Spanish) reference to the Virgin Mary.

Dorcas (Greek) gazelle.

Doreen (Irish) moody, sullen. (French) golden. (Greek) a form of Dora.
Doreena, Dorena, Dorene, Dorina, Dorine

Dores (Portuguese) a form of Dolores.

Doretta (American) a form of Dora, Dorothy.
Doretha, Dorette, Dorettie

Dori, Dory (American) familiar forms of Dora, Doria, Doris, Dorothy.
Dore, Dorey, Dorie, Dorree, Dorri, Dorrie, Dorry

Doria (Greek) a form of Dorian.
Dori

Dorian B☿ (Greek) from Doris, Greece.
Dorean, Doriana, Doriane, Doriann, Dorianna, Dorianne, Dorin, Dorina, Dorriane

Dorinda (Spanish) a form of Dora.

Doris (Greek) sea. Mythology: wife of Nereus and mother of the Nereids or sea nymphs.
Dori, Dorice, Dorisa, Dorise, Dorris, Dorrise, Dorrys, Dory, Dorys

Dorotea (Greek) a form of Dorothea.

Doroteia (Spanish) gift of God.

Dorotéia (Portuguese) a form of Doroteia.

Dorothea (Greek) a form of Dorothy. See also Thea.
Dorethea, Doroteya, Dorotha, Dorothia, Dorotthea, Dorthea, Dorthia

Dorothy (Greek) gift of God. See also Dasha, Dodie, Lolotea, Theodora.
Dasya, Do, Doa, Doe, Dolly, Doortje, Dorathy, Dordei, Dordi, Doretta, Dori, Dorika, Doritha,

*Dorka, Dorle, Dorlisa, Doro,
Dorolice, Dorosia, Dorota,
Dorothea, Dorothee, Dorothi,
Dorothie, Dorottya, Dorte, Dortha,
Dorthy, Dory, Dosi, Dossie, Dosya,
Dottie*

Dorrit (Greek) dwelling.
(Hebrew) generation.
Dorit, Dorita, Doritt

Dottie, Dotty (Greek) familiar
forms of Dorothy.
Dot, Dottee

Douglas **BG** (Scottish) dark river,
dark stream.

Drake **BG** (English) dragon;
owner of the inn with the dragon
trademark.

Draven **BG** (American) a combination of the letter D + Raven.

Drew **BG** (Greek) courageous;
strong. (Latin) a short form of
Drusilla.
Dru, Drue

Drinka (Spanish) a form of
Alexandria.
Dreena, Drena, Drina

Drusi (Latin) a short form of
Drusilla.
*Drucey, Druci, Drucie, Drucy,
Drusey, Drusie, Drusy*

Drusilla (Latin) descendant of
Drusus, the strong one. See also
Drew.
*Drewsila, Drucella, Drucill,
Drucilla, Druscilla, Druscille,
Drusi*

Duane **BG** (Irish) a form of
Dwayne.

Dulce (Latin) sweet.
*Delcina, Delcine, Douce, Doucie,
Dulcea, Dulcey, Dulci, Dulcia,
Dulciana, Dulcibel, Dulcibella,
Dulcie, Dulcine, Dulcinea, Dulcy,
Dulse, Dulsea*

Dulcina, Dulcinia (Spanish)
sweet.

Dulcinea (Spanish) sweet.
Literature: Don Quixote's love
interest.

Dunia (Hebrew) life.

Duscha (Russian) soul;
sweetheart; term of endearment.
Duschah, Dusha, Dushenka

Dusti (English) a familiar form of
Dustine.
Dustee, Dustie

Dustin **BG** (German, English) a
form of Dustine.

Dustine (German) valiant fighter.
(English) brown rock quarry.
*Dusteena, Dusti, Dustin, Dustina,
Dustyn*

Dusty **BG** (English) a familiar
form of Dustine.

Dwayne **BG** (Irish) dark.

Dyamond, Dymond (Latin)
forms of Diamond.
*Dyamin, Dyamon, Dyamone,
Dymin, Dymon, Dymonde,
Dymone, Dymonn*

Dyana (Latin) a form of Diana.
(Native American) deer.
Dyan, Dyane, Dyani, Dyann,
Dyanna, Dyanne

Dylan 🅱🅶 (Welsh) sea.
Dylaan, Dylaina, Dylana, Dylane,
Dylanee, Dylanie, Dylann, Dylanna,
Dylen, Dylin, Dyllan, Dylynn

Dyllis (Welsh) sincere.
Dilys, Dylis, Dylys

Dynasty (Latin) powerful ruler.
Dynastee, Dynasti, Dynastie

Dyshawna (American) a combi-
nation of the prefix Dy + Shawna.
Dyshanta, Dyshawn, Dyshonda,
Dyshonna

E

E 🅶🅱 (American) an initial used as
a first name.

Earlene (Irish) pledge. (English)
noblewoman.
Earla, Earlean, Earlecia, Earleen,
Earlena, Earlina, Earlinda, Earline,
Erla, Erlana, Erlene, Erlenne,
Erlina, Erlinda, Erline, Erlisha

Eartha (English) earthy.
Ertha

Easter (English) Easter time.
History: a name for a child born
on Easter.
Eastan, Eastlyn, Easton

Ebe (Greek) youthful like a flower.

Ebone, Ebonee (Greek) forms of
Ebony.
Abonee, Ebanee, Eboné, Ebonea,
Ebonne, Ebonnee

Eboni, Ebonie (Greek) forms of
Ebony.
Ebanie, Ebeni, Ebonni, Ebonnie

Ebony 🅶🅱 (Greek) a hard, dark
wood.
Abony, Eban, Ebanie, Ebany,
Ebbony, Ebone, Eboney, Eboni,
Ebonie, Ebonique, Ebonisha,
Ebonye, Ebonyi

Echo (Greek) repeated sound.
Mythology: the nymph who pined
for the love of Narcissus until
only her voice remained.
Echoe, Ecko, Ekko, Ekkoe

Eda (Irish, English) a short form
of Edana, Edith.

Edana (Irish) ardent; flame.
Eda, Edan, Edanna

Edda (German) a form of Hedda.
Etta

Eddy 🅱🅶 (American) a familiar
form of Edwina.
Eady, Eddi, Eddie, Edy

Edelia (Greek) remains young.

Edeline (English) noble; kind.
Adeline, Edelyne, Ediline, Edilyne

Edelma, Edelmira (Teutonic) of
noble heritage; known for her
noble heritage.

Eden GB (Babylonian) a plain. (Hebrew) delightful. Bible: the earthly paradise.
Eaden, Ede, Edena, Edene, Edenia, Edin, Edyn

Edén (Hebrew) a form of Eden.

Edgar BG (English) successful spearman.

Edgarda (Teutonic) defends her homes and land with a lance.

Edie (English) a familiar form of Edith.
Eadie, Edi, Edy, Edye, Eyde, Eydie

Edilia, Edilma (Greek) remains young.

Edith (English) rich gift. See also Dita.
Eadith, Eda, Ede, Edetta, Edette, Edie, Edit, Edita, Edite, Editha, Edithe, Editta, Ediva, Edyta, Edyth, Edytha, Edythe

Edna (Hebrew) rejuvenation. Religion: the wife of Enoch, according to the Book of Enoch.
Adna, Adnisha, Ednah, Edneisha, Edneshia, Ednisha, Ednita, Edona

Edrianna (Greek) a form of Adrienne.
Edria, Edriana, Edrina

Eduarda (Teutonic) attentive guardian of her domain.

Eduardo BG (Spanish) a form of Edward (see Boys' Names).

Edurne (Basque) snow.

Eduviges (Teutonic) fighting woman.

Eduvijis (German) fortunate in battle.

Edwin BG (English) prosperous friend.

Edwina (English) a form of Edwin. See also Winnie.
Eddy, Edina, Edweena, Edwena, Edwine, Edwyna, Edwynn

Effia (Ghanaian) born on Friday.

Effie (Greek) spoken well of. (English) a short form of Alfreda, Euphemia.
Effi, Effia, Effy, Ephie

Efigenia (Greek) woman of strong heritage.

Efigênia (Portuguese) a form of Efigenia.

Egda (Greek) shield-bearer.

Egeria (Greek) she who gives encouragement.

Egida (Spanish) born or having lived in Elade, Greece.

Egidia (Greek) warrior with a shield of goatskin.

Eileen GB (Irish) a form of Helen. See also Aileen, Ilene.
Eilean, Eileena, Eileene, Eilena, Eilene, Eiley, Eilie, Eilieh, Eilina, Eiline, Eilleen, Eillen, Eilyn, Eleen, Elene

Eira (Scandinavian) goddess-protectorate of health.

Ekaterina (Russian) a form of Katherine.
Ekaterine, Ekaterini

Ela (Polish) a form of Adelaide.

Eladia (Greek) born or having lived in Elade, Greece.

Elaina (French) a form of Helen.
Elainea, Elainia, Elainna

Elaine (French) a form of Helen. See also Lainey, Laine.
Eilane, Elain, Elaina, Elaini, Elan, Elana, Elane, Elania, Elanie, Elanit, Elauna, Elayna, Ellaine

Elaís (Spanish) a form of Elam.

Elam (Hebrew) highlands.

Elana (Greek) a short form of Eleanor. See also Ilana, Lana.
Elan, Elanee, Elaney, Elani, Elania, Elanie, Elanna, Elanni

Elata (Latin) elevated.

Elayna (French) a form of Elaina.
Elayn, Elaynah, Elayne, Elayni

Elba (Latin) a form of Alba.

Elberta (English) a form of Alberta.
Elbertha, Elberthina, Elberthine, Elbertina, Elbertine

Elbia (Spanish) a form of Elba.

Elcira (Teutonic) noble adornment.

Elda (German) she who battles.

Eldora (Spanish) golden, gilded.
Eldoree, Eldorey, Eldori, Eldoria, Eldorie, Eldory

Eleadora (Spanish) gift of the sun.

Eleanor GB (Greek) light.
History: Anna Eleanor Roosevelt was a U.S. delegate to the United Nations, a writer, and the thirty-second First Lady of the United States. See also Elana, Ella, Ellen, Leanore, Lena, Lenore, Leonore, Leora, Nellie, Nora, Noreen.
Elana, Elanor, Elanore, Eleanora, Eleanore, Elena, Eleni, Elenor, Elenorah, Elenore, Eleonor, Eleonore, Elianore, Elinor, Elinore, Elladine, Ellenor, Ellie, Elliner, Ellinor, Ellinore, Elna, Elnore, Elynor, Elynore

Eleanora (Greek) a form of Eleanor. See also Lena.
Elenora, Eleonora, Elianora, Ellenora, Ellenorah, Elnora, Elynora

Electa (Greek) blonde like the sun.

Electra (Greek) shining; brilliant. Mythology: the daughter of Agamemnon, leader of the Greeks in the Trojan War.
Elektra

Elena (Greek) a form of Eleanor. (Italian) a form of Helen.
Eleana, Eleen, Eleena, Elen, Elene, Elenitsa, Elenka, Elenna, Elenoa, Elenola, Ellena, Lena

Eleni (Greek) a familiar form of Eleanor.
Elenie, Eleny

Eleodora (Greek) she who came from the sun.

Eleora (Hebrew) the Lord is my light.
Eliora, Elira, Elora

Eleutería (Spanish) free.

Elexis (Greek) a form of Alexis.
Elexas, Elexes, Elexess, Elexeya, Elexia, Elexiah

Elexus (Greek) a form of Alexius, Alexus.
Elexius, Elexsus, Elexxus, Elexys

Elfrida (German) peaceful. See also Freda.
Elfrea, Elfreda, Elfredda, Elfreeda, Elfreyda, Elfrieda, Elfryda

Elga (Norwegian) pious. (German) a form of Helga.
Elgiva

Eli BG (Hebrew) uplifted. A short form of Elijah, Elisha.

Elia GB (Hebrew) a short form of Eliana.
Eliah

Eliana (Hebrew) my God has answered me. See also Iliana.
Elia, Eliane, Elianna, Ellianna, Liana, Liane

Eliane (Hebrew) a form of Eliana.
Elianne, Elliane, Ellianne

Elicia (Hebrew) a form of Elisha. See also Alicia.
Elecia, Elica, Elicea, Elicet, Elichia, Eliscia, Elisia, Elissia, Ellecia, Ellicia

Elida, Elide (Latin) forms of Alida.
Elidee, Elidia, Elidy

Eligia (Italian, Spanish) chosen one.

Elijah BG (Hebrew) a form of Eliyahu (see Boys' Names).

Elina (Greek, Italian) a form of Elena.

Elisa (Spanish, Italian, English) a short form of Elizabeth. See also Alisa, Ilisa.
Elecea, Eleesa, Elesa, Elesia, Elisia, Elisya, Ellisa, Ellisia, Ellissa, Ellissia, Ellissya, Ellisya, Elysa, Elysia, Elyssia, Elyssya, Elysya, Lisa

Elisabete (Portuguese) consecrated to God.

Elisabeth GB (Hebrew) a form of Elizabeth.
Elisabet, Elisabeta, Elisabethe, Elisabetta, Elisabette, Elisabith, Elisebet, Elisheba, Elisheva

Elise (French, English) a short form of Elizabeth, Elysia. See also Ilise, Liese, Lisette, Lissie.
Eilis, Eilise, Elese, Élise, Elisee, Elisie, Elisse, Elizé, Ellice, Ellise, Ellyce, Ellyse, Ellyze, Elsey, Elsie, Elsy, Elyce, Elyci, Elyse, Elyze, Lisel, Lisl, Lison

Elisea (Hebrew) God is salvation, protect my health.

Elisha BG (Hebrew) consecrated to God. (Greek) a form of Alisha. See also Ilisha, Lisha.
Eleacia, Eleasha, Eleesha, Eleisha, Elesha, Eleshia, Eleticia, Elicia, Elishah, Elisheva, Elishia, Elishua, Eliska, Ellesha, Ellexia, Ellisha, Elsha, Elysha, Elyshia

Elissa, Elyssa (Greek, English) forms of Elizabeth. Short forms of Melissa. See also Alissa, Alyssa, Lissa.
Elissah, Ellissa, Ellyssa, Ilissa, Ilyssa

Elita (Latin, French) chosen. See also Lida, Lita.
Elitia, Elitia, Elitie, Ellita, Ellitia, Ellitie, Ilida, Ilita, Litia

Eliza (Hebrew) a short form of Elizabeth. See also Aliza.
Eliz, Elizaida, Elizalina, Elize, Elizea

Elizabet (Hebrew) a form of Elizabeth.
Elizabete, Elizabette

Elizabeth ☀ GB (Hebrew) consecrated to God. Bible: the mother of John the Baptist. See also Bess, Beth, Betsy, Betty, Elsa, Ilse, Libby, Liese, Liesel, Lisa, Lisbeth, Lisette, Lissa, Lissie, Liz, Liza, Lizabeta, Lizabeth, Lizbeth, Lizina, Lizzy, Veta, Yelisabeta, Zizi.
Alizabeth, Eliabeth, Elisa, Elisabeth, Elise, Elissa, Eliza, Elizabee, Elizabet, Elizaveta, Elizebeth, Elka, Elsabeth, Elsbeth, Elschen, Elspeth, Elysabeth, Elzbieta, Elzsébet, Helsa, Ilizzabet, Lusa

Elizaveta (Polish, English) a form of Elizabeth.
Elisavet, Elisaveta, Elisavetta, Elisveta, Elizavet, Elizavetta, Elizveta, Elsveta, Elzveta

Elka (Polish) a form of Elizabeth.
Ilka

Elke (German) a form of Adelaide, Alice.
Elki, Ilki

Ella ☀ GB (English) elfin; beautiful fairy-woman. (Greek) a short form of Eleanor.
Ellah, Ellamae, Ellia, Ellie

Elle (Greek) a short form of Eleanor. (French) she.
El, Ele, Ell

Ellen (English) a form of Eleanor, Helen.
Elen, Elenee, Eleny, Elin, Elina, Elinda, Ellan, Ellena, Ellene, Ellie, Ellin, Ellon, Ellyn, Ellynn, Ellynne, Elyn

Ellice (English) a form of Elise.
Ellecia, Ellyce, Elyce

Ellie GB (English) a short form of Eleanor, Ella, Ellen.
Ele, Elie, Ellee, Elleigh, Elli

Elliot, Elliott BG (English) forms of Eli, Elijah.

Ellis BG (English) a form of Elias.

Elly (English) a short form of Eleanor, Ella, Ellen.

Elma (Turkish) sweet fruit.

Elmira (Arabic, Spanish) a form of Almira.
Elmeera, Elmera, Elmeria, Elmyra

Elnora (American) a combination of Ella + Nora.

Elodie (American) a form of Melody. (English) a form of Alodie.
Elodee, Elodia, Elody

Eloísa (German) a form of Louise.

Eloise (French) a form of Louise.
Elois, Eloisa, Eloisia

Elora (American) a short form of Elnora.
Ellora, Elloree, Elorie

Elpidia (Greek) she who waits faithfully, who lives her life waiting.

Elsa (German) noble. (Hebrew) a short form of Elizabeth. See also Ilse.
Ellsa, Ellse, Else, Elsia, Elsie, Elsje

Elsbeth (German) a form of Elizabeth.
Elsbet, Elzbet, Elzbieta

Elsie (German) a familiar form of Elsa, Helsa.
Ellsie, Ellsie, Ellsy, Elsi, Elsy

Elspeth (Scottish) a form of Elizabeth.
Elspet, Elspie

Elva (English) elfin. See also Alva, Alvina.
Elvia, Elvie

Elvina (English) a form of Alvina.
Elvenea, Elvinea, Elvinia, Elvinna

Elvira (Latin) white; blond. (German) closed up. (Spanish) elfin. Geography: the town in Spain that hosted a Catholic synod in 300 A. D.
Elva, Elvera, Elvire, Elwira, Vira

Elvisa (Teutonic) famous warrior.

Elvita (Spanish) truth.

Elyse (Latin) a form of Elysia.
Ellysa, Ellyse, Elyce, Elys, Elysee, Elysse

Elysia (Greek) sweet; blissful. Mythology: Elysium was the dwelling place of happy souls.
Elise, Elishia, Ellicia, Elycia, Elyssa, Ilysha, Ilysia

Elyssa (Latin) a form of Elysia.
Ellyssa

Emalee (Latin) a form of Emily.
Emaili, Emalea, Emaleigh, Emali, Emalia, Emalie

Emani (Arabic) a form of Iman.
Eman, Emane, Emaneé, Emanie, Emann

Emanuel BG (Hebrew) a form of Emanuelle.

Emanuelle (Hebrew) a form of
Emmanuelle.
Emanual, Emanuel, Emanuela,
Emanuella

Ember (French) a form of Amber.
Emberlee, Emberly

Emelia, Emelie (Latin) forms of
Emily.
Emellie

Emelinda (Teutonic) hard-
working and kind.

Emely (Latin) a form of Emily.
Emelly

Emerald (French) bright green
gemstone.
Emelda, Esmeralda

Emerenciana (Latin) she who
will be rewarded.

Emerita (Latin) she who God
rewards for her virtues.

Emerson BG (German, English)
child of Emery.

Emery BG (German) industrious
leader.
Emeri, Emerie

Emesta (Spanish) serious.

Emile BG (English) a form of
Emilee.

Emilee, Emilie (English) forms
of Emily.
Emile, Emilea, Emileigh, Émilie,
Emiliee, Emillee, Emillie,
Emmélie, Emmilee, Emylee

Emilia (Italian) a form of Amelia,
Emily.
Emalia, Emelia, Emila

Emilio BG (Italian, Spanish) a
form of Emil (see Boys' Names).

Emily ☀ GB (Latin) flatterer.
(German) industrious. See also
Amelia, Emma, Millie.
Eimile, Em, Emaily, Emalee,
Emeli, Emelia, Emelie, Emelita,
Emely, Emilee, Emiley, Emili,
Emilia, Emilie, Émilie, Emilis,
Emilka, Emillie, Emilly, Emmaline,
Emmaly, Emmélie, Emmey, Emmi,
Emmie, Emmilly, Emmily, Emmy,
Emmye, Emyle

Emilyann (American) a
combination of Emily + Ann.
Emileane, Emileann, Emileanna,
Emileanne, Emiliana, Emiliann,
Emilianna, Emilianne, Emillyane,
Emillyann, Emillyanna,
Emillyanne, Emliana, Emliann,
Emlianna, Emlianne

Emma ☀ GB (German) a short
form of Emily. See also Amy.
Em, Ema, Emmah, Emmy

Emmalee (American) a
combination of Emma + Lee. A
form of Emily.
Emalea, Emalee, Emilee,
Emmalea, Emmalei, Emmaleigh,
Emmaley, Emmali, Emmalia,
Emmalie, Emmaliese, Emmalyse,
Emylee

Emmaline (French) a form of Emily.
Emalina, Emaline, Emelina, Emeline, Emilienne, Emilina, Emiline, Emmalina, Emmalene, Emmeline, Emmiline

Emmalynn (American) a combination of Emma + Lynn.
Emelyn, Emelyne, Emelynne, Emilyn, Emilynn, Emilynne, Emlyn, Emlynn, Emlynne, Emmalyn, Emmalynne

Emmanuel BG (Hebrew) God is with us.

Emmanuela (Hebrew) a form of Emmanuelle.

Emmanuelle GB (Hebrew) a form of Emmanuel.
Emanuelle, Emmanuella

Emmy (German) a familiar form of Emma.
Emi, Emie, Emiy, Emmi, Emmie, Emmye, Emy

Emmylou (American) a combination of Emmy + Lou.
Emlou, Emmalou, Emmelou, Emmilou, Emylou

Emna (Teutonic) hard-working and kind.

Emory BG (German) a form of Emery.

Emperatriz (Latin) she who is the sovereign leader.

Ena (Irish) a form of Helen.
Enna

Enara (Basque) name given to a swallow.

Encarna, Encarnita (Spanish) forms of Encarnación.

Encarnación (Latin) alluding to the incarnation of Jesus in his mother, Mary.

Enedina (Greek) warm or indulgent.

Enid (Welsh) life; spirit.

Enma (Hebrew) a form of Emmanuela.

Enrica (Spanish) a form of Henrietta. See also Rica.
Enrieta, Enrietta, Enrika, Enriqua, Enriqueta, Enriquetta, Enriquette

Epifanía (Spanish) epiphany.

Eppie (English) a familiar form of Euphemia.
Effie, Effy, Eppy

Ercilia (Greek) she who is delicate, tender, kind.

Erendira, Erendiria (Spanish) one with a smile.

Eric BG (Scandinavian) ruler of all. (English) brave ruler. (German) a short form of Frederick (see Boys' Names).

Erica GB (Scandinavian) ruler of all. (English) brave ruler. See also Arica, Rica, Ricki.
Érica, Ericca, Ericha, Ericka, Errica

Ericka (Scandinavian) a form of Erica.
Erickah, Erricka

Erik BG (Scandinavian) a form of Eric.

Erika GB (Scandinavian) a form of Erica.
Erikaa, Erikah, Erikka, Errika, Eyka, Erykka, Eyrika

Erin ☆ GB (Irish) peace. History: another name for Ireland. See also Arin.
Earin, Earrin, Eran, Eren, Erena, Erene, Ereni, Eri, Erian, , Erine, Erinetta, Erinn, Errin, Eryn

Erina (Irish) a form of Erin.

Erinda (Spanish) a form of Erina.

Erinn (Irish) a form of Erin.
Erinna, Erinne

Erma (Latin) a short form of Ermine, Hermina. See also Irma.
Ermelinda

Ermenilda (German) powerful warrior.

Ermine (Latin) a form of Hermina.
Erma, Ermin, Ermina, Erminda, Erminie

Erminia (Latin) a form of Ermine.

Erna (English) a short form of Ernestine.

Ernestine (English) earnest, sincere.
Erna, Ernaline, Ernesia, Ernesta, Ernestina, Ernesztina

Eryn GB (Irish) a form of Erin.
Eiryn, Eryne, Erynn, Erynne

Escolástica (Latin) she who knows much and teaches.

Eshe (Swahili) life.
Eisha, Esha

Esmé (French) a familiar form of Esmeralda. A form of Amy.
Esma, Esme, Esmëe

Esmerada (Latin) shining, standing out. radiates purity and hope.

Esmeralda (Greek, Spanish) a form of Emerald.
Emelda, Esmé, Esmerelda, Esmerilda, Esmiralda, Ezmerelda, Ezmirilda

Esperanza (Spanish) hope. See also Speranza.
Esparanza, Espe, Esperance, Esperans, Esperansa, Esperanta, Esperanz, Esperenza

Essence (Latin) life; existence.
Essa, Essenc, Essencee, Essences, Essenes, Essense, Essynce

Essie (English) a short form of Estelle, Esther.
Essa, Essey, Essie, Essy

Estaquia (Spanish) possessor of a head of wheat.

Estebana (Spanish) crowned with laurels.

Estee (English) a short form of Estelle, Esther.
Esta, Estée, Esti

Estefani, Estefania, Estefany (Spanish) forms of Stephanie.
Estafania, Estefana, Estefane, Estefanía, Estefanie

Estela (French) a form of Estelle.

Estelinda (Teutonic) she who is noble and protects the village.

Estelle (French) a form of Esther. See also Stella, Trella.
Essie, Estee, Estel, Estele, Esteley, Estelina, Estelita, Estell, Estella, Estellina, Estellita, Esthella

Estephanie (Spanish) a form of Stephanie.
Estephania, Estephani, Estephany

Esterina (Greek) she who is strong and vital.

Esteva (Greek) crowned with laurels.

Esther (Persian) star. Bible: the Jewish captive whom Ahasuerus made his queen. See also Hester.
Essie, Estee, Ester, Esthur, Eszter, Eszti

Estralita (Spanish) a form of Estrella.

Estrella (French) star.
Estrela, Estrelinha, Estrell, Estrelle, Estrellita

Etel (Spanish) a short form of Etelvina.

Etelinda (German) noble one that protects her village.

Etelvina (German) she who is a loyal and noble friend.

Ethan **BG** (Hebrew) strong; firm.

Ethana (Hebrew) a form of Ethan.

Ethel (English) noble.
Ethelda, Ethelin, Etheline, Ethelle, Ethelyn, Ethelynn, Ethelynne, Ethyl

Etienne **BG** (French) a form of Stephen.

Étoile (French) star.

Etta (German) little. (English) a short form of Henrietta.
Etka, Etke, Etti, Ettie, Etty, Itke, Itta

Eudocia, Eudosia, Eudoxia (Greek) famous one, very knowledgeable.

Eudora (Greek) honored gift. See also Dora.

Eufrasia (Greek) she who is full of joy.

Eugene **BG** (Greek) born to nobility.

Eugenia (Greek) a form of Eugene. See also Gina.
Eugenie, Eugenina, Eugina, Evgenia

Eugênia (Portuguese) a form of Eugenia.

Eugenie (Greek) a form of Eugenia.
Eugenee, Eugénie

Eulalia (Greek) well spoken. See also Ula.
Eula, Eulalee, Eulalie, Eulalya, Eulia

Eulália (Portuguese) a form of Eulalia.

Eulogia (Greek) she who speaks eloquently.

Eumelia (Greek) she who sings well, the melodious one.

Eun (Korean) silver.

Eunice (Greek) happy; victorious. Bible: the mother of Saint Timothy. See also Unice.
Euna, Eunique, Eunise, Euniss

Eunomia (Greek) good order.

Euphemia (Greek) spoken well of, in good repute. History: a fourth-century Christian martyr.
Effam, Effie, Eppie, Eufemia, Euphan, Euphemie, Euphie

Eurídice (Greek) a form of Eurydice.

Eurydice (Greek) wide, broad. Mythology: the wife of Orpheus.
Euridice, Euridyce, Eurydyce

Eusebia (Greek) respectful, pious.

Eustacia (Greek) productive. (Latin) stable; calm. See also Stacey.
Eustasia

Eustaquia (Greek) well-built.

Eutimia (Spanish) she who is benevolent.

Eva GB (Greek) a short form of Evangelina. (Hebrew) a form of Eve. See also Ava, Chava.
Éva, Evah, Evalea, Evalee, Evike

Evaline (French) a form of Evelyn.
Evalin, Evalina, Evalyn, Evalynn, Eveleen, Evelene, Evelina, Eveline

Evan BG (Irish) young warrior.

Evangelina (Greek) bearer of good news.
Eva, Evangelene, Evangelia, Evangelica, Evangeline, Evangelique, Evangelyn, Evangelynn

Evania (Irish) a form of Evan.
Evana, Evanka, Evann, Evanna, Evanne, Evany, Eveania, Evvanne, Evvunea, Evyan

Evarista (Greek) excellent one.

Eve (Hebrew) life. Bible: the first woman created by God. (French) a short form of Evonne. See also Chava, Hava, Naeva, Vica, Yeva.
Eva, Evie, Evita, Evuska, Evyn, Ewa, Yeva

Evelia (Hebrew) she who generates life.

Evelin (English) a form of Evelyn.
Evelina, Eveline

Evelyn ⚝ **GB** (English) hazelnut.
Avalyn, Aveline, Evaleen, Evalene, Evaline, Evalyn, Evalynn, Evalynne, Eveleen, Evelin, Evelyna, Evelyne, Evelynn, Evelynne, Evline, Ewalina

Everett **BG** (German) courageous as a boar.

Everilda (German) she who fought with the wild boar.

Evette (French) a form of Yvette. A familiar form of Evonne. See also Ivette.
Evett

Evie (Hungarian) a form of Eve.
Evey, Evi, Evicka, Evike, Evka, Evuska, Evvie, Evvy, Evy, Ewa

Evita (Spanish) a form of Eve.

Evline (English) a form of Evelyn.
Evleen, Evlene, Evlin, Evlina, Evlyn, Evlynn, Evlynne

Evodia (Greek) she who always wants others to have a good trip.

Evonne (French) a form of Yvonne. See also Ivonne.
Evanne, Eve, Evenie, Evenne, Eveny, Evette, Evin, Evon, Evona, Evone, Evoni, Evonna, Evonnie, Evony, Evyn, Evynn, Eyona, Eyvone

Exal (Spanish) diminutive form of Exaltación.

Exaltación (Spanish) lifted up.

Ezmeralda (Spanish) emerald.

Ezra **BG** (Hebrew) a form of Ezri.

Ezri (Hebrew) helper; strong.
Ezra, Ezria

F

Fabia (Latin) bean grower.
Fabiana, Fabienne, Fabiola, Fabra, Fabria

Fabian **BG** (Latin) a form of Fabienne.

Fabiana (Latin) a form of Fabia.
Fabyana

Fabienne (Latin) a form of Fabia.
Fabian, Fabiann, Fabianne, Fabiene, Fabreanne

Fabiola, Faviola (Latin) forms of Fabia.
Fabiole, Fabyola, Faviana, Faviolha

Fabricia (Latin) artisan, daughter of artisans.

Facunda (Latin) eloquent speaker.

Faith ⚝ **GB** (English) faithful; fidelity. See also Faye, Fidelity.
Fayth, Faythe

Faizah (Arabic) victorious.

Falda (Icelandic) folded wings.
Faida, Fayda

Faline (Latin) catlike.
Faleen, Falena, Falene, Falin, Falina, Fallyn, Fallyne, Faylina, Fayline, Faylyn, Faylynn, Faylynne, Felenia, Felina

Fallon 🇬🇧 (Irish) grandchild of the ruler.
Falan, Falen, Fallan, Fallen, Fallonne, Falon, Falyn, Falynn, Falynne, Phalon

Falviana (Spanish) she who has blonde locks of hair.

Fancy (French) betrothed. (English) whimsical; decorative.
Fanchette, Fanchon, Fanci, Fancia, Fancie

Fannie, Fanny (American) familiar forms of Frances.
Fan, Fanette, Fani, Fania, Fannee, Fanney, Fanni, Fannia, Fany, Fanya

Fantasia (Greek) imagination.
Fantasy, Fantasya, Fantaysia, Fantazia, Fiantasi

Farah, Farrah (English) beautiful; pleasant.
Fara, Farra, Fayre

Faren, Farren (English) wanderer.
Faran, Fare, Farin, Faron, Farrahn, Farran, Farrand, Farrin, Farron, Farryn, Farye, Faryn, Feran, Ferin, Feron, Ferran, Ferren, Ferrin, Ferron, Ferryn

Fátim (Arabic) only daughter of Mahoma.

Fatima (Arabic) daughter of the Prophet. History: the daughter of Muhammad.
Fatema, Fathma, Fatimah, Fatime, Fatma, Fatmah, Fatme, Fattim

Fátima (Arabic) a form of Fatima.

Fausta, Faustina (Latin) fortunate or lucky.

Favia (Latin) she who raises beans.

Fawn (French) young deer.
Faun, Fawna, Fawne

Fawna (French) a form of Fawn.
Fauna, Fawnia, Fawnna

Faye (French) fairy; elf. (English) a form of Faith.
Fae, Fay, Fayann, Fayanna, Fayette, Fayina, Fey

Fayola (Nigerian) lucky.
Fayla, Feyla

Fe (Latin) trust or belief.

Febe (Greek) shining one.

Fedra (Greek) splendid one.

Felecia (Latin) a form of Felicia.
Flecia

Felecidade (Portuguese) happiness.

Felica (Spanish) a short form of Felicia.
Falisa, Felisa, Felisca, Felissa, Feliza

Felice (Latin) a short form of
Felicia.
*Felece, Felicie, Felise, Felize,
Felyce, Felysse*

Felicia (Latin) fortunate; happy.
See also Lecia, Phylicia.
*Falecia, Faleshia, Falicia, Fela,
Felecia, Felica, Felice, Felicidad,
Feliciona, Felicity, Felicya,
Felisea, Felisha, Felisia, Felisiana,
Felissya, Felita, Felixia, Felizia,
Felka, Fellcia, Felycia, Felysia,
Felyssia, Fleasia, Fleichia,
Fleishia, Flichia*

Feliciana (Spanish, Italian,
Ancient Roman) a form of Felix.

Felicity (English) a form of
Felicia.
*Falicity, Felicita, Felicitas, Félicité,
Feliciti, Felisita, Felisity*

Felipe **BG** (Spanish) a form of
Philip.

Felisha (Latin) a form of Felicia.
*Faleisha, Falesha, Falisha,
Falleshia, Feleasha, Feleisha,
Felesha, Felishia, Fellishia,
Felysha, Flisha*

Felix (Latin) fortunate; happy.

Femi (French) woman. (Nigerian)
love me.
Femie, Femmi, Femmie, Femy

Feodora (Greek) gift of God.
Fedora, Fedoria

Fermina (Spanish) strong.

Fern (English) fern. (German) a
short form of Fernanda.
*Ferne, Ferni, Fernlee, Fernleigh,
Fernley, Fernly*

Fernanda (German) daring,
adventurous. See also Andee,
Nan.
*Ferdie, Ferdinanda, Ferdinande,
Fern, Fernande, Fernandette,
Fernandina, Nanda*

Feronia (Latin) goddess of the
forest and fountains.

Fiala (Czech) violet.

Fidelia (Latin) a form of Fidelity.
Fidela, Fidele, Fidelina

Fidelity (Latin) faithful, true. See
also Faith.
Fidelia, Fidelita

Fifi **GB** (French) a familiar form
of Josephine.
Feef, Feefee, Fifine

Filippa (Italian) a form of
Philippa.
Felipa, Filipa, Filippina, Filpina

Filis (Greek) adorned with leaves.

Filomena (Italian) a form of
Philomena.
Fila, Filah, Filemon

Filotea (Greek) she who loves
God.

Fiona (Irish) fair, white.
Fionna

Fionnula (Irish) white
shouldered. See also Nola, Nuala.
*Fenella, Fenula, Finella, Finola,
Finula*

Fiorel (Latin) a form of Flor.

Fiorela (Italian) small flower.

Fiorella (Spanish) a form of
Fiorela.

Flair (English) style; verve.
Flaire, Flare

Flaminia (Latin) alluding to one
who belongs to a religious order.

Flannery (Irish) redhead.
Literature: Flannery O'Connor
was a renowned American writer.
Flan, Flann, Flanna

Flavia (Latin) blond, golden
haired.
*Flavere, Flaviar, Flavie, Flavien,
Flavienne, Flaviere, Flavio,
Flavyere, Fulvia*

Flávia (Portuguese) a form of
Flavia.

Flavie (Latin) a form of Flavia.
Flavi

Fleur (French) flower.
Fleure, Fleuree, Fleurette

Flo (American) a short form of
Florence.

Flor (Latin) a short form of Flora.

Flora (Latin) flower. A short form
of Florence. See also Lore.
*Fiora, Fiore, Fiorenza, Florann,
Florella, Florelle, Floren, Floria,
Floriana, Florianna, Florica,
Florimel*

Floramaría (Spanish) flower of
Mary.

Florence (Latin) blooming;
flowery; prosperous. History:
Florence Nightingale, a British
nurse, is considered the founder
of modern nursing. See also
Florida.
*Fiorenza, Flo, Flora, Florance,
Florencia, Florency, Florendra,
Florentia, Florentina, Florentyna,
Florenza, Floretta, Florette, Florie,
Florina, Florine, Floris, Flossie*

Floria (Basque) a form of Flora.
Flori, Florria

Florida (Spanish) a form of
Florence.
Floridia, Florinda, Florita

Florie (English) a familiar form of
Florence.
*Flore, Flori, Florri, Florrie, Florry,
Flory*

Florinia (Latin) blooming or
flowering.

Floris (English) a form of
Florence.
Florisa, Florise

Florisel (Spanish) a form of
Flora.

Flossie (English) a familiar form
of Florence.
Floss, Flossi, Flossy

Floyd BG (English) a form of
Lloyd.

Fola (Yoruba) honorable.

Fonda (Latin) foundation.
(Spanish) inn.
Fondea, Fonta

Fontanna (French) fountain.
*Fontaine, Fontana, Fontane,
Fontanne, Fontayne*

Forest BG (French) a form of
Forrest.

Forrest BG (French) forest;
woodsman.

Fortuna (Latin) fortune; fortunate.
Fortoona, Fortune

Fortunata (Latin) fortunate one.

Fran GB (Latin) a short form of
Frances.
Frain, Frann

Frances GB (Latin) a form of
Francis. See also Paquita.
*Fanny, Fran, Franca, France,
Francee, Francena, Francesca,
Francess, Francesta, Franceta,
Francetta, Francette, Francine,
Francisca, Françoise, Frankie,
Frannie, Franny*

Francesca GB (Italian) a form of
Frances.
*Franceska, Francessca, Francesta,
Franchesca, Franzetta*

Franchesca (Italian) a form of
Francesca.
*Cheka, Chekka, Chesca, Cheska,
Francheca, Francheka, Franchelle,
Franchesa, Francheska,
Franchessca, Franchesska*

Franci (Hungarian) a familiar
form of Francine.
Francey, Francie, Francy

Francine (French) a form of
Frances.
*Franceen, Franceine, Franceline,
Francene, Francenia, Franci,
Francin, Francina, Francyne*

Francis BG (Latin) free; from
France.
Francise, Franncia, Francys

Francisca (Italian) a form of
Frances.
*Franciska, Franciszka, Frantiska,
Franziska*

Françoise (French) a form of
Frances.

Frankie BG (American) a familiar
form of Frances.
*Francka, Francki, Franka, Frankey,
Franki, Frankia, Franky, Frankye*

Franklin BG (English) free
landowner.

Frannie, Franny (English)
familiar forms of Frances.
*Frani, Frania, Franney, Franni,
Frany*

Fraser BG (French) strawberry.
(English) curly haired.

Freda, Freida, Frida (German)
short forms of Alfreda, Elfrida,
Frederica, Sigfreda.
*Frayda, Fredda, Fredella, Fredia,
Fredra, Freeda, Freeha, Freia,
Frida, Frideborg, Frieda*

Freddi (English) familiar forms of
Frederica, Winifred.
*Fredda, Freddy, Fredi, Fredia,
Fredy, Frici*

Freddie 🅱🅶 (English) a form of
Freddi.

Fredel (Nahuatl) forever you.

Frederica (German) peaceful
ruler. See also Alfreda, Rica,
Ricki.
*Farica, Federica, Freda,
Fredalena, Fredaline, Freddi,
Freddie, Frederickina, Frederika,
Frederike, Frederina, Frederine,
Frederique, Fredith, Fredora,
Fredreca, Fredrica, Fredricah,
Fredricia, Freida, Fritzi, Fryderica*

Frederika (German) a form of
Frederica.
*Fredericka, Fredreka, Fredricka,
Fredrika, Fryderyka*

Frederike (German) a form of
Frederica.
Fredericke, Friederike

Frederique 🅶🅱 (French) a form
of Frederica.
Frédérique, Rike

Fredrick 🅱🅶 (German) a form of
Frederick (see Boys' Names).

Freja (Scandinavian) a form of
Freya.

Frescura (Spanish) freshness.

Freya (Scandinavian)
noblewoman. Mythology: the
Norse goddess of love.
Fraya, Freya

Freyra (Slavic) goddess of love.

Frine (Spanish) female toad.

Fritzi (German) a familiar form of
Frederica.
*Friezi, Fritze, Fritzie, Fritzinn,
Fritzline, Fritzy*

Fronde (Latin) leafy branch.

Fructuosa (Spanish) fruitful.

Fulgencia (Spanish) she who
excels because of her great
kindness.

G

G 🅱🅶 (American) an initial used as
a first name.

Gabina (Latin) she who is a native
of Gabio, an ancient city close to
Rome where Romulus was
raised.

Gabriel 🅱🅶 (French) devoted to
God.

Gabriele (French) forms of
Gabrielle.
Gabbriel, Gabbryel, Gabreal,

Gabreale, Gabreil, Gabrial, Gabryel

Gabriela GB (Italian) a form of Gabrielle.
Gabriala, Gabrielia, Gabrila

Gabriella ✾ GB (Italian) a form of Gabrielle.
Gabrialla, Gabriellia, Gabrilla, Gabryella

Gabrielle ✾ GB (French) a form of Gabriel.
Gabbrielle, Gabielle, Gabrealle, Gabriana, Gabriel, Gabriela, Gabriele, Gabriell, Gabriella, Gabrille, Gabrina, Gabriylle, Gabryell, Gabryelle, Gaby, Gavriella

Gabryel BG (French) a form of Gabriel.

Gaby (French) a familiar form of Gabrielle.
Gabbey, Gabbi, Gabbie, Gabby, Gabey, Gabi, Gabie, Gavi, Gavy

Gada (Hebrew) lucky.
Gadah

Gaea (Greek) planet Earth. Mythology: the Greek goddess of Earth.
Gaia, Gaiea, Gaya

Gaetana (Italian) from Gaeta. Geography: Gaeta is a city in southern Italy.
Gaetan, Gaétane, Gaetanne

Gagandeep BG (Sikh) sky's light.
Gagandip, Gagnadeep, Gagndeep

Gage BG (French) pledge.

Gail (Hebrew) a short form of Abigail. (English) merry, lively.
Gael, Gaela, Gaelle, Gaila, Gaile, Gale, Gayla, Gayle

Gala (Norwegian) singer.
Galla

Galatea (Greek) she with skin as white as milk.

Galen BG (Greek) healer; calm. (Irish) little and lively.
Gaelen, Gaellen, Galyn, Gaylaine, Gayleen, Gaylen, Gaylene, Gaylyn

Galena (Greek) healer; calm.

Galenia (Greek) healer.

Gali (Hebrew) hill; fountain; spring.
Galice, Galie

Galilah (Hebrew) important, exalted.

Galina (Russian) a form of Helen.
Gailya, Galayna, Galenka, Galia, Galiana, Galiena, Galinka, Galochka, Galya, Galyna

Ganesa (Hindi) fortunate. Religion: Ganesha was the Hindu god of wisdom.

Ganya BG (Hebrew) garden of the Lord. (Zulu) clever.
Gana, Gani, Gania, Ganice, Ganit

Garabina, Garabine (Spanish) purification.

Garaitz (Basque) victory.

Garbina, Garbine (Spanish) purification.

García (Latin) she who demonstrates her charm and grace.

Gardenia (English) Botany: a sweet-smelling flower.
Deeni, Denia, Gardena, Gardinia

Garett 🅱🅶 (Irish) a form of Garrett.

Garland 🅱🅶 (French) wreath of flowers.

Garnet (English) dark red gem.
Garnetta, Garnette

Garoa (Basque) fern.

Garrett 🅱🅶 (Irish) brave spear carrier.

Garrison 🅱🅶 (French) troops stationed at a fort; garrison.

Gary 🅱🅶 (German) mighty spear carrier. (English) a familiar form of Gerald.

Garyn (English) spear carrier.
Garan, Garen, Garra, Garryn

Gasha (Russian) a familiar form of Agatha.
Gashka

Gaspara (Spanish) treasurer.

Gaudencia (Spanish) happy, content.

Gavin 🅱🅶 (Welsh) white hawk.

Gavriella (Hebrew) a form of Gabrielle.
Gavila, Gavilla, Gavrid, Gavrieela, Gavriela, Gavrielle, Gavrila, Gavrilla

Gay (French) merry.
Gae, Gai, Gaye

Gayle (English) a form of Gail.
Gayla

Gayna (English) a familiar form of Guinevere.
Gaynah, Gayner, Gaynor

Gea (Greek) old name given to the earth.

Gechina (Basque) grace.

Geela (Hebrew) joyful.
Gela, Gila

Geena (American) a form of Gena.
Geania, Geeana, Geeanna

Gelya (Russian) angelic.

Gema, Gemma (Latin, Italian) jewel, precious stone. See also Jemma.
Gem, Gemmey, Gemmie, Gemmy

Gemini (Greek) twin.
Gemelle, Gemima, Gemina, Geminine, Gemmina

Gen (Japanese) spring. A short form of names beginning with "Gen."

Gena 🅶🅱 (French) a form of Gina. A short form of Geneva, Genevieve, Iphigenia.
Geanna, Geena, Geenah, Gen, Genae, Genah, Genai, Genea, Geneja, Geni, Genia, Genie

Gene BG (Greek) a short form of Eugene.

Geneen (Scottish) a form of Jeanine.
Geanine, Geannine, Gen, Genene, Genine, Gineen, Ginene

Genell (American) a form of Jenelle.

Generosa (Spanish) generous.

Genesis GB (Latin) origin; birth.
Genes, Genese, Genesha, Genesia, Genesiss, Genessa, Genesse, Genessie, Genessis, Genicis, Genises, Genysis, Yenesis

Geneva (French) juniper tree. A short form of Genevieve. Geography: a city in Switzerland.
Geena, Gen, Gena, Geneieve, Geneiva, Geneive, Geneve, Ginneva, Janeva, Jeaneva, Jeneva

Genevieve GB (German, French) a form of Guinevere. See also Gwendolyn.
Gen, Genaveeve, Genaveve, Genavie, Genavieve, Genavive, Geneva, Geneveve, Genevie, Geneviéve, Genevievre, Genevive, Genovieve, Genvieve, Ginette, Gineveve, Ginevieve, Ginevive, Guinevieve, Guinivive, Gwenevieve, Gwenivive, Jennavieve

Genevra (French, Welsh) a form of Guinevere.
Gen, Genever, Genevera, Ginevra

Genice (American) a form of Janice.
Gen, Genece, Geneice, Genesa, Genesee, Genessia, Genis, Genise

Genita (American) a form of Janita.
Gen, Genet, Geneta

Genna (English) a form of Jenna.
Gen, Gennae, Gennay, Genni, Gennie, Genny

Gennifer (American) a form of Jennifer.
Gen, Genifer, Ginnifer

Genovieve (French) a form of Genevieve.
Genoveva, Genoveve, Genovive

Georgeanna (English) a combination of Georgia + Anna.
Georgana, Georganna, Georgeana, Georgiana, Georgianna, Georgyanna, Giorgianna

Georgeanne (English) a combination of Georgia + Anne.
Georgann, Georganne, Georgean, Georgeann, Georgie, Georgyann, Georgyanne

Georgene (English) a familiar form of Georgia.
Georgeena, Georgeina, Georgena, Georgenia, Georgiena, Georgienne, Georgina, Georgine

Georgette (French) a form of Georgia.
Georgeta, Georgett, Georgetta, Georjetta

Georgia GB (Greek) farmer. Art: Georgia O'Keeffe was an American painter known especially for her paintings of flowers. Geography: a southern American state; a country in Eastern Europe. See also Jirina, Jorja.
Georgene, Georgette, Georgie, Giorgia

Georgianna (English) a form of Georgeanna.
Georgiana, Georgiann, Georgianne, Georgie, Georgieann, Georgionna

Georgie (English) a familiar form of Georgeanne, Georgia, Georgianna.
Georgi, Georgy, Giorgi

Georgina (English) a form of Georgia.
Georgena, Georgene, Georgine, Giorgina, Jorgina

Gerald BG (German) mighty spear carrier.

Geraldine (German) a form of Gerald. See also Dena, Jeraldine.
Geralda, Geraldina, Geraldyna, Geraldyne, Gerhardine, Geri, Gerianna, Gerianne, Gerrilee, Giralda

Geralyn (American) a combination of Geraldine + Lynn.
Geralisha, Geralynn, Gerilyn, Gerrilyn

Geranio (Greek) she is as beautiful as a geranium.

Gerardo BG (English) brave with a spear.
Gerardine

Gerda (Norwegian) protector. (German) a familiar form of Gertrude.
Gerta

Geri (American) a familiar form of Geraldine. See also Jeri.
Gerri, Gerrie, Gerry

Germaine (French) from Germany. See also Jermaine.
Germain, Germana, Germanee, Germani, Germanie, Germaya, Germine

Gertie (German) a familiar form of Gertrude.
Gert, Gertey, Gerti, Gerty

Gertrude (German) beloved warrior. See also Trudy.
Gerda, Gerta, Gertie, Gertina, Gertraud, Gertrud, Gertruda

Gertrudes, Gertrudis (Spanish) beloved warrior.

Gervaise BG (French) skilled with a spear.

Gervasi (Spanish) having to do with spears.

Gessica (Italian) a form of Jessica.
Gesica, Gesika, Gess, Gesse, Gessy

Geva (Hebrew) hill.
Gevah

Gezana, Gezane (Spanish) reference to the Incarnation.

Ghada (Arabic) young; tender.
Gada

Ghita (Italian) pearly.
Gita

Gianira (Greek) nymph from the sea.

Gianna (Italian) a short form of Giovanna. See also Jianna, Johana.
Geona, Geonna, Giana, Gianella, Gianetta, Gianina, Gianinna, Gianne, Giannee, Giannella, Giannetta, Gianni, Giannie, Giannina, Gianny, Gianoula

Gigi (French) a familiar form of Gilberte.
Geegee, G. G., Giggi

Gilana (Hebrew) joyful.
Gila, Gilah

Gilberte (German) brilliant; pledge; trustworthy. See also Berti.
Gigi, Gilberta, Gilbertina, Gilbertine, Gill

Gilda (English) covered with gold.
Gilde, Gildi, Gildie, Gildy

Gill (Latin, German) a short form of Gilberte, Gillian.
Gili, Gilli, Gillie, Gilly

Gillian GB (Latin) a form of Jillian.
Gila, Gilana, Gilenia, Gili, Gilian, Gill, Gilliana, Gilliane, Gilliann, Gillianna, Gillianne, Gillie, Gilly, Gillyan, Gillyane, Gillyann, Gillyanne, Gyllian, Lian

Gin (Japanese) silver. A short form of names beginning with "Gin."

Gina (Italian) a short form of Angelina, Eugenia, Regina, Virginia. See also Jina.
Gena, Gin, Ginah, Ginai, Ginna

Ginebra (Celtic) white as foam.

Gines (Greek) she who engenders life.

Ginette (English) a form of Genevieve.
Gin, Ginata, Ginett, Ginetta, Ginnetta, Ginnette

Ginger (Latin) flower; spice. A familiar form of Virginia.
Gin, Ginja, Ginjer, Ginny

Ginia (Latin) a familiar form of Virginia.
Gin

Ginnifer (English) white; smooth; soft. (Welsh) a form of Jennifer.
Gin, Ginifer

Ginny (English) a familiar form of Ginger, Virginia. See also Jin, Jinny.
Gin, Gini, Ginney, Ginni, Ginnie, Giny, Gionni, Gionny

Gioconda (Latin) she who engenders life.

Giordana (Italian) a form of Jordana.

Giorgianna (English) a form of Georgeanna.
Giorgina

Giovanna (Italian) a form of Jane.
Geovana, Geovanna, Geovonna, Giavanna, Giavonna, Giovana, Giovanne, Giovannica, Giovonna, Givonnie, Jeveny

Giovanni BG (Italian) a form of Giovanna.

Gisa (Hebrew) carved stone.
Gazit, Gissa

Gisela (German) a form of Giselle.
Gisella, Gissela, Gissella

Giselda (German, Teutonic) arrow; ray; token of happiness.

Giselle GB (German) pledge; hostage. See also Jizelle.
Ghisele, Gisel, Gisela, Gisele, Geséle, Giseli, Gisell, Gissell, Gisselle, Gizela, Gysell

Gissel, Gisselle (German) forms of Giselle.
Gissell

Gita (Yiddish) good. (Polish) a short form of Margaret.
Gitka, Gitta, Gituska

Gitana (Spanish) gypsy; wanderer.

Gitta (Irish) a short form of Bridget.
Getta

Giulia (Italian) a form of Julia.
Giulana, Giuliana, Giulianna, Giulliana, Guila, Guiliana, Guilietta

Giunia (Latin) she who was born in June.

Gizela (Czech) a form of Giselle.
Gizel, Gizele, Gizella, Gizelle, Gizi, Giziki, Gizus

Gladis (Irish) a form of Gladys.
Gladi, Gladiz

Gladys (Latin) small sword. (Irish) princess. (Welsh) a form of Claudia.
Glad, Gladis, Gladness, Gladwys, Glady, Gwladys

Glaucia (Portuguese) brave gift.

Glen BG (Irish) a form of Glenn.

Glenda (Welsh) a form of Glenna.
Glanda, Glennda, Glynda

Glenn BG (Irish) valley, glen.

Glenna (Irish) a form of Glenn. See also Glynnis.
Glenda, Glenetta, Glenina, Glenine, Glenne, Glennesha, Glennia, Glennie, Glenora, Gleny, Glyn

Glennesha (American) a form of Glenna.
Glenesha, Glenisha, Glennisha, Glennishia

Gloria GB (Latin) glory. History: Gloria Steinem, a leading American feminist, founded Ms. magazine.
Gloresha, Gloriah, Gloribel, Gloriela, Gloriella, Glorielle, Gloris, Glorisha, Glorvina, Glory

Glorianne (American) a combination of Gloria + Anne.
Gloriana, Gloriane, Gloriann, Glorianna

Glory (Latin) a form of Gloria.

Glynnis (Welsh) a form of Glenna.
Glenice, Glenis, Glenise, Glenyse, Glennis, Glennys, Glenwys, Glenys, Glenyss, Glinnis, Glinys, Glynesha, Glynice, Glynis, Glynisha, Glyniss, Glynitra, Glynys, Glynyss

Godalupe (Spanish) reference to the Virgin Mary.

Golda (English) gold. History: Golda Meir was a Russian-born politician who served as prime minister of Israel.
Goldarina, Golden, Goldie, Goldina

Goldie (English) a familiar form of Golda.
Goldi, Goldy

Goma (Swahili) joyful dance.

Graça (Portuguese) a form of Grace.

Grace ☆ (Latin) graceful.
Engracia, Graca, Gracia, Gracie, Graciela, Graciella, Gracinha, Graice, Grata, Gratia, Gray, Grayce, Grecia

Graceanne (English) a combination of Grace + Anne.
Graceann, Graceanna, Gracen, Graciana, Gracianna, Gracin, Gratiana

Gracia (Spanish) a form of Grace.
Gracea, Grecia

Gracie (English) a familiar form of Grace.
Gracee, Gracey, Graci, Gracy, Graecie, Graysie

Graham BG (English) grand home.

Grant BG (English) great; giving.

Grayson BG (English) bailiff's child.
Graison, Graisyn, Grasien, Grasyn, Graysen

Grazia (Latin) a form of Grace.
Graziella, Grazielle, Graziosa, Grazyna

Grecia (Latin) a form of Grace.

Greer (Scottish) vigilant.
Grear, Grier

Gregoria (Spanish) vigilant watchman.

Gregoriana (Spanish) a form of Gregoria.

Gregorina (Latin) watches over her group of people.

Gregory 🅱🅶 (Latin) vigilant watch guard.

Greta (German) a short form of Gretchen, Margaret.
Greatal, Greatel, Greeta, Gretal, Grete, Gretel, Gretha, Grethal, Grethe, Grethel, Gretta, Grette, Grieta, Gryta, Grytta

Gretchen (German) a form of Margaret.
Greta, Gretchin, Gretchyn

Gricelda (German) a form of Griselda.
Gricelle

Griffin 🅱🅶 (Latin) hooked nose.

Grisel (German) a short form of Griselda.
Grisell, Griselle, Grissel, Grissele, Grissell, Grizel

Grisela (Spanish) a form of Griselda.

Griselda (German) gray woman warrior. See also Selda, Zelda.
Gricelda, Grisel, Griseldis, Griseldys, Griselys, Grishilda, Grishilde, Grisselda, Grissely, Grizelda

Guadalupe 🅶🅱 (Arabic) river of black stones. See also Lupe.
Guadalup, Guadelupe, Guadlupe, Guadulupe, Gudalupe

Gudrun (Scandinavian) battler. See also Runa.
Gudren, Gudrin, Gudrinn, Gudruna

Guía (Spanish) guide.

Guillelmina (Italian, Spanish) resolute protector.

Guillerma (Spanish) a short form of Guillermina.
Guilla, Guillermina

Guinevere (French, Welsh) white wave; white phantom. Literature: the wife of King Arthur. See also Gayna, Genevieve, Genevra, Jennifer, Winifred, Wynne.
Generva, Genn, Ginette, Guenevere, Guenna, Guinivere, Guinna, Gwen, Gwenevere, Gwenivere, Gwynnevere

Guioma (Spanish) a form of Giuomar.

Guiomar (German) famous in combat.

Gunda (Norwegian) female warrior.
Gundala, Gunta

Gundelina (Teutonic) she who helps in battle.

Gundelinda (German) pious one in the battle.

Gundenia (German) fighter.

Gurit (Hebrew) innocent baby.

Gurjot 🅱🅶 (Sikh) light of the guru.

Gurleen (Sikh) follower of the guru.

Gurpreet BG (Punjabi) religion.
Gurprit

Gurvir BG (Sikh) guru's warrior.

Gusta (Latin) a short form of Augusta.
Gus, Gussi, Gussie, Gussy, Gusti, Gustie, Gusty

Gustava (Scandinavian) staff of the Goths.

Guy BG (Hebrew) valley. (German) warrior. (French) guide.

Gwen (Welsh) a short form of Guinevere, Gwendolyn.
Gwenesha, Gweness, Gweneta, Gwenetta, Gwenette, Gweni, Gwenisha, Gwenita, Gwenn, Gwenna, Gwennie, Gwenny

Gwenda (Welsh) a familiar form of Gwendolyn.
Gwinda, Gwynda, Gwynedd

Gwendolyn (Welsh) white wave; white browed; new moon. Literature: Gwendoloena was the wife of Merlin, the magician. See also Genevieve, Gwyneth, Wendy.
Guendolen, Gwen, Gwendalin, Gwenda, Gwendalee, Gwendaline, Gwendalyn, Gwendalynn, Gwendela, Gwendelyn, Gwendelynn, Gwendilyn, Gwendolen, Gwendolene, Gwendolin, Gwendoline, Gwendolyne,
Gwendolynn, Gwendolynne, Gwendylan, Gwyndolyn, Gwynndolen

Gwyn GB (Welsh) a short form of Gwyneth.
Gwinn, Gwinne, Gwynn, Gwynne

Gwyneth (Welsh) a form of Gwendolyn. See also Winnie, Wynne.
Gweneth, Gwenith, Gwenneth, Gwennyth, Gwenyth, Gwyn, Gwynneth

Gypsy (English) wanderer.
Gipsy, Gypsie, Jipsi

H GB (American) an initial used as a first name.

Habiba (Arabic) beloved.
Habibah, Habibeh

Hachi (Japanese) eight; good luck.
Hachiko, Hachiyo

Hada (Hebrew) she who radiates joy.

Hadara (Hebrew) adorned with beauty.
Hadarah

Hadasa (Hebrew) myrtle.

Hadassah (Hebrew) myrtle tree.
Hadas, Hadasah, Hadassa, Haddasa, Haddasah

Hadiya (Swahili) gift.
Hadaya, Hadia, Hadiyah, Hadiyyah

Hadley GB (English) field of heather.
Hadlea, Hadlee, Hadleigh, Hadli, Hadlie, Hadly

Hadriane (Greek, Latin) a form of Adrienne.
Hadriana, Hadrianna, Hadrianne, Hadriene, Hadrienne

Haeley (English) a form of Hailey.
Haelee, Haeleigh, Haeli, Haelie, Haelleigh, Haelli, Haellie, Haely

Hagar (Hebrew) forsaken; stranger. Bible: Sarah's handmaiden, the mother of Ishmael.
Haggar

Haidee (Greek) modest.
Hady, Haide, Haidi, Haidy, Haydee, Haydy

Haiden BG (English) heather-covered hill.
Haden, Hadyn, Haeden, Haidn, Haidyn

Hailee (English) a form of Hayley.
Haile, Hailei, Haileigh, Haillee

Hailey ☆ GB (English) a form of Hayley.
Haeley, Haiely, Hailea, Hailley, Hailly, Haily

Haili, Hailie (English) forms of Hayley.
Haille, Hailli, Haillie

Hakeem BG (Arabic) a form of Hakim (see Boys' Names).

Haldana (Norwegian) half-Danish.

Halee GB (English) a form of Haley.
Hale, Halea, Haleah, Haleh, Halei

Haleigh (English) a form of Haley.

Haley ☆ GB (Scandinavian) heroine. See also Hailey, Hayley.
Halee, Haleigh, Hali, Halley, Hallie, Haly, Halye

Hali GB (English) a form of Haley.

Halia (Hawaiian) in loving memory.

Halie (English) a form of Haley.
Haliegh

Halimah (Arabic) gentle; patient.
Halima, Halime

Halina (Hawaiian) likeness. (Russian) a form of Helen.
Haleen, Haleena, Halena, Halinka

Halla (African) unexpected gift.
Hala, Hallah, Halle

Halley GB (English) a form of Haley.
Hally, Hallye

Hallie GB (Scandinavian) a form of Haley.
Hallee, Hallei, Halleigh, Halli

Halona (Native American) fortunate.
Halonah, Haloona, Haona

Halsey GB (English) Hall's island.
Halsea, Halsie

Hama (Japanese) shore.

Hana, Hanah (Japanese) flower.
(Arabic) happiness. (Slavic)
forms of Hannah.
*Hanae, Hanan, Haneen, Hanicka,
Hanin, Hanita, Hanka*

Hanako (Japanese) flower child.

Hania (Hebrew) resting place.
*Haniya, Hanja, Hannia, Hanniah,
Hanya*

Hanna GB (Hebrew) a form of
Hannah.

Hannah ☆ GB (Hebrew)
gracious. Bible: the mother of
Samuel. See also Anci, Anezka,
Ania, Anka, Ann, Anna, Annalie,
Anneka, Chana, Nina, Nusi.
*Hana, Hanna, Hanneke, Hannele,
Hanni, Hannon, Honna*

Hanni (Hebrew) a familiar form
of Hannah.
Hani, Hanne, Hannie, Hanny

Happy (English) happy.
Happi

Hara GB (Hindi) tawny. Religion:
another name for the Hindu god
Shiva, the destroyer.

Harlee, Harleigh, Harlie
(English) forms of Harley.
Harlei, Harli

Harley BG (English) meadow of
the hare. See also Arleigh.
Harlee, Harleey, Harly

Harleyann (English) a combi-
nation of Harley + Ann.
*Harlann, Harlanna, Harlanne,
Harleen, Harlene, Harleyanna,
Harleyanne, Harliann, Harlianna,
Harlianne, Harlina, Harline*

Harmony (Latin) harmonious.
*Harmene, Harmeni, Harmon,
Harmonee, Harmonei, Harmoni,
Harmonia, Harmonie*

Harpreet GB (Punjabi) devoted
to God.
Harprit

Harriet (French) ruler of the
household. (English) a form of
Henrietta. Literature: Harriet
Beecher Stowe was an American
writer noted for her novel *Uncle
Tom's Cabin*.
*Harri, Harrie, Harriett, Harrietta,
Harriette, Harriot, Harriott, Hattie*

Harrison BG (English) child of
Harry.

Haru (Japanese) spring.

Harvir BG (Sikh) God's warrior.

Hasana (Swahili) she arrived
first. Culture: a name used for the
first-born female twin. See also
Huseina.
*Hasanna, Hasna, Hassana,
Hassna, Hassona*

Hasina (Swahili) good.
Haseena, Hasena, Hassina

Hateya (Moquelumnan) footprints.

Hattie (English) familiar forms of Harriet, Henrietta.
Hatti, Hatty, Hetti, Hettie, Hetty

Hausu (Moquelumnan) like a bear yawning upon awakening.

Hava (Hebrew) a form of Chava. See also Eve.
Havah, Havvah

Haven GB (English) a form of Heaven.
Havan, Havana, Havanna, Havannah, Havyn

Haviva (Hebrew) beloved.
Havalee, Havelah, Havi, Hayah

Hayden BG (English) a form of Haiden.
Hayde, Haydin, Haydn, Haydon

Hayfa (Arabic) shapely.

Haylee, Hayleigh, Haylie (English) forms of Hayley.
Hayle, Haylea, Haylei, Hayli, Haylle, Hayllie

Hayley GB (English) hay meadow. See also Hailey, Haley.
Hailee, Haili, Haylee, Hayly

Hazel (English) hazelnut tree; commanding authority.
Hazal, Hazaline, Haze, Hazeline, Hazell, Hazelle, Hazen, Hazyl

Heath BG (English) a form of Heather.

Heather GB (English) flowering heather.
Heatherlee, Heatherly

Heaven GB (English) place of beauty and happiness. Bible: where God and angels are said to dwell.
Haven, Heavan, Heavenly, Heavin, Heavon, Heavyn, Hevean, Heven, Hevin

Hebe (Greek) youthful like a flower.

Hecuba (Greek) wife of Priam, king of Troy.

Hedda (German) battler. See also Edda, Hedy.
Heda, Hedaya, Hedia, Hedvick, Hedvig, Hedvika, Hedwig, Hedwiga, Heida, Hetta

Hedy (Greek) delightful; sweet. (German) a familiar form of Hedda.
Heddey, Heddi, Heddie, Heddy, Hede, Hedi

Heidi, Heidy (German) short forms of Adelaide.
Heida, Heide, Heidee, Heidie, Heydy, Hidee, Hidi, Hidie, Hidy, Hiede, Hiedi, Hydi

Helda (German) she who battles.

Helen GB (Greek) light. See also Aileen, Aili, Alena, Eileen, Elaina, Elaine, Eleanor, Ellen, Galina, Ila, Ilene, Ilona, Jelena, Leanore,

Leena, Lelya, Lenci, Lene, Liolya,
Nellie, Nitsa, Olena, Onella,
Yalena, Yelena.
Elana, Ena, Halina, Hela, Hele,
Helena, Helene, Helle, Hellen,
Helli, Hellin, Hellon, Hellyn,
Helon

Helena (Greek) a form of Helen.
See also Ilena.
Halena, Halina, Helaina, Helana,
Helania, Helayna, Heleana,
Heleena, Helenia, Helenka,
Helenna, Helina, Hellanna,
Hellena, Hellenna, Helona,
Helonna

Helene (French) a form of Helen.
Helaine, Helanie, Helayne,
Heleen, Heleine, Hèléne, Helenor,
Heline, Hellenor

Helga (German) pious.
(Scandinavian) a form of Olga.
See also Elga.

Heli (Spanish) a form of Heliana.

Helia (Greek) as if she were the
sun.

Heliana (Greek) she who offers
herself to God.

Heliena (Greek) sun.

Helki BG (Native American)
touched.
Helkey, Helkie, Helky

Helma (German) a short form of
Wilhelmina.
Halma, Helme, Helmi, Helmine,
Hilma

Heloísa (German) a form of
Eloísa.

Heloise (French) a form of Louise.
Héloïse, Hlois

Helsa (Danish) a form of Elizabeth.
Helse, Helsey, Helsi, Helsie,
Helsy

Heltu (Moquelumnan) like a bear
reaching out.

Helvecia (Latin) member of the
Helvetians, ancient inhabitants of
Switzerland; happy friend.

Helvia (Latin) she who has
blonde locks of hair.

Henna (English) a familiar form
of Henrietta.
Hena, Henaa, Henah, Heni,
Henia, Henny, Henya

Henrietta (English) ruler of the
household. See also Enrica, Etta,
Yetta.
Harriet, Hattie, Hatty, Hendrika,
Heneretta, Henka, Henna,
Hennrietta, Hennriette, Henretta,
Henrica, Henrie, Henrieta,
Henriete, Henriette, Henrika,
Henrique, Henriquetta, Henryetta,
Hetta, Hettie

Hera (Greek) queen; jealous.
Mythology: the queen of heaven
and the wife of Zeus.

Hercilia, Hersilia (Greek) she
who is delicate, tender, kind.

Hermelinda (German) she who
is the shield of strength.

Hermenegilda (Spanish) she who offers sacrifices to God.

Hermia (Greek) messenger.

Hermilda (German) battle of force.

Hermina (Latin) noble. (German) soldier. See also Erma, Ermine, Irma.
Herma, Hermenia, Hermia, Herminna

Herminda (Greek) announcer.

Hermínia (Portuguese) a form of Hermina.

Hermione (Greek) earthy.
Hermalina, Hermia, Hermina, Hermine, Herminia

Hermosa (Spanish) beautiful.

Hernanda (Spanish) bold voyager.

Hertha (English) child of the earth.
Heartha, Hirtha

Herundina (Latin) like a swallow.

Hester (Dutch) a form of Esther.
Hessi, Hessie, Hessye, Hesther, Hettie

Hestia (Persian) star. Mythology: the Greek goddess of the hearth and home.
Hestea, Hesti, Hestie, Hesty

Heta (Native American) racer.

Hetta (German) a form of Hedda. (English) a familiar form of Henrietta.

Hettie (German) a familiar form of Henrietta, Hester.
Hetti, Hetty

Higinia (Greek) she who has and enjoys good health.

Hilary, Hillary GB (Greek) cheerful, merry. See also Alair.
Hilaree, Hilari, Hilaria, Hilarie, Hilery, Hiliary, Hillaree, Hillari, Hillarie, Hilleary, Hilleree, Hilleri, Hillerie, Hillery, Hillianne, Hilliary, Hillory

Hilda (German) a short form of Brunhilda, Hildegarde.
Helle, Hilde, Hildey, Hildie, Hildur, Hildy, Hulda, Hylda

Hildegarda (German) she who hopes to fight.

Hildegarde (German) fortress.
Hilda, Hildagard, Hildagarde, Hildegard, Hildred

Hildegunda (German) heroic fighter.

Hinda (Hebrew) hind; doe.
Hindey, Hindie, Hindy, Hynda

Hipatia (Greek) best.

Hipólita (Greek) she who unties her horse and readies herself for battle.

Hisa (Japanese) long lasting.
Hisae, Hisako, Hisay

Hiti (Eskimo) hyena.
Hitty

Hoa (Vietnamese) flower; peace.
Ho, Hoai

Hogolina (Teutonic) having clear thoughts and great intelligence.

Hola (Hopi) seed-filled club.

Holden BG (English) hollow in the valley.

Holley (English) a form of Holly.
Holleah, Hollee

Holli (English) a form of Holly.

Hollie GB (English) a form of Holly.
Holeigh, Holleigh

Hollis BG (English) near the holly bushes.
Hollise, Hollyce, Holyce

Holly GB (English) holly tree.
Holley, Hollye

Hollyann (English) a combination of Holly + Ann.
Holliann, Hollianna, Hollianne, Hollyanne, Hollyn

Hollyn (English) a short form of Hollyann.
Holin, Holeena, Hollina, Hollynn

Honey (English) sweet. (Latin) a familiar form of Honora.
Honalee, Hunney, Hunny

Hong (Vietnamese) pink.

Honora (Latin) honorable. See also Nora, Onora.
Honey, Honner, Honnor, Honnour, Honor, Honorah, Honorata, Honore, Honoree, Honoria,
Honorina, Honorine, Honour, Honoure

Honoratas (Spanish) honor.

Hope GB (English) hope.
Hopey, Hopi, Hopie

Hortense (Latin) gardener. See also Ortensia.
Hortencia, Hortensia

Hoshi (Japanese) star.
Hoshie, Hoshiko, Hoshiyo

Houston BG (English) hill town. Geography: a city in Texas.

Hua (Chinese) flower.

Huanquyi (Mapuche) announcer; she who has a loud voice, shouted.

Huata (Moquelumnan) basket carrier.

Hugo BG (Latin) a form of Hugh (see Boys' Names).

Hugolina (Teutonic) having clear thoughts and great intelligence.

Huilen, Huillen, Hullen (Araucanian) spring.

Humildad (Latin) humility.

Hunter BG (English) hunter.
Hunta, Huntar, Huntter

Huong (Vietnamese) flower.

Huseina (Swahili) a form of Hasana.

Hyacinth (Greek) Botany: a plant with colorful, fragrant flowers. See also Cynthia, Jacinda.
Giacinta, Hyacintha, Hyacinthe, Hyacinthia, Hyacinthie, Hycinth, Hycynth

Hydi, Hydeia (German) forms of Heidi.
Hyde, Hydea, Hydee, Hydia, Hydie, Hydiea

Hye (Korean) graceful.

I

Ian 🅑🅖 (Hebrew) God is gracious.
Iaian, Iain, Iana, Iann, Ianna, Iannel, Iyana

Ianthe (Greek) violet flower.
Iantha, Ianthia, Ianthina

Iara (Tupi) she is a lady.

Iberia (Latin) she who is a native of Iberia or comes from the Iberian peninsula.

Icess (Egyptian) a form of Isis.
Ices, Icesis, Icesse, Icey, Icia, Icis, Icy

Ida (German) hard working. (English) prosperous.
Idah, Idaia, Idalia, Idalis, Idaly, Idamae, Idania, Idarina, Idarine, Idaya, Ide, Idelle, Idette, Idys

Idalina (English) a combination of Ida + Lina.
Idaleena, Idaleene, Idalena, Idalene, Idaline

Idalis (English) a form of Ida.
Idalesse, Idalise, Idaliz, Idallas, Idallis, Idelis, Idelys, Idialis

Idara (Latin) well-organized woman.

Ideashia (American) a combination of Ida + Iesha.
Idasha, Idaysha, Ideesha, Idesha

Idelgunda (German) combative when fighting.

Idelia, Idelina (German) she who is noble.

Idelle (Welsh) a form of Ida.
Idell, Idella, Idil

Idoia (Spanish) reference to the Virgin Mary.

Idoya (Spanish) pond, an important place of worship of the Virgin Mary.

Idumea (Latin) red.

Idurre (Spanish) reference to the Virgin Mary.

Iesha (American) a form of Aisha.
Ieachia, Ieaisha, Ieasha, Ieashe, Ieesha, Ieeshia, Ieisha, Ieishia, Iescha, Ieshah, Ieshea, Iesheia, Ieshia, Iiesha, Iisha

Ifigenia (Greek) having great strength and vitality; woman of strong, vital roots.

Ifiginia (Spanish) a form of Ifigenia.

Ignacia (Latin) fiery, ardent.
Ignacie, Ignasha, Ignashia, Ignatia, Ignatzia

Ikia (Hebrew) God is my salvation. (Hawaiian) a form of Isaiah.
Ikaisha, Ikea, Ikeea, Ikeia, Ikeisha, Ikeishi, Ikeishia, Ikesha, Ikeshia, Ikeya, Ikeyia, Ikiea, Ikiia

Ila (Hungarian) a form of Helen.

Ilana (Hebrew) tree.
Ilaina, Ilane, Ilani, Ilania, Ilainie, Illana, Illane, Illani, Ilania, Illanie, Ilanit

Ilchahueque (Mapuche) young, virginal woman.

Ilda (German) heroine in battle.

Ildegunda (German) she who knows how to fight.

Ileana (Hebrew) a form of Iliana.
Ilea, Ileah, Ileane, Ileanna, Ileanne, Illeana

Ilena (Greek) a form of Helena.
Ileana, Ileena, Ileina, Ilina, Ilyna

Ilene (Irish) a form of Helen. See also Aileen, Eileen.
Ileen, Ileene, Iline, Ilyne

Iliana (Greek) from Troy.
Ileana, Ili, Ilia, Iliani, Illiana, Illiani, Illianna, Illyana, Illyanna

Ilima (Hawaiian) flower of Oahu.

Ilisa (Scottish, English) a form of Alisa, Elisa.
Ilicia, Ilissa, Iliza, Illisa, Illissa, Illysa, Illyssa, Ilycia, Ilysa, Ilysia, Ilyssa, Ilyza

Ilise (German) a form of Elise.
Ilese, Illytse, Ilyce, Ilyse

Ilisha (Hebrew) a form of Alisha, Elisha. See also Lisha.
Ileshia, Ilishia, Ilysha, Ilyshia

Ilka (Hungarian) a familiar form of Ilona.
Ilke, Milka, Milke

Ilona (Hungarian) a form of Helen.
Ilka, Illona, Illonia, Illonya, Ilonka, Ilyona

Ilse (German) a form of Elizabeth. See also Elsa.
Ilsa, Ilsey, Ilsie, Ilsy

Iluminada (Spanish) illuminated.

Ima (Japanese) presently. (German) a familiar form of Amelia.

Imaculada (Portuguese) immaculate.

Imala (Native American) strong-minded.

Iman GB (Arabic) believer.
Aman, Imana, Imane, Imani

Imani GB (Arabic) a form of Iman.
Amani, Emani, Imahni, Imanie, Imanii, Imonee, Imoni

Imelda (German) warrior.
Imalda, Irmhilde, Melda

Imena (African) dream.
Imee, Imene

Imogene (Latin) image, likeness.
*Emogen, Emogene, Imogen,
Imogenia, Imojean, Imojeen,
Innogen, Innogene*

Imperia (Latin) imperial.

Imperio (Latin) head of state, ruler.

Ina (Irish) a form of Agnes.
Ena, Inanna, Inanne

Indamira, Indemira (Arabic)
guest of the princess.

India (Hindi) from India.
*Indea, Indeah, Indee, Indeia,
Indeya, Indi, Indiah, Indian,
Indiana, Indianna, Indie, Indieya,
Indiya, Indy, Indya*

Indigo (Latin) dark blue color.
Indiga, Indygo

Indira (Hindi) splendid. History:
Indira Nehru Gandhi was an Indian
politician and prime minister.
Indiara, Indra, Indre, Indria

Ines, Inés, Inez (Spanish) forms
of Agnes. See also Ynez.
Inesa, Inesita, Inésita, Inessa

Inês (Portuguese) a form of Ines.

Inga (Scandinavian) a short form
of Ingrid.
*Ingaberg, Ingaborg, Inge,
Ingeberg, Ingeborg, Ingela*

Ingrid (Scandinavian) hero's
daughter; beautiful daughter.
Inga, Inger

Inmaculada (Latin) she who is
pure and clean, without
blemishes.

Inoa (Hawaiian) name.

**Inocencia, Inoceneia,
Inocenta** (Spanish) innocence.

Invención (Latin) invention.

Ioana (Romanian) a form of Joan.
Ioani, Ioanna

Iola (Greek) dawn; violet colored.
(Welsh) worthy of the Lord.
Iole, Iolee, Iolia

Iolana (Hawaiian) soaring like a
hawk.

Iolanthe (English) a form of
Yolanda. See also Jolanda.
Iolanda, Iolande

Iona (Greek) violet flower.
*Ione, Ioney, Ioni, Ionia, Iyona,
Iyonna*

Iphigenia (Greek) sacrifice.
Mythology: the daughter of the
Greek leader Agamemnon. See
also Gena.

Ipi (Mapuche) harvester; careful.

Iratze (Basque) reference to the
Virgin Mary.

Irene GB (Greek) peaceful.
Mythology: the goddess of peace.
See also Orina, Rena, Rene,

Yarina.
Irén, Irien, Irina, Jereni

Iridia (Latin) belonging to Iris.

Iriel (Hebrew) a form of Uriel.

Irimia (Spanish) name of the place where the Miño river starts.

Irina (Russian) a form of Irene.
Eirena, Erena, Ira, Irana, Iranda, Iranna, Irena, Irenea, Irenka, Iriana, Irin, Irinia, Irinka, Irona, Ironka, Irusya, Iryna, Irynka, Rina

Iris GB (Greek) rainbow. Mythology: the goddess of the rainbow and messenger of the gods.
Irisa, Irisha, Irissa, Irita, Irys, Iryssa

Irma (Latin) a form of Erma.
Irmina, Irminia

Irmã (Portuguese) a form of Irma.

Irma de la Paz (Spanish) peaceful Irma.

Irta (Greek) pearl.

Irune (Basque) reference to the holy trinity.

Irupe (Guarani) like the flower of the same name.

Irupé (Guarani) refers to the aquatic plant of the same name.

Isabeau (French) a form of Isabel.

Isabel ☀ GB (Spanish) consecrated to God. See also Bel, Belle, Chavella, Ysabel.
Isabal, Isabeau, Isabeli, Isabelita, Isabella, Isabelle, Ishbel, Isobel, Issie, Izabel, Izabele, Izabella

Isabelina (Hebrew) she who loves God.

Isabella ☀ GB (Italian) a form of Isabel.
Isabela, Isabelia, Isabello

Isabelle GB (French) a form of Isabel.
Isabele, Isabell

Isadora (Latin) gift of Isis.
Isidora

Isaiah BG (Hebrew) God is my salvation.

Isaldina (German) powerful warrior, she who controls harshly.

Isamar GB (Hebrew) a form of Itamar.

Isaura (Greek) native of Isauria, ancient region in Asia Minor.

Isberga (German) she who protects, sword in hand.

Isela (Scottish) a form of Isla.
Isel

Iselda (German) she who remains faithful.

Iseult (Welsh) fair lady. Literature: Also known as Isolde, a princess in the Arthurian legends; a heroine in the medieval romance *Tristan and Isolde*. See also Yseult.

Isha (American) a form of Aisha.
Ishae, Ishana, Ishanaa, Ishanda, Ishanee, Ishaney, Ishani, Ishanna, Ishaun, Ishawna, Ishaya, Ishenda, Ishia, Iysha

Ishi (Japanese) rock.
Ishiko, Ishiyo, Shiko, Shiyo

Isis (Egyptian) supreme goddess. Mythology: the goddess of nature and fertility.
Icess, Issis, Isys

Isla (Scottish) Geography: the River Isla is in Scotland.
Isela

Isleta (Spanish) small island.

Ismelda (German) she who uses the sword in battle.

Ismenia (Greek) she who words anxiously.

Isobel (Spanish) a form of Isabel.
Isobell, Isobella, Isobelle

Isoka (Benin) gift from god.
Soka

Isolde (Welsh) fair lady. Literature: Also known as Iseult, a princess in the Arthurian legends; a heroine in the medieval romance *Tristan and Isolde*. See also Yseult.
Isolda, Isolt, Izolde

Isolina (German) powerful warrior, she who controls harshly.

Issie (Spanish) a familiar form of Isabel.
Isa, Issi, Issy, Iza

Ita (Irish) thirsty.

Italia (Italian) from Italy.
Itali, Italie, Italy, Italya

Italina (Italian) native of the land between two seas.

Itamar (Hebrew) palm island.
Isamar, Isamari, Isamaria, Ithamar, Ittamar

Itatay (Guarani) hand bell.

Itati (Guarani) refers to the dedication of the virgin of Itatí.

Itatí (Guarani) white rock; refers to the dedication of the virgin of Itatí.

Itsaso (Basque) sea.

Itzel (Spanish) protected.
Itcel, Itchel, Itesel, Itsel, Itssel, Itza, Itzallana, Itzayana, Itzell, Ixchel

Iva (Slavic) a short form of Ivana.
Ivah

Ivan BG (Russian) a form of John.

Ivana (Slavic) God is gracious. See also Yvanna.
Iva, Ivanah, Ivania, Ivanka, Ivanna, Ivannia, Ivany

Iverem (Tiv) good fortune; blessing.

Iverna (Latin) from Ireland.
Ivernah

Ivette (French) a form of Yvette. See also Evette.
Ivet, Ivete, Iveth, Ivetha, Ivett, Ivetta

Ivey GB (English) a form of Ivy.

Ivón (Spanish) a form of Ivonne.

Ivonne (French) a form of Yvonne. See also Evonne.
Ivon, Ivona, Ivone, Ivonna, Iwona, Iwonka, Iwonna, Iwonne

Ivory (Latin) made of ivory.
Ivoory, Ivori, Ivorie, Ivorine, Ivree

Ivria (Hebrew) from the land of Abraham.
Ivriah, Ivrit

Ivy GB (English) ivy tree.
Ivey, Ivie

Iyabo (Yoruba) mother has returned.

Iyana, Iyanna (Hebrew) forms of Ian.
Iyanah, Iyannah, Iyannia

Izabella (Spanish) a form of Isabel.
Izabela, Izabell, Izabellah, Izabelle, Izobella

Izar (Basque) star.

Izarbe (Aragonese) Virgin Mary of the Pyrenees mountains.

Izarra, Izarre (Basque) star.

Izazkun (Basque) reference to the Virgin Mary.

Izusa (Native American) white stone.

J BG (American) an initial used as a first name.

Jabel (Hebrew) flowing stream.

Jabrea, Jabria (American) combinations of the prefix Ja + Brea.
Jabreal, Jabree, Jabreea, Jabreena, Jabrelle, Jabreona, Jabri, Jabriah, Jabriana, Jabrie, Jabriel, Jabrielle, Jabrienna, Jabrina

Jacalyn (American) a form of Jacqueline.
Jacalynn, Jacolyn, Jacolyne, Jacolynn

Jace BG (Greek) a form of Jacey.

Jacelyn (American) a form of Jocelyn.
Jaceline, Jacelyne, Jacelynn, Jacilyn, Jacilyne, Jacilynn, Jacylyn, Jacylyne, Jacylynn

Jacey GB (Greek) a familiar form of Jacinda. (American) a combination of the initials J. + C.

Jaci, Jacie (Greek) forms of
Jacey.
*Jacci, Jacia, Jacie, Jaciel, Jaici,
Jaicie*

Jacinda, Jacinta (Greek)
beautiful, attractive. (Spanish)
forms of Hyacinth.
*Jacenda, Jacenta, Jacey,
Jacinthe, Jacintia, Jacynthe,
Jakinda, Jaxine*

Jacinthe (Spanish) a form of
Jacinda.
Jacinte, Jacinth, Jacintha

Jackalyn (American) a form of
Jacqueline.
*Jackalene, Jackalin, Jackaline,
Jackalynn, Jackalynne, Jackelin,
Jackeline, Jackelyn, Jackelynn,
Jackelynne, Jackilin, Jackilyn,
Jackilynn, Jackilynne, Jackolin,
Jackoline, Jackolyn, Jackolynn,
Jackolynne*

Jackeline, Jackelyn
(American) forms of Jacqueline.
*Jackelin, Jackelline, Jackellyn,
Jockeline*

Jacki (American) a familiar form
of Jacqueline.

Jackie 🅱🅶 (American) a familiar
form of Jacqueline.
*Jackee, Jackey, Jackia,
Jackielee, Jacky, Jackye*

Jacklyn (American) a form of
Jacqueline.
*Jacklin, Jackline, Jacklyne,
Jacklynn, Jacklynne*

Jackquel (French) a short form
of Jacqueline.
*Jackqueline, Jackquetta,
Jackquiline, Jackquilyn,
Jackquilynn, Jackquilynne*

Jackson 🅱🅶 (English) child of
Jack.

Jaclyn 🅶🅱 (American) a short
form of Jacqueline.
*Jacleen, Jaclin, Jacline, Jaclyne,
Jaclynn*

Jacob 🅱🅶 (Hebrew) supplanter,
substitute.

Jacobi (Hebrew) a form of Jacob.
*Coby, Jacoba, Jacobee, Jacobette,
Jacobia, Jacobina, Jacoby,
Jacolbi, Jacolbia, Jacolby*

Jacoby 🅱🅶 (Hebrew) a form of
Jacobi.

Jacqualine (French) a form of
Jacqueline.
*Jacqualin, Jacqualine, Jacqualyn,
Jacqualyne, Jacqualynn*

Jacquelin (French) a form of
Jacqueline.
Jacquelina

Jacqueline (French) supplanter,
substitute; little Jacqui.
*Jacalyn, Jackalyn, Jackeline,
Jacki, Jacklyn, Jackquel, Jaclyn,
Jacqueena, Jacqueine, Jacquel,
Jacqueleen, Jacquelene,
Jacquelin, Jacquelyn,
Jacquelynn, Jacquena, Jacquene,
Jacquenetta, Jacquenette,
Jacqui, Jacquiline, Jacquine,*

*Jakelin, Jaquelin, Jaqueline,
Jaquelyn, Jocqueline*

Jacquelyn, Jacquelynn
(French) forms of Jacqueline.
*Jackquelyn, Jackquelynn,
Jacquelyne, Jacquelynne*

Jacques BG (French) a form of
Jacob, James.

Jacqui (French) a short form of
Jacqueline.
*Jacquay, Jacqué, Jacquee,
Jacqueta, Jacquete, Jacquetta,
Jacquette, Jacquie, Jacquise,
Jacquita, Jaquay, Jaqui, Jaquie,
Jaquiese, Jaquina, Jaquita*

Jacquiline (French) a form of
Jacqueline.
*Jacquil, Jacquilin, Jacquilyn,
Jacquilyne, Jacquilynn*

Jacqulin, Jacqulyn (American)
forms of Jacqueline.
*Jackquilin, Jacqul, Jacqulin,
Jacqulyne, Jacqulynn,
Jacqulynne, Jacquoline*

Jacy (Greek) a familiar form of
Jacinda. (American) a combi-
nation of the initials J. + C.
*Jace, Jac-E, Jacee, Jaci, Jacie,
Jacylin, Jaice, Jaicee*

Jacynthe (Spanish) a form of
Jacinda.
*Jacynda, Jacynta, Jacynth,
Jacyntha*

Jada ☆ **GB** (Spanish) a form of
Jade.
*Jadah, Jadda, Jadae, Jadzia,
Jadziah, Jaeda, Jaedra, Jayda*

Jade GB (Spanish) jade.
*Jadea, Jadeann, Jadee, Jaden,
Jadera, Jadi, Jadie, Jadienne,
Jady, Jadyn, Jaedra, Jaida,
Jaide, Jaiden, Jayde, Jayden*

Jadelyn (American) a
combination of Jade + Lynn.
*Jadalyn, Jadelaine, Jadeline,
Jadelyne, Jadelynn, Jadielyn*

Jaden BG (Spanish) a form of
Jade.
*Jadeen, Jadena, Jadene, Jadeyn,
Jadin, Jadine, Jaeden, Jaedine*

Jadyn GB (Spanish) a form of
Jade.
Jadynn, Jaedyn, Jaedynn

Jae (Latin) jaybird. (French) a
familiar form of Jacqueline.
Jaea, Jaey, Jaya

Jael GB (Hebrew) mountain goat;
climber. See also Yael.
*Jaela, Jaelee, Jaeli, Jaelie,
Jaelle, Jahla, Jahlea*

Jaelyn, Jaelynn (American)
combinations of Jae + Lynn.
*Jaeleen, Jaelin, Jaelinn, Jaelyn,
Jailyn, Jalyn, Jalynn, Jayleen,
Jaylyn, Jaylynn, Jaylynne*

Jaffa (Hebrew) a form of Yaffa.
Jaffice, Jaffit, Jafit, Jafra

Jaha (Swahili) dignified.
Jahaida, Jahaira, Jaharra, Jahayra, Jahida, Jahira, Jahitza

Jai 🅱🅶 (Tai) heart. (Latin) a form of Jaye.

Jaida, Jaide (Spanish) forms of Jade.
Jaidah, Jaidan

Jaiden 🅱🅶 (Spanish) a form of Jade.
Jaidey, Jaidi, Jaidin, Jaidon

Jaidyn (Spanish) a form of Jade.

Jailyn (American) a form of Jaelyn.
Jaileen, Jailen, Jailene, Jailin, Jailine

Jaime 🅱🅶 (French) I love.
Jaima, Jaimee, Jaimey, Jaimie, Jaimini, Jaimme, Jaimy, Jamee

Jaimee 🅶🅱 (French) a form of Jaime.

Jaimie 🅶🅱 (French) a form of Jaime.
Jaimi, Jaimmie

Jaira (Spanish) Jehovah teaches.
Jairah, Jairy

Jakeisha (American) a combination of Jakki + Aisha.
Jakeisia, Jakesha, Jakisha

Jakelin (American) a form of Jacqueline.
Jakeline, Jakelyn, Jakelynn, Jakelynne

Jakki (American) a form of Jacki.
Jakala, Jakea, Jakeela, Jakeida, Jakeita, Jakela, Jakelia, Jakell, Jakena, Jaketta, Jakevia, Jaki, Jakia, Jakiah, Jakira, Jakita, Jakiya, Jakiyah, Jakke, Jakkia

Jaleel 🅱🅶 (Hindi) a form of Jalil (see Boys' Names).

Jaleesa (American) a form of Jalisa.
Jaleasa, Jalece, Jalecea, Jaleesah, Jaleese, Jaleesia, Jaleisa, Jaleisha, Jaleisya

Jalen 🅱🅶 (American) a form of Jalena.

Jalena (American) a combination of Jane + Lena.
Jalaina, Jalana, Jalani, Jalanie, Jalayna, Jalean, Jaleen, Jaleena, Jaleene, Jalen, Jalene, Jalina, Jaline, Jallena, Jalyna, Jelayna, Jelena, Jelina, Jelyna

Jalesa, Jalessa (American) forms of Jalisa.
Jalese, Jalesha, Jaleshia, Jalesia

Jalia, Jalea (American) combinations of Jae + Leah.
Jaleah, Jalee, Jaleea, Jaleeya, Jaleia, Jalitza

Jalila (Arabic) great.
Jalile

Jalisa, Jalissa (American) combinations of Jae + Lisa.
Jaleesa, Jalesa, Jalise, Jalisha, Jalisia, Jalysa

Jalyn, Jalynn (American) combinations of Jae + Lynn. See also Jaylyn.
Jaelin, Jaeline, Jaelyn, Jaelyne, Jaelynn, Jaelynne, Jalin, Jaline, Jalyne, Jalynne

Jalysa (American) a form of Jalisa.
Jalyse, Jalyssa, Jalyssia

Jamaal BG (Arabic) a form of Jamal.

Jamaica (Spanish) Geography: an island in the Caribbean.
Jameca, Jamecia, Jameica, Jameika, Jameka, Jamica, Jamika, Jamoka, Jemaica, Jemika, Jemyka

Jamal BG (Arabic) beautiful.

Jamani (American) a form of Jami.
Jamana

Jamar BG (American) a form of Jamaria.

Jamarcus BG (American) a combination of the prefix Ja + Marcus.

Jamaria (American) combinations of Jae + Maria.
Jamar, Jamara, Jamarea, Jamaree, Jamari, Jamarie, Jameira, Jamerial, Jamira

Jamecia (Spanish) a form of Jamaica.

Jamee (French) a form of Jaime.

Jameika, Jameka (Spanish) forms of Jamaica.
Jamaika, Jamaka, Jamecka, Jamekia, Jamekka

James BG (Hebrew) supplanter, substitute. (English) a form of Jacob.

Jamesha (American) a form of Jami.
Jameisha, Jamese, Jameshia, Jameshyia, Jamesia, Jamesica, Jamesika, Jamesina, Jamessa, Jameta, Jametta, Jamiesha, Jamisha, Jammesha, Jammisha

Jameson BG (English) son of James.

Jamey (English) a form of Jami, Jamie.

Jami, Jamie GB (Hebrew, English) supplanter, substitute.
Jama, Jamani, Jamay, Jamesha, Jamey, Jamia, Jamii, Jamis, Jamise, Jammie, Jamy, Jamye, Jayme, Jaymee, Jaymie

Jamia (English) a form of Jami, Jamie.
Jamea, Jamiah, Jamiea, Jamiya, Jamiyah, Jamya, Jamyah

Jamica (Spanish) a form of Jamaica.
Jamika

Jamil BG (Arabic) a form of Jamal.

Jamila (Arabic) beautiful. See also Yamila.
Jahmela, Jahmelia, Jahmil, Jahmilla, Jameela, Jameelah, Jameeliah, Jameila, Jamela, Jamelia, Jameliah, Jamell, Jamella, Jamelle, Jamely, Jamelya, Jamiela, Jamielee, Jamilah, Jamilee, Jamilia, Jamiliah, Jamilla, Jamillah, Jamille, Jamillia, Jamilya, Jamyla, Jemeela, Jemelia, Jemila, Jemilla

Jamilynn (English) a combination of Jami + Lynn.
Jamielin, Jamieline, Jamielyn, Jamielyne, Jamielynn, Jamielynne, Jamilin, Jamiline, Jamilyn, Jamilyne, Jamilynne

Jamison 🇧🇬 (English) child of James.

Jammie (American) a form of Jami.
Jammi, Jammice, Jammise

Jamonica (American) a combination of Jami + Monica.
Jamoni

Jamylin (American) a form of Jamilynn.
Jamylin, Jamyline, Jamylyn, Jamylyne, Jamylynn, Jamylynne, Jaymylin, Jaymyline, Jaymylyn, Jaymylyne, Jaymylynn, Jaymylynne

Jan 🇧🇬 (Dutch, Slavic) a form of John. (English) a short form of Jane, Janet, Janice.
Jania, Jandy

Jana 🇬🇧 (Hebrew) gracious, merciful. (Slavic) a form of Jane. See also Yana.
Janalee, Janalisa, Janna, Janne

Janae 🇬🇧 (American) a form of Jane.
Janaé, Janaea, Janaeh, Janah, Janai, Janea, Janee, Janée, Jannae, Jenae, Jennae

Janai (American) a form of Janae.
Janaiah, Janaira, Janaiya

Janalynn (American) a combination of Jana + Lynn.
Janalin, Janaline, Janalyn, Janalyne, Janalynne

Janan (Arabic) heart; soul.
Jananee, Janani, Jananie, Janann, Jananni

Janay (American) a form of Jane.
Janaya, Janaye, Jannay, Jenay, Jenaya, Jennay, Jennaya, Jennaye

Jane 🇬🇧 (Hebrew) God is gracious. See also Chavon, Jean, Joan, Juanita, Seana, Shana, Shawna, Sheena, Shona, Shunta, Sinead, Zaneta, Zanna, Zhana.
Jaine, Jan, Jana, Janae, Janay, Janelle, Janessa, Janet, Jania, Janice, Janie, Janika, Janine, Janis, Janka, Jannie, Jasia, Jayna, Jayne, Jenica

Janel (French) a form of Janelle.
Janiel, Jannel, Jaynel

Janell **GB** (French) a form of
Janelle.
Jannell, Janyll, Jaynell

Janelle **GB** (French) a form of
Jane.
*Janel, Janela, Janele, Janelis,
Janell, Janella, Janelli, Janellie,
Janelly, Janely, Janelys, Janielle,
Janille, Jannelle, Jannellies,
Jaynelle*

Janesha (American) a form of
Janessa.
*Janeisha, Janeshia, Janiesha,
Janisha, Janishia, Jannesha,
Jannisha, Janysha, Jenesha,
Jenisha, Jennisha*

Janessa **GB** (American) a form
of Jane.
*Janeesa, Janesa, Janesea,
Janesha, Janesia, Janeska,
Janessi, Janessia, Janiesa,
Janissa, Jannesa, Jannessa,
Jannisa, Jannissa, Janyssa,
Jenesa, Jenessa, Jenissa,
Jennisa, Jennissa*

Janet (English) a form of Jane.
See also Jessie, Yanet.
*Jan, Janeta, Janete, Janeth,
Janett, Janette, Jannet, Janot,
Jante, Janyte*

Janeth (English) a form of Janet.
Janetha, Janith, Janneth

Janette **GB** (French) a form of
Janet.
Janett, Janetta

Jannette (French) a form of
Janet.
Jannett, Jannetta

Janice (Hebrew) God is gracious.
(English) a familiar form of Jane.
See also Genice.
*Jan, Janece, Janecia, Janeice,
Janiece, Janizzette, Jannice,
Janniece, Janyce, Jenice,
Jhanice, Jynice*

Janie (English) a familiar form of
Jane.
*Janey, Jani, Janiyh, Jannie,
Janny, Jany*

Janika (Slavic) a form of Jane.
*Janaca, Janeca, Janecka,
Janeika, Janeka, Janica, Janick,
Janicka, Janieka, Janikka,
Janikke, Janique, Janka, Jankia,
Jannica, Jannick, Jannika,
Janyca, Jenica, Jenicka, Jenika,
Jeniqua, Jenique, Jennica,
Jennika, Jonika*

Janine **GB** (French) a form of
Jane.
*Janean, Janeann, Janeanne,
Janeen, Janenan, Janene,
Janina, Jannen, Jannina,
Jannine, Jannyne, Janyne,
Jeannine, Jeneen, Jenine*

Janis **GB** (English) a form of
Jane.
*Janees, Janese, Janesey,
Janess, Janesse, Janise, Jannis,
Jannise, Janys, Jenesse, Jenis,
Jennise, Jennisse*

Janita (American) a form of Juanita. See also Genita.
Janitra, Janitza, Janneta, Jaynita, Jenita, Jennita

Janna (Arabic) harvest of fruit. (Hebrew) a short form of Johana.
Janaya, Janaye, Jannae, Jannah, Jannai

Jannie (English) a familiar form of Jan, Jane.
Janney, Janny

Jaquan 🅱🅶 (American) a combination of the prefix Ja + Quan (see Boys' Names).

Jaquana (American) a combination of Jacqueline + Anna.
Jaqua, Jaquai, Jaquanda, Jaquania, Jaquanna

Jaquelen (American) a form of Jacqueline.
Jaquala, Jaquera, Jaqulene, Jaquonna

Jaquelin, Jaqueline (French) forms of Jacqueline.
Jaqualin, Jaqualine, Jaquelina, Jaquline, Jaquella

Jaquelyn (French) a form of Jacqueline.
Jaquelyne, Jaquelynn, Jaquelynne

Jardena (Hebrew) a form of Jordan. (French, Spanish) garden.
Jardan, Jardana, Jardane, Jarden, Jardenia, Jardin, Jardine, Jardyn, Jardyne

Jared 🅱🅶 (Hebrew) a form of Jordan.

Jarian (American) a combination of Jane + Marian.

Jarita (Arabic) earthen water jug.
Jara, Jaretta, Jari, Jaria, Jarica, Jarida, Jarietta, Jarika, Jarina, Jaritta, Jaritza, Jarixa, Jarnita, Jarrika, Jarrine

Jarod 🅱🅶 (Hebrew) a form of Jared.

Jarred 🅱🅶 (Hebrew) a form of Jared.

Jarrett 🅱🅶 (English) a form of Garrett, Jared.

Jas 🅱🅶 (American) a short form of Jasmine.
Jase, Jass, Jaz, Jazz, Jazze, Jazzi

Jasia (Polish) a form of Jane.
Jaisha, Jasa, Jasea, Jasha, Jashae, Jashala, Jashona, Jashonte, Jasie, Jassie, Jaysa

Jaskaran 🅱🅶 (Sikh) sings praises to the Lord.

Jaskarn 🅱🅶 (Sikh) a form of Jaskaran.

Jasleen 🅶🅱 (Latin) a form of Jocelyn.
Jaslene, Jaslien, Jaslin, Jasline

Jaslyn (Latin) a form of Jocelyn.
Jaslynn, Jaslynne

Jasmain (Persian) a short form of Jasmine.
Jasmaine, Jasmane, Jassmain, Jassmaine

Jasmarie (American) a combination of Jasmine + Marie.
Jasmari

Jasmeet BG (Persian) a form of Jasmine.

Jasmin GB (Persian) a form of Jasmine.
Jasimin, Jasman, Jasmeen, Jasmen, Jasmon, Jassmin, Jassminn

Jasmine ☀ GB (Persian) jasmine flower. See also Jessamine, Yasmin.
Jas, Jasma, Jasmain, Jasme, Jasmeet, Jasmene, Jasmin, Jasmina, Jasminne, Jasmira, Jasmit, Jasmyn, Jassma, Jassmin, Jassmine, Jassmit, Jassmon, Jassmyn, Jazmin, Jazmyn, Jazzmin

Jasmyn, Jasmyne (Persian) forms of Jasmine.
Jasmynn, Jasmynne, Jassmyn

Jasone (Basque) assumption.

Jasper BG (Punjabi) a form of Jaspreet.

Jaspreet BG (Punjabi) virtuous.
Jaspar, Jasparit, Jasparita, Jasper, Jasprit, Jasprita, Jasprite

Jatara (American) a combination of Jane + Tara.
Jataria, Jatarra, Jatori, Jatoria

Javana (Malayan) from Java.
Naván, Javanna, Javanne, Javona, Javonna, Jawana, Jawanna, Jawn

Javiera (Spanish) owner of a new house. See also Xaviera.
Javeera, Viera

Javon BG (Malayan) a form of Javona.

Javona, Javonna (Malayan) forms of Javana.
Javon, Javonda, Javone, Javoni, Javonne, Javonni, Javonya

Javonte BG (American) a form of Javan (see Boys' Names).

Jay BG (French) blue jay.

Jaya (Hindi) victory.
Jaea, Jaia

Jaycee (American) a combination of the initials J. + C.
Jacee, Jacey, Jaci, Jacie, Jacy, Jayce, Jaycey, Jayci, Jaycie, Jaycy

Jayda (Spanish) a form of Jada.
Jaydah, Jeyda

Jayde GB (Spanish) a form of Jade.
Jayd

Jaydee (American) a combination of the initials J. + D.
Jadee, Jadey, Jadi, Jadie, Jady, Jaydey, Jaydi, Jaydie, Jaydy

Jayden 🅱🅶 (Spanish) a form of Jade.
Jaydeen, Jaydene, Jaydin, Jaydn, Jaydon

Jaye (Latin) jaybird.
Jae, Jay

Jayla 🅶🅱 (American) a short form of Jaylene.
Jaylaa, Jaylah, Jayli, Jaylia, Jayliah, Jaylie

Jaylen 🅱🅶 (American) a form of Jaylene.

Jaylene (American) forms of Jaylyn.
Jayelene, Jayla, Jaylan, Jayleana, Jaylee, Jayleen, Jayleene, Jaylen, Jaylenne

Jaylin 🅱🅶 (American) a form of Jaylyn.
Jayline, Jaylinn

Jaylon 🅱🅶 (American) a form of Jaylen.

Jaylyn 🅱🅶 (American) a combination of Jaye + Lynn. See also Jalyn.
Jaylene, Jaylin, Jaylyne

Jaylynn (American) a form of Jaylyn.
Jaylynne

Jayme 🅶🅱 (English) a form of Jami.

Jaymee, Jaymi (English) forms of Jami.

Jaymie (English) a form of Jami.
Jaymi, Jaymia, Jaymine, Jaymini

Jayna (Hebrew) a form of Jane.
Jaynae, Jaynah, Jaynna

Jayne (Hindi) victorious. (English) a form of Jane.
Jayn, Jaynie, Jaynne

Jaynie (English) a familiar form of Jayne.
Jaynee, Jayni

Jazlyn (American) a combination of Jazmin + Lynn.
Jasleen, Jazaline, Jazalyn, Jazleen, Jazlene, Jazlin, Jazline, Jazlon, Jazlynn, Jazlynne, Jazzalyn, Jazzleen, Jazzlene, Jazzlin, Jazzline, Jazzlyn, Jazzlynn, Jazzlynne

Jazmin (Persian) a form of Jasmine.
Jazmaine, Jazman, Jazmen, Jazmín, Jazminn, Jazmon, Jazzmit

Jazmine 🅶🅱 (Persian) a form of Jasmine.

Jazmyn, Jazmyne (Persian) forms of Jasmine.
Jazmynn, Jazmynne, Jazzmyn, Jazzmyne

Jazzmin, Jazzmine (Persian) forms of Jasmine.
Jazzman, Jazzmeen, Jazzmen, Jazzmene, Jazzmenn, Jazzmon

Jean 🅑🅖 (Scottish) a form of Jeanne.

Jeanne (Scottish) God is gracious. See also Kini.
Jeana, Jeanann, Jeancie, Jeane, Jeaneia, Jeanette, Jeaneva, Jeanice, Jeanie, Jeanine, Jeanmaria, Jeanmarie, Jeanna, Jeanné, Jeannie, Jeannita, Jeannot, Jeantelle

Jeana, Jeanna (Scottish) forms of Jean.
Jeanae, Jeannae, Jeannia

Jeanette 🅖🅑 (French) a form of Jean.
Jeanet, Jeanete, Jeanett, Jeanetta, Jeanita, Jenet, Jenett, Jenette, Jinetta, Jinette

Jeanie, Jeannie (Scottish) familiar forms of Jean.
Jeannee, Jeanney, Jeani, Jeanny, Jeany

Jeanine, Jenine (Scottish) forms of Jean. See also Geneen.
Jeaneane, Jeaneen, Jeanene, Jeanina, Jeannina, Jeannine, Jennine

Jeannett (French) a form of Jean.
Jeannete, Jeannetta, Jeannette, Jeannita, Jennet, Jennett, Jennetta, Jennette, Jennita

Jedidiah 🅑🅖 (Hebrew) friend of God, beloved of God.

Jefferson 🅑🅖 (English) child of Jeff.

Jeffery 🅑🅖 (English) a form of Jeffrey.

Jeffrey 🅑🅖 (English) divinely peaceful.

Jelena (Russian) a form of Helen. See also Yelena.
Jalaine, Jalane, Jalani, Jalanna, Jalayna, Jalayne, Jaleen, Jaleena, Jaleene, Jalena, Jalene, Jelaina, Jelaine, Jelana, Jelane, Jelani, Jelanni, Jelayna, Jelayne, Jelean, Jeleana, Jeleen, Jeleena, Jelene

Jelisa (American) a combination of Jean + Lisa.
Jalissa, Jelesha, Jelessa, Jelise, Jelissa, Jellese, Jellice, Jelysa, Jelyssa, Jillisa, Jillissa, Julissa

Jem 🅖🅑 (Hebrew) a short form of Jemima.
Gem, Jemi, Jemia, Jemiah, Jemie, Jemm, Jemmi, Jemmy

Jemima (Hebrew) dove.
Jamim, Jamima, Jem, Jemimah, Jemma

Jemina, Jenima (Hebrew) dove.

Jemma (Hebrew) a short form of Jemima. (English) a form of Gemma.
Jemmia, Jemmiah, Jemmie, Jemmy

Jena, Jenae (Arabic) forms of Jenna.
Jenah, Jenai, Jenal, Jenay, Jenaya, Jenea

Jenara (Latin) dedicated to the god, Janus.

Jendaya (Zimbabwean) thankful.
Daya, Jenda, Jendayah

Jenelle (American) a combination of Jenny + Nelle.
Genell, Jeanell, Jeanelle, Jenall, Jenalle, Jenel, Jenela, Jenele, Jenell, Jenella, Jenille, Jennel, Jennell, Jennella, Jennelle, Jennielle, Jennille, Jinelle, Jinnell

Jenessa (American) a form of Jenisa.
Jenesa, Jenese, Jenesia, Jenessia, Jennesa, Jennese, Jennessa, Jinessa

Jenica (Romanian) a form of Jane.
Jeneca, Jenika, Jenikka, Jennica, Jennika

Jenifer, Jeniffer (Welsh) forms of Jennifer.
Jenefer

Jenilee (American) a combination of Jennifer + Lee.
Jenalea, Jenalee, Jenaleigh, Jenaly, Jenelea, Jenelee, Jeneleigh, Jenely, Jenelly, Jenileigh, Jenily, Jennalee, Jennely, Jennielee, Jennilea, Jennilee, Jennilie

Jenisa (American) a combination of Jennifer + Nisa.
Jenessa, Jenisha, Jenissa, Jenisse, Jennisa, Jennise,

Jennisha, Jennissa, Jennisse, Jennysa, Jennyssa, Jenysa, Jenyse, Jenyssa, Jenysse

Jenka (Czech) a form of Jane.

Jenna ☆ 🇬🇧 (Arabic) small bird. (Welsh) a short form of Jennifer. See also Gen.
Jena, Jennae, Jennah, Jennai, Jennat, Jennay, Jennaya, Jennaye, Jhenna

Jenni, Jennie (Welsh) familiar forms of Jennifer.
Jeni, Jenne, Jenné, Jennee, Jenney, Jennia, Jennier, Jennita, Jennora, Jensine

Jennifer ☆ 🇬🇧 (Welsh) white wave; white phantom. A form of Guinevere. See also Gennifer, Ginnifer, Yenifer.
Jen, Jenifer, Jeniffer, Jenipher, Jenna, Jennafer, Jenni, Jenniferanne, Jenniferlee, Jenniffe, Jenniffer, Jenniffier, Jennifier, Jennilee, Jenniphe, Jennipher, Jenny, Jennyfer

Jennilee (American) a combination of Jenny + Lee.
Jennalea, Jennalee, Jennielee, Jennilea, Jennilie, Jinnalee

Jennilyn, Jennilynn (American) combinations of Jenni + Lynn.
Jennalin, Jennaline, Jennalyn, Jenalynann, Jenelyn, Jenilyn, Jennalyne, Jennalynn, Jennalynne, Jennilin, Jenniline, Jennilyne, Jennilynne

Jenny GB (Welsh) a familiar form of Jennifer.
Jenney, Jenni, Jennie, Jeny, Jinny

Jennyfer (Welsh) a form of Jennifer.
Jenyfer

Jeraldine (English) a form of Geraldine.
Jeraldeen, Jeraldene, Jeraldina, Jeraldyne, Jeralee, Jeri

Jeremiah BG (Hebrew) God will uplift.

Jeremy BG (English) a form of Jeremiah.

Jereni (Russian) a form of Irene.
Jerena, Jerenae, Jerina

Jeri, Jerri, Jerrie (American) short forms of Jeraldine. See also Geri.
Jera, Jerae, JeRae, Jeree, Jeriel, Jerilee, Jerinda, Jerra, Jerrah, Jerrece, Jerree, Jerriann, Jerrilee, Jerrine, Jerry, Jerrylee, Jerryne, Jerzy

Jerica (American) a combination of Jeri + Erica.
Jereca, Jerecka, Jerice, Jericka, Jerika, Jerrica, Jerrice, Jeryka

Jerilyn (American) a combination of Jeri + Lynn.
Jeralin, Jeraline, Jeralyn, Jeralyne, Jeralynn, Jeralynne, Jerelin, Jereline, Jerelyn, Jerelyne, Jerelynn, Jerelynne, Jerilin, Jeriline, Jerilyne, Jerilynn,
Jerilynne, Jerrilin, Jerriline, Jerrilyn, Jerrilyne, Jerrilynn, Jerrilynne, Jerrylea

Jermaine BG (French) a form of Germaine.
Jermain, Jerman, Jermanay, Jermanaye, Jermane, Jermanee, Jermani, Jermanique, Jermany, Jermayne, Jermecia, Jermia, Jermice, Jermicia, Jermika, Jermila

Jerónima (Greek) she who has a sacred name.

Jerrica (American) a form of Jerica.
Jerreka, Jerricah, Jerricca, Jerricha, Jerricka, Jerrieka, Jerrika

Jerry BG (American) a form of Jeri.

Jerusalén (Hebrew) vision of peace.

Jerusha (Hebrew) inheritance.
Jerushah, Yerusha

Jesabel (Hebrew) God's oath.

Jesenia, Jessenia GB (Arabic) flower.
Jescenia, Jessennia, Jessenya

Jesica, Jesika (Hebrew) forms of Jessica.
Jesicca, Jesikah, Jesikkah

Jésica (Slavic) a form of Jessica.

Jess BG (Hebrew) a short form of Jessie.

Jessa (American) a short form of Jessalyn, Jessamine, Jessica.
Jesa, Jesha, Jessah

Jessalyn (American) a combination of Jessica + Lynn.
Jesalin, Jesaline, Jesalyn, Jesalyne, Jesalynn, Jesalynne, Jesilin, Jesiline, Jesilyn, Jesilyne, Jesilynn, Jesilynne, Jessa, Jessalin, Jessaline, Jessalyne, Jessalynn, Jessalynne, Jesselin, Jesseline, Jesselyn, Jesselyne, Jesselynn, Jesselynne, Jesslyn

Jessamine (French) a form of Jasmine.
Jessa, Jessamin, Jessamon, Jessamy, Jessamyn, Jessemin, Jessemine, Jessimin, Jessimine, Jessmin, Jessmine, Jessmon, Jessmy, Jessmyn

Jesse B☐ (Hebrew) a form of Jessie.
Jese, Jesi, Jesie

Jesseca (Hebrew) a form of Jessica.

Jessi G☐ (Hebrew) a form of Jessie.

Jessica ☀ G☐ (Hebrew) wealthy. Literature: a name perhaps invented by Shakespeare for a character in his play *The Merchant of Venice*. See also Gessica, Yessica.
Jesica, Jesika, Jessa, Jessaca, Jessca, Jesscia, Jesseca, Jessia, Jessicah, Jessicca, Jessicia,

Jessicka, Jessika, Jessiqua, Jessy, Jessyca, Jessyka, Jezeca, Jezica, Jezika, Jezyca

Jessie B☐ (Hebrew) a short form of Jessica. (Scottish) a form of Janet.
Jescie, Jesey, Jessé, Jessee, Jessey, Jessi, Jessia, Jessiya, Jessye

Jessika G☐ (Hebrew) a form of Jessica.
Jessieka

Jesslyn (American) a short form of Jessalyn.
Jessilyn, Jessilynn, Jesslin, Jesslynn, Jesslynne

Jessy B☐ (Hebrew, Scottish) a form of Jessie.

Jessyca, Jessyka (Hebrew) forms of Jessica.

Jesus B☐ (Hebrew) a form of Joshua.

Jesusa (Spanish) Jehovah is salvation.

Jésusa (Hebrew, Spanish) God is my salvation.

Jetta (English) jet black mineral. (American) a familiar form of Jevette.
Jeta, Jetia, Jetje, Jette, Jettie

Jevette (American) a combination of Jean + Yvette.
Jetta, Jeva, Jeveta, Jevetta

Jewel (French) precious gem.
Jewelann, Jewelia, Jeweliana,
Jeweliann, Jewelie, Jewell,
Jewelle, Jewellee, Jewellene,
Jewellie, Juel, Jule

Jezebel (Hebrew) unexalted;
impure. Bible: the wife of King
Ahab.
Jesibel, Jessabel, Jessebel, Jez,
Jezabel, Jezabella, Jezabelle,
Jezebell, Jezebella, Jezebelle

Jianna (Italian) a form of Giana.
Jiana, Jianina, Jianine, Jianni,
Jiannini

Jibon (Hindi) life.

Jill GB (English) a short form of
Jillian.
Jil, Jilli, Jillie, Jilly

Jillaine (Latin) a form of Jillian.
Jilaine, Jilane, Jilayne, Jillana,
Jillane, Jillann, Jillanne, Jillayne

Jilleen (Irish) a form of Jillian.
Jileen, Jilene, Jiline, Jillene,
Jillenne, Jilline, Jillyn

Jillian GB (Latin) youthful. See
also Gillian.
Jilian, Jiliana, Jiliann, Jilianna,
Jilianne, Jilienna, Jilienne, Jill,
Jillaine, Jilliana, Jilliane, Jilliann,
Jillianne, Jileen, Jillien, Jillienne,
Jillion, Jilliyn

Jimi (Hebrew) supplanter,
substitute.
Jimae, Jimaria, Jimee, Jimella,
Jimena, Jimia, Jimiah, Jimie,

Jimiyah, Jimmeka, Jimmet,
Jimmi, Jimmia, Jimmie

Jimisha (American) a combination of Jimi + Aisha.
Jimica, Jimicia, Jimmicia, Jimysha

Jimmie BG (Hebrew) a form of
Jimi.

Jimmy BG (English) a familiar
form of Jim (see Boys' Names).

Jin BG (Japanese) tender.
(American) a short form of
Ginny, Jinny.

Jina (Swahili) baby with a name.
(Italian) a form of Gina.
Jena, Jinae, Jinan, Jinda, Jinna,
Jinnae

Jinny (Scottish) a familiar form of
Jenny. (American) a familiar
form of Virginia. See also Ginny.
Jin, Jinnee, Jinney, Jinni, Jinnie

Jirina (Czech) a form of Georgia.
Jirah, Jireh

Jizelle (American) a form of
Giselle.
Jessel, Jezel, Jezell, Jezella,
Jezelle, Jisel, Jisela, Jisell, Jisella,
Jiselle, Jissel, Jissell, Jissella,
Jisselle, Jizel, Jizella, Joselle

Jo GB (American) a short form of
Joanna, Jolene, Josephine.
Joangie, Joetta, Joette, Joey

Joan (Hebrew) God is gracious.
History: Joan of Arc was a
fifteenth-century heroine and
resistance fighter. See also Ioana,
Jean, Juanita, Siobhan.
*Joane, Joaneil, Joanel, Joanelle,
Joanie, Joanmarie, Joann,
Joannanette, Joanne, Joannel,
Joanny, Jonni*

Joana (English) a form of Joanna.

Joanna GB (English) a form of
Joan. See also Yoanna.
*Janka, Jhoana, Jo, Jo-Ana,
Joandra, Joanka, Joananna, Jo-
Anie, Joanka, Jo-Anna, Joannah,
Jo-Annie, Joeana, Joeanna,
Johana, Johanna, Johannah*

Joanie, Joannie (Hebrew)
familiar forms of Joan.
*Joanee, Joani, Joanni, Joenie,
Johanie, Johnnie, Joni*

Joanne (English) a form of Joan.
*Joanann, Joananne, Joann, Jo-
Ann, Jo-Anne, Joayn, Joeann,
Joeanne*

Joanny (Hebrew) a familiar form
of Joan.
Joany

Joaquina (Hebrew) God will
establish.
Joaquine

Jobeth (English) a combination
of Jo + Beth.

Joby BG (Hebrew) afflicted.
(English) a familiar form of
Jobeth.
*Jobey, Jobi, Jobie, Jobina,
Jobita, Jobrina, Jobye, Jobyna*

Jocacia (American) a combination of Joy + Acacia.

Jocelin, Joceline (Latin) forms
of Jocelyn.
Jocelina, Jocelinn

Jocelín (Latin) a form of Jocelin.

Jocelyn ☀ GB (Latin) joyous.
See also Yocelin, Yoselin.
*Jacelyn, Jasleen, Jocelin, Jocelle,
Jocelyne, Jocelynn, Joci, Jocia,
Jocilyn, Jocilynn, Jocinta, Joclyn,
Joclynn, Josalyn, Joscelin, Joselin,
Joselyn, Joshlyn, Josilin, Jossalin,
Josselyn, Joycelyn*

Jocelyne (Latin) a form of Jocelyn.
Joceline, Jocelynne, Joclynne

Jocosa, Jocose (Latin) jubilant.

Jodi, Jodie GB (American)
familiar forms of Judith.

Jody BG (American) a familiar
form of Judith.
*Jodee, Jodele, Jodell, Jodelle,
Jodevea, Jodey, Jodia, Jodiee,
Jodilee, Jodi-Lee, Jodilynn, Jodi-
Lynn, Joedi, Joedy*

Jodiann (American) a
combination of Jodi + Ann.
*Jodene, Jodi-Ann, Jodianna,
Jodi-Anna, Jodianne, Jodi-Anne,
Jodine, Jodyann, Jody-Ann,*

Jodyanna, Jody-Anna, Jodyanne, Jody-Anne, Jodyne

Joe BG (Latin) a form of Joy.

Joel BG (Hebrew) God is willing.

Joelle BG (Hebrew) a form of Joel.
Joela, Joele, Joelee, Joeli, Joelia, Joelie, Joell, Joella, Joëlle, Joelli, Joelly, Joely, Joyelle

Joelynn (American) a combination of Joelle + Lynn.
Joeleen, Joelene, Joeline, Joellen, Joellyn, Joelyn, Joelyne

Joey BG (French) a familiar form of Josephine. (American) a form of Jo.

Johana, Johanna, Johannah (German) forms of Joana.
Janna, Joahna, Johanah, Johanka, Johanne, Johnna, Johonna, Jonna, Joyhanna, Joyhannah

Johanie, Johannie (Hebrew) forms of Joanie.
Johani, Johanni, Johanny, Johany

John BG (Hebrew) God is gracious.

Johnna, Jonna (American) forms of Johana, Joanna.
Jahna, Jahnaya, Jhona, Jhonna, Johna, Johnda, Johnnielynn, Johnnie-Lynn, Johnnquia, Joncie, Jonda, Jondrea, Jontel, Jutta

Johnnessa (American) a combination of Johnna + Nessa.
Jahnessa, Johneatha, Johnecia, Johnesha, Johnetra, Johnisha, Johnishi, Johnnise, Jonyssa

Johnnie BG (Hebrew) a form of Joanie.
Johni, Johnie, Johnni, Johnny

Johnny BG (Hebrew) a form of Johnnie.

Joi GB (Latin) a form of Joy.
Joia, Joie

Jokla (Swahili) beautiful robe.

Jolanda (Greek) a form of Yolanda. See also Iolanthe.
Jola, Jolan, Jolán, Jolande, Jolander, Jolanka, Jolánta, Jolantha, Jolanthe

Joleen, Joline (English) forms of Jolene.
Joleena, Joleene, Jolleen, Jollene

Jolene GB (Hebrew) God will add, God will increase. (English) a form of Josephine.
Jo, Jolaine, Jolana, Jolane, Jolanna, Jolanne, Jolanta, Jolayne, Jole, Jolean, Joleane, Joleen, Jolena, Joléne, Jolenna, Jolin, Jolina, Jolinda, Joline, Jolinn, Jolinna, Jolleane, Jolleen, Jolline

Jolie (French) pretty.
Jole, Jolea, Jolee, Joleigh, Joley, Joli, Jolibeth, Jollee, Jollie, Jolly, Joly, Jolye

Jolisa (American) a combination of Jo + Lisa.
Joleesa, Joleisha, Joleishia, Jolieasa, Jolise, Jolisha, Jolisia, Jolissa, Jolysa, Jolyssa, Julissa

Jolynn (American) a combination of Jo + Lynn.
Jolyn, Jolyne, Jolynne

Jon 🅱🅶 (Hebrew) a form of John. A short form of Jonathan.

Jonah 🅱🅶 (Hebrew) dove.

Jonatan 🅱🅶 (Hebrew) a form of Jonathan.

Jonatha (Hebrew) gift of God.
Johnasha, Johnasia, Jonesha, Jonisha

Jonathan 🅱🅶 (Hebrew) gift of God.

Jonelle (American) a combination of Joan + Elle.
Jahnel, Jahnell, Jahnelle, Johnel, Johnell, Johnella, Johnelle, Jonel, Jonell, Jonella, Jonyelle, Jynell, Jynelle

Jonesha, Jonisha (American) forms of Jonatha.
Joneisha, Jonesa, Joneshia, Jonessa, Jonisa, Jonishia, Jonneisha, Jonnesha, Jonnessia

Joni (American) a familiar form of Joan.
Jona, Jonae, Jonai, Jonann, Jonati, Joncey, Jonci, Joncie, Jonice, Jonie, Jonilee, Joni-lee, Jonis, Jony

Jonika (American) a form of Janika.
Johnica, Johnique, Johnquia, Johnnica, Johnnika, Joneeka, Joneika, Jonica, Joniqua, Jonique

Jonina (Hebrew) dove. See also Yonina.
Jona, Jonita, Jonnina

Jonita (Hebrew) a form of Jonina. See also Yonita.
Johnetta, Johnette, Johnita, Johnittia, Jonati, Jonetia, Jonetta, Jonette, Jonit, Jonnita, Jonta, Jontae, Jontaé, Jontaya

Jonni, Jonnie (American) familiar forms of Joan.
Jonny

Jonquil (Latin, English) Botany: an ornamental plant with fragrant yellow flowers.
Jonquelle, Jonquie, Jonquill, Jonquille

Jontel (American) a form of Johnna.
Jontaya, Jontell, Jontelle, Jontia, Jontila, Jontrice

Jora 🅶🅱 (Hebrew) autumn rain.
Jorah

Jordan ✶ **BG** (Hebrew)
descending. See also Jardena.
Jordain, Jordaine, Jordana,
Jordane, Jordann, Jordanna,
Jordanne, Jordany, Jordea,
Jordee, Jorden, Jordi, Jordian,
Jordie, Jordin, Jordon, Jordyn,
Jori, Jorie, Jourdan

Jordana, Jordanna (Hebrew)
forms of Jordan. See also
Giordana, Yordana.
Jordannah, Jordina, Jordonna,
Jourdana, Jourdanna

Jorden **BG** (Hebrew) a form of
Jordan.
Jordenne

Jordin (Hebrew) a form of
Jordan.
Jordine

Jordon **BG** (Hebrew) a form of
Jordan.

Jordyn **GB** (Hebrew) a form of
Jordan.
Jordyne, Jordynn, Jordynne

Jorge **BG** (Spanish) a form of
George (see Boys' Names).

Jorgelina (Greek) she who
works well in the countryside.

Jori, Jorie (Hebrew) familiar
forms of Jordan.
Jorai, Jorea, Joree, Jorée, Jorey,
Jorian, Jorin, Jorina, Jorine,
Jorita, Jorre, Jorrey, Jorri,
Jorrian, Jorrie, Jorry, Jory

Joriann (American) a
combination of Jori + Ann.
Jori-Ann, Jorianna, Jori-Anna,
Jorianne, Jori-Anne, Jorriann,
Jorrianna, Jorrianne, Jorryann,
Jorryanna, Jorryanne, Joryann,
Joryanna, Joryanne

Jorja (American) a form of
Georgia.
Jeorgi, Jeorgia, Jorgana, Jorgi,
Jorgia, Jorgina, Jorjana, Jorji

Josalyn (Latin) a form of Jocelyn.
Josalene, Josalin, Josalind,
Josaline, Josalynn, Joshalyne

Joscelin, Joscelyn (Latin)
forms of Jocelyn.
Josceline, Joscelyne, Joscelynn,
Joscelynne, Joselin, Joseline,
Joselyn, Joselyne, Joselynn,
Joselynne, Joshlyn

Jose **BG** (Spanish) a form of
Joseph.

Josee **GB** (American) a familiar
form of Josephine.
Joesee, Josey, Josi, Josina, Josy,
Jozee

Josée (American) a familiar form
of Josephine.

Josefina (Spanish) a form of
Josephine.
Josefa, Josefena, Joseffa,
Josefine

Joselin, Joseline (Latin) forms
of Jocelyn.
Joselina, Joselinne, Josielina

Joselín (Latin) a form of Joselin.

Joselle (American) a form of Jizelle.
Joesell, Jozelle

Joselyn, Joslyn (Latin) forms of Jocelyn.
Joselene, Joselyne, Joselynn, Joshely, Josiline, Josilyn

Joseph B G (Hebrew) God will add, God will increase.

Josephine G B (French) a form of Joseph. See also Fifi, Pepita, Yosepha.
Fina, Jo, Joey, Josee, Josée, Josefina, Josepha, Josephe, Josephene, Josephin, Josephina, Josephyna, Josephyne, Josette, Josey, Josie, Jozephine, Jozie, Sefa

Josette (French) a familiar form of Josephine.
Joesette, Josetta, Joshetta, Jozette

Josey (Hebrew) a familiar form of Josephine.
Josi, Josse, Jossee, Jossie, Josy, Josye

Joshann (American) a combination of Joshlyn + Ann.
Joshana, Joshanna, Joshanne

Joshlyn (Latin) a form of Jocelyn. (Hebrew) God is my salvation.
Joshalin, Joshalyn, Joshalynn, Joshalynne, Joshelle, Joshleen, Joshlene, Joshlin, Joshline, Joshlyne, Joshlynn, Joshlynne

Joshua B G (Hebrew) God is my salvation.

Josiah B G (Hebrew) fire of the Lord.

Josiane, Josianne (American) combinations of Josie + Anne.
Josian, Josie-Ann, Josieann

Josie (Hebrew) a familiar form of Josephine.

Josilin, Joslin (Latin) forms of Jocelyn.
Josielina, Josiline, Josilyn, Josilyne, Josilynn, Josilynne, Joslin, Josline, Joslyn, Joslyne, Joslynn, Joslynne

Jossalin (Latin) a form of Jocelyn.
Jossaline, Jossalyn, Jossalynn, Jossalynne, Josselyn, Josslin, Jossline

Josselyn (Latin) a form of Jocelyn.
Josselen, Josselin, Josseline, Jossellen, Jossellin, Jossellyn, Josselyne, Josselynn, Josselynne, Josslyn, Josslyne, Josslynn, Josslynne

Josune (Spanish) named for Jesus.

Jourdan (Hebrew) a form of Jordan.
Jourdain, Jourdann, Jourdanne, Jourden, Jourdian, Jourdon, Jourdyn

Jovana (Latin) a form of Jovanna.
Jeovana, Jouvan, Jovan,
Jovanah, Jovena, Jovian, Jowan,
Jowana

Jovani BG (Italian) a form of
Jovannie.

Jovanna (Latin) majestic.
(Italian) a form of Giovanna.
Mythology: Jove, also known as
Jupiter, was the supreme Roman
god.
Jeovanna, Jovado, Joval, Jovana,
Jovann, Jovannie, Jovena,
Jovina, Jovon, Jovonda, Jovonia,
Jovonna, Jovonnah, Jovonne,
Jowanna

Jovanni BG (Italian) a form of
Jovannie.

Jovannie (Italian) a familiar form
of Jovanna.
Jovanee, Jovani, Jovanie,
Jovanne, Jovanni, Jovanny,
Jovonnie

Jovita (Latin) jovial.
Joveda, Joveta, Jovetta, Jovida,
Jovitta

Joy GB (Latin) joyous.
Joya, Joye, Joyeeta, Joyella,
Joyia, Joyous, Joyvina

Joyanne (American) a
combination of Joy + Anne.
Joyan, Joyann, Joyanna

Joyce (Latin) joyous. A short
form of Joycelyn.
Joice, Joycey, Joycie, Joyous,
Joysel

Joycelyn (American) a form of
Jocelyn.
Joycelin, Joyceline, Joycelyne,
Joycelynn, Joycelynne

Joyceta (Spanish) a form of
Joyce.

Joylyn (American) a combination
of Joy + Lynn.
Joyleen, Joylene, Joylin, Joyline,
Joylyne, Joylynn, Joy-Lynn,
Joylynne

Jozie (Hebrew) a familiar form of
Josephine.
Jozee, Jozée, Jozi, Jozy

Juan BG (Spanish) a form of John.

Juana (Spanish) a short form of
Juanita.
Juanell, Juaney, Juanika, Juanit,
Juanna, Juannia

Juana del Pilar (Spanish) a
form of Juana.

Juandalyn (Spanish) a form of
Juanita.
Jualinn, Juandalin, Juandaline,
Juandalyne, Juandalynn,
Juandalynne

Juaneta (Spanish) God is
gracious.

Juanita (Spanish) a form of Jane,
Joan. See also Kwanita, Nita,
Waneta, Wanika.
Juana, Juandalyn, Juaneice,
Juanequa, Juanesha, Juanice,
Juanicia, Juaniqua, Juanisha,
Juanishia

Juci (Hungarian) a form of Judy.
Jucika

Judith (Hebrew) praised.
Mythology: the slayer of
Holofernes, according to ancient
Jewish legend. See also Yehudit,
Yudita.
*Giuditta, Ioudith, Jodi, Jodie,
Jody, Jude, Judine, Judit, Judita,
Judite, Juditha, Judithe, Judy,
Judyta, Jutka*

Judy GB (Hebrew) a familiar
form of Judith.
Juci, Judi, Judie, Judye

Judyann (American) a combi-
nation of Judy + Ann.
*Judana, Judiann, Judianna,
Judianne, Judyanna, Judyanne*

Jula (Polish) a form of Julia.
Julca, Julcia, Juliska, Julka

Julene (Basque) a form of Julia.
See also Yulene.
*Julena, Julina, Juline, Julinka,
Juliska, Julleen, Jullena, Jullene,
Julyne*

Julia ☆ GB (Latin) youthful. See
also Giulia, Jill, Jillian, Sulia,
Yulia.
*Iulia, Jula, Julea, Juleah, Julene,
Juliah, Juliana, Juliann, Julica,
Julie, Juliea, Juliet, Julija, Julina,
Juline, Julisa, Julissa, Julita,
Juliya, Julka, Julyssa*

Julian BG (English) a form of
Juliann.

Juliana (Czech, Spanish,
Hungarian) a form of Julia.
*Julieana, Juliena, Julliana,
Julyana, Yuliana*

Juliann (English) a form of Julia.
*Julean, Julian, Juliane, Julien,
Juliene, Jullian*

Julianna GB (Czech, Spanish,
Hungarian) a form of Julia.
Julieanna, Jullianna, Julyanna

Julianne GB (English) a form of
Julia.
*Juleann, Julieann, Julie-Ann,
Julieanne, Julie-Anne, Julienn,
Julienne*

Julie GB (English) a form of
Julia.
*Juel, Jule, Julee, Juli, Julie-Lynn,
Julie-Mae, Julle, Jullee, Jullie,
Jully, July*

Julien BG (English) a form of
Juliann.

Juliet GB (French) a form of
Julia.
Julet, Julieta, Jullet, Julliet

Juliette (French) a form of Julia.
Juliett, Julietta, Jullietta

Julio BG (Hispanic) a form of
Julius.

Julisa, Julissa (Latin) forms of
Julia.
Julis, Julisha, Julysa, Julyssa

Julita (Spanish) a form of Julia.
Julitta, Julyta

Julius BG (Greek, Latin) youthful, downy bearded.

Jumaris (American) a combination of Julie + Maris.

Jun BG (Chinese) truthful.

June (Latin) born in the sixth month.
Juna, Junea, Junel, Junell, Junella, Junelle, Junette, Juney, Junia, Junie, Juniet, Junieta, Junietta, Juniette, Junina, Junita

Juno (Latin) queen. Mythology: the supreme Roman goddess.

Justa (Latin) she who lives for and according to the law of God.

Justice GB (Latin) just, righteous.
Justis, Justise, Justiss, Justisse, Justus, Justyce, Justys

Justin BG (Latin) just, righteous.

Justina GB (Italian) a form of Justine.
Jestena, Jestina, Justinna, Justyna

Justine GB (Latin) just, righteous.
Giustina, Jestine, Juste, Justi, Justice, Justie, Justina, Justinn, Justy, Justyn, Justyne, Justynn, Justynne

Justiniana (Spanish) just, fair.

Justyn BG (Latin) a form of Justine.

Juvencia, Juventina (Latin) youth.

Juwan BG (American) a form of Jajuan (see Boys' Names).

K

K GB (American) an initial used as a first name.

Kacey, Kacy GB (Irish) brave. (American) forms of Casey. Combinations of the initials K. + C.
K. C., Kace, Kacee, Kaci, Kacie, Kaicee, Kaicey, Kasey, Kasie, Kaycee, Kayci, Kaycie

Kachina (Native American) sacred dancer.
Kachine

Kaci, Kacie GB (American) forms of Kacey, Kacy.
Kasci, Kaycie, Kaysie

Kacia (Greek) a short form of Acacia.
Kaycia, Kaysia

Kade BG (Scottish) wetlands. (American) a combination of the initials K. + D.

Kadedra (American) a combination of Kady + Dedra.
Kadeadra, Kadedrah, Kadedria, Kadeedra, Kadeidra, Kadeidre, Kadeidria

Kadeem BG (Arabic) servant.

Kadejah (Arabic) a form of
Kadijah.
Kadeija, Kadeijah, Kadejá, Kadejia

Kadelyn (American) a combination of Kady + Lynn.

Kaden 🅱🅶 (Arabic) a form of
Kadin (see Boys' Names).

Kadesha (American) a combi-
nation of Kady + Aisha.
*Kadeesha, Kadeeshia, Kadeesia,
Kadeesiah, Kadeezia, Kadesa,
Kadesheia, Kadeshia, Kadesia,
Kadessa, Kadezia*

Kadie (English) a form of Kady.
Kadi, Kadia, Kadiah

Kadijah (Arabic) trustworthy.
*Kadajah, Kadeeja, Kadeejah,
Kadija*

Kadisha (American) a form of
Kadesha.
*Kadiesha, Kadieshia, Kadishia,
Kadisia, Kadysha, Kadyshia*

Kady (English) a form of Katy. A
combination of the initials K. +
D. See also Cady.
*K. D., Kade, Kadee, Kadey, Kadie,
Kadya, Kadyn, Kaidi, Kaidy,
Kayde, Kaydee, Kaydey, Kaydi,
Kaydie, Kaydy*

Kae (Greek, Teutonic, Latin) a
form of Kay.

Kaedé (Japanese) maple leaf.

Kaela (Hebrew, Arabic) beloved,
sweetheart. A short form of Kalila,
Kelila.
*Kaelah, Kaelea, Kaeleah, Kaelee,
Kaeli, Kayla*

Kaelee, Kaeli (American) forms
of Kaela.
*Kaelei, Kaeleigh, Kaeley, Kaelia,
Kaelie, Kaelii, Kaelly, Kaely, Kaelye*

Kaelin (American) a form of
Kaelyn.
*Kaeleen, Kaelene, Kaelina,
Kaelinn, Kalan*

Kaelyn 🅶🅱 (American) a combi-
nation of Kae + Lynn. See also
Caelin, Kaylyn.
*Kaelan, Kaelen, Kaelin, Kaelynn,
Kaelynne*

Kaetlyn (Irish) a form of Kaitlin.
Kaetlin, Kaetlynn

Kagami (Japanese) mirror.

Kahlil 🅱🅶 (Arabic) a form of
Khalíl (see Boys' Names).

Kahsha (Native American) fur robe.
Kasha, Kashae, Kashia

Kai 🅱🅶 (Hawaiian) sea. (Hopi,
Navajo) willow tree.
Kae, Kaie

Kaia (Greek) earth. Mythology:
Gaea was the earth goddess.
Kaiah, Kaija

Kaila (Hebrew) laurel; crown.
*Kailah, Kailea, Kaileah, Kailee,
Kailey, Kayla*

Kailee, Kailey (American) familiar forms of Kaila. Forms of Kaylee.
Kaile, Kaileh, Kaileigh, Kaili, Kailia, Kailie, Kailli, Kaillie, Kaily, Kailya

Kailyn GB (American) a form of Kaitlin.
Kailan, Kaileen, Kaileena, Kailen, Kailena, Kailene, Kaileyne, Kailin, Kailina, Kailon

Kailynn (American) a form of Kailyn.
Kailynne

Kairos (Greek) last, final, complete. Mythology: the last goddess born to Jupiter.
Kaira, Kairra

Kaishawn (American) a combination of Kai + Shawna.
Kaeshun, Kaisha, Kaishala, Kaishon

Kaitlin GB (Irish) pure. See also Katelin.
Kaetlyn, Kailyn, Kailynn, Kaitlan, Kaitland, Kaitleen, Kaitlen, Kaitlind, Kaitlinn, Kaitlinne, Kaitlon, Kaytlin

Kaitlyn ☆ (Irish) a form of Caitlyn.

Kaitlynn (Irish) a form of Caitlyn.
Kaitelynne, Kaitlynne

Kaiya (Japanese) forgiveness.
Kaiyah, Kaiyia

Kala GB (Arabic) a short form of Kalila. A form of Cala.
Kalah, Kalla, Kallah

Kalama BG (Hawaiian) torch.

Kalani GB (Hawaiian) chieftain; sky.
Kailani, Kalanie, Kaloni

Kalare (Latin, Basque) bright; clear.

Kalea (Hawaiian) bright; clear.
Kahlea, Kahleah, Kailea, Kaileah, Kaleah, Kaleeia, Kaleia, Kalia, Kallea, Kalleah, Kaylea, Kayleah, Khalea, Khaleah

Kaleb BG (Hebrew) a form of Caleb.

Kalee, Kalie (American) forms of Caley, Kaylee.
Kalei

Kalei (Hawaiian) flower wreath.
Kahlei, Kailei, Kallei, Kaylei, Khalei

Kaleigh, Kaley GB (American) forms of Caley, Kaylee.
Kalley, Kalleigh, Kally, Kaly

Kalena (Hawaiian) pure. See also Kalina.
Kaleen, Kaleena, Kalene, Kalenea, Kalenna

Kalere (Swahili) short woman.
Kaleer

Kali GB (Hindi) the black one.
(Hawaiian) hesitating. Religion: a
form of the Hindu goddess Devi.
See also Cali.
*Kalee, Kaleigh, Kaley, Kalie,
Kallee, Kalley, Kalli, Kallie, Kally,
Kallye, Kaly*

Kalia (Hawaiian) a form of Kalea.
Kaliah, Kaliea, Kalieya

Kalifa (Somali) chaste; holy.

Kalila (Arabic) beloved,
sweetheart. See also Kaela.
*Kahlila, Kala, Kaleela, Kalilla,
Kaylil, Kaylila, Kelila, Khalila,
Khalilah, Khalillah, Kylila, Kylilah,
Kylillah*

Kalina (Slavic) flower. (Hawaiian)
a form of Karen. See also Kalena.
*Kalin, Kalinna, Kalyna, Kalynah,
Kalynna*

Kalinda (Hindi) sun.
*Kaleenda, Kalindi, Kalynda,
Kalyndi*

Kalisa (American) a combination
of Kate + Lisa.
Kalise, Kalissa, Kalysa, Kalyssa

Kalisha (American) a
combination of Kate + Aisha.
Kaleesha, Kaleisha, Kalishia

Kaliska (Moquelumnan) coyote
chasing deer.

Kallan (Slavic) stream, river.
*Kalahn, Kalan, Kalen, Kallen,
Kallon, Kalon*

Kalle BG (Finnish) a form of
Carol.
Kaille, Kaylle

Kalli, Kallie (Greek) forms of
Callie. Familiar forms of Kalliope,
Kallista, Kalliyan.
Kalle, Kallee, Kalley, Kallita, Kally

Kalliope (Greek) a form of
Calliope.
Kalli, Kallie, Kallyope

Kallista (Greek) a form of
Callista.
*Kalesta, Kalista, Kallesta, Kalli,
Kallie, Kallysta, Kaysta*

Kalliyan (Cambodian) best.
Kalli, Kallie

Kaltha (English) marigold, yellow
flower.

Kaluwa (Swahili) forgotten one.
Kalua

Kalyca (Greek) rosebud.
Kalica, Kalika, Kaly

Kalyn GB (American) a form of
Kaylyn.
*Kalin, Kallen, Kallin, Kallon,
Kallyn, Kalyne*

Kalynn GB (American) a forms of
Kalyn.
Kalynne

Kama (Sanskrit) loved one.
Religion: the Hindu god of love.

Kamala (Hindi) lotus.
Kamalah, Kammala

Kamali (Mahona) spirit guide; protector.
Kamalie

Kamaria (Swahili) moonlight.
Kamar, Kamara, Kamarae, Kamaree, Kamari, Kamariah, Kamarie, Kamariya, Kamariyah, Kamarya

Kamata (Moquelumnan) gambler.

Kambria (Latin) a form of Cambria.
Kambra, Kambrie, Kambriea, Kambry

Kamea (Hawaiian) one and only; precious.
Kameah, Kameo, Kamiya

Kameke (Swahili) blind.

Kameko (Japanese) turtle child. Mythology: the turtle symbolizes longevity.

Kameron BG (American) a form of Cameron.
Kameran, Kamri

Kami GB (Japanese) divine aura. (Italian, North African) a short form of Kamila, Kamilah. See also Cami.
Kamie, Kammi, Kammie, Kammy, Kammye, Kamy

Kamil BG (Arabic) a form of Kamal (see Boys' Names).

Kamila (Slavic) a form of Camila. See also Millie.
Kameela, Kamela, Kamelia, Kamella, Kami, Kamilah, Kamilia, Kamilka, Kamilla, Kamille, Kamma, Kammilla, Kamyla

Kamilah (North African) perfect.
Kameela, Kameelah, Kami, Kamillah, Kammilah

Kamiya (Hawaiian) a form of Kamea.
Kamia, Kamiah, Kamiyah

Kamri (American) a short form of Kameron. See also Camri.
Kamree, Kamrey, Kamrie, Kamry, Kamrye

Kamryn (American) a short form of Kameron. See also Camryn.
Kameryn, Kamren, Kamrin, Kamron, Kamrynn

Kanani (Hawaiian) beautiful.
Kana, Kanae, Kanan

Kanda (Native American) magical power.

Kandace, Kandice GB (Greek) glittering white; glowing. (American) forms of Candace, Candice.
Kandas, Kandess, Kandi, Kandis, Kandise, Kandiss, Kandus, Kandyce, Kandys, Kandyse

Kandi (American) a familiar form of Kandace, Kandice. See also Candi.
Kandhi, Kandia, Kandie, Kandy, Kendi, Kendie, Kendy, Kenndi, Kenndie, Kenndy

Kandra (American) a form of
Kendra. See also Candra.
Kandrea, Kandree, Kandria

Kane BG (Japanese) two right
hands.

Kaneisha, Kanisha (American)
forms of Keneisha.
*Kaneasha, Kanecia, Kaneesha,
Kanesah, Kanesha, Kaneshea,
Kaneshia, Kanessa, Kaneysha,
Kaniece, Kanishia*

Kanene (Swahili) a little
important thing.

Kani (Hawaiian) sound.

Kanika (Mwera) black cloth.
Kanica, Kanicka

Kannitha (Cambodian) angel.

Kanoa BG (Hawaiian) free.

Kanya (Hindi) virgin. (Tai) young
lady. Religion: a form of the
Hindu goddess Devi.
Kanea, Kania, Kaniya, Kanyia

Kapri (American) a form of Capri.
*Kapre, Kapree, Kapria, Kaprice,
Kapricia, Kaprisha, Kaprisia*

Kapua (Hawaiian) blossom.

Kapuki (Swahili) first-born
daughter.

Kara GB (Greek, Danish) pure.
*Kaira, Kairah, Karah, Karalea,
Karaleah, Karalee, Karalie, Kari,
Karra*

Karah (Greek, Danish) a form of
Kara. (Irish, Italian) a form of
Cara.
Karrah

Karalynn (English) a combination
of Kara + Lynn.
*Karalin, Karaline, Karalyn,
Karalyne, Karalynne*

Kareem BG (Arabic) noble;
distinguished.

Karel BG (American) a form of
Karelle.

Karelle (American) a form of
Carol.
Karel, Kareli, Karell, Karely

Karen GB (Greek) pure. See also
Carey, Carina, Caryn.
*Kaaren, Kalina, Karaina, Karan,
Karena, Karin, Karina, Karine,
Karna, Karon, Karren, Karron,
Karyn, Kerron, Koren*

Karena (Scandinavian) a form of
Karen.
*Kareen, Kareena, Kareina,
Karenah, Karene, Karreen,
Karreena, Karrena, Karrene*

Karessa (French) a form of
Caressa.

Kari GB (Greek) pure. (Danish) a
form of Caroline, Katherine. See
also Carey, Cari, Carrie.
*Karee, Karey, Karia, Kariah, Karie,
Karrey, Karri, Karrie, Karry, Kary*

Kariane, Karianne (American)
combinations of Kari + Ann.
*Karian, Kariana, Kariann,
Karianna*

Karida (Arabic) untouched, pure.
Kareeda, Karita

Karilynn (American) a
combination of Kari + Lynn.
*Kareelin, Kareeline, Kareelinn,
Kareelyn, Kareelyne, Kareelynn,
Kareelynne, Karilin, Kariline,
Karilinn, Karilyn, Karilyne,
Karilynne, Karylin, Karyline,
Karylinn, Karylyn, Karylyne,
Karylynn, Karylynne*

Karimah (Arabic) generous.
*Kareema, Kareemah, Karima,
Karime*

Karin (Scandinavian) a form of
Karen.
*Kaarin, Kareen, Karina, Karine,
Karinne, Karrin, Kerrin*

Karina GB (Russian) a form of
Karen.
*Kaarina, Karinna, Karrina,
Karryna, Karyna, Karynna*

Karine (Russian) a form of Karen.
Karrine, Karryne, Karyne

Karis (Greek) graceful.
*Karess, Karice, Karise, Karisse,
Karris, Karys, Karyss*

Karissa (Greek) a form of
Carissa.
*Karese, Karesse, Karisa, Karisha,
Karishma, Karisma, Karissimia,*

*Kariza, Karrisa, Karrissa, Karysa,
Karyssa, Kerisa*

Karla GB (German) a form of
Carla. (Slavic) a short form of
Karoline.
*Karila, Karilla, Karle, Karlene,
Karlicka, Karlinka, Karlisha,
Karlisia, Karlitha, Karlla, Karlon,
Karlyn*

Karlee, Karleigh (American)
forms of Karley, Karly. See also
Carlee.
Karlea, Karleah, Karlei

Karlene, Karlyn (American)
forms of Karla. See also Carleen.
*Karleen, Karlen, Karlena, Karlign,
Karlin, Karlina, Karlinna, Karlyan,
Karlynn, Karlynne*

Karley, Karly GB (Latin) little
and strong. (American) forms of
Carly.
*Karlee, Karley, Karlie, Karlyan,
Karlye*

Karli, Karlie (American) forms of
Karley, Karly. See also Carli.

Karlotte (American) a form of
Charlotte.
*Karlita, Karletta, Karlette,
Karlotta*

Karma (Hindi) fate, destiny;
action.

Karmel BG (Hebrew) a form of
Carmela.
*Karmeita, Karmela, Karmelina,
Karmella, Karmelle, Karmiella,
Karmielle, Karmyla*

Karmen (Latin) song.
Karman, Karmencita, Karmin, Karmina, Karmine, Karmita, Karmon, Karmyn, Karmyne

Karolane (American) a combination of Karoll + Anne.
Karolan, Karolann, Karolanne, Karol-Anne

Karolina, Karoline (Slavic) forms of Caroline. See also Carolina.
Karaleen, Karalena, Karalene, Karalin, Karaline, Karileen, Karilena, Karilene, Karilin, Karilina, Kariline, Karleen, Karlen, Karlena, Karlene, Karling, Karoleena, Karolena, Karolinka, Karroleen, Karrolena, Karrolene, Karrolin, Karroline

Karoll (Slavic) a form of Carol.
Karel, Karilla, Karily, Karol, Karola, Karole, Karoly, Karrol, Karyl, Kerril

Karolyn (American) a form of Carolyn.
Karalyn, Karalyna, Karalynn, Karalynne, Karilyn, Karilyna, Karilynn, Karilynne, Karlyn, Karlynn, Karlynne, Karolyna, Karolynn, Karolynne, Karrolyn, Karrolyna, Karrolynn, Karrolynne

Karri, Karrie (American) forms of Carrie.
Kari, Karie, Karry, Kary

Karsen, Karsyn (English) child of Kar. Forms of Carson.
Karson

Karuna (Hindi) merciful.

Karyn (American) a form of Karen.
Karyne, Karynn, Karynna, Kerrynn, Kerrynne

Kasa (Hopi) fur robe.

Kasandra (Greek) a form of Kassandra.
Kasander, Kasandria, Kasandra, Kasaundra, Kasondra, Kasoundra

Kasey, Kasie 🇬🇧 (Irish) brave. (American) forms of Casey, Kacey.
Kaisee, Kaisie, Kasci, Kascy, Kasee, Kasi, Kassee, Kassey, Kasy, Kasya, Kaysci, Kaysea, Kaysee, Kaysey, Kaysi, Kaysie, Kaysy

Kashawna (American) a combination of Kate + Shawna.
Kasha, Kashae, Kashana, Kashanna, Kashauna, Kashawn, Kasheana, Kasheanna, Kasheena, Kashena, Kashonda, Kashonna

Kashmir (Sanskrit) Geography: a region located between India and Pakistan.
Cashmere, Kashmear, Kashmere, Kashmia, Kashmira, Kasmir, Kasmira, Kazmir, Kazmira

Kasi (Hindi) from the holy city.

Kasia (Polish) a form of Katherine. See also Cassia.
Kashia, Kasiah, Kasian, Kasienka, Kasja, Kaska, Kassa, Kassia, Kassya, Kasya

Kasinda (Umbundu) our last baby.

Kassandra GB (Greek) a form of Cassandra.
Kassandr, Kassandre, Kassandré, Kassaundra, Kassi, Kassondra, Kassondria, Kassundra, Kazandra, Khrisandra, Krisandra, Krissandra

Kassi, Kassie (American) familiar forms of Kassandra, Kassidy. See also Cassie.
Kassey, Kassia, Kassy

Kassidy GB (Irish) clever. (American) a form of Cassidy.
Kassadee, Kassadi, Kassadie, Kassadina, Kassady, Kasseday, Kassedee, Kassi, Kassiddy, Kassidee, Kassidi, Kassidie, Kassity, Kassydi

Katalina (Irish) a form of Caitlin. See also Catalina.
Kataleen, Kataleena, Katalena, Katalin, Katalyn, Katalynn

Katarina (Czech) a form of Katherine.
Kata, Katareena, Katarena, Katarin, Katarine, Katarinna, Katarinne, Katarrina, Kataryna, Katarzyna, Katinka, Katrika, Katrinka

Kate GB (Greek) pure. (English) a short form of Katherine.
Kait, Kata, Katee, Kati, Katica, Katie, Katka, Katy, Katya

Katee, Katey (English) familiar forms of Kate, Katherine.

Katelin (Irish) a form of Caitlin. See also Kaitlin.
Kaetlin, Katalin, Katelan, Kateland, Kateleen, Katelen, Katelene, Katelind, Kateline, Katelinn, Katelun, Kaytlin

Katelyn ☀ GB (Irish) a form of Caitlin.
Kaetlyn, Katelyne, Kaytlyn

Katelynn (Irish) a forms of Katelyn.
Kaetlynn, Kaetlynne, Katelynne, Kaytlynn, Katlynne

Katerina GB (Slavic) a form of Katherine.
Katenka, Katerine, Katerini, Katerinka

Katharine (Greek) a form of Katherine.
Katharaine, Katharin, Katharina, Katharyn

Katherine ☀ GB (Greek) pure. See also Carey, Catherine, Ekaterina, Kara, Karen, Kari, Kasia, Katerina, Yekaterina.
Ekaterina, Ekatrinna, Kasienka, Kasin, Kat, Katarina, Katchen, Kate, Katee, Kathann, Kathanne, Katharine, Kathereen, Katheren, Katherene, Katherenne, Katherin, Katherina, Katheryn, Katheryne, Kathi, Kathleen, Kathrine, Kathryn, Kathy, Kathyrine, Katia, Katina, Katlaina, Katoka, Katreeka, Katrina, Kay, Kitty

Kathi (English) a form of Kathy. See also Cathi.

Kathleen (Irish) a form of
Katherine. See also Cathleen.
*Katheleen, Kathelene, Kathi,
Kathileen, Kathlean, Kathleena,
Kathleene, Kathlene, Kathlin,
Kathlina, Kathlyn, Kathlyne,
Kathlynn, Kathy, Katleen*

Kathrine GB (Greek) a form of
Katherine.
*Kathreen, Kathreena, Kathrene,
Kathrin, Kathrina*

Kathryn GB (English) a form of
Katherine.
*Kathren, Kathryne, Kathrynn,
Kathrynne*

Kathy GB (English) familiar forms
of Katherine, Kathleen. See also
Cathi.
*Kaethe, Katha, Kathe, Kathee,
Kathey, Kathie, Katka, Katla, Kató*

Kati (Estonian) a familiar form of
Kate.
Katja, Katya, Katye

Katia GB (Russian) a form of
Katherine.
Cattiah, Katiya, Kattia, Kattiah

Katie (English) a familiar form of
Kate.
*Katee, Kati, Kãtia, Katti, Kattie,
Katy, Kayte, Kaytee, Kaytie*

Katilyn (Irish) a form of Katlyn.
Katilin, Katilynn

Katlin GB (Irish) a form of Katlyn.
Katlina, Katline

Katlyn (Greek) pure. (Irish) a
form of Katelin.
*Kaatlain, Katilyn, Katland, Katlin,
Katlynd, Katlyne, Katlynn,
Katlynne*

Katriel (Hebrew) God is my
crown.
*Katrelle, Katri, Katrie, Katry,
Katryel*

Katrina (German) a form of
Katherine. See also Catrina, Trina.
*Katreen, Katreena, Katrene, Katri,
Katrice, Katricia, Katrien, Katrin,
Katrine, Katrinia, Katriona,
Katryn, Katryna, Kattrina,
Kattryna, Katus, Katuska*

Katy (English) a familiar form of
Kate. See also Cady.
Kady, Katey, Katty, Kayte

Katya (Russian) a form of Katia
Katyah

Kaulana (Hawaiian) famous.
Kaula, Kauna, Kahuna

Kaveri (Hindi) Geography: a
sacred river in India.

Kavindra (Hindi) poet.

Kawena (Hawaiian) glow.
Kawana, Kawona

Kay GB (Greek) rejoicer.
(Teutonic) a fortified place.
(Latin) merry. A short form of
Katherine.
Caye, Kae, Kai, Kaye, Kayla

Kaya (Hopi) wise child.
(Japanese) resting place.
Kaja, Kayah, Kayia

Kaycee GB (American) a
combination of the initials K. + C.
*Kayce, Kaysee, Kaysey, Kaysi,
Kaysie, Kaysii*

Kaydee (American) a combi-
nation of the initials K. + D.
*Kayda, Kayde, Kayden, Kaydi,
Kaydie*

Kayden BG (American) a form of
Kaydee.

Kayla ☆ GB (Arabic, Hebrew)
laurel; crown. A form of Kaela,
Kaila. See also Cayla.
*Kaylah, Kaylea, Kaylee, Kayleen,
Kaylene, Kaylia, Keila, Keyla*

Kaylah (Arabic, Hebrew) a form
of Kayla.
Kayleah, Kaylia, Keylah

Kaylan GB (Hebrew) a form of
Kayleen.
*Kaylana, Kayland, Kaylani,
Kaylann*

Kaylee ☆ GB (American) a form
of Kayla. See also Caeley, Kalee.
*Kailee, Kayle, Kayleigh, Kayley,
Kayli, Kaylie*

Kayleen, Kaylene (Hebrew)
beloved, sweetheart. Forms of
Kayla.
*Kaylan, Kayleena, Kayleene,
Kaylen, Kaylena*

Kayleigh (American) a form of
Kaylee.
Kaylei

Kaylen (Hebrew) a form of
Kayleen.
*Kaylean, Kayleana, Kayleanna,
Kaylenn*

Kayley, Kayli, Kaylie
(American) forms of Kaylee.

Kaylin GB (American) a form of
Kaylyn.
Kaylon BG (American) a form of
Kaylin.

Kaylyn GB (American) a
combination of Kay + Lynn. See
also Kaelyn.
*Kalyn, Kayleen, Kaylene, Kaylin,
Kaylyna, Kaylyne*

Kaylynn (American) a
combination of Kay + Lynn.
Kalynn, Kaylynne

Kaytlin, Kaytlyn (Irish) forms of
Kaitlin.
*Kaytlan, Kaytlann, Kaytlen,
Kaytlyne, Kaytlynn, Kaytlynne*

Keaira (Irish) a form of Keara.
*Keair, Keairah, Keairra, Keairre,
Keairrea*

Keala (Hawaiian) path.

Keana, Keanna GB (German)
bold; sharp. (Irish) beautiful.
*Keanah, Keanne, Keanu, Keenan,
Keeyana, Keeyanah, Keeyanna,
Keeyona. Keeyonna, Keiana,
Keianna, Keona, Keonna*

Keandra, Keondra (American) forms of Kenda.
Keandrah, Keandre, Keandrea, Keandria, Kedeana, Kedia, Keonda, Keondre, Keondria

Keanu 🅱🅶 (German, Irish) a form of Keana.

Keara (Irish) dark; black. Religion: an Irish saint.
Keaira, Kearah, Kearia, Kearra, Keera, Keerra, Keiara, Keiarah, Keiarra, Keira, Kera

Kearsten, Keirsten (Greek) forms of Kirstin.
Kearstin, Kearston, Kearstyn, Keirstan, Keirstein, Keirstin, Keirston, Keirstyn, Keirstynne

Keaton 🅱🅶 (English) where hawks fly.

Keegan 🅱🅶 (Irish) little; fiery.

Keeley, Keely 🅶🅱 (Irish) forms of Kelly.
Kealee, Kealey, Keali, Kealie, Keallie, Kealy, Keela, Keelan, Keele, Keelee, Keeleigh, Keeli, Keelia, Keelie, Keellie, Keelye, Keighla, Keilee, Keileigh, Keiley, Keilly, Kiela, Kiele, Kieley, Kielly, Kiely

Keelyn (Irish) a form of Kellyn.
Kealyn, Keelin, Keilan, Kielyn

Keena (Irish) brave.
Keenya, Kina

Keenan 🅱🅶 (German, Irish) a form of Keana.

Keesha (American) a form of Keisha.
Keesa, Keeshae, Keeshana, Keeshanne, Keeshawna, Keeshonna, Keeshya, Keiosha

Kei (Japanese) reverent.

Keiana, Keianna (Irish) forms of Keana. (American) forms of Kiana.
Keiann, Keiannah, Keionna

Keiki (Hawaiian) child.
Keikana, Keikann, Keikanna, Keikanne

Keiko (Japanese) happy child.

Keila (Arabic, Hebrew) a form of Kayla.
Keilah, Kela, Kelah

Keilani (Hawaiian) glorious chief.
Kaylani, Keilan, Keilana, Keilany, Kelana, Kelanah, Kelane, Kelani, Kelanie

Keira (Irish) a form of Keara.
Keiara, Keiarra, Keirra, Keirrah, Kera, Keyeira

Keisha (American) a short form of Keneisha.
Keasha, Keashia, Keesha, Keishaun, Keishauna, Keishawn, Kesha, Keysha, Kiesha, Kisha, Kishanda

Keita (Scottish) woods; enclosed place.
Keiti

Kekona (Hawaiian) second-born child.

Kelcey, Kelci, Kelcie (Scottish)
forms of Kelsey.
Kelse, Kelcee, Kelcy

Kelila (Hebrew) crown, laurel.
See also Kaela, Kayla, Kalila.
Kelilah, Kelula

Kellen **BG** (Irish) a form of
Kellyn.

Kelley **GB** (Irish) a form of Kelly.

Kelli, Kellie **GB** (Irish) familiar
forms of Kelly.
*Keleigh, Keli, Kelia, Keliah, Kelie,
Kellee, Kelleigh, Kellia, Kellisa*

Kelly **GB** (Irish) brave warrior.
See also Caeley.
*Keeley, Keely, Kelley, Kelley, Kelli,
Kellie, Kellye*

Kellyanne (Irish) a combination
of Kelly + Anne.
Kelliann, Kellianne, Kellyann

Kellyn (Irish) a combination of
Kelly + Lynn.
*Keelyn, Kelleen, Kellen, Kellene,
Kellina, Kelline, Kellynn, Kellynne*

Kelsea **GB** (Scottish) a form of
Kelsey.
*Kelcea, Kelcia, Kelsa, Kelsae,
Kelsay, Kelse*

Kelsey **GB** (Scandinavian,
Scottish) ship island. (English) a
form of Chelsea.
*Kelcey, Kelda, Kellsee, Kellsei,
Kellsey, Kellsie, Kellsy, Kelsea,
Kelsei, Kelsey, Kelsi, Kelsie,
Kelsy, Kelsye*

Kelsi, Kelsie, Kelsy **GB**
(Scottish) forms of Chelsea.
Kalsie, Kelci, Kelcie, Kellsi

Kelton **BG** (English) keel town;
port.

Kelvin **BG** (Irish, English) narrow
river. Geography: a river in
Scotland.

Kenda (English) water baby.
(Dakota) magical power.
Keandra, Kendra, Kennda

Kendal **GB** (English) a form of
Kendall.
*Kendahl, Kendale, Kendalie,
Kendalin, Kendalyn, Kendalynn,
Kendel, Kendele, Kendil, Kindal*

Kendall **GB** (English) ruler of the
valley.
*Kendal, Kendalla, Kendalle,
Kendell, Kendelle, Kendera,
Kendia, Kendyl, Kinda, Kindall,
Kindi, Kindle, Kynda, Kyndal,
Kyndall, Kyndel*

Kendra **GB** (English) a form of
Kenda.
*Kandra, Kendrah, Kendre,
Kendrea, Kendreah, Kendria,
Kenndra, Kentra, Kentrae, Kindra,
Kyndra*

Kendrick **BG** (Irish) child of
Henry. (Scottish) royal chieftain.

Kendyl (English) a form of
Kendall.
Kendyle, Kendyll

Keneisha (American) a combination of the prefix Ken + Aisha.
Kaneisha, Keisha, Keneesha, Kenesha, Keneshia, Kenisha, Kenneisha, Kennesha, Kenneshia, Keosha, Kineisha

Kenenza (English) a form of Kennice.
Kenza

Kenia 🄶🄱 (Hebrew) a form of Kenya.
Keniya, Kennia

Kenisha (American) a form of Keneisha.
Kenisa, Kenise, Kenishia, Kenissa, Kennisa, Kennisha, Kennysha

Kenna 🄶🄱 (Irish) a short form of Kennice.

Kennedy 🄶🄱 (Irish) helmeted chief. History: John F. Kennedy was the thirty-fifth U.S. president.
Kenedee, Kenedey, Kenedi, Kenedie, Kenedy, Kenidee, Kenidi, Kenidie, Kenidy, Kennadee, Kennadi, Kennadie, Kennady, Kennedee, Kennedey, Kennedi, Kennedie, Kennidee, Kennidi, Kennidy, Kynnedi

Kenneth 🄱🄶 (Irish) beautiful. (English) royal oath.

Kennice (English) beautiful.
Kanice, Keneese, Kenenza, Kenese, Kennise

Kenny 🄱🄶 (Scottish) a familiar form of Kenneth.

Kent 🄱🄶 (Welsh) white; bright. Geography: a region in England.

Kentrell 🄱🄶 (English) king's estate.

Kenya 🄶🄱 (Hebrew) animal horn. Geography: a country in Africa.
Keenya, Kenia, Kenja, Kenyah, Kenyana, Kenyatta, Kenyia

Kenyatta (American) a form of Kenya.
Kenyata, Kenyatah, Kenyatte, Kenyattia, Kenyatta, Kenyette

Kenzie 🄶🄱 (Scottish) light skinned. (Irish) a short form of Mackenzie.
Kenzea, Kenzee, Kenzey, Kenzi, Kenzia, Kenzy, Kinzie

Keon 🄱🄶 (Irish) a form of Ewan (see Boys' Names).

Keona, Keonna (Irish) forms of Keana.
Keiona, Keionna, Keoana, Keoni, Keonia, Keonnah, Keonni, Keonnia

Keosha (American) a short form of Keneisha.
Keoshae, Keoshi, Keoshia, Keosia

Kerani (Hindi) sacred bells. See also Rani.
Kera, Kerah, Keran, Kerana

Keren (Hebrew) animal's horn.
Kerrin, Keryn

Kerensa (Cornish) a form of Karenza.
Karensa, Karenza, Kerenza

Keri, Kerri, Kerrie GB (Irish) forms of Kerry.
Keriann, Kerianne, Kerriann, Kerrianne

Kerry GB (Irish) dark haired. Geography: a county in Ireland.
Keary, Keiry, Keree, Kerey, Keri, Kerri, Kerrie, Kerryann, Kerryanne, Kery, Kiera, Kierra

Kerstin (Scandinavian) a form of Kirsten.
Kerstan, Kerste, Kerstein, Kersten, Kerstie, Kerstien, Kerston, Kerstyn, Kerstynn

Kesare (Latin) long haired. (Russian) a form of Caesar (see Boys' Names).

Kesha (American) a form of Keisha.
Keshah, Keshal, Keshala, Keshan, Keshana, Keshara, Keshawn, Keshawna, Keshawnna

Keshia (American) a form of Keisha. A short form of Keneisha.
Kecia, Keishia, Keschia, Keshea, Kesia, Kesiah, Kessia, Kessiah

Kesi (Swahili) born during difficult times.

Kessie (Ashanti) chubby baby.
Kess, Kessa, Kessey, Kessi

Kesse GB (Ashanti) a form of Kessie.

Keven BG (Irish) a form of Kevyn.

Kevin BG (Irish) beautiful.

Kevon BG (Irish) a form of Kevyn.

Kevyn BG (Irish) beautiful.
Keva, Kevan, Keven, Kevia, Keviana, Kevinna, Kevina, Kevion, Kevionna, Kevon, Kevona, Kevone, Kevonia, Kevonna, Kevonne, Kevonya, Kevynn

Keyana GB (American) a form of Kiana.
Keya, Keyanah, Keyanda, Keyandra

Keyanna (American) a form of Kiana.
Keyannah

Keyara (Irish) a form of Kiara.
Keyarah, Keyari, Keyarra, Keyera, Keyerah, Keyerra

Keyona (American) a form of Kiana.
Keyonda, Keyondra

Keyonna GB (American) a form of Kiana.
Keyonnia, Keyonnie

Keysha (American) a form of Keisha.
Keyosha, Keyoshia, Keyshana, Keyshanna, Keyshawn, Keyshawna, Keyshia, Keyshla, Keyshona, Keyshonna

Keziah (Hebrew) cinnamon-like spice. Bible: one of the daughters of Job.
Kazia, Kaziah, Ketzi, Ketzia, Ketziah, Kezi, Kezia, Kizzy

Khadijah GB (Arabic)
trustworthy. History:
Muhammed's first wife.
*Khadaja, Khadajah, Khadeeja,
Khadeejah, Khadeja, Khadejah,
Khadejha, Khadija, Khadije,
Khadijia, Khadijiah*

Khalida (Arabic) immortal,
everlasting.
*Khali, Khalia, Khaliah, Khalidda,
Khalita*

Khrissa (American) a form of
Chrissa. (Czech) a form of Krista.
*Khrishia, Khryssa, Krisha, Krisia,
Krissa, Krysha, Kryssa*

Khristina (Russian, Scandinavian)
a form of Kristina, Christina.
*Khristeen, Khristen, Khristin,
Khristine, Khyristya, Khristyana,
Khristyna, Khrystyne*

Ki (Korean) arisen.

Kia GB (African) season's
beginning. (American) a short
form of Kiana.
Kiah

Kiana GB (American) a combi-
nation of the prefix Ki + Ana.
*Keanna, Keiana, Keyana, Keyona,
Khiana, Khianah, Khianna, Ki,
Kiahna, Kiane, Kiani, Kiania,
Kianna, Kiandra, Kiandria,
Kiauna, Kiaundra, Kiyana, Kyana*

Kianna (American) a form of
Kiana.
Kiannah, Kianne, Kianni

Kiara GB (Irish) little and dark.
*Keyara, Kiarra, Kieara, Kiearah,
Kiearra, Kyara*

Kiaria, Kiarra, Kichi (Japanese)
fortunate.

Kiele GB (Hawaiian) gardenia;
fragrant blossom.
Kiela, Kieley, Kieli, Kielli, Kielly

Kiera, Kierra (Irish) forms of
Kerry.
Kierana, Kieranna, Kierea

Kieran BG (Irish) little and dark;
little Keir.

Kiersten GB (Scandinavian) a
form of Kirsten.
*Keirstan, Kerstin, Kierstan,
Kierston, Kierstyn, Kierstynn*

Kierstin (Scandinavian) a form of
Kirsten.

Kiki GB (Spanish) a familiar form
of names ending in "queta."

Kiku (Japanese) chrysanthemum.
Kiko

Kiley GB (Irish) attractive; from
the straits.
*Kilea, Kilee, Kileigh, Kili, Kilie,
Kylee, Kyli, Kylie*

Kim GB (Vietnamese) needle.
(English) a short form of
Kimberly.
Kima, Kimette, Kym

Kimana (Shoshone) butterfly.
Kiman, Kimani

Kimber (English) a short form of
Kimberly.
Kimbra

Kimberlee, Kimberley (English)
forms of Kimberly.
*Kimbalee, Kimberlea, Kimberlei,
Kimberleigh, Kimbley*

Kimberly ☆ GB (English) chief,
ruler.
*Cymberly, Cymbre, Kim, Kimba,
Kimbely, Kimber, Kimbereley,
Kimberely, Kimberlee, Kimberli,
Kimberlie, Kimberlyn, Kimbery,
Kimbria, Kimbrie, Kimbry, Kimmie,
Kymberly*

Kimberlyn (English) a form of
Kimberly.
Kimberlin, Kimberlynn

Kimi (Japanese) righteous.
*Kimia, Kimika, Kimiko, Kimiyo,
Kimmi, Kimmie, Kimmy*

Kimmie (English) a familiar form
of Kimberly.
*Kimee, Kimme, Kimmee, Kimmi,
Kimmy, Kimy*

Kina (Hawaiian) from China.

Kineisha (American) a form of
Keneisha.
*Kineesha, Kinesha, Kineshia,
Kinisha, Kinishia*

Kineta (Greek) energetic.
Kinetta

Kini GB (Hawaiian) a form of
Jean.
Kina

Kinsey GB (English) offspring;
relative.
*Kinsee, Kinsley, Kinza, Kinze,
Kinzee, Kinzey, Kinzi, Kinzie,
Kinzy*

Kinsley (American) a form of
Kinsey.
Kinslee, Kinslie, Kinslyn

Kioko (Japanese) happy child.
Kiyo, Kiyoko

Kiona (Native American) brown
hills.
Kionah, Kioni, Kionna

Kira GB (Persian) sun. (Latin)
light.
*Kirah, Kiri, Kiria, Kiro, Kirra,
Kirrah, Kirri*

Kiran GB (Hindi) ray of light.

Kirby BG (Scandinavian) church
village. (English) cottage by the
water.
Kirbee, Kirbi

Kirima (Eskimo) hill.

Kirsi (Hindi) amaranth blossoms.
Kirsie

Kirsta (Scandinavian) a form of
Kirsten.

Kirsten GB (Greek) Christian; anointed. (Scandinavian) a form of Christine.
Karsten, Kearsten, Keirstan, Kerstin, Kiersten, Kirsteni, Kirsta, Kirstan, Kirstene, Kirstie, Kirstin, Kirston, Kirsty, Kirstyn, Kjersten, Kursten, Kyersten, Kyrsten, Kyrstin

Kirstie, Kirsty (Scandinavian) familiar forms of Kirsten.
Kerstie, Kirsta, Kirste, Kirstee, Kirstey, Kirsti, Kjersti, Kyrsty

Kirstin (Scandinavian) a form of Kirsten.
Karstin, Kirsteen, Kirstien, Kirstine

Kirstyn (Greek) a form of Kirsten.
Kirstynn

Kisa (Russian) kitten.
Kisha, Kiska, Kissa, Kiza

Kishi (Japanese) long and happy life.

Kissa (Ugandan) born after twins.

Kita (Japanese) north.

Kitra (Hebrew) crowned.

Kitty (Greek) a familiar form of Katherine.
Ketter, Ketti, Ketty, Kit, Kittee, Kitteen, Kittey, Kitti, Kittie

Kiwa (Japanese) borderline.

Kiyana (American) a form of Kiana.
Kiya, Kiyah, Kiyan, Kiyani, Kiyanna, Kiyenna

Kizzy (American) a familiar form of Keziah.
Kezi, Kissie, Kizzi, Kizzie

Klara (Hungarian) a form of Clara.
Klára, Klari, Klarika

Klarise (German) a form of Klarissa.
Klarice, Kláris, Klaryce

Klarissa (German) clear, bright. (Italian) a form of Clarissa.
Klarisa, Klarise, Klarrisa, Klarrissa, Klarrissia, Klarisza, Klarysa, Klaryssa, Kleresa

Klaudia (American) a form of Claudia.
Klaudija

Kloe (American) a form of Chloe.
Khloe, Kloee, Kloey, Klohe, Kloie

Kodi BG (American) a form of Codi.
Kodee, Kodey, Kodie, Kody, Kodye, Koedi

Kody BG (American) a form of Kodi.

Koffi (Swahili) born on Friday.
Kaffe, Kaffi, Koffe, Koffie

Koko (Japanese) stork. See also Coco.

Kolby BG (American) a form of Colby.
Kobie, Koby, Kolbee, Kolbey, Kolbi, Kolbie

Kolina (Swedish) a form of Katherine. See also Colleen.
Koleén, Koleena, Kolena, Kolene, Koli, Kolleen, Kollena, Kollene, Kolyn, Kolyna

Kona BG (Hawaiian) lady. (Hindi) angular.
Koni, Konia

Konstance (Latin) a form of Constance.
Konstantina, Konstantine, Konstanza, Konstanze

Kora (Greek) a form of Cora.
Korah, Kore, Koren, Koressa, Koretta, Korra

Koral (American) a form of Coral.
Korel, Korele, Korella, Korilla, Korral, Korrel, Korrell, Korrelle

Korey BG (American) a form of Kori.

Kori GB (American) a short form of Korina. See also Corey, Cori.
Koree, Korey, Koria, Korie, Korri, Korrie, Korry, Kory

Korina (Greek) a form of Corina.
Koreena, Korena, Koriana, Korianna, Korine, Korinna, Korreena, Korrina, Korrinna, Koryna, Korynna

Korine (Greek) a form of Korina.
Koreen, Korene, Koriane, Korianne, Korin, Korinn, Korinne, Korrin, Korrine, Korrinne, Korryn, Korrynne, Koryn, Koryne, Korynn

Kornelia (Latin) a form of Cornelia.
Karniela, Karniella, Karnis, Kornelija, Kornelis, Kornelya, Korny

Kortney GB (English) a form of Courtney.
Kortnay, Kortnee, Kortni, Kortnie, Kortny

Kory BG (American) a form of Kori.

Kosma (Greek) order; universe.
Cosma

Kosta (Latin) a short form of Constance.
Kostia, Kostusha, Kostya

Koto (Japanese) harp.

Kourtney GB (American) a form of Courtney.
Kourtnay, Kourtne, Kourtnee, Kourtnei, Kourtneigh, Kourtni, Kourtny, Kourtynie

Kris BG (American) a short form of Kristine. A form of Chris.
Khris, Krissy

Krissy (American) a familiar form of Kris.
Krissey, Krissi, Krissie

Krista GB (Czech) a form of Christina. See also Christa.
Khrissa, Khrista, Khryssa, Khrysta, Krissa, Kryssa, Krysta

Kristal (Latin) a form of Crystal.
Kristale, Kristall, Kristill, Kristl, Kristle, Kristy

Kristan (Greek) a form of Kristen.
*Kristana, Kristanna, Kristanne,
Kriston, Krystan, Krystane*

Kristen GB (Greek) Christian;
anointed. (Scandinavian) a form
of Christine.
*Christen, Kristan, Kristene,
Kristien, Kristin, Kristyn, Krysten*

Kristi, Kristie (Scandinavian)
short forms of Kristine.
Christi

Kristian BG (Greek) Christian;
anointed. Forms of Christian.
*Khristian, Kristian, Kristiane,
Kristiann, Kristi-Ann, Kristianna,
Kristianne, Kristi-Anne,
Kristienne, Kristyan, Kristyana,
Kristy-Ann, Kristy-Anne*

Kristiana (Greek) a form of
Kristian.

Kristin GB (Scandinavian) a form
of Kristen. See also Cristen.
Kristiin, Krystin

Kristina GB (Greek) Christian;
anointed. (Scandinavian) a form
of Christina. See also Cristina.
*Khristina, Kristena, Kristeena,
Kristina, Kristinka, Krystina*

Kristine GB (Scandinavian) a
form of Christine.
*Kris, Kristeen, Kristene, Kristi,
Kristie, Kristy, Krystine, Krystyne*

Kristopher BG (Greek) a form of
Christopher.

Kristy GB (American) a familiar
form of Kristine, Krystal. See also
Cristy.
*Kristi, Kristia, Kristie, Krysia,
Krysti*

Kristyn GB (Greek) a form of
Kristen.
Kristyne, Kristynn

Krysta (Polish) a form of Krista.
Krystah, Krystka

Krystal GB (American) clear,
brilliant glass.
*Kristabel, Kristal, Krystalann,
Krystalanne, Krystale, Krystall,
Krystalle, Krystel, Krystil, Krystle,
Krystol*

Krystalee (American) a
combination of Krystal + Lee.
*Kristalea, Kristaleah, Kristalee,
Krystalea, Krystaleah, Krystlea,
Krystleah, Krystlee, Krystlelea,
Krystleleah, Krystlelee*

Krystalynn (American) a
combination of Krystal + Lynn.
*Kristaline, Kristalyn, Kristalynn,
Kristilyn, Kristilynn, Kristlyn,
Krystaleen, Krystalene, Krystalin,
Krystalina, Krystallyn, Krystalyn,
Krystalynne*

Krystel (Latin) a form of Krystal.
*Kristel, Kristell, Kristelle,
Krystelle*

Krysten (Greek) a form of
Kristen.
Krystene, Krystyn, Krystyne

Krystian BG (Greek) a form of
Christian.
*Krystianne, Krysty-Ann, Krystyan,
Krystyanne, Krysty-Anne,
Krystyen*

Krystiana (Greek) a form of
Krystian.
*Krystiana, Kristianna, Kristyana,
Krystyanna*

Krystin (Czech) a form of Kristin.

Krystina (Greek) a form of
Kristina.
*Krysteena, Krystena, Krystyna,
Krystynka*

Krystle (American) a form of
Krystal.
Krystl, Krystyl

Kudio (Swahili) born on Monday.

Kuma (Japanese) bear. (Tongan)
mouse.

Kumiko (Japanese) girl with
braids.
Kumi

Kumuda (Sanskrit) lotus flower.

Kuniko (Japanese) child from the
country.

Kunto (Twi) third-born.

Kuri (Japanese) chestnut.

Kusa (Hindi) God's grass.

Kwanita (Zuni) a form of Juanita.

Kwashi (Swahili) born on
Sunday.

Kwau (Swahili) born on
Thursday.

Kyana (American) a form of
Kiana.
*Kyanah, Kyani, Kyann, Kyanna,
Kyanne, Kyanni, Kyeana,
Kyeanna*

Kyara (Irish) a form of Kiara.
*Kiyara, Kiyera, Kiyerra, Kyarah,
Kyaria, Kyarie, Kyarra, Kyera,
Kyerra*

Kyla GB (Irish) attractive.
(Yiddish) crown; laurel.
Khyla, Kylah, Kylea, Kyleah, Kylia

Kyle BG (Irish) attractive.
*Kial, Kiele, Kylee, Kyleigh,
Kylene, Kylie*

Kylee GB (Irish) a familiar form
of Kyle.
Kylea, Kyleah, Kylie, Kyliee

Kyleigh (Irish) a form of Kyle.
Kyliegh

Kylene (Irish) a form of Kyle.
Kyleen, Kylen, Kylyn, Kylynn

Kyler BG (English) a form of Kyle.

Kylie ☆ GB (West Australian
Aboriginal) curled stick;
boomerang. (Irish) a familiar
form of Kyle.
*Keiley, Keilley, Keilly, Keily, Kiley,
Kye, Kylee, Kyley, Kyli, Kyllie*

Kym GB (English, Vietnamese) a
form of Kim.

Kymberly (English) a form of Kimberly.
Kymber, Kymberlee, Kymberleigh, Kymberley, Kymberli, Kymberlie, Kymberlyn, Kymberlynn, Kymberlynne

Kyndal (English) a form of Kendall.
Kyndahl, Kyndel, Kyndle, Kyndol

Kyndall GB (English) a form of Kendall.
Kyndalle, Kyndell, Kyndelle

Kynthia (Greek) a form of Cynthia.
Kyndi

Kyoko (Japanese) mirror.

Kyra (Greek) ladylike. A form of Cyrilla.
Keera, Keira, Kira, Kyrah, Kyrene, Kyria, Kyriah, Kyriann, Kyrie

L

L BG (American) an initial used as a first name.

Lacey, Lacy GB (Latin) cheerful. (Greek) familiar forms of Larissa.
Lacee, Laci, Lacie, Lacye

Lachandra (American) a combination of the prefix La + Chandra.
Lachanda, Lachandice

Laci, Lacie (Latin) forms of Lacey.
Lacia, Laciann, Lacianne

Lacrecia (Latin) a form of Lucretia.
Lacrasha, Lacreash, Lacreasha, Lacreashia, Lacreisha, Lacresha, Lacreshia, Lacresia, Lacretia, Lacricia, Lacriesha, Lacrisah, Lacrisha, Lacrishia, Lacrissa

Lada (Russian) Mythology: the Slavic goddess of beauty.

Ladasha (American) a combination of the prefix La + Dasha.
Ladaesha, Ladaisa, Ladaisha, Ladaishea, Ladaishia, Ladashiah, Ladaseha, Ladashia, Ladasia, Ladassa, Ladaysha, Ladesha, Ladisha, Ladosha

Ladeidra (American) a combination of the prefix La + Deidra.
Ladedra, Ladiedra

Ladonna (American) a combination of the prefix La + Donna.
Ladan, Ladana, Ladon, Ladona, Ladonne, Ladonya

Laela (Arabic, Hebrew) a form of Leila.
Lael, Laelle

Laelia (Latin) she who is talkative.

Lahela (Hawaiian) a form of Rachel.

Laica (Greek) pure, secular.

Laila (Arabic) a form of Leila.
Lailah, Laili, Lailie

Laine, Layne BG (French) short forms of Elaine.
Lain, Laina, Lainah, Lainee, Lainna, Layna

Lainey, Layney (French) familiar forms of Elaine.
Laini, Lainie, Laynee, Layni, Laynie

Lajila (Hindi) shy, coy.

Lajuana (American) a combination of the prefix La + Juana.
Lajuanna, Lawana, Lawanna, Lawanza, Lawanze, Laweania

Laka (Hawaiian) attractive; seductive; tame. Mythology: the goddess of the hula.

Lakayla (American) a combination of the prefix La + Kayla.
Lakala, Lakaya, Lakeila, Lakela, Lakella

Lakeisha (American) a combination of the prefix La + Keisha. See also Lekasha.
Lakaiesha, Lakaisha, Lakasha, Lakashia, Lakaysha, Lakaysia, Lakeasha, Lakecia, Lakeesh, Lakeesha, Lakeeshia, Lakesha, Lakeshia, Lakeysha, Lakezia, Lakicia, Lakieshia, Lakisha

Laken GB (American) a short form of Lakendra.
Lakena

Lakendra (American) a combination of the prefix La + Kendra.
Lakanda, Lakedra, Laken, Lakenda

Lakenya (American) a combination of the prefix La + Kenya.
Lakeena, Lakeenna, Lakeenya, Lakena, Lakenia, Lakinja, Lakinya, Lakwanya, Lekenia, Lekenya

Lakesha, Lakeshia, Lakisha (American) forms of Lakeisha.
Lakecia, Lakeesha, Lakesa, Lakese, Lakeseia, Lakeshya, Lakesi, Lakesia, Lakeyshia, Lakiesha

Laketa (American) a combination of the prefix La + Keita.
Lakeeta, Lakeetah, Lakeita, Lakeitha, Lakeithia, Laketha, Laketia, Laketta, Lakieta, Lakietha, Lakita, Lakitia, Lakitra, Lakitri, Lakitta

Lakia (Arabic) found treasure.
Lakiea, Lakkia

Lakin, Lakyn (American) short forms of Lakendra.
Lakyna, Lakynn

Lakota BG (Dakota) a tribal name.
Lakoda, Lakohta, Lakotah

Lakresha (American) a form of Lucretia.
Lacresha, Lacreshia, Lacresia, Lacretia, Lacrisha, Lakreshia, Lakrisha, Lekresha, Lekresia

Lakya (Hindi) born on Thursday.
Lakeya, Lakeyah, Lakieya, Lakiya, Lakyia

Lala (Slavic) tulip.
Lalah, Lalla

Lalasa (Hindi) love.

Laleh (Persian) tulip.
Lalah

Lali (Spanish) a form of Lulani.
Lalia, Lalli, Lally

Lalita (Greek) talkative. (Sanskrit) charming; candid.

Lallie (English) babbler.
Lalli, Lally

Lamar B G (German) famous throughout the land. (French) sea, ocean.

Lamesha (American) a combination of the prefix La + Mesha.
Lamees, Lameesha, Lameise, Lameisha, Lameshia, Lamisha, Lamishia, Lemisha

Lamia (German) bright land.
Lama, Lamiah

Lamis (Arabic) soft to the touch.
Lamese, Lamise

Lamonica (American) a combination of the prefix La + Monica.
Lamoni, Lamonika

Lamont B G (Scandinavian) lawyer.

Lamya (Arabic) dark lipped.
Lama

Lan (Vietnamese) flower.

Lana (Latin) woolly. (Irish) attractive, peaceful. A short form of Alana, Elana. (Hawaiian) floating; bouyant.
Lanae, Lanai, Lanata, Lanay, Laneah, Laneetra, Lanette, Lanna, Lannah

Lanca (Latin) blessed, fortunate one.

Lance B G (German) a short form of Lancelot (see Boys' Names).

Landa (Basque) another name for the Virgin Mary.

Landin B G (English) a form of Landon.

Landon B G (English) open, grassy meadow.
Landan, Landen, Landin, Landyn, Landynne

Landra (German, Spanish) counselor.
Landrea

Landrada (Spanish) counselor.

Lane B G (English) narrow road.
Laina, Laney, Layne

Laneisha (American) a combination of the prefix La + Keneisha.
Laneasha, Lanecia, Laneesha, Laneise, Laneishia, Lanesha, Laneshe, Laneshea, Laneshia, Lanesia, Lanessa, Lanesse, Lanisha, Lanishia

Laney (English) a familiar form of Lane.
Lanie, Lanni, Lanny, Lany

Lani GB (Hawaiian) sky; heaven. A short form of Atalanta, 'Aulani, Leilani.
Lanee, Lanei, Lania, Lanie, Lanita, Lanney, Lanni, Lannie

Laporsha (American) a combination of the prefix La + Porsha.
Laporcha, Laporche, Laporscha, Laporsche, Laporschia, Laporshe, Laporshia, Laportia

Laqueena (American) a combination of the prefix La + Queenie.
Laqueen, Laquena, Laquenetta, Laquinna

Laquinta (American) a combination of the prefix La + Quintana.
Laquanta, Laqueinta, Laquenda, Laquenta, Laquinda

Laquisha (American) a combination of the prefix La + Queisha.
Laquasha, Laquaysha, Laqueisha, Laquesha, Laquiesha

Laquita (American) a combination of the prefix La + Queta.
Laqeita, Laqueta, Laquetta, Laquia, Laquiata, Laquieta, Laquitta, Lequita

Lara GB (Greek) cheerful. (Latin) shining; famous. Mythology: a Roman nymph. A short form of Laraine, Larissa, Laura.
Larae, Larah, Laretta, Larette

Laraine (Latin) a form of Lorraine.
Lara, Laraene, Larain, Larane, Larayn, Larayne, Laraynna, Larein, Lareina, Lareine, Laren, Larenn, Larenya, Lauraine, Laurraine

Larina (Greek) seagull.
Larena, Larine

Larisa (Greek) a form of Larissa.
Lareesa, Lareese, Laresa, Laris, Larise, Larisha, Larrisa, Larysa, Laurisa

Larissa (Greek) cheerful. See also Lacey.
Lara, Laressa, Larisa, Larissah, Larrissa, Larryssa, Laryssa, Laurissa, Laurissah

Lark (English) skylark.

Larry BG (Latin) a familiar form of Lawrence.

Lashae, Lashay (American) combinations of the prefix La + Shay.
Lasha, Lashai, Lashaia, Lashaya, Lashaye, Lashea

Lashana (American) a combination of the prefix La + Shana.
Lashanay, Lashane, Lashanna, Lashannon, Lashona, Lashonna

Lashanda (American) a combination of the prefix La + Shanda.
Lashandra, Lashanta, Lashante

Lashawna (American) a combination of the prefix La + Shawna.
Lashaun, Lashauna, Lashaune, Lashaunna, Lashaunta, Lashawn, Lashawnd, Lashawnda, Lashawndra, Lashawne, Lashawnia, Leshawn, Leshawna

Lashonda (American) a combination of the prefix La + Shonda.
Lachonda, Lashaunda, Lashaundra, Lashon, Lashond, Lashonde, Lashondia, Lashondra, Lashonta, Lashunda, Lashundra, Lashunta, Lashunte, Leshande, Leshandra, Leshondra, Leshundra

Latanya (American) a combination of the prefix La + Tanya.
Latana, Latandra, Latania, Latanja, Latanna, Latanua, Latonshia

Latara (American) a combination of the prefix La + Tara.

Latasha (American) a combination of the prefix La + Tasha.
Latacha, Latacia, Latai, Lataisha, Latashia, Latasia, Lataysha, Letasha, Letashia, Letasiah

Latavia (American) a combination of the prefix La + Tavia.

Lateefah (Arabic) pleasant. (Hebrew) pat, caress.
Lateefa, Latifa, Latifah, Latipha

Latesha (American) a form of Leticia.
Lataeasha, Lateasha, Lateashia, Latecia, Lateicia, Lateisha, Latesa, Lateshia, Latessa, Lateysha, Latisa, Latissa, Leteisha, Leteshia

Latia (American) a combination of the prefix La + Tia.
Latea, Lateia, Lateka

Latika (Hindi) elegant.
Lateeka, Lateka

Latisha (Latin) joy. (American) a combination of the prefix La + Tisha.
Laetitia, Laetizia, Latashia, Lateasha, Lateashia, Latecia, Lateesha, Lateicia, Lateisha, Latice, Laticia, Latiesha, Latishia, Latishya, Latissha, Latitia, Latysha

Latona (Latin) Mythology: the powerful goddess who bore Apollo and Diana.
Latonna, Latonnah

Latonya (American) a combination of the prefix La + Tonya. (Latin) a form of Latona.
Latoni, Latonia

Latoria (American) a combination of the prefix La + Tori.
Latoira, Latorio, Latorja, Latorray, Latorreia, Latory, Latorya, Latoyra, Latoyria

Latosha (American) a combination of the prefix La + Tosha.
Latoshia, Latoshya, Latosia

Latoya (American) a combination of the prefix La + Toya.
Latoia, Latoiya, LaToya, Latoye, Latoyia, Latoyita, Latoyo

Latrice (American) a combination of the prefix La + Trice.
Latrece, Latreece, Latreese, Latresa, Latrese, Latressa, Letreece, Letrice

Latricia (American) a combination of the prefix La + Tricia.
Latrecia, Latresh, Latresha, Latreshia, Latrica, Latrisha, Latrishia

Laura GB (Latin) crowned with laurel.
Lara, Laurah, Lauralee, Laurelen, Laurella, Lauren, Lauricia, Laurie, Laurka, Laury, Lauryn, Lavra, Lolly, Lora, Loretta, Lori, Lorinda, Lorna, Loura

Laurel (Latin) laurel tree.
Laural, Laurell, Laurelle, Lorel, Lorelle

Lauren ☆ GB (English) a form of Laura.
Lauran, Laureen, Laurena, Laurene, Laurien, Laurin, Laurine, Lawren, Loren, Lorena

Laurence GB (Latin) crowned with laurel.
Laurencia, Laurens, Laurent, Laurentana, Laurentina, Lawrencia

Laurianna (English) a combination of Laurie + Anna.
Laurana, Laurann, Laureana, Laureanne, Laureen, Laureena, Laurian, Lauriana, Lauriane, Laurianna, Laurie Ann, Laurie Anne, Laurina

Laurie GB (English) a familiar form of Laura.
Lari, Larilia, Laure, Lauré, Lauri, Lawrie

Laurinda, Laurita (Spanish) crowned with laurels.

Laury GB (English) a familiar form of Laura.

Lauryn (English) a familiar form of Laura.
Laurynn

Laveda (Latin) cleansed, purified.
Lavare, Lavetta, Lavette

Lavelle (Latin) cleansing.
Lavella

Lavena (Irish, French) joy. (Latin) a form of Lavina.

Laverne (Latin) springtime. (French) grove of alder trees. See also Verna.
Laverine, Lavern, Laverna, La Verne

Laviana (Latin) native of Rome.

Lavina (Latin) purified; woman of Rome. See also Vina.
Lavena, Lavenia, Lavinia, Lavinie, Levenia, Levinia, Livinia, Louvinia, Lovina, Lovinia

Lavonna (American) a combination of the prefix La + Yvonne.
Lavon, Lavonda, Lavonder, Lavondria, Lavone, Lavonia, Lavonica, Lavonn, Lavonne, Lavonnie, Lavonya

Lawan (Tai) pretty.
Lawanne

Lawanda (American) a combination of the prefix La + Wanda.
Lawonda, Lawynda

Lawrence 🅱🅶 (Latin) crowned with laurel.

Layce (American) a form of Lacey.
Laycee, Layci, Laycia, Laycie, Laysa, Laysea, Laysie

Layla (Hebrew, Arabic) a form of Leila.
Laylah, Layli, Laylie

Layton 🅱🅶 (English) a form of Leighton (see Boys' Names).

Le (Vietnamese) pearl.

Lea (Hawaiian) Mythology: the goddess of canoe makers. (Hebrew) a form of Leah.

Leah ☀ 🅶🅱 (Hebrew) weary. Bible: the first wife of Jacob. See also Lia.
Lea, Léa, Lee, Leea, Leeah, Leia

Leala (French) faithful, loyal.
Lealia, Lealie, Leial

Lean, Leann (English) forms of Leeann, Lian.
Leane

Leandra (Latin) like a lioness.
Leanda, Leandre, Leandrea, Leandria, Leeanda, Leeandra

Leanna, Leeanna (English) forms of Liana.
Leana, Leeana, Leianna

Leanne 🅶🅱 (English) a form of Leeann, Lian.

Leanore (Greek) a form of Eleanor. (English) a form of Helen.
Leanora, Lanore

Lecia (Latin) a short form of Felecia.
Leasia, Leecia, Leesha, Leesia, Lesha, Leshia, Lesia

Leda (Greek) lady. Mythology: the queen of Sparta and the mother of Helen of Troy.
Ledah, Lyda, Lydah

Ledicia (Latin) great joy.

Lee 🅱🅶 (Chinese) plum. (Irish) poetic. (English) meadow. A short form of Ashley, Leah.
Lea, Leigh

Leeann, Leeanne (English) combinations of Lee + Ann. Forms of Lian.
Leane, Leean, Leian, Leiann, Leianne

Leena (Estonian) a form of Helen. (Greek, Latin, Arabic) a form of Lina.

Leeza (Hebrew) a short form of Aleeza. (English) a form of Lisa, Liza.
Leesa

Lefitray (Mapuche) sound, the speed of sound, rapid sound.

Leflay (Mapuche) lethargic woman without energies, lacking in curiosity.

Lei **BG** (Hawaiian) a familiar form of Leilani.

Leigh **GB** (English) a form of Leah.
Leighann, Leighanne

Leigha (English) a form of Leigh.
Leighanna

Leiko (Japanese) arrogant.

Leila (Hebrew) dark beauty; night. (Arabic) born at night. See also Laela, Layla, Lila.
Laila, Leela, Leelah, Leilah, Leilia, Lela, Lelah, Leland, Lelia, Leyla

Leilani (Hawaiian) heavenly flower; heavenly child.
Lailanee, Lailani, Lailanie, Lailany, Lailoni, Lani, Lei, Leilany, Leiloni, Leilony, Lelani, Lelania

Leira (Basque) reference to the Virgin Mary.

Lekasha (American) a form of Lakeisha.
Lekeesha, Lekeisha, Lekesha,

Lekeshia, Lekesia, Lekicia, Lekisha

Leland **BG** (Hebrew) a form of Leila.

Leli (Swiss) a form of Magdalen.
Lelie

Lelia (Greek) fair speech. (Hebrew, Arabic) a form of Leila.
Leliah, Lelika, Lelita, Lellia

Lelica (Latin) talkative.

Lelya (Russian) a form of Helen.

Lena (Hebrew) dwelling or lodging. (Latin) temptress. (Norwegian) illustrious. (Greek) a short form of Eleanor. Music: Lena Horne, a well-known African American singer and actress.
Lenah, Lene, Lenee, Leni, Lenka, Lenna, Lennah, Lina, Linah

Lenci (Hungarian) a form of Helen.
Lency

Lene (German) a form of Helen.
Leni, Line

Leneisha (American) a combination of the prefix Le + Keneisha.
Lenece, Lenesha, Leniesha, Lenieshia, Leniesia, Leniessia, Lenisa, Lenise, Lenisha, Lennise, Lennisha, Lynesha

Lenia (German) a form of Leona.
Lenayah, Lenda, Lenea, Leneen, Lenna, Lennah, Lennea, Leny

Lenis (Latin) half, soft, silky.

Lenita (Latin) gentle.
Leneta, Lenette, Lennette

Lenore (Greek, Russian) a form of Eleanor.
Lenni, Lenor, Lenora, Lenorah

Leocadia (Greek) she who shines because of her whiteness.

Leocricia (Greek) she who judges her village well.

Leona (German) brave as a lioness. See also Lona.
Lenia, Leoine, Leola, Leolah, Leonae, Leonah, Leondra, Leone, Leonelle, Leonia, Leonice, Leonicia, Leonie, Leonissa, Leonna, Leonne, Liona

Leonarda, Leoncia Leonela (Latin) strong and fierce as a lion.

Leonie (German) a familiar form of Leona.
Leoni, Léonie, Leony

Leonilda (German) fighter.

Leonore (Greek) a form of Eleanor. See also Nora.
Leonor, Leonora, Leonorah, Léonore

Leontina (German) strong as a lion.

Leontine (Latin) like a lioness.
Leona, Leonine, Leontyne, Léontyne

Leopolda (German) princess of the village.

Leopoldina (Spanish) a form of Leopoldo.

Leopoldo (Italian) a form of Leopold (see Boys' Names).

Leora (Hebrew) light. (Greek) a familiar form of Eleanor. See also Liora.
Leorah, Leorit

Leotie (Native American) prairie flower.

Lera (Russian) a short form of Valera.
Lerka

Lesbia (Greek) native of the Greek island of Lesbos.

Lesley 🇬🇧 (Scottish) gray fortress.
Leslea, Leslee, Leslie, Lesly, Lezlee, Lezley

Leslie ☀★ 🇬🇧 (Scottish) a form of Lesley.
Leslei, Lesleigh, Lesli, Lesslie, Lezli

Lesly 🇬🇧 (Scottish) a form of Lesley.
Leslye, Lessly, Lezly

Lester 🇧🇬 (Latin) chosen camp. (English) from Leicester, England.

Leta (Latin) glad. (Swahili) bringer. (Greek) a short form of Aleta.
Lita, Lyta

Leticia (Latin) joy. See also
Latisha, Tisha.
*Laticia, Leisha, Leshia, Let, Leta,
Letesa, Letesha, Leteshia, Letha,
Lethia, Letice, Letichia, Letisha,
Letishia, Letisia, Letissa, Letita,
Letitia, Letiticia, Letiza, Letizia,
Letty, Letycia, Loutitia*

Letty (English) a familiar form of
Leticia.
Letta, Letti, Lettie

Levana (Hebrew) moon; white.
(Latin) risen. Mythology: the
goddess of newborn babies.
*Lévana, Levania, Levanna,
Levenia, Lewana, Livana*

Levani (Fijian) anointed with oil.

Levi BG (Hebrew) a form of Levia.

Levia (Hebrew) joined, attached.
Leevya, Levi, Levie

Levina (Latin) flash of lightning.
Levene

Levona (Hebrew) spice; incense.
*Leavonia, Levonat, Levonna,
Levonne, Livona*

Lewana (Hebrew) a form of
Levana.
Lebhanah, Lewanna

Lewis BG (Welsh) a form of
Llewellyn. (English) a form of
Louis (see Boys' Names).

Lexandra (Greek) a short form of
Alexandra.
Lisandra

Lexi (Greek) a familiar form of
Alexandra.

Lexia (Greek) a familiar form of
Alexandra.
*Leska, Lesya, Lexa, Lexane,
Lexina, Lexine*

Lexie GB (Greek) a familiar form
of Alexandra.
Leksi, Lexey, Lexy

Lexis (Greek) a short form of
Alexius, Alexus.
Laexis, Lexius, Lexsis, Lexxis

Lexus GB (Greek) a short form of
Alexis.
Lexuss, Lexxus, Lexyss

Leya (Spanish) loyal. (Tamil) the
constellation Leo.
Leyah, Leyla

Lia GB (Greek) bringer of good
news. (Hebrew, Dutch, Italian)
dependent. See also Leah.
Lía, Liah

Liam BG (Irish) a form of
William.

Lian (Chinese) graceful willow.
(Latin) a short form of Gillian,
Lillian.
*Lean, Leeann, Liane, Liann,
Lianne*

Liana, Lianna GB (Latin) youth.
(French) bound, wrapped up;
tree covered with vines. (English)
meadow. (Hebrew) short forms
of Eliana.
Leanna

Liane, Lianne (Hebrew) short forms of Eliane. (English) forms of Lian.
Leeanne

Liban 🅱🅶 (Hawaiian) a form of Laban (see Boys' Names).

Libby (Hebrew) a familiar form of Elizabeth.
Ibby, Lib, Libbee, Libbey, Libbie

Libera, Líbera (Latin) she who bestows abundance.

Liberada (Latin) liberated.

Liberata (Latin) she who loves liberty.

Liberia, Liberta (Spanish) freedom.

Libertad (Latin) she who has the skills to act in good faith.

Liberty (Latin) free.
Liberti, Libertie

Libia (Latin) comes from the desert.

Libitina (Latin) she who is wanted.

Libna (Latin) whiteness.

Liboria (Latin) she who was born in Libor, the name of several ancient cities in Spain and Portugal.

Librada (Latin) liberated.

Lican (Mapuche) flint stone.

Licia (Greek) a short form of Alicia.
Licha, Lishia, Lisia, Lycia

Lida (Greek) happy. (Slavic) loved by people. (Latin) a short form of Alida, Elita.
Leeda, Lidah, Lidochka, Lyda

Lide (Latin, Basque) life.

Lidia (Greek) a form of Lydia.
Lidea, Lidi, Lidija, Lidiya, Lidka, Lidya

Lídia (Portuguese) a form of Lidia.

Lien (Chinese) lotus.
Lienne

Liesabet (German) a short form of Elizabeth.
Liesbeth, Lisbete

Liese (German) a familiar form of Elise, Elizabeth.
Liesa, Lieschen, Lise

Liesel (German) a familiar form of Elizabeth.
Leesel, Leesl, Leezel, Leezl, Liesl, Liezel, Liezl, Lisel

Ligia (Greek) Mythology: name of a mermaid.

Lígia (Portuguese) a form of Ligia.

Lila (Arabic) night. (Hindi) free will of God. (Persian) lilac. A short form of Dalila, Delilah, Lillian.
Lilah, Lilia, Lyla, Lylah

Lilac (Sanskrit) lilac; blue purple.

Lilia (Persian) a form of Lila.
Lili

Lilian (Latin) a form of Lillian.
Liliane, Liliann, Lilianne

Lilián (Spanish) a form of Lilian.

Lílian (Portuguese) a form of Lilian.

Liliana (Latin) a form of Lillian.
Lileana, Lilliana, Lilianna, Lilliana, Lillianna

Lilibeth (English) a combination of Lily + Beth.
Lilibet, Lillibeth, Lillybeth, Lilybet, Lilybeth

Lilith (Arabic) of the night; night demon. Mythology: the first wife of Adam, according to ancient Jewish legends.
Lillis, Lily

Lillian ✻ (Latin) lily flower.
Lian, Lil, Lila, Lilas, Lileane, Lilia, Lilian, Liliana, Lilias, Liliha, Lilja, Lilla, Lilli, Lillia, Lilliane, Lilliann, Lillianne, Lillyann, Lis, Liuka

Lillyann (English) a combination of Lily + Ann. (Latin) a form of Lillian.
Lillyan, Lillyanne, Lily, Lilyan, Lilyana, Lilyann, Lilyanna, Lilyanne

Lilvina (Latin, German) friend of the Iris.

Lily ✻ (Latin, Arabic) a familiar form of Lilith, Lillian, Lillyann.
Lil, Líle, Lili, Lilie, Lilijana, Lilika, Lilike, Liliosa, Lilium, Lilka, Lille, Lilli, Lillie, Lilly

Limber (Tiv) joyful.

Lin GB (Chinese) beautiful jade. (English) a form of Lynn.
Linh, Linn

Lina (Greek) light. (Arabic) tender. (Latin) a form of Lena.

Lincoln BG (English) settlement by the pool.

Linda GB (Spanish) pretty.
Lind, Lindy, Linita, Lynda

Lindsay GB (English) a form of Lindsey.
Lindsi, Linsay, Lyndsay

Lindsey GB (English) linden tree island; camp near the stream.
Lind, Lindsea, Lindsee, Lindsi, Linsey, Lyndsey, Lynsey

Lindsi (American) a familiar form of Lindsay, Lindsey.
Lindsie, Lindsy, Lindze, Lindzee, Lindzey, Lindzy

Lindy (Spanish) a familiar form of Linda.
Linde, Lindee, Lindey, Lindi, Lindie

Linette (Welsh) idol. (French) bird.
Lanette, Linet, Linnet, Linnetta, Linnette, Lyannette, Lynette

Ling (Chinese) delicate, dainty.

Linnea (Scandinavian) lime tree.
Botany: the national flower of
Sweden.
*Lin, Linae, Linea, Linnae, Linnaea,
Linneah, Lynea, Lynnea*

Linsey (English) a form of
Lindsey.
*Linsea, Linsee, Linsi, Linsie, Linsy,
Linzee, Linzey, Linzi, Linzie, Linzy,
Linzzi, Lynsey*

Liolya (Russian) a form of Helen.

Lionela (Greek) little lion.

Liora (Hebrew) light. See also
Leora.

Lirit (Hebrew) poetic; lyrical,
musical.

Liron BG (Hebrew) my song.
Leron, Lerone, Lirone

Lisa GB (Hebrew) consecrated to
God. (English) a short form of
Elizabeth.
*Leeza, Liesa, Liisa, Lise, Lisenka,
Lisette, Liszka, Litsa, Lysa*

Lisbeth (English) a short form of
Elizabeth.
Lisbet

Lise GB (German) a form of Lisa.

Lisette GB (French) a form of
Lisa. (English) a familiar form of
Elise, Elizabeth.
*Liset, Liseta, Lisete, Liseth, Lisett,
Lisetta, Lisettina, Lizet, Lizette,
Lysette*

Lisha (Arabic) darkness before
midnight. (Hebrew) a short form
of Alisha, Elisha, Ilisha.
Lishe

Lissa (Greek) honey bee. A short
form of Elissa, Elizabeth, Melissa,
Millicent.
Lyssa

Lissette (French) a form of Lisa.
(English) a familiar form of Elise,
Elizabeth.
Lisset, Lissete, Lissett

Lissie (American) a familiar form
of Allison, Elise, Elizabeth.
Lissee, Lissey, Lissi, Lissy, Lissye

Lita (Latin) a familiar form of
names ending in "lita."
Leta, Litah, Litta

Litonya (Moquelumnan) darting
hummingbird.

Liv (Latin) a short form of Livia,
Olivia.

Livana (Hebrew) a form of
Levana.
Livna, Livnat

Livia (Hebrew) crown. A familiar
form of Olivia. (Latin) olive.
Levia, Liv, Livie, Livy, Livya, Livye

Liviya (Hebrew) brave lioness;
royal crown.
Leviya, Levya, Livya

Livona (Hebrew) a form of
Levona.

Liz (English) a short form of Elizabeth.

Liza (American) a short form of Elizabeth.
Leeza, Lizela, Lizka, Lyza

Lizabeta (Russian) a form of Elizabeth.
Lizabetah, Lizaveta, Lizonka

Lizabeth (English) a short form of Elizabeth.
Lisabet, Lisabeth, Lisabette, Lizabette

Lizbeth GB (English) a short form of Elizabeth.
Lizbet, Lizbett

Lizet, Lizette (French) forms of Lisette.
Lizet, Lizete, Lizeth, Lizett, Lizzet, Lizzeth, Lizzette

Lizina (Latvian) a familiar form of Elizabeth.

Lizzy (American) a familiar form of Elizabeth.
Lizzie, Lizy

Llanquipan (Mapuche) fallen branch; solitary lioness; retiring soul; lady who distances herself from the noise of the world.

Llanquiray (Mapuche) flowered pearl; fallen flower, fallen petals.

Llesenia (Spanish) gypsy female lead in a 1970s soap opera.

Lloyd BG (Welsh) gray haired; holy.

Lluvia (Spanish) rain.

Logan BG (Irish) meadow.
Logann, Loganne, Logen, Loghan, Logun, Logyn, Logynn

Loida, Loída (Greek) example of faith and piousness.

Lois (German) famous warrior.

Lola (Spanish) a familiar form of Carlotta, Dolores, Louise.
Lolah, Lolita

Lolita (Spanish) sorrowful. A familiar form of Lola.
Lita, Lulita

Lolly (English) sweet; candy. A familiar form of Laura.

Lolotea (Zuni) a form of Dorothy.

Lomasi (Native American) pretty flower.

Lona (Latin) lioness. (English) solitary. (German) a short form of Leona.
Loni, Lonna

London BG (English) fortress of the moon. Geography: the capital of the United Kingdom.
Landyn, Londen, Londun, Londyn

Loni (American) a form of Lona.
Lonee, Lonie, Lonni, Lonnie

Lora (Latin) crowned with laurel. (American) a form of Laura.
Lorah, Lorane, Lorann, Lorra, Lorrah, Lorrane

Lorda (Spanish) shrine of the Virgin Mary.

Lore (Basque) flower. (Latin) a short form of Flora.
Lor

Lorelei (German) alluring. Mythology: the siren of the Rhine River who lured sailors to their deaths. See also Lurleen.
Loralee, Loralei, Lorali, Loralie, Loralyn, Loreal, Lorelea, Loreley, Loreli, Lorilee, Lorilyn

Lorelle (American) a form of Laurel.

Loren GB (American) a form of Lauren.
Loreen, Lorena, Lorin, Lorne, Lorren, Lorrin, Lorryn, Loryn, Lorynn, Lorynne

Lorena GB (English) a form of Lauren.
Lorene, Lorenea, Lorenia, Lorenna, Lorina, Lorrina, Lorrine, Lurana

Lorenza (Latin) a form of Laura.
Laurencia, Laurentia, Laurentina

Loreta (Spanish) a form of Loreto.

Loreto (Italian) a form of Loretta.

Loretta (English) a familiar form of Laura.
Larretta, Lauretta, Laurette, Loretah, Lorette, Lorita, Lorretta, Lorrette

Lori GB (Latin) crowned with laurel. (French) a short form of Lorraine. (American) a familiar form of Laura.
Loree, Lorey, Loria, Lorianna, Lorianne, Lorie, Lorree, Lorri, Lorrie, Lory

Lorin (American) a form of Loren.
Lorine

Lorinda (Spanish) a form of Laura.

Loris BG (Latin) thong. (Dutch) clown. (Greek) a short form of Chloris.
Laurice, Laurys, Lorice

Lorna (Latin) crowned with laurel. Literature: probably coined by Richard Blackmore in his novel *Lorna Doone*.
Lorrna

Lorraine (Latin) sorrowful. (French) from Lorraine, a former province of France. See also Rayna.
Laraine, Lorain, Loraine, Lorayne, Lorein, Loreine, Lori, Lorine, Lorrain, Lorraina, Lorrayne, Lorreine

Lotte (German) a short form of Charlotte.
Lotie, Lotta, Lottchen, Lottey, Lottie, Lotty, Loty

Lotus (Greek) lotus.

Lou BG (American) a short form of Louise, Luella.
Lu

Louam (Ethiopian) sleep well.

Louisa (English) a familiar form of Louise. Literature: Louisa May Alcott was an American writer and reformer best known for her novel *Little Women*.
Aloisa, Eloisa, Heloisa, Lou, Louisian, Louisane, Louisina, Louiza, Lovisa, Luisa, Luiza, Lujza, Lujzika

Louise **GB** (German) famous warrior. See also Alison, Eloise, Heloise, Lois, Lola, Ludovica, Luella, Lulu.
Loise, Lou, Louisa, Louisette, Louisiane, Louisine, Lowise, Loyce, Loyise, Luise

Lourdes **GB** (French) from Lourdes, France. Religion: a place where the Virgin Mary was said to have appeared.

Louredes (Spanish) shrine of the Virgin Mary.

Love (English) love, kindness, charity.
Lovely, Lovewell, Lovey, Lovie, Lovy, Luv, Luvvy

Lovisa (German) a form of Louisa.

Lúa (Latin) moon.

Luann (Hebrew, German) graceful woman warrior. (Hawaiian) happy; relaxed. (American) a combination of Louise + Ann.
Louann, Louanne, Lu, Lua, Luan, Luane, Luanna, Luanne, Luanni, Luannie

Luanna (German) a form of Luann.
Lewanna, Louanna, Luana, Luwana

Lubov (Russian) love.
Luba, Lubna, Lubochka, Lyuba, Lyubov

Luca **BG** (Latin) a form of Lucy.

Lucas **BG** (German, Irish, Danish, Dutch) a form of Lucius (see Boys' Names).

Lucelia (Spanish) a combination of Luz and Celia.

Lucena (Spanish) bringer of light.

Lucerne (Latin) lamp; circle of light. Geography: the Lake of Lucerne is in Switzerland.
Lucerna, Lucero

Lucero (Latin) a form of Lucerne.

Lucetta (English) a familiar form of Lucy.
Lucette

Lucia (Italian, Spanish) a form of Lucy.
Lúcia, Lucía, Luciana, Lucianna

Lucie (French) a familiar form of Lucy.

Lucille (English) a familiar form of Lucy.
Lucila, Lucile, Lucilla

Lucinda (Latin) a form of Lucy. See also Cindy.

Lucine (Arabic) moon. (Basque) a form of Lucy.
Lucienne, Lucina, Lucyna, Lukene, Lusine, Luzine

Lucita (Spanish) a form of Lucy.
Lusita

Lucretia (Latin) rich; rewarded.
Lacrecia, Lucrece, Lucréce, Lucrecia, Lucreecia, Lucresha, Lucreshia, Lucrezia, Lucrisha, Lucrishia

Lucrezia (Italian) a form of Lucretia. History: Lucrezia Borgia was the Duchess of Ferrara and a patron of learning and the arts.

Lucy (Latin) light; bringer of light.
Luca, Luce, Lucetta, Luci, Lucia, Lucida, Lucie, Lucija, Lucika, Lucille, Lucinda, Lucine, Lucita, Luciya, Lucya, Luzca, Luzi

Ludmilla (Slavic) loved by the people. See also Mila.
Ludie, Ludka, Ludmila, Lyuba, Lyudmila

Ludovica (German) a form of Louise.
Ludovika, Ludwiga

Luella (English) elf. (German) a familiar form of Louise.
Loella, Lou, Louella, Ludella, Luelle, Lula, Lulu

Luis ⒷⒼ (Spanish) a form of Louis (see Boys' Names).

Luisa ⒼⒷ (Spanish) a form of Louisa.

Luisina (Teutonic) celebrated warrior; celebrated; very well known.

Luke ⒷⒼ (Latin) a form of Lucius (see Boys' Names).

Lulani ⒷⒼ (Polynesian) highest point of heaven.

Lulu (Arabic) pearl. (English) soothing, comforting. (Native American) hare. (German) a familiar form of Louise, Luella.
Loulou, Lula, Lulie

Luna (Latin) moon.
Lunetta, Lunette, Lunneta, Lunnete

Lupa (Latin) wolf.

Lupe (Latin) wolf. (Spanish) a short form of Guadalupe.
Lupi, Lupita, Luppi

Lupita (Latin) a form of Lupe.

Lurdes (Portuguese, Spanish) a form of Lourdes.

Lurleen, Lurlene (Scandinavian) war horn. (German) forms of Lorelei.
Lura, Lurette, Lurline

Lusa (Finnish) a form of Elizabeth.

Lusela (Moquelumnan) like a bear swinging its foot when licking it.

Lutgarda (German) she who protects her village.

Luvena (Latin, English) little; beloved.
Lovena, Lovina, Luvenia, Luvina

Luyu BG (Moquelumnan) like a pecking bird.

Luz GB (Spanish) light. Religion: Nuestra Señora de Luz-Our Lady of the Light-is another name for the Virgin Mary.
Luzi, Luzija

Luzia (Portuguese) a form of Lucia.

Lycoris (Greek) twilight.

Lyda (Greek) a short form of Lidia, Lydia.

Lydia GB (Greek) from Lydia, an ancient land in Asia. (Arabic) strife.
Lidia, Lidija, Lidiya, Lyda, Lydie, Lydië

Lyla (French) island. (English) a form of Lyle (see Boys' Names). (Arabic, Hindi, Persian) a form of Lila.
Lila, Lilah

Lynda (Spanish) pretty. (American) a form of Linda.
Lyndah, Lynde, Lyndi, Lynnda

Lyndell (English) a form of Lynelle.
Lyndall, Lyndel, Lyndella

Lyndi (Spanish) a familiar form of Lynda.
Lyndee, Lindie, Lyndy, Lynndie, Lynndy

Lyndsay GB (American) a form of Lindsay.
Lyndsaye

Lyndsey (English) linden tree island; camp near the stream. (American) a form of Lindsey.
Lyndsea, Lyndsee, Lyndsi, Lyndsie, Lyndsy, Lyndzee, Lyndzey, Lyndzi, Lyndzie, Lynndsie

Lynelle (English) pretty.
Linel, Linell, Linnell, Lyndell, Lynel, Lynell, Lynella, Lynnell

Lynette (Welsh) idol. (English) a form of Linette.
Lynett, Lynetta, Lynnet, Lynnette

Lynn, Lynne GB (English) waterfall; pool below a waterfall.
Lin, Lina, Linley, Linn, Lyn, Lynlee, Lynley, Lynna, Lynnae, Lynnea

Lynnell (English) a form of Lynelle.
Linnell, Lynnelle

Lynsey (American) a form of Lyndsey.
Lynnsey, Lynnzey, Lynsie, Lynsy, Lynzee, Lynzey, Lynzi, Lynzie, Lynzy

Lyra (Greek) lyre player.
Lyre, Lyric, Lyrica, Lyrie, Lyris

Lysandra (Greek) liberator.
Lisandra, Lysandre, Lytle

Lysanne (American) a combination of Lysandra + Anne.
Lisanne, Lizanne

M

M GB (American) an initial used as a first name.

Mab (Irish) joyous. (Welsh) baby. Literature: queen of the fairies.
Mabry

Mabel (Latin) lovable. A short form of Amabel.
Mabelle, Mable, Mabyn, Maible, Maybel, Maybeline, Maybelle, Maybull

Macarena (Spanish) she who carries the sword; name for the Virgin Mary.

Macaria (Greek) having a long life.

Macawi (Dakota) generous; motherly.

Macayla (American) a form of Michaela.
Macaela, Macaila, Macala, Macalah, Macaylah, Macayle, Macayli, Mackayla

Macey (Polish) a familiar form of Macia.
Macee

Machaela (Hebrew) a form of Michaela.
Machael, Machaelah, Machaelie, Machaila, Machala, Macheala

Machiko (Japanese) fortunate child.
Machi

Macia (Polish) a form of Miriam.
Macelia, Macey, Machia, Macie, Macy, Masha, Mashia

Macie, Macy GB (Polish) familiar forms of Macia.
Maci, Macye

Maciela (Latin) very slender, skeletal.

Mackenna (American) a form of Mackenzie.
Mackena, Makenna, Mckenna

Mackenzie ☀ GB (Irish) child of the wise leader. See also Kenzie.
Macenzie, Mackenna, Mackensi, Mackensie, Mackenze, Mackenzee, Mackenzey, Mackenzi, Mackenzia, Mackenzy, Mackenzye, Mackinsey, Mackynze, Makenzie, McKenzie, Mckinzie, Mekenzie, Mykenzie

Mackinsey (Irish) a form of Mackenzie.
Mackinsie, Mackinze, Mackinzee, Mackinzey, Mackinzi, Mackinzie

Macra (Greek) she who grows.

Mada (English) a short form of Madaline, Magdalen.
Madda, Mahda

Madaline (English) a form of Madeline.
Mada, Madailéin, Madaleen,

Madaleine, Madalene, Madalin, Madaline

Madalyn (Greek) a form of Madeline.
Madalyne, Madalynn, Madalynne

Maddie (English) a familiar form of Madeline.
Maddi, Maddy, Mady, Maidie, Maydey

Maddison **GB** (English) a form of Madison.
Maddisan, Maddisen, Maddisson, Maddisyn, Maddyson

Madelaine (French) a form of Madeline.
Madelane, Madelayne

Madeleine (French) a form of Madeline.
Madalaine, Madalayne, Madelaine, Madelein, Madeliene

Madelena (English) a form of Madeline.
Madalaina, Madalena, Madalina, Maddalena, Madelaina, Madeleina, Madelina, Madelyna

Madeline ☆ **GB** (Greek) high tower. See also Lena, Lina, Maud.
Madaline, Madalyn, Maddie, Madel, Madelaine, Madeleine, Madelena, Madelene, Madelia, Madella, Madelle, Madelon, Madelyn, Madge, Madilyn, Madlen, Madlin, Madline, Madlyn, Madolyn, Maida

Madelón (Spanish) a form of Magdalen.

Madelyn (Greek) a form of Madeline.
Madelyne, Madelynn, Madelynne, Madilyn, Madlyn, Madolyn

Madena, Madia, Madina (Greek) from the high tower.

Madge (Greek) a familiar form of Madeline, Margaret.
Madgi, Madgie, Mady

Madilyn (Greek) a form of Madeline.
Madilen, Madiline, Madilyne, Madilynn

Madisen **GB** (English) a form of Madison.
Madisan, Madisin, Madissen, Madisun

Madison ☆ **GB** (English) good; child of Maud.
Maddison, Madisen, Madisson, Madisyn, Madyson, Mattison

Madisyn (English) a form of Madison.
Madissyn, Madisynn, Madisynne

Madolyn (Greek) a form of Madeline.
Madoline, Madolyne, Madolynn, Madolynne

Madonna (Latin) my lady.
Madona

Madrona (Spanish) mother.
Madre, Madrena

Madyson (English) a form of
Madison.
Madysen, Madysun

Mae (English) a form of May.
History: Mae Jemison was the first
African American woman in
space.
*Maelea, Maeleah, Maelen,
Maelle, Maeona*

Maegan (Irish) a form of Megan.
Maegen, Maeghan, Maegin

Maeko (Japanese) honest child.
Mae, Maemi

Maeve (Irish) joyous. Mythology:
a legendary Celtic queen. See also
Mavis.
Maevi, Maevy, Maive, Mayve

Mafalda (Spanish) a form of
Matilde.

Magali, Magaly (Hebrew) from
the high tower.
Magalie, Magally

Magalí (French) a form of
Magali.

Magan, Magen (Greek) forms
of Megan.
Maggen, Maggin

Magda (Czech, Polish, Russian) a
form of Magdalen.
Mahda, Makda

Magdalen (Greek) high tower.
Bible: Magdala was the home of
Saint Mary Magdalen. See also
Madeline, Malena, Marlene.
Mada, Magda, Magdala,
*Magdaleen, Magdalena,
Magdalene, Magdaline,
Magdalyn, Magdalynn,
Magdelane, Magdelene,
Magdeline, Magdelyn, Magdlen,
Magdolna, Maggie, Magola,
Maighdlin, Mala, Malaine*

Magdalena (Greek) a form of
Magdalen.
*Magdalina, Magdelana,
Magdelena, Magdelina*

Magena (Native American)
coming moon.

Maggie (Greek) pearl. (English)
a familiar form of Magdalen,
Margaret.
*Mag, Magge, Maggee, Maggi,
Maggia, Maggie, Maggiemae,
Maggy, Magi, Magie, Mags*

Maggy, Meggy (English) forms
of Maggie.
Maggey, Magy

Magnolia (Latin) flowering tree.
See also Nollie.
Nola

Mahal (Filipino) love.

Mahala (Arabic) fat, marrow;
tender. (Native American)
powerful woman.
*Mahalah, Mahalar, Mahalla,
Mahela, Mahila, Mahlah,
Mahlaha, Mehala, Mehalah*

Mahalia (American) a form of
Mahala.
*Mahaley, Mahaliah, Mahalie,
Mahayla, Mahaylah, Mahaylia,*

Mahelea, Maheleah, Mahelia,
Mahilia, Mehalia

Maharene (Ethiopian) forgive us.

Mahesa (Hindi) great lord.
Religion: a name for the Hindu
god Shiva.
Maheesa, Mahisa

Mahila (Sanskrit) woman.

Mahina (Hawaiian) moon glow.

Mahira (Hebrew) energetic.
Mahri

Mahogony (Spanish) rich;
strong.
Mahagony, Mahoganey,
Mahogani, Mahoganie,
Mahogany, Mahogney, Mahogny,
Mohogany, Mohogony

Mai (Japanese) brightness.
(Vietnamese) flower. (Navajo)
coyote.

Maia (Greek) mother; nurse.
(English) kinswoman; maiden.
Mythology: the loveliest of the
Pleiades, the seven daughters of
Atlas, and the mother of Hermes.
See also Maya.
Maiah, Maie, Maiya

Maiara (Tupi) wise.

Maida (English) maiden. (Greek)
a short form of Madeline.
Maidel, Mayda, Maydena

Maija (Finnish) a form of Mary.
Maiji, Maikki

Maika (Hebrew) a familiar form
of Michaela.
Maikala, Maikka, Maiko

Maira **GB** (Irish) a form of Mary.
Maairah, Mair, Mairi, Mairim,
Mairin, Mairona, Mairwen

Maire (Irish) a form of Mary.

Maisie (Scottish) familiar forms
of Margaret.
Maisa, Maise, Maisey, Maisi,
Maisy, Maizie, Maycee, Maysie,
Mayzie, Mazey, Mazie, Mazy,
Mazzy, Mysie, Myzie

Maita (Spanish) a form of
Martha.
Maitia

Maite (Spanish) a form of Maita.

Maitea (Spanish) dearly loved.

Maiten (Spanish) a form of
Malen.

Maitena (Spanish) a form of
Maite.

Maitlyn (American) a
combination of Maita + Lynn.
Maitlan, Maitland, Maitlynn,
Mattilyn

Maiya (Greek) a form of Maia.
Maiyah

Maja (Arabic) a short form of
Majidah.
Majal, Majalisa, Majalyn,
Majalynn

Majesta (Latin) majesty.

Majidah (Arabic) splendid.
Maja, Majida

Makaela, Makaila (American)
forms of Michaela.
*Makaelah, Makaelee, Makaella,
Makaely, Makail, Makailah,
Makailee, Makailla, Makaillah,
Makealah, Makell*

Makala (Hawaiian) myrtle.
(Hebrew) a form of Michaela.
*Makalae, Makalah, Makalai,
Makalea, Makalee, Makaleh,
Makaleigh, Makaley, Makalia,
Makalie, Makalya, Makela,
Makelah, Makell, Makella*

Makana (Hawaiian) gift, present.

Makani 🅱🅶 (Hawaiian) wind.

Makara (Hindi) Astrology:
another name for the zodiac sign
Capricorn.

Makayla ☀ (American) a form
of Michaela.
*Macayla, Makaylah, Makaylee,
Makayleigh, Makayli, Makaylia,
Makaylla, Makell, Makyla,
Makylah, Mckayla, Mekayla,
Mikayla*

Makell 🅶🅱 (American) a short
form of Makaela, Makala,
Makayla.
Makele, Makelle, Mckell, Mekel

Makenna 🅶🅱 (American) a form
of Mackenna.
Makena, Makennah, Mikenna

Makenzie 🅶🅱 (Irish) a form of
Mackenzie.
*Makense, Makensey, Makensie,
Makenze, Makenzee, Makenzey,
Makenzi, Makenzy, Makenzye,
Makinzey, Makynzey, Mekenzie,
Mykenzie*

Mala (Greek) a short form of
Magdalen.
Malana, Malee, Mali

Malana (Hawaiian) bouyant,
light.

Malaya (Filipino) free.
*Malayaa, Malayah, Malayna,
Malea, Maleah*

Malen (Swedish) a form of
Malena.

Malena (Swedish) a familiar
form of Magdalen.
*Malenna, Malin, Malina, Maline,
Malini, Malinna*

Malha (Hebrew) queen.
*Maliah, Malkah, Malkia, Malkiah,
Malkie, Malkiya, Malkiyah,
Miliah*

Mali (Tai) jasmine flower.
(Tongan) sweet. (Hungarian) a
short form of Malika.
Malea, Malee, Maley

Malia (Hawaiian, Zuni) a form of
Mary. (Spanish) a form of Maria.
*Malea, Maleah, Maleeya,
Maleeyah, Maleia, Maliah,
Maliasha, Malie, Maliea, Maliya,
Maliyah, Malli, Mally*

Malik BG (Hungarian, Arabic) a form of Malika.

Malika (Hungarian) industrious. (Arabic) queen.
Malak, Maleeka, Maleka, Mali, Maliaka, Malik, Malikah, Malikee, Maliki, Malikia, Malky

Malina (Hebrew) tower. (Native American) soothing. (Russian) raspberry.
Malin, Maline, Malina, Malinna, Mallie

Malinda (Greek) a form of Melinda.
Malinde, Malinna, Malynda

Malini (Hindi) gardener.
Maliny

Malissa (Greek) a form of Melissa.
Malisa, Malisah, Malyssa

Mallalai (Pashto) beautiful.

Malley (American) a familiar form of Mallory.
Mallee, Malli, Mallie, Mally, Maly

Mallorie (French) a form of Mallory.
Malerie, Mallari, Mallerie, Malloreigh, Mallori

Mallory GB (German) army counselor. (French) unlucky.
Maliri, Mallary, Mallauri, Mallery, Malley, Malloree, Mallorey, Mallorie, Malorie, Malory,
Malorym, Malree, Malrie, Mellory

Malorie, Malory (German) forms of Mallory.
Malarie, Maloree, Malori, Melorie, Melory

Malva (English) a form of Melba.
Malvi, Malvy

Malvina (Scottish) a form of Melvina. Literature: a name created by the eighteenth-century Romantic poet James Macpherson.
Malvane, Malvi

Mamie (American) a familiar form of Margaret.
Mame, Mamee, Mami, Mammie, Mamy, Mamye

Mamo BG (Hawaiian) saffron flower; yellow bird.

Mana (Hawaiian) psychic; sensitive.
Manal, Manali, Manna, Mannah

Manar (Arabic) guiding light.
Manayra

Manda (Spanish) woman warrior. (Latin) a short form of Amanda.
Mandy

Mandara (Hindi) calm.

Mandeep BG (Punjabi) enlightened.

Mandisa (Xhosa) sweet.

Mandy GB (Latin) lovable. A familiar form of Amanda, Manda, Melinda.
Mandee, Mandi, Mandie

Manela (Catalonian) a form of Manuela.

Manette (French) a form of Mary.

Mangena (Hebrew) song, melody.
Mangina

Mani (Chinese) a mantra repeated in Tibetan Buddhist prayer to impart understanding.
Manee

Manila (Latin) woman with small hands.

Manjot BG (Indian) light of the mind.

Manka (Polish, Russian) a form of Mary.

Manoela (Hebrew) God is with us.

Manola (Spanish) a form of Manuela.

Manon (French) a familiar form of Marie.
Mannon

Manón (Spanish) a form of Manon.

Manpreet GB (Punjabi) mind full of love.
Manprit

Manque (Mapuche) condor; the main woman; woman of unyielding character.

Mansi (Hopi) plucked flower.
Mancey, Manci, Mancie, Mansey, Mansie, Mansy

Manuela (Spanish) a form of Emmanuelle.
Manuala, Manuelita, Manuella, Manuelle

Manya (Russian) a form of Mary.

Mar (Spanish) sea.

Mara (Hebrew) melody. (Greek) a short form of Amara. (Slavic) a form of Mary.
Mahra, Marae, Marah, Maralina, Maraline, Marra

Marabel (English) a form of Mirabel.
Marabella, Marabelle

Maranda (Latin) a form of Miranda.

Maraya (Hebrew) a form of Mariah.
Mareya

Marcel BG (French) a form of Marcellus (see Boys' Names).

Marcela (Latin) a form of Marcella.
Marcele, Marcelen, Marcelia, Marcelina, Marceline, Maricela

Marcelen (English) a form of Marcella.
Marcelen, Marcelin, Marcelina,

Marceline, Marcellin, Marcellina,
Marcelline, Marcelyn, Marcilen

Marceliana (Latin) a form of
Marcela.

Marcella (Latin) martial, warlike.
Mythology: Mars was the god of
war.
Mairsil, Marca, Marce, Marceil,
Marcela, Marcelen, Marcell,
Marcelle, Marcello, Marcena,
Marchella, Marchelle, Marci,
Marcia, Marcie, Marciella,
Marcile, Marcilla, Marcille,
Marella, Marsella, Marselle,
Marsiella

Marcena (Latin) a form of
Marcella, Marcia.
Maracena, Marceen, Marcene,
Marcenia, Marceyne, Marcina

Marci, Marcie (English) familiar
forms of Marcella, Marcia.
Marca, Marcee, Marcita, Marcy,
Marsi, Marsie

Marcia (Latin) martial, warlike.
See also Marquita.
Marcena, Marchia, Marci,
Marciale, Marcie, Marcsa,
Marsha, Martia

Márcia (Portuguese) a form of
Marcia.

Marciann (American) a
combination of Marci + Ann.
Marciane, Marcianna,
Marcianne, Marcyane,
Marcyanna, Marcyanne

Marcilynn (American) a
combination of Marci + Lynn.
Marcilen, Marcilin, Marciline,
Marcilyn, Marcilyne, Marcilynne,
Marcylen, Marcylin, Marcyline,
Marcylyn, Marcylyne, Marcylynn,
Marcylynne

Marco BG (Italian) a form of
Marcus.

Marcus BG (Latin) martial,
warlike.

Marcy (English) a form of Marci.
Marsey, Marsy

Mardi (French) born on Tuesday.
(Aramaic) a familiar form of
Martha.

Mare (Irish) a form of Mary.
Mair, Maire

Marelda (German) renowned
warrior.
Marella, Marilda

Maren GB (Latin) sea. (Aramaic)
a form of Mary. See also Marina.
Marin, Marine, Marinn, Miren

Maresa, Maressa (Latin) forms
of Marisa.
Maresha, Meresa

Maretta (English) a familiar form
of Margaret.
Maret, Marette

Margaret 🆖 (Greek) pearl.
History: Margaret Hilda Thatcher
served as British prime minister.
See also Gita, Greta, Gretchen,
Marjorie, Markita, Meg, Megan,
Peggy, Reet, Rita.
*Madge, Maergrethe, Maggie,
Maisie, Mamie, Maretta, Marga,
Margalo, Marganit, Margara,
Maretha, Margarett, Margarette,
Margarida, Margarit, Margarita,
Margaro, Margaux, Marge,
Margeret, Margeretta,
Margerette, Margery, Margetta,
Margiad, Margie, Margisia,
Margit, Margo, Margot, Margret,
Marguerite, Meta*

Margarit (Greek) a form of
Margaret.
*Margalide, Margalit, Margalith,
Margarid, Margaritt, Margerit*

Margarita (Italian, Spanish) a
form of Margaret.
*Margareta, Margaretta,
Margarida, Margaritis,
Margaritta, Margeretta,
Margharita, Margherita,
Margrieta, Margrita, Marguarita,
Marguerita, Margurita*

Margaux (French) a form of
Margaret.
Margeaux

Marge (English) a short form of
Margaret, Marjorie.
Margie

Margery (English) a form of
Margaret.
Margerie, Margorie

Margie (English) a familiar form
of Marge, Margaret.
Margey, Margi, Margy

Margit (Hungarian) a form of
Margaret.
Marget, Margette, Margita

Margo, Margot (French) forms
of Margaret.
Mago, Margaro

Margret (German) a form of
Margaret.
*Margreta, Margrete, Margreth,
Margrett, Margretta, Margrette,
Margrieta, Margrita*

Marguerite (French) a form of
Margaret.
*Margarete, Margaretha,
Margarethe, Margarite,
Margerite, Marguaretta,
Marguarette, Marguarite,
Marguerette, Margurite*

Mari (Japanese) ball. (Spanish) a
form of Mary.

Maria ☆ 🆖 (Hebrew) bitter;
sea of bitterness. (Italian,
Spanish) a form of Mary.
*Maie, Malia, Marea, Mareah,
Mariabella, Mariae, Mariesa,
Mariessa, Mariha, Marija,
Mariya, Mariyah, Marja, Marya*

María (Hebrew) a form of Maria.

María de la Concepción (Spanish) Mary of the conception.

María de la Paz (Spanish) Mary of peace.

María de las Nieves (Spanish) Mary of the snows.

María de las Victorias (Spanish) victorious Mary.

María de los Angeles (Spanish) angelic Mary.

María de los Milagros (Spanish) miraculous Mary.

María del Mar (Spanish) Mary of the sea.

María Inmaculada (Spanish) immaculate Mary.

María José (Latin) name composed of María and José.

María Noel (Latin) name composed of María and Noel.

Mariah GB (Hebrew) a form of Mary. See also Moriah.
Maraia, Maraya, Mariyah, Marriah, Meriah

Mariam GB (Hebrew) a form of Miriam.
Mariama, Mariame, Mariem, Meryam

Marian GB (English) a form of Maryann.
Mariana, Mariane, Mariann, Marianne, Mariene, Marion, Marrian, Marriann

Marián (Spanish) a short form of Mariana.

Mariana, Marianna (Spanish) forms of Marian.
Marriana, Marrianna, Maryana, Maryanna

Mariane, Marianne GB (English) forms of Marian.
Marrianne, Maryanne

Marianela (Spanish) a combination of Mariana and Estela.

Mariángeles (Spanish) a combination of María and Ángeles.

Maribel (French) beautiful. (English) a combination of Maria + Bell.
Marabel, Marbelle, Mariabella, Maribella, Maribelle, Maridel, Marybel, Marybella, Marybelle

Marice (Italian) a form of Mary. See also Maris.
Marica, Marise, Marisse

Maricela (Latin) a form of Marcella.
Maricel, Mariceli, Maricelia, Maricella, Maricely

Maricruz (Spanish) a combination of María and Cruz.

Maridel (English) a form of Maribel.

Marie GB (French) a form of Mary.
Maree, Marietta, Marrie

Mariel, Marielle (German, Dutch) forms of Mary.
Marial, Marieke, Marielana, Mariele, Marieli, Marielie, Marieline, Mariell, Mariellen, Marielsie, Mariely, Marielys

Mariela, Mariella (German, Dutch) forms of Mary.

Marieta (Hebrew) a form of María.

Marietta (Italian) a familiar form of Marie.
Maretta, Marette, Mariet, Mariette, Marrietta

Marieve (American) a combination of Mary + Eve.

Marigold (English) Mary's gold. Botany: a plant with yellow or orange flowers.
Marygold

Marika (Dutch, Slavic) a form of Mary.
Marica, Marieke, Marija, Marijke, Marikah, Marike, Marikia, Marikka, Mariska, Mariske, Marrika, Maryk, Maryka, Merica, Merika

Mariko (Japanese) circle.

Marilee (American) a combination of Mary + Lee.
Marili, Marilie, Marily, Marrilee, Marylea, Marylee, Merrilee, Merrili, Merrily

Marilena (Spanish) a combination of María and Elena.

Marilina (Latin) a combination of María and Elina.

Marilla (Hebrew, German) a form of Mary.
Marella, Marelle

Marilou (American) a form of Marylou.
Marilu, Mariluz

Marilú (Spanish) a combination of María and Luz.

Marilyn (Hebrew) Mary's line of descendants. See also Merilyn.
Maralin, Maralyn, Maralyne, Maralynn, Maralynne, Marelyn, Marilin, Marillyn, Marilyne, Marilynn, Marilynne, Marlyn, Marolyn, Marralynn, Marrilin, Marrilyn, Marrilynn, Marrilynne, Marylin, Marylinn, Marylyn, Marylyne, Marylynn, Marylynne

Marina 🇬🇧 (Latin) sea. See also Maren.
Mareena, Marena, Marenka, Marinae, Marinah, Marinda, Marindi, Marinka, Marinna, Marrina, Maryna, Merina, Mirena

Mariña (Latin) a form of Marina.

Marinés (Spanish) a combination of María and Inés.

Marini (Swahili) healthy; pretty.

Mario 🇧🇬 (Italian) a form of Marino (see Boys' Names).

Mariola (Italian) a form of María.

Marion **GB** (French) a form of Mary.
Marrian, Marrion, Maryon, Maryonn

Marión (Spanish) a form of María.

Maris (Latin) sea. (Greek) a short form of Amaris, Damaris. See also Marice.
Maries, Marise, Marris, Marys, Maryse, Meris

Marisa (Latin) sea.
Maresa, Mariesa, Mariessa, Marisela, Marissa, Marita, Mariza, Marrisa, Marrissa, Marysa, Maryse, Maryssa, Merisa

Marisabel (Spanish) a combination of María and Isabel.

Marisabela (Spanish) a form of Marisabel.

Marisel (Spanish) a combination of María and Isabel.

Marisela **GB** (Latin) a form of Marisa.
Mariseli, Marisella, Marishelle, Marissela

Marisha (Russian) a familiar form of Mary.
Mareshah, Marishenka, Marishka, Mariska

Marisol (Spanish) sunny sea.
Marise, Marizol, Marysol

Marissa ☆ **GB** (Latin) a form of Maris, Marisa.
Maressa, Marisa, Marisha,

Marissah, Marisse, Marizza, Marrissa, Marrissia, Maryssa, Merissa, Morissa

Marit (Aramaic) lady.
Marita, Marite

Marita (Spanish) a form of Marisa. (Aramaic) a form of Marit.
Marité, Maritha

Maritza (Arabic) blessed.
Maritsa, Maritssa

Mariyan (Arabic) purity.
Mariya, Mariyah, Mariyana, Mariyanna

Marja (Finnish) a form of Mary.
Marjae, Marjatta, Marjie

Marjan (Persian) coral. (Polish) a form of Mary.
Marjaneh, Marjanna

Marjie (Scottish) a familiar form of Marjorie.
Marje, Marjey, Marji, Marjy

Marjolaine **GB** (French) marjoram.

Marjorie (Greek) a familiar form of Margaret. (Scottish) a form of Mary.
Majorie, Marge, Margeree, Margerey, Margerie, Margery, Margorie, Margory, Marjarie, Marjary, Marjerie, Marjery, Marjie, Marjorey, Marjori, Marjory

Mark **BG** (Latin) a form of Marcus.

Markayla (American) a combination or Mary + Kayla.
Marka, Markaiah, Markaya, Markayel, Markeela, Markel

Markeisha (English) a combination of Mary + Keisha.
Markasha, Markeisa, Markeisia, Markesha, Markeshia, Markesia, Markiesha, Markisha, Markishia, Marquesha

Markell 🅱🅶 (Latin) a form of Mark.

Markita (Czech) a form of Margaret.
Marka, Markeah, Markeda, Markee, Markeeta, Marketa, Marketta, Marki, Markia, Markie, Markieta, Markita, Markitha, Markketta, Merkate

Marla (English) a short form of Marlena, Marlene.
Marlah, Marlea, Marleah

Marlana (English) a form of Marlena.
Marlaena, Marlaina, Marlainna, Marlania, Marlanna, Marlayna, Marleana

Marlee (English) a form of Marlene.
Marlea, Marleah, Marleigh

Marlen 🅶🅱 (Greek, Slavic) a form of Marlene.

Marlena (German) a form of Marlene.
Marla, Marlaina, Marlana,

Marlanna, Marleena, Marlina, Marlinda, Marlyna, Marna

Marlene (Greek) high tower. (Slavic) a form of Magdalen.
Marla, Marlaine, Marlane, Marlayne, Marlee, Marleen, Marleene, Marlen, Marlena, Marlenne, Marley, Marlin, Marline, Marlyne

Marley 🅶🅱 (English) a familiar form of Marlene.
Marlee, Marli, Marlie, Marly

Marlis (English) a combination of Maria + Lisa.
Marles, Marlisa, Marlise, Marlys, Marlyse, Marlyssa

Marlo (English) a form of Mary.
Marlow, Marlowe

Marlon 🅱🅶 (English) a form of Marlo.

Marlyn 🅶🅱 (Hebrew) a short form of Marilyn. (Greek, Slavic) a form of Marlene.
Marlynn, Marlynne

Marmara (Greek) sparkling, shining.
Marmee

Marni (Hebrew) a form of Marnie.
Marnia, Marnique

Marnie (Hebrew) a short form of Marnina.
Marna, Marnay, Marne, Marnee, Marney, Marni, Marnisha, Marnja, Marny, Marnya, Marnye

Marnina (Hebrew) rejoice.

Maroula (Greek) a form of Mary.

Marquesa (Spanish) she who works with a hammer.

Marquez BG (Portuguese) a form of Marques (see Boys' Names).

Marquilla (Spanish) bitter.

Marquis BG (French) a form of Marquise.

Marquise BG (French) noblewoman.
Markese, Marquees, Marquese, Marquice, Marquies, Marquiese, Marquis, Marquisa, Marquisee, Marquisha, Marquisse, Marquiste

Marquisha (American) a form of Marquise.
Marquiesha, Marquisia

Marquita (Spanish) a form of Marcia.
Marquatte, Marqueda, Marquedia, Marquee, Marqueita, Marquet, Marqueta, Marquetta, Marquette, Marquia, Marquida, Marquietta, Marquitra, Marquitia, Marquitta

Marrim (Chinese) tribal name in Manpur state.

Marsala (Italian) from Marseilles, France.
Marsali, Marseilles

Marsha (English) a form of Marcia.
Marcha, Marshae, Marshay, Marshel, Marshele, Marshell, Marshia, Marshiela

Marshall BG (French) caretaker of the horses; military title.

Marta (English) a short form of Martha, Martina.
Martá, Martä, Marte, Martia, Marttaha, Merta

Martha (Aramaic) lady; sorrowful. Bible: a friend of Jesus. See also Mardi.
Maita, Marta, Martaha, Marth, Marthan, Marthe, Marthy, Marti, Marticka, Martita, Mattie, Matty, Martus, Martuska, Masia

Marti GB (English) a familiar form of Martha, Martina.
Martie, Marty

Martin BG (Latin, French) a form of Martinus (see Boys' Names)

Martina GB (Latin) martial, warlike. See also Tina.
Marta, Martel, Martella, Martelle, Martene, Marthena, Marthina, Marthine, Marti, Martine, Martinia, Martino, Martisha, Martosia, Martoya, Martricia, Martrina, Martyna, Martyne, Martynne

Martine GB (Latin) a form of Martina.

Martiniana (Latin) she who was consecrated to the god Mars; born in May.

Martirio (Spanish) martyrdom.

Martiza (Arabic) blessed.

Maru (Japanese) round.

Maruca (Spanish) a form of Mary.
Maruja, Maruska

Marvella (French) marvelous.
*Marva, Marvel, Marvela,
Marvele, Marvelle, Marvely,
Marvetta, Marvette, Marvia,
Marvina*

Mary ★ GB (Hebrew) bitter; sea
of bitterness. Bible: the mother of
Jesus. See also Maija, Malia,
Maren, Mariah, Marjorie, Maura,
Maureen, Miriam, Mitzi, Moira,
Mollie, Muriel.
*Maira, Maire, Manette, Manka,
Manon, Manya, Mara, Mare,
Maree, Maren, Marella, Marelle,
Mari, Maria, Maricara, Marice,
Marie, Mariel, Mariela, Marika,
Marilla, Marilyn, Marion,
Mariquilla, Mariquita, Marisha,
Marja, Marjan, Marlo, Maroula,
Maruca, Marye, Maryla, Marynia,
Masha, Mavra, Mendi, Mérane,
Meridel, Mhairie, Mirja, Molara,
Morag, Moya*

Marya (Arabic) purity; bright
whiteness.
Maryah

Maryam (Hebrew) a form of
Miriam.
Maryama

Maryann, Maryanne (English)
combinations of Mary + Ann.
*Marian, Marryann, Maryan,
Meryem*

Marybeth (American) a combination of Mary + Beth.
Maribeth, Maribette

Maryellen (American) a combination of Mary + Ellen.
Mariellen

Maryjane (American) a combination of Mary + Jane.

Maryjo (American) a combination of Mary + Jo.
Marijo, Maryjoe

Marykate (American) a combination of Mary + Kate.
Mary-Kate

Marylou (American) a combination of Mary + Lou.
Marilou, Marylu

Maryssa (Latin) a form of Marissa.
Maryse, Marysia

Masago (Japanese) sands of time.

Masani (Luganda) gap toothed.

Masha (Russian) a form of Mary.
Mashka, Mashenka

Mashika (Swahili) born during
the rainy season.
Masika

Mason BG (French) stone
worker.

Massimo BG (Italian) greatest.

Matana (Hebrew) gift.
Matat

Mathena (Hebrew) gift of God.

Mathew BG (Hebrew) a form of Matthew.

Mathieu BG (French) a form of Matthew.

Mathilde (German) a form of Matilda.
Mathilda

Matilda (German) powerful battler. See also Maud, Tilda, Tillie.
Máda, Mahaut, Maitilde, Malkin, Mat, Matelda, Mathilde, , Mattie, Matty, Matusha, Matylda

Matilde (German) a form of Matilda.

Matrika (Hindi) mother. Religion: a name for the Hindu goddess Shakti in the form of the letters of the alphabet.
Matrica

Matsuko (Japanese) pine tree.

Mattea (Hebrew) gift of God.
Matea, Mathea, Mathia, Matia, Matte, Matthea, Matthia, Mattia, Matya

Matthew BG (Hebrew) gift of God.

Mattie, Matty (English) familiar forms of Martha, Matilda.
Matte, Mattey, Matti, Mattye

Matusha (Spanish) a form of Matilda.
Matuja, Matuxa

Maud, Maude (English) short forms of Madeline, Matilda. See also Madison.
Maudie, Maudine, Maudlin

Maura (Irish) dark. A form of Mary, Maureen. See also Moira.
Maurah, Maure, Maurette, Mauricette, Maurita

Maureen (French) dark. (Irish) a form of Mary.
Maura, Maurene, Maurine, Mo, Moreen, Morena, Morene, Morine, Morreen, Moureen

Maurelle (French) dark; elfin.
Mauriel, Mauriell, Maurielle

Mauricia (Spanish) a form of Mauro.

Mauricio BG (Spanish) a form of Maurice (see Boys' Names).

Maurise (French) dark skinned; moor; marshland.
Maurisa, Maurissa, Maurita, Maurizia

Mauro (Latin) a short form of Maurice (see Boys' Names).

Mausi (Native American) plucked flower.

Mauve (French) violet colored.

Maverick BG (American) independent.

Mavis (French) thrush, songbird. See also Maeve.
Mavies, Mavin, Mavine, Mavon, Mavra

Max ⓑⓖ (Latin) a short form of Maxine.

Maxie (English) a familiar form of Maxine.
Maxi, Maxy

Máxima (Latin) great one.

Maxime ⓑⓖ (Latin) a form of Maxine.

Maximiana (Spanish) a form of Máxima.

Maximiliana (Latin) eldest of all.

Maxine ⓖⓑ (Latin) greatest.
Max, Maxa, Maxeen, Maxena, Maxene, Maxie, Maxima, Maxime, Maximiliane, Maxina, Maxna, Maxyne

Maxwell ⓑⓖ (English) great spring.

May (Latin) great. (Arabic) discerning. (English) flower; month of May. See also Mae, Maia.
Maj, Mayberry, Maybeth, Mayday, Maydee, Maydena, Maye, Mayela, Mayella, Mayetta, Mayrene

Maya ☆ (Hindi) God's creative power. (Greek) mother; grandmother. (Latin) great. A form of Maia.
Mayam, Mya

Maybeline (Latin) a familiar form of Mabel.

Maygan, Maygen (Irish) forms of Megan.
Mayghan, Maygon

Maylyn (American) a combination of May + Lynn.
Mayelene, Mayleen, Maylen, Maylene, Maylin, Maylon, Maylynn, Maylynne

Mayoree (Tai) beautiful.
Mayra, Mayree, Mayariya

Mayra (Tai) a form of Mayoree.

Maysa (Arabic) walks with a proud stride.

Maysun (Arabic) beautiful.

Mayte (Spanish) a combination of María and Teresa.

Mazel (Hebrew) lucky.
Mazal, Mazala, Mazella

Mc Kenna ⓖⓑ (American) a form of Mackenna.

Mc Kenzie ⓖⓑ (Irish) a form of Mackenzie.

Mckay ⓑⓖ (Scottish) child of Kay.

Mckayla ⓖⓑ (American) a form of Makayla.
Mckaela, Mckaila, Mckala, Mckaylah, Mckayle, Mckaylee, Mckayleh, Mckayleigh, Mckayli, Mckaylia, Mckaylie

Mckell ⓖⓑ (American) a form of Makell.
Mckelle

Mckenna **GB** (American) a form of Mackenna.
Mckena, Mckennah, Mckinna, Mckinnah

Mckenzie **GB** (Scottish) a form of Mackenzie.
Mckennzie, Mckensee, Mckensey, McKensi, Mckensi, Mckensie, Mckensy, Mckenze, Mckenzee, Mckenzey, Mckenzi, Mckenzy, Mckenzye, Mekensie, Mekenzi, Mekenzie

Mckinley **BG** (Irish) daughter of the learned ruler.
Mckinlee, Mckinleigh, Mckinlie, Mckinnley

Mckinzie (American) a form of Mackenzie.
Mckinsey, Mckinze, Mckinzea, Mckinzee, Mckinzi, Mckinzy, Mckynze, Mckynzie

Mead, Meade **BG** (Greek) honey wine.

Meagan (Irish) a form of Megan.
Maegan, Meagain, Meagann, Meagen, Meagin, Meagnah, Meagon

Meaghan **GB** (Welsh) a form of Megan.
Maeghan, Meaghann, Meaghen, Meahgan

Meara (Irish) mirthful.

Mecha (Latin) a form of Mercedes.

Meda (Native American) prophet; priestess.

Medea (Greek) ruling. (Latin) middle. Mythology: a sorceress who helped Jason get the Golden Fleece.
Medeia

Medina (Arabic) History: the site of Muhammed's tomb.
Medinah

Medora (Greek) mother's gift. Literature: a character in Lord Byron's poem *The Corsair*.

Meena (Hindi) blue semiprecious stone; bird. (Greek, German, Dutch) a form of Mena.

Meg (English) a short form of Margaret, Megan.

Megan ✵ **GB** (Greek) pearl; great. (Irish) a form of Margaret.
Maegan, Magan, Magen, Meagan, Meaghan, Magen, Maygan, Maygen, Meg, Megane, Megann, Megean, Megen, Meggan, Meggen, Meggie, Meghan, Megyn, Meygan

Megane (Irish) a form of Megan.
Magana, Meganna, Meganne

Megara (Greek) first. Mythology: Heracles's first wife.

Meggie (English) a familiar form of Margaret, Megan.
Meggi, Meggy

Meghan GB (Welsh) a form of Megan.
Meeghan, Meehan, Megha, Meghana, Meghane, Meghann, Meghanne, Meghean, Meghen, Mehgan, Mehgen

Mehadi (Hindi) flower.

Mehira (Hebrew) speedy; energetic.
Mahira

Mehitabel (Hebrew) benefited by trusting God.
Mehetabel, Mehitabelle, Hetty, Hitty

Mehri (Persian) kind; lovable; sunny.

Mei (Hawaiian) great. (Chinese) a short form of Meiying.
Meiko

Meira (Hebrew) light.
Meera

Meit (Burmese) affectionate.

Meiying (Chinese) beautiful flower.
Mei

Meka GB (Hebrew) a familiar form of Michaela.

Mekayla (American) a form of Michaela.
Mekaela, Mekaila, Mekayela, Mekaylia

Mel BG (Portuguese, Spanish) sweet as honey.

Mela (Hindi) religious service. (Polish) a form of Melanie.

Melana (Russian) a form of Melanie.
Melanna, Melashka, Melenka, Milana

Melanie ✩ GB (Greek) dark skinned.
Malania, Malanie, Meila, Meilani, Meilin, Melaine, Melainie, Melana, Melane, Melanee, Melaney, Melani, Melania, Mélanie, Melanka, Melanney, Melannie, Melany, Melanya, Melasya, Melayne, Melenia, Mella, Mellanie, Melonie, Melya, Milena, Milya

Melantha (Greek) dark flower.

Melba (Greek) soft; slender. (Latin) mallow flower.
Malva, Melva

Mele (Hawaiian) song; poem.

Melesse (Ethiopian) eternal.
Mellesse

Melia (German) a short form of Amelia.
Melcia, Melea, Meleah, Meleia, Meleisha, Meli, Meliah, Melida, Melika, Mema

Melina (Latin) canary yellow. (Greek) a short form of Melinda.
Melaina, Meleana, Meleena, Melena, Meline, Melinia, Melinna, Melynna

Melinda (Greek) honey. See also
Linda, Melina, Mindy.
*Maillie, Malinda, Melinde,
Melinder, Mellinda, Melynda,
Melyne, Milinda, Milynda,
Mylenda, Mylinda, Mylynda*

Meliora (Latin) better.
*Melior, Meliori, Mellear, Melyor,
Melyora*

Melisa (Greek) a form of Melissa.
*Melesa, Mélisa, Melise, Melisha,
Melishia, Melisia, Meliza,
Melizah, Mellisa, Melosa, Milisa,
Mylisa, Mylisia*

Melisande (French) a form of
Melissa, Millicent.
*Lisandra, Malisande, Malissande,
Malyssandre, Melesande,
Melisandra, Melisandre,
Mélisandré, Melisenda,
Melissande, Melissandre,
Mellisande, Melond, Melysande,
Melyssandre*

Melissa ⭐ GB (Greek) honey
bee. See also Elissa, Lissa,
Melisande, Millicent.
*Malissa, Mallissa, Melessa,
Meleta, Melisa, Mélissa, Melisse,
Melissia, Mellie, Mellissa, Melly,
Melyssa, Milissa, Millie, Milly,
Missy, Molissia, Mollissa,
Mylissa, Mylissia*

Melita (Greek) a form of Melissa.
(Spanish) a short form of
Carmelita (see Carmelit).
*Malita, Meleeta, Melitta,
Melitza, Melletta, Molita*

Melitona (Greek) she who was
born in Malta.

Melly (American) a familiar form
of names beginning with "Mel."
See also Millie.
Meli, Melie, Melli, Mellie

Melody (Greek) melody. See also
Elodie.
*Meladia, Melodee, Melodey,
Melodi, Melodia, Melodie,
Melodyann, Melodye*

Melonie (American) a form of
Melanie.
*Melloney, Mellonie, Mellony,
Melonee, Meloney, Meloni,
Melonie, Melonnie, Melony*

Melosa (Spanish) sweet; tender.

Melosia (Spanish) sweet.

Melusina (Greek) she who is
sweet as honey.

Melvina (Irish) armored chief.
See also Malvina.
*Melevine, Melva, Melveen,
Melvena, Melvene, Melvonna*

Melyne (Greek) a short form of
Melinda.
Melyn, Melynn, Melynne

Melyssa (Greek) a form of
Melissa.

Mena (German, Dutch) strong.
(Greek) a short form of
Philomena. History: Menes is
believed to be the first king of
Egypt.
Menah

Mendi (Basque) a form of Mary.
Menda, Mendy

Meranda (Latin) a form of
Miranda.
*Merana, Merandah, Merandia,
Merannda*

Mérane (French) a form of Mary.
Meraine, Merrane

Mercé (Spanish) a form of
Mercedes.

Mercedes (Latin) reward,
payment. (Spanish) merciful.
*Mercades, Mercadez, Mercadie,
Meceades, Merced, Mercede,
Mercedees, Mercedeez,
Mercedez, Mercedies, Mercedis,
Mersade, Mersades*

Merces (Latin) favors, graces;
skills.

Mercia (English) a form of
Marcia. History: an ancient
British kingdom.

Mercy (English) compassionate,
merciful. See also Merry.
*Mercey, Merci, Mercie, Mercille,
Mersey*

Meredith GB (Welsh) protector
of the sea.
*Meredeth, Meredithe, Meredy,
Meredyth, Meredythe, Meridath,
Merideth, Meridie, Meridith,
Merridie, Merridith, Merry*

Meri (Finnish) sea. (Irish) a short
form of Meriel.

Meriel (Irish) shining sea.
Meri, Merial, Meriol, Meryl

Merilyn (English) a combination
of Merry + Lynn. See also
Marilyn.
*Merelyn, Merlyn, Merralyn,
Merrelyn, Merrilyn*

Merissa (Latin) a form of
Marissa.
Merisa, Merisha

Merle BG (Latin, French)
blackbird.
*Merl, Merla, Merlina, Merline,
Merola, Murle, Myrle, Myrleen,
Myrlene, Myrline*

Merry (English) cheerful, happy.
A familiar form of Mercy,
Meredith.
*Merie, Merree, Merri, Merrie,
Merrielle, Merrilee, Merrili,
Merrilyn, Merris, Merrita*

Meryl (German) famous. (Irish)
shining sea. A form of Meriel,
Muriel.
*Meral, Merel, Merrall, Merrell,
Merril, Merrile, Merrill, Merryl,
Meryle, Meryll*

Mesha (Hindi) another name for
the zodiac sign Aries.
Meshal

Meta (German) a short form of
Margaret.
Metta, Mette, Metti

Mhairie (Scottish) a form of
Mary.
Mhaire, Mhairi, Mhari, Mhary

Mia ☆ (Italian) mine. A familiar form of Michaela, Michelle.
Mea, Meah, Miah

Micaela (Hebrew) a form of Michaela.
Macaela, Micaella, Micaila, Micala, Miceala

Micah **BG** (Hebrew) a short form of Michael. Bible: one of the Old Testament prophets.
Meecah, Mica, Micha, Mika, Myca, Mycah

Micayla, Michayla (Hebrew) forms of Michaela.
Micayle, Micaylee, Michaylah

Michael **BG** (Hebrew) who is like God?

Michaela **GB** (Hebrew) a form of Michael.
Machaela, Maika, Makaela, Makaila, Makala, Makayla, Mia, Micaela, Micayla, Michael, Michaelann, Michala, Michayla, Michealia, Michaelina, Michaeline, Michaell, Michaella, Michaelyn, Michaila, Michal, Michala, Micheal, Micheala, Michelia, Michelina, Michelle, Michely, Michelyn, Micheyla, Micheline, Micki, Miguela, Mikaela, Mikala, Misha, Mycala, Mychael, Mychal

Michal **BG** (Hebrew) a form of Michaela, Michele.

Michala (Hebrew) a form of Michaela.
Michalann, Michale, Michalene,

Michalin, Mchalina, Michalisha, Michalla, Michalle, Michayla, Michayle, Michela

Micheal **BG** (Hebrew) a form of Michael.

Michel **BG** (French) a form of Michelle.

Michele **GB** (Italian) a form of Michaela.
Michaelle, Michal, Michela

Michelle ☆ **GB** (French) a form of Michael. See also Shelley.
Machealle, Machele, Machell, Machella, Machelle, Mechelle, Meichelle, Meschell, Meshell, Meshelle, Mia, Michel, Michéle, Michell, Michella, Michellene, Michellyn, Mischel, Mischelle, Mishael, Mishaela, Mishayla, Mishell, Mishelle, Mitchele, Mitchelle

Michi (Japanese) righteous way.
Miche, Michee, Michiko

Mickael **BG** (Hebrew) a form of Mikaela.

Micki (American) a familiar form of Michaela.
Mickee, Mickeeya, Mickia, Mickie, Micky, Mickya, Miquia

Micol (Hebrew) she who is queen.

Midori (Japanese) green.

Mieko (Japanese) prosperous.
Mieke

Mielikki (Finnish) pleasing.

Miette (French) small; sweet.

Migina (Omaha) new moon.

Mignon (French) dainty, petite; graceful.
Mignonette, Minnionette, Minnonette, Minyonette, Minyonne

Miguel 🅱🅶 (Portuguese, Spanish) a form of Michael.

Miguela (Spanish) a form of Michaela.
Micquel, Miguelina, Miguelita, Miquel, Miquela, Miquella

Mika 🅶🅱 (Japanese) new moon. (Russian) God's child. (Native American) wise racoon. (Hebrew) a form of Micah. (Latin) a form of Dominica.
Mikah, Mikka

Mikael 🅱🅶 (Hebrew) a form of Mikaela.

Mikaela (Hebrew) a form of Michaela.
Mekaela, Mekala, Mickael, Mickaela, Mickala, Mickalla, Mickeel, Mickell, Mickelle, Mikael, Mikail, Mikaila, Mikal, Mikalene, Mikalovna, Mikalyn, Mikayla, Mikea, Mikeisha, Mikeita, Mikel, Mikela, Mikele, Mikell, Mikella, Mikesha, Mikeya, Mikhaela, Mikie, Mikiela, Mikkel, Mikyla, Mykaela

Mikala (Hebrew) a form of Michaela.
Mickala, Mikalah, Mikale, Mikalea, Mikalee, Mikaleh

Mikayla (American) a form of Mikaela.
Mekayla, Mickayla, Mikala, Mikayle, Mikyla

Mikel 🅱🅶 (Hebrew) a form of Mikaela.

Mikhaela (American) a form of Mikaela.
Mikhail, Mikhaila, Mikhala, Mikhalea, Mikhayla, Mikhelle

Miki 🅶🅱 (Japanese) flower stem.
Mikia, Mikiala, Mikie, Mikita, Mikiyo, Mikki, Mikkie, Mikkiya, Mikko, Miko

Mila (Russian) dear one. (Italian, Slavic) a short form of Camila, Ludmilla.
Milah, Milla

Milada (Czech) my love.
Mila, Milady

Milagres (Latin) wonder, miracle; prodigy.

Milagros (Spanish) miracle.
Mila, Milagritos, Milagro, Milagrosa, Mirari

Milana (Italian) from Milan, Italy. (Russian) a form of Melana.
Milan, Milane, Milani, Milanka, Milanna, Milanne

Milba, Milburga (German) kind protector.

Milca, Milcal (Hebrew) queen.

Mildereda (German) she who speaks soft, kind words.

Mildred (English) gentle counselor.
Mil, Mila, Mildrene, Mildrid, Millie, Milly

Mildreda (German) counselor.

Milena (Greek, Hebrew, Russian) a form of Ludmilla, Magdalen, Melanie.
Mila, Milène, Milenia, Milenny, Milini, Millini

Mileta (German) generous, merciful.

Milia (German) industrious. A short form of Amelia, Emily.
Mila, Milka, Milla, Milya

Miliani (Hawaiian) caress.
Milanni, Miliany

Mililani BG (Hawaiian) heavenly caress.
Milliani

Milissa (Greek) a form of Melissa.
Milessa, Milisa, Millisa, Millissa

Milka (Czech) a form of Amelia.
Milica, Milika

Millaray (Mapuche) golden or silver flower; fragrant, pleasant flower; subtle essence of fragrance.

Millicent (English) industrious. (Greek) a form of Melissa. See also Lissa, Melisande.
Melicent, Meliscent, Mellicent, Mellisent, Melly, Milicent, Milisent, Millie, Milliestone, Millisent, Milly, Milzie, Missy

Millie, Milly (English) familiar forms of Amelia, Camille, Emily, Kamila, Melissa, Mildred, Millicent.
Mili, Milla, Millee, Milley, Millie, Mylie

Milva (German) kind protector.

Mima (Burmese) woman.
Mimma

Mimi (French) a familiar form of Miriam.

Mina GB (German) love. (Persian) blue sky. (Arabic) harbor. (Japanese) south. A short form of names ending in "mina."
Meena, Mena, Min

Minal (Native American) fruit.

Minda (Hindi) knowledge.

Mindy (Greek) a familiar form of Melinda.
Mindee, Mindi, Mindie, Mindyanne, Mindylee, Myndy

Mine (Japanese) peak; mountain range.
Mineko

Minerva (Latin) wise. Mythology: the goddess of wisdom.
Merva, Minivera, Minnie, Myna

Minette (French) faithful defender.
Minnette, Minnita

Minia (German) great, strong.

Minka (Polish) a short form of Wilhelmina.

Minna (German) a short form of Wilhelmina.
Mina, Minka, Minnie, Minta

Minnie (American) a familiar form of Mina, Minerva, Minna, Wilhelmina.
Mini, Minie, Minne, Minni, Minny

Minowa (Native American) singer.
Minowah

Minta (English) Literature: originally coined by playwright Sir John Vanbrugh in his comedy *The Confederacy*.
Minty

Minya (Osage) older sister.

Mio (Japanese) three times as strong.

Mira (Latin) wonderful. (Spanish) look, gaze. A short form of Almira, Amira, Marabel, Mirabel, Miranda.
Mirae, Mirra, Mirah

Mirabel (Latin) beautiful.
Mira, Mirabell, Mirabella, Mirabelle, Mirable

Miracle GB (Latin) wonder, marvel.

Mirana (Spanish) a form of Miranda.

Miranda GB (Latin) strange; wonderful; admirable. Literature: the heroine of Shakespeare's *The Tempest*. See also Randi.
Maranda, Marenda, Meranda, Mira, Miran, Miranada, Mirandia, Mirinda, Mirindé, Mironda, Mirranda, Muranda, Myranda

Mireille (Hebrew) God spoke. (Latin) wonderful.
Mireil, Mirel, Mirella, Mirelle, Mirelys, Mireya, Mireyda, Mirielle, Mirilla, Myrella, Myrilla

Mireya (Hebrew) a form of Mireille.
Mireea, Miriah, Miryah

Miri (Gypsy) a short form of Miriam.
Miria, Miriah

Miriam GB (Hebrew) bitter; sea of bitterness. Bible: the original form of Mary. See also Macia, Mimi, Mitzi.
Mairwen, Mariam, Maryam, Miram, Mirham, Miri, Miriain, Miriama, Miriame, Mirian, Mirit, Mirjam, Mirjana, Mirriam, Mirrian, Miryam, Miryan, Myriam

Mirta, Mirtha (Greek) crown of myrtle.

Mirya (French) she who has earned everyone's admiration.

Misael BG (Hebrew) a form of Michael.

Misha GB (Russian) a form of Michaela.
Mischa, Mishae

Missy (English) a familiar form of Melissa, Millicent.
Missi, Missie

Misty GB (English) shrouded by mist.
Missty, Mistee, Mistey, Misti, Mistie, Mistin, Mistina, Mistral, Mistylynn, Mystee, Mysti, Mystie

Mitchell BG (English) a form of Michael.

Mitra (Hindi) Religion: god of daylight. (Persian) angel.
Mita

Mituna (Moquelumnan) like a fish wrapped up in leaves.

Mitzi (German) a form of Mary, Miriam.
Mieze, Mitzee, Mitzie, Mitzy

Miwa (Japanese) wise eyes.
Miwako

Miya (Japanese) temple.
Miyah, Miyana, Miyanna

Miyo (Japanese) beautiful generation.
Miyoko, Miyuko

Miyuki (Japanese) snow.

Moana (Hawaiian) ocean; fragrance.

Mocha (Arabic) chocolate-flavored coffee.
Moka

Modesty (Latin) modest.
Modesta, Modeste, Modestia, Modestie, Modestina, Modestine, Modestus

Moema (Tupi) sweet.

Moesha (American) a short form of Monisha.
Myesha

Mohala (Hawaiian) flowers in bloom.
Moala

Mohamed BG (Arabic) a form of Muhammad (see Boys' Names).

Moira (Irish) great. A form of Mary. See also Maura.
Moirae, Moirah, Moire, Moya, Moyra, Moyrah

Molara (Basque) a form of Mary.

Mollie (Irish) a form of Molly.
Moli, Molie, Molli

Molly ☀ GB (Irish) a familiar form of Mary.
Moll, Mollee, Molley, Mollissa

Mona GB (Irish) noble. (Greek) a short form of Monica, Ramona, Rimona.
Moina, Monah, Mone, Monea, Monna, Moyna

Monet (French) Art: Claude Monet was a leading French impressionist remembered for his paintings of water lilies.
Monae, Monay, Monee

Monica GB (Greek) solitary.
(Latin) advisor.
*Mona, Monca, Monee, Monia,
Monic, Mónica, Monice, Monicia,
Monicka, Monika, Monique,
Monise, Monn, Monnica,
Monnie, Monya*

Monifa (Yoruba) I have my luck.

Monika (German) a form of
Monica.
*Moneka, Monieka, Monike,
Monnika*

Monique (French) a form of
Monica.
*Moneeke, Moneik, Moniqua,
Moniquea, Moniquie, Munique*

Monisha (American) a combination of Monica + Aisha.
Moesha, Moneisha, Monishia

Monita (Spanish) noble.

Montana GB (Spanish) mountain.
Geography: a U.S. state.
Montanna

Montrell BG (French) a form of
Montreal (see Boys' Names).

Mora (Spanish) blueberry.
Morae, Morea, Moria, Morita

Morela (Polish) apricot.
Morelia, Morelle

Morena (Irish) a form of Maureen.

Morgan ☆ GB (Welsh)
seashore. Literature: Morgan le
Fay was the half-sister of King
Arthur.
*Morgance, Morgane,
Morganetta, Morganette,
Morganica, Morgann, Morganne,
Morgen, Morghan, Morgyn,
Morrigan*

Morgana (Welsh) a form of
Morgan.
Morganna

Morganda (Spanish) a form of
Morgana.

Morghan (Welsh) a form of
Morgan.
Morghen, Morghin, Morghyn

Moriah GB (Hebrew) God is my
teacher. (French) dark skinned.
Bible: the mountain on which the
Temple of Solomon was built. See
also Mariah.
*Moria, Moriel, Morit, Morria,
Morriah*

Morie (Japanese) bay.

Morowa (Akan) queen.

Morrisa (Latin) dark skinned;
moor; marshland.
Morisa, Morissa, Morrissa

Moselle (Hebrew) drawn from
the water. (French) a white wine.
Mozelle

Moses BG (Hebrew) drawn out
of the water. (Egyptian) child.

Mosi BG (Swahili) first-born.

Moswen BG (Tswana) white.

Mouna (Arabic) wish, desire.
Moona, Moonia, Mounia, Muna, Munia

Mrena (Slavic) white eyes.
Mren

Mumtaz (Arabic) distinguished.

Munira (Arabic) she who is the source of light.

Mura (Japanese) village.

Muriel (Arabic) myrrh. (Irish) shining sea. A form of Mary. See also Meryl.
Merial, Meriel, Meriol, Merrial, Merriel, Muire, Murial, Muriell, Murielle

Musetta (French) little bagpipe.
Musette

Muslimah (Arabic) devout believer.

Mya GB (Burmese) emerald. (Italian) a form of Mia.
My, Myah, Myia, Myiah

Myesha (American) a form of Moesha.
Myeisha, Myeshia, Myiesha, Myisha

Mykaela, Mykayla (American) forms of Mikaela.
Mykael, Mykaila, Mykal, Mykala, Mykaleen, Mykel, Mykela, Mykyla

Myla (English) merciful.

Mylene (Greek) dark.
Mylaine, Mylana, Mylee, Myleen

Myles BG (Latin) soldier. (German) a form of Miles (see Boys' Names).

Myra (Latin) fragrant ointment.
Mayra, Myrena, Myria

Myranda (Latin) a form of Miranda.
Myrandah, Myrandia, Myrannda

Myriam GB (American) a form of Miriam.
Myriame, Myryam

Myrna (Irish) beloved.
Merna, Mirna, Morna, Muirna

Myrtle (Greek) dark green shrub.
Mertis, Mertle, Mirtle, Myrta, Myrtia, Myrtias, Myrtice, Myrtie, Myrtilla, Myrtis

N BG (American) an initial used as a first name.

Nabila (Arabic) born to nobility.
Nabeela, Nabiha, Nabilah

Nadal (Catalonian) a form of Natividad.

Nadda (Arabic) generous; dewy.
Nada

Nadette (French) a short form of Bernadette.

Nadia (French, Slavic) hopeful.
Nadea, Nadenka, Nadezhda, Nadiah, Nadie, Nadija, Nadijah, Nadine, Nadiya, Nadiyah, Nadja, Nadjae, Nadjah, Nadka, Nadusha, Nady, Nadya

Nadine 🇬🇧 (French, Slavic) a form of Nadia.
Nadean, Nadeana, Nadeen, Nadena, Nadene, Nadien, Nadin, Nadina, Nadyne, Naidene, Naidine

Nadira (Arabic) rare, precious.
Naadirah, Nadirah

Naeva (French) a form of Eve.
Nahvon

Nafuna (Luganda) born feet first.

Nagida (Hebrew) noble; prosperous.
Nagda, Nageeda

Nahid (Persian) Mythology: another name for Venus, the goddess of love and beauty.

Nahimana (Dakota) mystic.

Naiara (Spanish) reference to the Virgin Mary.

Naida (Greek) water nymph.
Naiad, Naiya, Nayad, Nyad

Naila (Arabic) successful.
Nailah

Nairi (Armenian) land of rivers. History: a name for ancient Armenia.
Naira, Naire, Nayra

Naís (Spanish) a form of Inés.

Naiya (Greek) a form of Naida.
Naia, Naiyana, Naja, Najah, Naya

Najam (Arabic) star.
Naja, Najma

Najila (Arabic) brilliant eyes.
Naja, Najah, Najia, Najja, Najla

Nakeisha (American) a combination of the prefix Na + Keisha.
Nakeesha, Nakesha, Nakeshea, Nakeshia, Nakeysha, Nakiesha, Nakisha, Nekeisha

Nakeita (American) a form of Nikita.
Nakeeta, Nakeitha, Nakeithra, Nakeitra, Nakeitress, Nakeitta, Nakeittia, Naketta, Nakieta, Nakitha, Nakitia, Nakitta, Nakyta

Nakia 🇬🇧 (Arabic) pure.
Nakea, Nakeia, Nakeya, Nakeyah, Nakeyia, Nakiah, Nakiaya, Nakiea, Nakiya, Nakiyah, Nekia

Nakita (American) a form of Nikita.
Nakkita, Naquita

Nalani (Hawaiian) calm as the heavens.
Nalanie, Nalany

Ñambi (Guarani) curative herb.

Nami (Japanese) wave.
Namika, Namiko

Nan (German) a short form of Fernanda. (English) a form of Ann.
Nana, Nanice, Nanine, Nanna, Nanon

Nana (Hawaiian) spring.

Naná (Greek) she who is very young.

Nanci (English) a form of Nancy.
Nancie, Nancsi, Nansi

Nancy **GB** (English) gracious. A familiar form of Nan.
Nainsi, Nance, Nancee, Nancey, Nanci, Nancine, Nancye, Nanette, Nanice, Nanncey, Nanncy, Nanouk, Nansee, Nansey, Nanuk

Nanette (French) a form of Nancy.
Nan, Nanete, Nannette, Nettie, Nineta, Ninete, Ninetta, Ninette, Nini, Ninita, Ninnetta, Ninnette, Nynette

Nani (Greek) charming. (Hawaiian) beautiful.
Nanni, Nannie, Nanny

Nantilde (German) daring in combat.

Naolin (Spanish) sun god of the Mexican people.

Naomi (Hebrew) pleasant, beautiful. Bible: Ruth's mother-in-law.
Naoma, Naomia, Naomie,
Naomy, Navit, Neoma, Neomi, Noami, Noemi, Noma, Nomi, Nyomi

Naomí (Hebrew) a form of Naomi.

Naomie (Hebrew) a form of Naomi.
Naome, Naomee, Noemie

Napea (Latin) from the valleys.

Nara (Greek) happy. (English) north. (Japanese) oak.
Narah

Narcissa (Greek) daffodil. Mythology: Narcissus was the youth who fell in love with his own reflection.
Narcessa, Narcisa, Narcisse, Narcyssa, Narissa, Narkissa

Narda (Latin) fervently devoted.

Narelle (Australian) woman from the sea.
Narel

Nari (Japanese) thunder.
Narie, Nariko

Narmada (Hindi) pleasure giver.

Naroa (Basque) tranquil, peaceful.

Nashawna (American) a combination of the prefix Na + Shawna.
Nashan, Nashana, Nashanda, Nashaun, Nashauna, Nashaunda, Nashauwna, Nashawn, Nasheena, Nashounda, Nashuana

Nashota (Native American) double; second-born twin.

Nastasia (Greek) a form of Anastasia.
Nastasha, Nastashia, Nastasja, Nastassa, Nastassia, Nastassiya, Nastassja, Nastassya, Nastasya, Nastazia, Nastisija, Nastka, Nastusya, Nastya

Nasya (Hebrew) miracle.
Nasia, Nasyah

Nata (Sanskrit) dancer. (Latin) swimmer. (Native American) speaker; creator. (Polish, Russian) a form of Natalie. See also Nadia.
Natia, Natka, Natya

Natacha (Russian) a form of Natasha.
Natachia, Natacia, Naticha

Natalee, Natali (Latin) forms of Natalie.
Natale, Nataleh, Nataleigh, Nattlee

Natalí (Spanish) a form of Natalia.

Natalia (Russian) a form of Natalie. See also Talia.
Nacia, Natala, Natalea, Nataliia, Natalija, Natalina, Nataliya, Nataliyah, Natalja, Natalka, Natallea, Natallia, Natalya, Nathalia, Natka

Natália (Hungarian, Portuguese) a form of Natalie.

Natalie ☀ 🇬🇧 (Latin) born on Christmas day. See also Nata, Natasha, Noel, Talia.
Nat, Natalee, Natali, Natalia, Nataliee, Nataline, Natalle, Natallie, Nataly, Natelie, Nathalie, Nathaly, Natie, Natilie, Natlie, Nattalie, Nattilie

Nataline (Latin) a form of Natalie.
Natalene, Nataléne, Natalyn

Natalle (French) a form of Natalie.
Natale

Nataly (Latin) a form of Natalie.
Nathaly, Natally, Natallye

Natane (Arapaho) daughter.
Natanne

Natania (Hebrew) gift of God.
Natanya, Natée, Nathania, Nathenia, Netania, Nethania

Natara (Arabic) sacrifice.
Natori, Natoria

Natasha 🇬🇧 (Russian) a form of Natalie. See also Stacey, Tasha.
Nahtasha, Natacha, Natasa, Natascha, Natashah, Natashea, Natashenka, Natashia, Natashiea, Natashja, Natashka, Natasia, Natassia, Natassija, Natassja, Natasza, Natausha, Natawsha, Natesha, Nateshia, Nathasha, Nathassa, Natisha, Natishia, Natosha, Netasha, Notosha

Natesa (Hindi) cosmic dancer.
Religion: another name for the
Hindu god Shiva.
Natisa, Natissa

Nathália (Portuguese) a form of
Natalie.

Nathalie, Nathaly (Latin) forms
of Natalie.
*Nathalee, Nathali, Nathalia,
Nathalya*

Nathan BG (Hebrew) a short
form of Nathaniel.

Nathaniel BG (Hebrew) gift of
God.

Natie (English) a familiar form of
Natalie.
Nati, Natti, Nattie, Natty

Natividad (Spanish) nativity.

Natori GB (Arabic) a form of
Natara.

Natosha (Russian) a form of
Natasha.
*Natoshia, Natoshya, Netosha,
Notosha*

Nava (Hebrew) beautiful;
pleasant.
Navah, Naveh, Navit

Navdeep BG (Sikh) new light.

Nayara (Basque) swallow.

Nayeli (Zapotec) I love you.

Nayely (Irish) a form of Neila.
*Naeyli, Nayelia, Nayelli, Nayelly,
Nayla*

Nazarena (Hebrew) native of
Nazareth.

Nazaria (Spanish) dedicated to
God.

Neala (Irish) a form of Neila.
*Nayela, Naylea, Naylia, Nealia,
Neela, Neelia, Neila*

Necha (Spanish) a form of Agnes.
Necho

Neci BG (Hungarian) fiery,
intense.
Necia, Necie

Neda (Slavic) born on Sunday.
Nedah, Nedi, Nedia, Neida

Nedda (English) prosperous
guardian.
Neddi, Neddie, Neddy

Neely (Irish) a familiar form of
Neila, Nelia.
*Nealee, Nealie, Nealy, Neelee,
Neeley, Neeli, Neelie, Neili,
Neilie*

Neema (Swahili) born during
prosperous times.

Neena (Spanish) a form of Nina.
Neenah, Nena

Neftali (Hebrew) she who fights
and ends up victorious.

Neila (Irish) champion. See also
Neala, Neely.
*Nayely, Neilah, Neile, Neilia,
Neilla, Neille*

Nekeisha (American) a form of Nakeisha.
Nechesa, Neikeishia, Nekesha, Nekeshia, Nekiesha, Nekisha, Nekysha

Nekia (Arabic) a form of Nakia.
Nekeya, Nekiya, Nekiyah, Nekya, Nekiya

Nelia (Spanish) yellow. (Latin) a familiar form of Cornelia.
Neelia, Neely, Neelya, Nela, Neli, Nelka, Nila

Nélida (Greek) compassionate, merciful.

Nelle (Greek) stone.

Nellie, Nelly GB (English) familiar forms of Cornelia, Eleanor, Helen, Prunella.
Nel, Neli, Nell, Nella, Nelley, Nelli, Nellianne, Nellice, Nellis, Nelma

Nelson BG (English) child of Neil (see Boys' Names).

Nemesia (Greek) she who administers justice.

Nenet (Egyptian) born near the sea. Mythology: Nunet was the goddess of the sea.

Neola (Greek) youthful.
Neolla

Neona (Greek) new moon.

Nereida (Greek) a form of Nerine.
Nereyda, Nereyida, Nerida

Nerine (Greek) sea nymph.
Nereida, Nerina, Nerita, Nerline

Nerissa (Greek) sea nymph. See also Rissa.
Narice, Narissa, Nerice, Nerisa, Nerisse, Nerrisa, Nerys, Neryssa

Nessa (Scandinavian) promontory. (Greek) a short form of Agnes. See also Nessie.
Nesa, Nesha, Neshia, Nesiah, Nessia, Nesta, Nevsa, Neysa, Neysha, Neyshia

Nessie (Greek) a familiar form of Agnes, Nessa, Vanessa.
Nese, Neshie, Nesho, Nesi, Ness, Nessi, Nessy, Nest, Neys

Nestor BG (Greek) traveler; wise.

Neta (Hebrew) plant, shrub. See also Nettie.
Netia, Netta, Nettia

Netis (Native American) trustworthy.

Nettie (French) a familiar form of Annette, Nanette, Antoinette.
Neti, Netie, Netta, Netti, Netty, Nety

Neva (Spanish) snow. (English) new. Geography: a river in Russia.
Neiva, Neve, Nevia, Neyva, Nieve, Niva, Nivea, Nivia

Nevada GB (Spanish) snow. Geography: a western U.S. state.
Neiva, Neva

Neves (Portuguese) a form of Nieves.

Nevina (Irish) worshipper of the saint.
Neveen, Nevein, Nevena, Neveyan, Nevin, Nivena

Neylan (Turkish) fulfilled wish.
Neya, Neyla

Neza (Slavic) a form of Agnes.

Ngoc GB (Vietnamese) jade.

Nia GB (Irish) a familiar form of Neila. Mythology: Nia Ben Aur was a legendary Welsh woman.
Neya, Niah, Niajia, Niya, Nya

Niabi (Osage) fawn.

Nicanora (Spanish) victorious army.

Niceta (Spanish) victorious one.

Nichelle (American) a combination of Nicole + Michelle. Culture: Nichelle Nichols was the first African American woman featured in a television drama (*Star Trek*).
Nichele, Nichell, Nishelle

Nichole (French) a form of Nicole.
Nichol, Nichola, Nicholle

Nicki (French) a familiar form of Nicole.
Nicci, Nickey, Nickeya, Nickia, Nickie, Nickiya, Nicky, Niki

Nickolas BG (Greek) a form of Nicholas (see Boys' Names).

Nickole (French) a form of Nicole.
Nickol

Nico BG (Greek) a short form of Nicholas (see Boys' Names).

Nicola GB (Italian) a form of Nicole.
Nacola, Necola, Nichola, Nickola, Nicolea, Nicolla, Nikkola, Nikola, Nikolia, Nykola

Nicolas BG (Italian) a form of Nicholas (see Boys' Names).

Nicolasa (Spanish) victorious people.

Nicole ☆ GB (French) a form of Nicholas (see Boys' Names). See also Colette, Cosette, Nikita.
Nacole, Necole, Nica, Nichole, Nicia, Nicki, Nickole, Nicol, Nicola, Nicolette, Nicoli, Nicolie, Nicoline, Nicolle, Nikayla, Nikelle, Nikki, Niquole, Nocole, Nycole

Nicoleta (Greek) winner over all.

Nicolette GB (French) a form of Nicole.
Nicholette, Nicoletta, Nicollete, Nicollette, Nikkolette, Nikoleta, Nikoletta, Nikolette

Nicoline (French) a familiar form of Nicole.
Nicholine, Nicholyn, Nicoleen, Nicolene, Nicolina, Nicolyn, Nicolyne, Nicolynn, Nicolynne, Nikolene, Nikolina, Nikoline

Nicolle (French) a form of
Nicole.
Nicholle

Nida (Omaha) Mythology: an
elflike creature.
Nidda

Nidia (Latin) nest.
Nidi, Nidya

Niesha (American) pure.
(Scandinavian) a form of Nissa.
*Neisha, Neishia, Neissia, Nesha,
Neshia, Nesia, Nessia, Niessia,
Nisha, Nyesha*

Nieves (Latin) refers to the
blessed Virgin Mary.

Nige (Latin) dark night.
Nigea, Nigela, Nija, Nijae, Nijah

Nigel 🅱🅶 (Latin) dark night.

Nika (Russian) belonging to God.
Nikka

Nikayla, Nikelle (American)
forms of Nicole.
Nikeille, Nikel, Nikela, Nikelie

Nike 🅱🅶 (Greek) victorious.
Mythology: the goddess of victory.

Niki 🅶🅱 (Russian) a short form of
Nikita. (American) a familiar
form of Nicole.
Nikia, Nikiah

Nikita 🅶🅱 (Russian) victorious
people.
*Nakeita, Nakita, Niki, Nikitah,
Nikitia, Nikitta, Nikki, Nikkita,
Niquita, Niquitta*

Nikki 🅶🅱 (American) a familiar
form of Nicole, Nikita.
*Nicki, Nikia, Nikkea, Nikkey,
Nikkia, Nikkiah, Nikkie, Nikko,
Nikky*

Nikko 🅱🅶 (American) a form of
Nikki.

Niko 🅱🅶 (Hungarian) a form of
Nicholas (see Boys' Names).

Nikola 🅱🅶 (French) a form of
Nikole. (Italian) a form of Nicola.

Nikole (French) a form of Nicole.
*Nikkole, Nikkolie, Nikola, Nikole,
Nikolena, Nicolia, Nikolina,
Nikolle*

Nila 🅶🅱 (Latin) Geography: the
Nile River is in Africa. (Irish) a
form of Neila.
Nilah, Nilesia, Nyla

Nilda (Spanish) a short form of
Brunilda.

Nili (Hebrew) Botany: a pea plant
that yields indigo.

Nima (Hebrew) thread. (Arabic)
blessing.
Nema, Niama, Nimali

Nimia (Latin) she who has a lot of
ambition.

Nina 🅶🅱 (Hebrew) a familiar
form of Hannah. (Spanish) girl.
(Native American) mighty.
*Neena, Ninah, Ninacska, Ninja,
Ninna, Ninon, Ninosca, Ninoshka*

Ninfa (Greek) young wife.

Ninon (French) a form of Nina.

Niobe (Greek) she who rejuvenates.

Nirel (Hebrew) light of God.
Nirali, Nirelle

Nirveli (Hindi) water child.

Nisa (Arabic) woman.

Nisha (American) a form of Niesha, Nissa.
Niasha, Nishay

Nishi (Japanese) west.

Nissa (Hebrew) sign, emblem. (Scandinavian) friendly elf; brownie. See also Nyssa.
Nisha, Nisse, Nissie, Nissy

Nita (Hebrew) planter. (Choctaw) bear. (Spanish) a short form of Anita, Juanita.
Nitai, Nitha, Nithai, Nitika

Nitara (Hindi) deeply rooted.

Nitasha (American) a form of Natasha.
Nitasia, Niteisha, Nitisha, Nitishia

Nitsa (Greek) a form of Helen.

Nituna (Native American) daughter.

Nitza (Hebrew) flower bud.
Nitzah, Nitzana, Nitzanit, Niza, Nizah

Nixie (German) water sprite.

Niya (Irish) a form of Nia.
Niyah, Niyana, Niyia, Nyia

Nizana (Hebrew) a form of Nitza.
Nitzana, Nitzania, Zana

Noah BG (Hebrew) peaceful, restful.

Noe BG (Czech, French) a form of Noah.

Noel BG (Latin) Christmas. See also Natalie.
Noël, Noela, Noelani, Noele, Noeleen, Noelene, Noelia, Noeline, Noelle, Noelyn, Noelynn, Nohely, Noleen, Novelenn, Novelia, Nowel, Noweleen, Nowell

Noelani (Hawaiian) beautiful one from heaven.
Noela

Noelle (French) Christmas.
Noell, Noella, Noelleen, Noelly, Noellyn

Noemi (Hebrew) a form of Naomi.
Noam, Noemie, Noemy, Nohemi, Nomi

Noemí (Hebrew) a form of Noemi.

Noemie (Hebrew) a form of Noemi.

Noemy (Hebrew) a form of Noemi.
Noamy

Noga (Hebrew) morning light.

Nohely (Latin) a form of Noel.
*Noeli, Noelie, Noely, Nohal,
Noheli*

Nokomis (Dakota) moon
daughter.

Nola (Latin) small bell. (Irish)
famous; noble. A short form of
Fionnula.
Nuala

Nolan 🅱🅶 (Irish) famous; noble.

Noleta (Latin) unwilling.
Nolita

Nollie 🅱🅶 (English) a familiar
form of Magnolia.
Nolia, Nolle, Nolley, Nolli, Nolly

Noma (Hawaiian) a form of
Norma.

Nominanda (Latin) she who will
be elected.

Nona (Latin) ninth.
*Nonah, Noni, Nonia, Nonie,
Nonna, Nonnah, Nonya*

Noor (Aramaic) a form of Nura.
Noorie, Nour, Nur

Nora 🅶🅱 (Greek) light. A familiar
form of Eleanor, Honora,
Leonore.
Norah, Noreen

Noreen (Irish) a form of Eleanor,
Nora. (Latin) a familiar form of
Norma.
*Noorin, Noreena, Noreene,
Noren, Norena, Norene, Norina,
Norine, Nureen*

Norell (Scandinavian) from the
north.
*Narell, Narelle, Norela, Norelle,
Norely*

Nori (Japanese) law, tradition.
Noria, Norico, Noriko, Norita

Norma (Latin) rule, precept.
Noma, Noreen, Normi, Normie

Norman 🅱🅶 (French) Norseman.

Nova (Latin) new. A short form of
Novella, Novia. (Hopi) butterfly
chaser. Astronomy: a star that
releases bright bursts of energy.

Novella (Latin) newcomer.
Nova, Novela

Novia (Spanish) sweetheart.
Nova, Novka, Nuvia

Nu (Burmese) tender.
(Vietnamese) girl.
Nue

Nuala (Irish) a short form of
Fionnula.
Nola, Nula

Nubia (Latin) cloud.

Nuela (Spanish) a form of
Amelia.

Numa, Numas (Greek) she who
lays down rules and establishes
laws.

Numeria (Latin) she who
elaborates, who enumerates.

Nuna (Native American) land.

Nuncia (Latin) she who leaves messages, who informs.

Nunciata (Latin) messenger.
Nunzia

Nunila (Spanish) ninth daughter.

Nura (Aramaic) light.
Noor, Noora, Noorah, Noura, Nurah

Nuria (Aramaic) the Lord's light.
Nuri, Nuriel, Nurin

Nurita (Hebrew) Botany: a flower with red and yellow blossoms.
Nurit

Nuru BG (Swahili) daylight.

Nusi (Hungarian) a form of Hannah.

Nuwa (Chinese) mother goddess. Mythology: another name for Nü-gua, the creator of mankind.

Nya (Irish) a form of Nia.
Nyaa, Nyah, Nyia

Nycole (French) a form of Nicole.
Nychelle, Nycolette, Nycolle

Nydia (Latin) nest.
Nyda

Nyesha (American) a form of Niesha.
Nyeisha, Nyeshia

Nyla (Latin, Irish) a form of Nila.
Nylah

Nyoko (Japanese) gem, treasure.

Nyomi (Hebrew) a form of Naomi.
Nyome, Nyomee, Nyomie

Nyree (Maori) sea.
Nyra, Nyrie

Nyssa (Greek) beginning. See also Nissa.
Nisha, Nissi, Nissy, Nyasia, Nysa

Nyusha (Russian) a form of Agnes.
Nyushenka, Nyushka

O

Oba BG (Yoruba) chief, ruler.

Obdulia (Latin) she who takes away sadness and pain.

Obelia (Greek) needle.

Oceana (Greek) ocean. Mythology: Oceanus was the god of the ocean.
Ocean, Oceananna, Oceane, Oceania, Oceanna, Oceanne, Oceaonna, Oceon

Octavia GB (Latin) eighth. See also Tavia.
Octabia, Octaviah, Octaviais, Octavice, Octavie, Octavienne, Octavio, Octavious, Octavise, Octavya, Octivia, Otavia, Ottavia

Octaviana (Spanish) a form of Octavia.

Octavio BG (Latin) a form of
Octavia.

Odalis, Odalys (Spanish) a form
of Odilia.

Odeda (Hebrew) strong;
courageous.

Odele (Greek) melody, song.
Odelet, Odelette, Odell, Odelle

Odelia (Greek) ode; melodic.
(Hebrew) I will praise God.
(French) wealthy. See also
Odetta.
*Oda, Odeelia, Odeleya, Odelina,
Odelinda, Odelyn, Odila, Odile*

Odella (English) wood hill.
Odela, Odelle, Odelyn

Odera (Hebrew) plough.

Odessa (Greek) odyssey, long
voyage.
*Adesha, Adeshia, Adessa,
Adessia, Odessia*

Odetta (German, French) a form
of Odelia.
Oddetta, Odette

Odilia (Greek, Hebrew, French) a
form of Odelia.

Odina (Algonquin) mountain.

Ofelia (Greek) a form of Ophelia.
Ofeelia, Ofilia

Ofélia (Portuguese) a form of
Ophelia.

Ofira (Hebrew) gold.
Ofarrah, Ophira

Ofra (Hebrew) a form of Aphra.
Ofrat

Ogin (Native American) wild rose.

Ohanna (Hebrew) God's gracious
gift.

Okalani (Hawaiian) heaven.
Okilani

Oki (Japanese) middle of the
ocean.
Okie

Oksana (Latin) a form of Osanna.
Oksanna

Ola GB (Greek) a short form of
Olesia. (Scandinavian) ancestor.

Olalla (Spanish) well-spoken one.

Olathe (Native American)
beautiful.
Olathia

Olaya (Greek) she who speaks
well.

Oleda (Spanish) a form of Alida.
See also Leda.
Oleta, Olida, Olita

Olena (Russian) a form of Helen.
*Oleena, Olenka, Olenna, Olenya,
Olya*

Olesia (Greek) a form of
Alexandra.
*Cesya, Ola, Olecia, Oleesha,
Oleishia, Olesha, Olesya, Olexa,
Olice, Olicia, Olisha, Olishia,
Ollicia*

Oletha (Scandinavian) nimble.
Oleta, Yaletha

Olethea (Latin) truthful. See also
Alethea.
Oleta

Olga (Scandinavian) holy. See also
Helga, Olivia.
*Olenka, Olia, Olja, Ollya, Olva,
Olya*

Oliana (Polynesian) oleander.

Olina (Hawaiian) filled with
happiness.

Olinda (Latin) scented. (Spanish)
protector of property. (Greek) a
form of Yolanda.

Olisa (Ibo) God.

Olive (Latin) olive tree.
Oliff, Oliffe, Olivet, Olivette

Oliver **BG** (Latin) olive tree.
(Scandinavian) kind; affectionate.

Oliveria (Latin) affectionate.

Olivia ✵ **GB** (Latin) a form of
Olive. (English) a form of Olga.
See also Liv, Livia.
*Alivia, Alyvia, Olevia, Oliva,
Olivea, Oliveia, Olivetta, Olivi,
Olivianne, Olivya, Oliwia, Ollie,
Olva, Olyvia*

Olívia (Portuguese) a form of
Olivia.

Olivier **BG** (French) a form of
Oliver.

Ollie **BG** (English) a familiar form
of Olivia.
Olla, Olly, Ollye

Olwen (Welsh) white footprint.
*Olwenn, Olwin, Olwyn, Olwyne,
Olwynne*

Olympia (Greek) heavenly.
Olimpia, Olympe, Olympie

Olyvia (Latin) a form of Olivia.

Oma (Hebrew) reverent.
(German) grandmother. (Arabic)
highest.

Omaira (Arabic) red.
*Omar, Omara, Omarah, Omari,
Omaria, Omarra*

Omar **BG** (Arabic) a form of
Omaira.

Omega (Greek) last, final, end.
Linguistics: the last letter in the
Greek alphabet.

Ona (Latin, Irish) a form of Oona,
Una. (English) river.

Onatah (Iroquois) daughter of the
earth and the corn spirit.

Onawa (Native American) wide
awake.
Onaja, Onajah

Ondine (Latin) a form of Undine.
Ondene, Ondina, Ondyne

Ondrea (Czech) a form of Andrea.
*Ohndrea, Ohndreea, Ohndreya,
Ohndria, Ondraya, Ondreana,
Ondreea, Ondreya, Ondria,
Ondrianna, Ondriea*

Oneida (Native American) eagerly awaited.
Onida, Onyda

Onella (Hungarian) a form of Helen.

Onesha (American) a combination of Ondrea + Aisha.
Oneshia, Onesia, Onessa, Onessia, Onethia, Oniesha, Onisha

Oni (Yoruba) born on holy ground.
Onnie

Onora (Latin) a form of Honora.
Onoria, Onorine, Ornora

Oona (Latin, Irish) a form of Una.
Ona, Onna, Onnie, Oonagh, Oonie

Opa (Choctaw) owl. (German) grandfather.

Opal (Hindi) precious stone.
Opale, Opalina, Opaline

Ophelia (Greek) helper. Literature: Hamlet's love interest in the Shakespearean play *Hamlet*.
Filia, Ofelia, Ophélie, Ophilia, Phelia

Oprah (Hebrew) a form of Orpah.
Ophra, Ophrah, Opra

Ora (Latin) prayer. (Spanish) gold. (English) seacoast. (Greek) a form of Aura.
Orah, Orlice, Orra

Orabella (Latin) a form of Arabella.
Orabel, Orabela, Orabelle

Oraida (Arabic) eloquent; she who speaks well.

Oralee (Hebrew) the Lord is my light. See also Yareli.
Areli, Orali, Oralit, Orelie, Orlee, Orli, Orly

Oralia (French) a form of Aurelia. See also Oriana.
Oralis, Oriel, Orielda, Orielle, Oriena, Orlena, Orlene

Orea (Greek) mountains.
Oreal, Oria, Oriah

Orela (Latin) announcement from the gods; oracle.
Oreal, Orella, Orelle, Oriel, Orielle

Orenda (Iroquois) magical power.

Oretha (Greek) a form of Aretha.
Oreta, Oretta, Orette

Orfilia (German) female wolf.

Oriana (Latin) dawn, sunrise. (Irish) golden.
Orane, Orania, Orelda, Orelle, Ori, Oria, Orian, Oriane, Orianna, Orieana, Oryan

Orieta (Spanish) a form of Oriana.

Orina (Russian) a form of Irene.
Orya, Oryna

Orinda (Hebrew) pine tree.
(Irish) light skinned, white.
Orenda

Orino (Japanese) worker's field.
Ori

Oriole (Latin) golden; black-and-orange bird.
Auriel, Oriel, Oriell, Oriella, Oriola

Orion **BG** (Greek) child of fire.
Mythology: a giant hunter who was killed by Artemis.

Orla (Irish) golden woman.
Orlagh, Orlie, Orly

Orlanda (German) famous throughout the land.
Orlandia, Orlantha, Orlenda, Orlinda

Orlenda (Russian) eagle.

Orli (Hebrew) light.
Orlice, Orlie, Orly

Ormanda (Latin) noble.
(German) mariner.
Orma

Ornella (Latin) she who is like a flowery ash tree.

Ornice (Hebrew) cedar tree.
(Irish) pale; olive colored.
Orna, Ornah, Ornat, Ornette, Ornit

Orpah (Hebrew) runaway. See also Oprah.
Orpa, Orpha, Orphie

Orquidea (Spanish) orchid.
Orquidia

Orquídea (Italian) a form of Orquidea.

Orsa (Latin) a short form of Orseline. See also Ursa.
Orsaline, Orse, Orsel, Orselina, Orseline, Orsola

Ortensia (Italian) a form of Hortense.

Orva (French) golden; worthy.
(English) brave friend.

Osanna (Latin) praise the Lord.
Oksana, Osana

Oscar **BG** (Scandinavian) divine spear carrier.

Osen (Japanese) one thousand.

Oseye (Benin) merry.

Osma (English) divine protector.
Ozma

Otilde (Spanish) a form of Otilia.

Otilia (Czech) a form of Otilie.

Otilie (Czech) lucky heroine.
Otila, Otka, Ottili, Otylia

Ova (Latin) egg.

Ovia (Latin, Danish) egg.

Ovidia (German) she who takes care of the sheep.

Owen **BG** (Irish) born to nobility; young warrior. (Welsh) a form of Evan.

Owena (Welsh) a form of Owen.

Oya BG (Moquelumnan) called forth.

Oz BG (Hebrew) strength.

Ozara (Hebrew) treasure, wealth.

P

P BG (American) an initial used as a first name.

Pabla (Spanish) little.

Paca (Spanish) a short form of Pancha. See also Paka.

Pacífica (Spanish) derived from the name of the Pacific Ocean.

Padget BG (French) a form of Page.
Padgett, Paget, Pagett

Padma (Hindi) lotus.

Page GB (French) young assistant.
Pagen, Pagi, Payge

Paige ☀ GB (English) young child.
Payge

Paisley (Scottish) patterned fabric first made in Paisley, Scotland.
Paislay, Paislee, Paisleyann, Paisleyanne, Paizlei, Paizleigh, Paizley, Pasley, Pazley

Paiton (English) warrior's town.
Paiten, Paityn, Paityne, Paiyton, Paten, Patton

Paka (Swahili) kitten. See also Paca.

Pakuna (Moquelumnan) deer bounding while running downhill.

Palaciada, Palaciata (Greek) she who has a sumptuous mansion.

Paladia (Spanish) a form of Pallas.

Palas (Greek) goddess of wisdom and war.

Palba (Basque) blond.

Palila (Polynesian) bird.

Palixena (Greek) she who returns from the foreign land.

Pallas (Greek) wise. Mythology: another name for Athena, the goddess of wisdom.

Palma (Latin) palm tree.
Pallma, Palmira

Palmera (Spanish) palm tree.

Palmira (Spanish) a form of Palma.
Pallmirah, Pallmyra, Palmer, Palmyra

Paloma GB (Spanish) dove. See also Aloma.
Palloma, Palometa, Palomita, Paluma, Peloma

Pamela (Greek) honey.
Pam, Pama, Pamala, Pamalla,
Pamelia, Pamelina, Pamella,
Pamila, Pamilla, Pammela,
Pammi, Pammie, Pammy, Pamula

Panambi (Guarani) butterfly.

Pancha (Spanish) free; from
France.
Paca, Panchita

Pancracia (Greek) she who has
all the power.

Pandita (Hindi) scholar.

Pandora (Greek) all-gifted.
Mythology: a woman who opened
a box out of curiosity and
released evil into the world. See
also Dora.
Pandi, Pandorah, Pandorra,
Pandorrah, Pandy, Panndora,
Panndorah, Panndorra,
Panndorrah

Pansy (Greek) flower; fragrant.
(French) thoughtful.
Pansey, Pansie

Panthea (Greek) all the gods.
Pantheia, Pantheya

Panya (Swahili) mouse; tiny baby.
(Russian) a familiar form of
Stephanie.
Panyia

Panyin (Fante) older twin.

Paola GB (Italian) a form of
Paula.
Paoli, Paolina

Papina (Moquelumnan) vine
growing on an oak tree.

Paquita (Spanish) a form of
Frances.
Paqua

Pardeep BG (Sikh) mystic light.

Pari (Persian) fairy eagle.

Paris GB (French) Geography: the
capital of France. Mythology: the
Trojan prince who started the
Trojan War by abducting Helen.
Parice, Paries, Parisa, Parise,
Parish, Parisha, Pariss, Parissa,
Parisse, Parris, Parys, Parysse

Parker BG (English) park keeper.
Park, Parke

Parmenia (Greek) constant,
faithful.

Parmenias (Spanish) a form of
Parmenia.

Parris (French) a form of Paris.
Parrise, Parrish, Parrisha, Parrys,
Parrysh

Partenia (Greek) she who is as
pure as a virgin.

Parthenia (Greek) virginal.
Partheenia, Parthenie, Parthinia,
Pathina

Parveneh (Persian) butterfly.

Pascal BG (French) born on
Easter or Passover.
Pascalette, Pascaline, Pascalle,
Paschale, Paskel

Pascale GB (French) a form of Pascal.

Pascua, Pascualina (Hebrew) she who was born during the Easter festivities.

Pascuala (Spanish) born during the Easter season.

Pascuas (Hebrew) sacrificed for the good of the village.

Pasha BG (Greek) sea.
Palasha, Pascha, Pasche, Pashae, Pashe, Pashel, Pashka, Pasia, Passia

Passion (Latin) passion.
Pashion, Pashonne, Pasion, Passionaé, Passionate, Passionette

Pastora (German) shepherdess.

Pasua (Swahili) born by cesarean section.

Pat BG (Latin) a short form of Patricia, Patsy.

Pati (Moquelumnan) fish baskets made of willow branches.

Patia (Gypsy, Spanish) leaf. (Latin, English) a familiar form of Patience, Patricia.

Patience (English) patient.
Paciencia, Patia, Patiance, Patient, Patince, Patishia

Patra (Greek, Latin) a form of Petra.

Patrice GB (French) a form of Patricia.
Patrease, Patrece, Patreece, Patreese, Patreice, Patriece, Patryce, Pattrice

Patricia GB (Latin) noblewoman. See also Payton, Peyton, Tricia, Trisha, Trissa.
Pat, Patia, Patresa, Patrica, Patrice, Patricea, Patriceia, Patrichea, Patriciana, Patricianna, Patricja, Patricka, Patrickia, Patrisha, Patrishia, Patrisia, Patrissa, Patrizia, Patrizzia, Patrycia, Patrycja, Patsy, Patty

Patrick BG (Latin) noble. Religion: the patron saint of Ireland.

Patsy (Latin) a familiar form of Patricia.
Pat, Patsey, Patsi

Patty (English) a familiar form of Patricia.
Patte, Pattee, Patti, Pattie

Paul BG (Latin) small.

Paula (Latin) a form of Paul. See also Pavla, Polly.
Paliki, Paola, Paulane, Paulann, Paule, Paulette, Paulina, Pauline, Paulla, Pavia

Paulette (Latin) a familiar form of Paula.
Paulet, Paulett, Pauletta, Paulita, Paullett, Paulletta, Paullette

Paulina (Slavic) a form of Paula.
Paulena, Paulene, Paulenia,

Pauliana, Paulianne, Paullena,
Paulyna, Pawlina, Polena, Polina,
Polinia

Pauline (French) a form of Paula.
Pauleen, Paulene, Paulien, Paulin,
Paulyne, Paulynn, Pouline

Pausha (Hindi) lunar month of
Capricorn.

Pavla (Czech, Russian) a form of
Paula.
Pavlina, Pavlinka

Paxton BG (Latin) peaceful town.
Paxtin, Paxtynn

Payge (English) a form of Paige.

Payton GB (Irish) a form of
Patricia.
Paydon, Paytan, Payten, Paytin,
Paytn, Paytton

Paz GB (Spanish) peace.

Pazi (Ponca) yellow bird.

Pazia (Hebrew) golden.
Paza, Pazice, Pazit

Peace (English) peaceful.

Pearl (Latin) jewel.
Pearle, Pearleen, Pearlena,
Pearlene, Pearlette, Pearlina,
Pearline, Pearlisha, Pearlyn, Perl,
Perla, Perle, Perlette, Perlie,
Perline, Perlline

Pedra (Portuguese) rock.

Peggy (Greek) a familiar form of
Margaret.
Peg, Pegeen, Pegg, Peggey,
Peggi, Peggie, Pegi

Peke (Hawaiian) a form of
Bertha.

Pela (Polish) a short form of
Penelope.
Pele

Pelagia (Greek) sea.
Pelage, Pelageia, Pelagie, Pelga,
Pelgia, Pellagia

Pelipa (Zuni) a form of Philippa.

Pemba (Bambara) the power that
controls all life.

Penda (Swahili) loved.

Penelope (Greek) weaver.
Mythology: the clever and loyal
wife of Odysseus, a Greek hero.
Pela, Pen, Penelopa, Penna,
Pennelope, Penny, Pinelopi

Penélope (Greek) a form of
Penelope.

Peni (Carrier) mind.

Peninah (Hebrew) pearl.
Penina, Peninit, Peninnah, Penny

Penny (Greek) a familiar form of
Penelope, Peninah.
Penee, Peni, Penney, Penni,
Pennie

Peony (Greek) flower.
Peonie

Pepita (Spanish) a familiar form
of Josephine.
Pepa, Pepi, Peppy, Peta

Pepper (Latin) condiment from
the pepper plant.

Perah (Hebrew) flower.

Perdita (Latin) lost. Literature: a character in Shakespeare's play *The Winter's Tale.*
Perdida, Perdy

Peregrina (Latin) pilgrim, traveler.

Perfecta (Spanish) flawless.

Peri (Greek) mountain dweller. (Persian) fairy or elf.
Perita

Perla (Latin) a form of Pearl.
Pearla

Perlie (Latin) a familiar form of Pearl.
Pearley, Pearlie, Pearly, Perley, Perli, Perly, Purley, Purly

Perlita (Spanish) a form of Perla.

Pernella (Greek, French) rock. (Latin) a short form of Petronella.
Parnella, Pernel, Pernell, Pernelle

Perpetua (Spanish) continuous.

Perri (Greek, Latin) small rock; traveler. (French) pear tree. (Welsh) child of Harry.
Perre, Perrey, Perriann, Perrie, Perrin, Perrine, Perry

Perry BG (Greek, French, Welsh) a form of Perri.

Persephone (Greek) Mythology: the goddess of the underworld.
Persephanie, Persephany, Persephonie

Perseveranda (Latin) she who perseveres on the good road.

Persis (Latin) from Persia.
Perssis, Persy

Peta (Blackfoot) golden eagle.

Peter BG (Greek, Latin) small rock.

Petra (Greek, Latin) small rock. A short form of Petronella.
Patra, Pet, Peta, Petena, Peterina, Petraann, Petrice, Petrina, Petrine, Petrova, Petrovna, Pier, Pierce, Pietra

Petronella (Greek) small rock. (Latin) of the Roman clan Petronius.
Pernella, Peternella, Petra, Petrona, Petronela, Petronella, Petronelle, Petronia, Petronija, Petronilla, Petronille

Petula (Latin) seeker.
Petulah

Petunia (Native American) flower.

Peyeche (Mapuche) unforgettable woman, remembered; popular, sought-after.

Peyton BG (Irish) a form of Patricia.
Peyden, Peydon, Peyten, Peytyn

Phaedra (Greek) bright.
Faydra, Phae, Phaidra, Phe, Phedre

Phallon (Irish) a form of Fallon.
Phalaine, Phalen, Phallan, Phallie,
Phalon, Phalyn

Phebe (Greek) a form of Phoebe.
Pheba, Pheby

Pheodora (Greek, Russian) a
form of Feodora.
Phedora, Phedorah, Pheodorah,
Pheydora, Pheydorah

Philana (Greek) lover of
mankind.
Phila, Philanna, Philene, Philiane,
Philina, Philine

Philantha (Greek) lover of
flowers.

Philicia (Latin) a form of
Phylicia.
Philecia, Philesha, Philica,
Philicha, Philycia

Philip 🅑🅖 (Greek) lover of
horses.

Philippa (Greek) a form of
Philip. See also Filippa.
Phil, Philipa, Philippe, Phillipina,
Phillippine, Phillie, Philly, Pippa,
Pippy

Philomena (Greek) love song;
loved one. Bible: a first-century
saint. See also Filomena, Mena.
Philoméne, Philomina

Phoebe (Greek) shining.
Phaebe, Phebe, Pheobe, Phoebey

Phylicia (Latin) fortunate; happy.
(Greek) a form of Felicia.
Philicia, Phylecia, Phylesha,

Phylesia, Phylica, Phylisha,
Phylisia, Phylissa, Phyllecia,
Phyllicia, Phyllisha, Phyllisia,
Phyllissa, Phyllyza

Phyllida (Greek) a form of
Phyllis.
Fillida, Philida, Phillida, Phillyda

Phyllis (Greek) green bough.
Filise, Fillys, Fyllis, Philis, Phillis,
Philliss, Philys, Philyss, Phylis,
Phyllida, Phyllis, Phylliss, Phyllys

Pia (Latin, Italian) devout.
Pía

Piedad (Spanish) devoted; pious.

Pier (French) a form of Petra.
Pierette, Pierrette, Pierra, Pierre

Pierce 🅑🅖 (English) a form of
Petra.

Pierre 🅑🅖 (French) a form of
Pier.

Pilar (Spanish) pillar, column.
Peelar, Pilár, Pillar

Pili (Spanish) a form of Pilar.

Pilmayquen (Araucanian)
swallow.

Pimpinela (Latin) fickle one.

Ping (Chinese) duckweed.
(Vietnamese) peaceful.

Pinga (Eskimo) Mythology: the
goddess of game and the hunt.

Piper (English) pipe player.

Pippa (English) a short form of Phillipa.

Pippi (French) rosy cheeked.
Pippen, Pippie, Pippin, Pippy

Piro (Mapuche) snows.

Pita (African) fourth daughter.

Pitrel (Mapuche) very small woman.

Plácida (Latin) she who is gentle and peaceful.

Placidia (Latin) serene.
Placida

Pleasance (French) pleasant.
Pleasence

Polimnia (Greek) a form of Polyhymnia, one of the nine Muses; she who inspires hymns.

Polixena (Greek) welcoming one.

Polla (Arabic) poppy.
Pola

Polly (Latin) a familiar form of Paula.
Paili, Pali, Pauli, Paulie, Pauly, Poll, Pollee, Polley, Polli, Pollie

Pollyam (Hindi) goddess of the plague. Religion: the Hindu name invoked to ward off bad spirits.

Pollyanna (English) a combination of Polly + Anna. Literature: an overly optimistic heroine created by Eleanor Porter.

Poloma (Choctaw) bow.

Pomona (Latin) apple. Mythology: the goddess of fruit and fruit trees.

Poni (African) second daughter.

Popea (Greek) venerable mother.

Poppy (Latin) poppy flower.
Popi, Poppey, Poppi, Poppie

Pora, Poria (Hebrew) fruitful.

Porcha (Latin) a form of Portia.
Porchae, Porchai, Porche, Porchia, Porcia

Porscha, Porsche (German) forms of Portia.
Porcsha, Porcshe, Porschah, Porsché, Porschea, Porschia, Pourche

Porsha (Latin) a form of Portia.
Porshai, Porshay, Porshe, Porshea, Porshia

Portia (Latin) offering. Literature: the heroine of Shakespeare's play *The Merchant of Venice*.
Porcha, Porscha, Porsche, Porsha, Portiea

Prabhjot 🅱🅶 (Sikh) the light of God.

Praxedes (Greek) she who has firm intentions.

Práxedes (Greek) a form of Praxedes.

Preciosa (Latin) she who possesses great valor and is invaluable.

Precious (French) precious; dear.
Pracious, Preciouse, Precisha, Prescious, Preshious, Presious

Presencia (Spanish) presence.

Presentación (Latin) she who expresses herself.

Presley GB (English) priest's meadow.
Preslea, Preslee, Preslei, Presli, Preslie, Presly, Preslye, Pressley, Presslie, Pressly

Presta (Spanish) hurry, quick.

Preston BG (English) priest's estate.

Prima (Latin) first, beginning; first child.
Prema, Primalia, Primetta, Primina, Priminia

Primavera (Italian, Spanish) spring.

Primitiva (Latin) first of all.

Primrose (English) primrose flower.
Primula

Princess (English) daughter of royalty.
Princcess, Princes, Princesa, Princessa, Princetta, Princie, Princilla

Priscilla (Latin) ancient.
Cilla, Piri, Precila, Precilla, Prescilla, Presilla, Pressilia, Pricila, Pricilla, Pris, Prisca, Priscela, Priscella, Priscila, Priscilia, Priscill, Priscille, Priscillia, Prisella, Prisila, Prisilla, Prissila, Prissilla, Prissy, Pryscylla, Prysilla

Prissy (Latin) a familiar form of Priscilla.
Prisi, Priss, Prissi, Prissie

Priya (Hindi) beloved; sweet natured.
Pria

Procopia (Latin) declared leader.

Promise (Latin) promise, pledge.
Promis, Promiss, Promys, Promyse

Proserpina (Greek) she who wants to annihilate.

Próspera (Greek) prosperous.

Pru (Latin) a short form of Prudence.
Prue

Prudence (Latin) cautious; discreet.
Pru, Prudencia, Prudens, Prudy

Prudenciana (Spanish) modest and honest.

Prudy (Latin) a familiar form of Prudence.
Prudee, Prudi, Prudie

Prunella (Latin) brown; little plum. See also Nellie.
Prunela

Psyche (Greek) soul. Mythology: a beautiful mortal loved by Eros, the Greek god of love.

Pua (Hawaiian) flower.

Pualani (Hawaiian) heavenly flower.
Puni

Puebla (Spanish) taken from the name of the Mexican city.

Pura (English) a form of Purity.

Purificación (Spanish) a form of Pura.

Purity (English) purity.
Pureza, Purisima

Pyralis (Greek) fire. *Pyrene*

Qadira (Arabic) powerful.
Kadira

Qamra (Arabic) moon.
Kamra

Qitarah (Arabic) fragrant.

Quaashie BG (Ewe) born on Sunday.

Quadeisha (American) a combination of Qadira + Aisha.
Qudaisha, Quadaishia, Quadajah, Quadasha, Quadasia, Quadayshia, Quadaza, Quadejah, Quadesha, Quadeshia, Quadiasha, Quaesha

Quaneisha (American) a combination of the prefix Qu + Niesha.
Quaneasa, Quanece, Quanecia, Quaneice, Quanesha, Quanisha, Quansha, Quarnisha, Queisha, Qwanisha, Qynisha

Quanesha (American) a form of Quaneisha.
Quamesha, Quaneesha, Quaneshia, Quanesia, Quanessa, Quanessia, Quannesha, Quanneshia, Quannezia, Quayneshia, Quinesha

Quanika (American) a combination of the prefix Qu + Nika.
Quanikka, Quanikki, Quaniqua, Quanique, Quantenique, Quawanica, Queenika, Queenique

Quanisha (American) a form of Quaneisha.
Quaniesha, Quanishia, Quaynisha, Queenisha, Quenisha, Quenishia

Quartilla (Latin) fourth.
Quantilla

Qubilah (Arabic) agreeable.

Queen (English) queen. See also Quinn.
Queena, Queenie, Quenna

Queenie (English) a form of Queen.
Queenation, Queeneste, Queeny

Queisha (American) a short form of Quaneisha.
Qeysha, Queshia, Queysha

Quenby BG (Scandinavian) feminine.

Quenisha (American) a combination of Queen + Aisha.
Queneesha, Quenesha, Quennisha, Quensha, Quinesha, Quinisha

Quenna (English) a form of Queen.
Quenell, Quenessa

Quentin BG (Latin) fifth. (English) queen's town.

Querida (Spanish) dear; beloved.

Querima, Querina (Arabic) generous one.

Quesara (Latin) youthful.

Questa (French) searcher.

Queta (Spanish) a short form of names ending in "queta" or "quetta."
Quenetta, Quetta

Quetromán (Mapuche) mute condor; restrained soul; prudence.

Quiana (American) a combination of the prefix Qu + Anna.
Quian, Quianah, Quianda, Quiane,

Quiani, Quianita, Quianna, Quianne, Quionna

Quíbele (Turkish) goddess mother.

Quiliana (Spanish) substantial; productive.

Quillen (Spanish) woman of the heights.

Quimey (Mapuche) beautiful.

Quinby (Scandinavian) queen's estate.

Quincy BG (Irish) fifth.
Quincee, Quincey, Quinci, Quincia, Quincie

Quinella (Latin) a form of Quintana.

Quinesburga (Anglo-Saxon) royal strength.

Quinesha, Quinisha (American) forms of Quenisha.
Quineshia, Quinessa, Quinessia, Quinisa, Quinishia, Quinnesha, Quinneshia, Quinnisha, Quneasha, Quonesha, Quonisha, Quonnisha

Quinetta (Latin) a form of Quintana.
Queenetta, Queenette, Quinette, Quinita, Quinnette

Quinn BG (German, English) queen. See also Queen.
Quin, Quinna, Quinne, Quynn

Quinshawna (American) a combination of Quinn + Shauna. *Quinshea*

Quintana (Latin) fifth. (English) queen's lawn. See also Quinella, Quinetta.
Quinntina, Quinta, Quintanna, Quintara, Quintarah, Quintia, Quintila, Quintilla, Quintina, Quintona, Quintonice

Quintessa (Latin) essence. See also Tess.
Quintaysha, Quintesa, Quintesha, Quintessia, Quintice, Quinticia, Quintisha, Quintosha

Quintiliana (Spanish) born in the fifth month of the year.

Quinton 🅱🅶 (Latin) a form of Quentin.

Quintrell (American) a combination of Quinn + Trella.
Quintela, Quintella, Quintrelle

Quintruy (Mapuche) investigator; woman of initiative and curiosity; leader.

Quintuqueo (Mapuche) she who searches for wisdom; woman of experience, having the gifts of knowledge, counseling, and perfection.

Quinturay (Mapuche) she who has a flower; she whose goal is to find the nectar and the essence of the flower.

Quionia (Greek) she who is fertile.

Quirina (Latin) she who carries the lance.

Quirita (Latin) citizen.

Quiterie (Latin, French) tranquil.
Quita

Qwanisha (American) a form of Quaneisha.
Qwanechia, Qwanesha, Qwanessia, Qwantasha

R

R 🅱🅶 (American) an initial used as a first name.

Rabecca (Hebrew) a form of Rebecca.
Rabecka, Rabeca, Rabekah

Rabi 🅱🅶 (Arabic) breeze.
Rabia, Rabiah

Rachael (Hebrew) a form of Rachel.
Rachaele, Rachaell, Rachail, Rachalle

Racheal (Hebrew) a form of Rachel.

Rachel ☆ 🅶🅱 (Hebrew) female sheep. Bible: the second wife of Jacob. See also Lahela, Rae, Rochelle.
Racha, Rachael, Rachal, Racheal, Rachela, Rachelann, Rachele, Rachelle, Racquel, Raechel, Rahel, Rahela, Rahil, Raiche, Raquel,

Rashel, Rashelle, Ray, Raycene,
Raychel, Raychelle, Rey, Ruchel

Rachelle (French) a form of
Rachel. See also Shelley.
Rachalle, Rachell, Rachella,
Raechell, Raechelle, Raeshelle,
Rashel, Rashele, Rashell, Rashelle,
Raychell, Rayshell, Ruchelle

Racquel (French) a form of
Rachel.
Rackel, Racquell, Racquella,
Racquelle

Radegunda (German) she who
counsels regarding battling.

Radella (German) counselor.

Radeyah (Arabic) content, satisfied.
Radeeyah, Radhiya, Radiah,
Radiyah

Radinka (Slavic) full of life;
happy, glad.

Radmilla (Slavic) worker for the
people.

Rae (English) doe. (Hebrew) a
short form of Rachel.
Raeh, Raeneice, Raeneisha,
Raesha, Ray, Raye, Rayetta,
Rayette, Rayma, Rey

Raeann (American) a
combination of Rae + Ann. See
also Rayanne.
Raea, Raean, Raeanna,
Raeannah, Raeona, Reanna,
Raeanne

Raechel (Hebrew) a form of
Rachel.
Raechael, Raechal, Raechele,
Raechell, Raechyl

Raeden (Japanese) Mythology:
Raiden was the god of thunder
and lightning.
Raeda, Raedeen

Raegan GB (Irish) a form of
Reagan.
Raegen, Raegene, Raegine,
Raegyn

Raelene (American) a
combination of Rae + Lee.
Rael, Raela, Raelani, Raele,
Raeleah, Raelee, Raeleen,
Raeleia, Raeleigh, Raeleigha,
Raelein, Raelene, Raelennia,
Raelesha, Raelin, Raelina, Raelle,
Raelyn, Raelynn

Raelyn, Raelynn (American)
forms of Raelene.
Raelynda, Raelyne, Raelynne

Raena (German) a form of Raina.
Raenah, Raenia, Raenie, Raenna,
Raeonna, Raeyauna, Raeyn,
Raeyonna

Raeven (English) a form of
Raven.
Raevin, Raevion, Raevon,
Raevonna, Raevyn, Raevynne,
Raewyn, Raewynne, Raivan,
Raiven, Raivin, Raivyn

Rafa (Arabic) happy; prosperous.

Rafael BG (Spanish) a form of
Raphael.

Rafaela (Hebrew) a form of
Raphaela.
Rafaelia, Rafaella

Ragan (Irish) a form of Reagan.
*Ragean, Rageane, Rageen,
Ragen, Ragene, Rageni, Ragenna,
Raggan, Raygan, Raygen,
Raygene, Rayghan, Raygin*

Ragine (English) a form of Regina.
Raegina, Ragin, Ragina, Raginee

Ragnild (Scandinavian) battle
counsel.
*Ragna, Ragnell, Ragnhild, Rainell,
Renilda, Renilde*

Raheem BG (Punjabi)
compassionate God.
Raheema, Rahima

Ráidah (Arabic) leader.

Raimunda (Spanish) wise
defender.

Raina (German) mighty. (English)
a short form of Regina. See also
Rayna.
*Raeinna, Raena, Raheena, Rain,
Rainah, Rainai, Raine, Rainea,
Rainna, Reanna*

Rainbow (English) rainbow.
*Rainbeau, Rainbeaux, Rainbo,
Raynbow*

Raine GB (Latin) a short form of
Regina. A form of Raina, Rane.
*Rainee, Rainey, Raini, Rainie,
Rainy, Reyne*

Raingarda (German) prudent
defender.

Raisa (Russian) a form of Rose.
*Raisah, Raissa, Raiza, Raysa,
Rayza, Razia*

Raizel (Yiddish) a form of Rose.
Rayzil, Razil, Reizel, Resel

Raja (Arabic) hopeful.
Raia, Rajaah, Rajae, Rajah, Rajai

Raku (Japanese) pleasure.

Raleigh BG (Irish) a form of Riley.
Ralea, Raleiah, Raley

Ralph BG (English) wolf counselor.

Rama (Hebrew) lofty, exalted.
(Hindi) godlike. Religion: an
incarnation of the Hindu god
Vishnu.
Ramah

Raman GB (Spanish) a form of
Ramona.

Ramandeep (Sikh) covered by
the light of the Lord's love.

Ramira (Spanish) judicious.

Ramla (Swahili) fortuneteller.
Ramlah

Ramona (Spanish) mighty; wise
protector. See also Mona.
*Raman, Ramonda, Raymona,
Romona, Romonda*

Ramsey BG (English) ram's island.
Ramsha, Ramsi, Ramsie, Ramza

Ran (Japanese) water lily.
(Scandinavian) destroyer.
Mythology: the Norse sea goddess
who destroys.

Rana (Sanskrit) royal. (Arabic) gaze, look.
Rahna, Rahni, Rani

Ranait (Irish) graceful; prosperous.
Rane, Renny

Randall BG (English) protected.
Randa, Randah, Randal, Randalee, Randel, Randell, Randelle, Randi, Randilee, Randilynn, Randlyn, Randy, Randyl

Randi GB (English) a familiar form of Miranda, Randall.
Rande, Randee, Randeen, Randene, Randey, Randie, Randii

Randy BG (English) a form of Randi.

Rane (Scandinavian) queen.
Raine

Rani GB (Sanskrit) queen. (Hebrew) joyful. A short form of Kerani.
Rahni, Ranee, Raney, Rania, Ranie, Ranice, Ranique, Ranni, Rannie

Ranita (Hebrew) song; joyful.
Ranata, Ranice, Ranit, Ranite, Ranitta, Ronita

Raniyah (Arabic) gazing.
Ranya, Ranyah

Rapa (Hawaiian) moonbeam.

Raphael BG (Hebrew) God has healed.

Raphaela (Hebrew) healed by God.
Rafaella, Raphaella, Raphaelle

Raphaelle (French) a form of Raphaela.
Rafaelle, Raphael, Raphaele

Raquel GB (French) a form of Rachel.
Rakel, Rakhil, Rakhila, Raqueal, Raquela, Raquella, Raquelle, Rickelle, Rickquel, Ricquel, Ricquelle, Rikell, Rikelle, Rockell

Raquildis (German) fighting princess.

Rasha (Arabic) young gazelle.
Rahshea, Rahshia, Rashae, Rashai, Rashea, Rashi, Rashia

Rashawn BG (American) a form of Rashawna.

Rashawna (American) a combination of the prefix Ra + Shawna.
Rashana, Rashanae, Rashanah, Rashanda, Rashane, Rashani, Rashanna, Rashanta, Rashaun, Rashauna, Rashaunda, Rashaundra, Rashaune, Rashawn, Rashawnda, Rashawnna, Rashon, Rashona, Rashonda, Rashunda

Rasheed BG (Arabic) a form of Rashad (see Boys' Names).

Rashel, Rashelle (American) forms of Rachel.
Rashele, Rashell, Rashella

Rashida GB (Swahili, Turkish) righteous.
Rahshea, Rahsheda, Rahsheita, Rashdah, Rasheda, Rashedah, Rasheeda, Rasheedah, Rasheeta, Rasheida, Rashidah, Rashidi

Rashieka (Arabic) descended from royalty.
Rasheeka, Rasheika, Rasheka, Rashika, Rasika

Rasia (Greek) rose.

Ratana (Tai) crystal.
Ratania, Ratanya, Ratna, Rattan, Rattana

Ratri (Hindi) night. Religion: the goddess of the night.

Ratrudis (German) faithful counselor.

Raula (French) wolf counselor.
Raoula, Raulla, Raulle

Raven GB (English) blackbird.
Raeven, Raveen, Raveena, Raveenn, Ravena, Ravene, Ravenn, Ravenna, Ravennah, Ravenne, Raveon, Ravin, Ravon, Ravyn, Rayven, Revena

Ravin (English) a form of Raven.
Ravi, Ravina, Ravine, Ravinne, Ravion

Ravyn (English) a form of Raven.
Ravynn

Rawnie (Gypsy) fine lady.
Rawan, Rawna, Rhawnie

Ray BG (Hebrew) a short form of Raya.

Raya (Hebrew) friend.
Raia, Raiah, Raiya, Ray, Rayah

Rayanne (American) a form of Raeann.
Rayane, Ray-Ann, Rayan, Rayana, Rayann, Rayanna, Rayeanna, Rayona, Rayonna, Reyan, Reyana, Reyann, Reyanna, Reyanne

Raychel, Raychelle (Hebrew) forms of Rachel.
Raychael, Raychele, Raychell, Raychil

Rayén (Araucanian, Mapuche) flower.

Raylene (American) forms of Raylyn.
Ralina, Rayel, Rayele, Rayelle, Rayleana, Raylee, Rayleen, Rayleigh, Raylena, Raylin, Raylinn, Raylona, Raylyn, Raylynn, Raylynne

Raymonde (German) wise protector.
Rayma, Raymae, Raymie

Rayna (Scandinavian) mighty. (Yiddish) pure, clean. (English) king's advisor. (French) a familiar form of Lorraine. See also Raina.
Raynah, Rayne, Raynell, Raynelle, Raynette, Rayona, Rayonna, Reyna

Rayven (English) a form of
Raven.
*Rayvan, Rayvana, Rayvein,
Rayvenne, Rayveona, Rayvin,
Rayvon, Rayvonia*

Rayya (Arabic) thirsty no longer.

Razi **BG** (Aramaic) secretive.
*Rayzil, Rayzilee, Raz, Razia,
Raziah, Raziela, Razilee, Razili*

Raziya (Swahili) agreeable.

Rea (Greek) poppy flower.
Reah

Reagan **GB** (Irish) little ruler.
Reagen, Reaghan, Reagine

Reanna (German, English) a form
of Raina. (American) a form of
Raeann.
Reannah

Reanne (American) a form of
Raeann, Reanna.
*Reana, Reane, Reann, Reannan,
Reanne, Reannen, Reannon,
Reeana*

Reba (Hebrew) fourth-born child.
A short form of Rebecca. See also
Reva, Riva.
Rabah, Reeba, Rheba

Rebeca (Hebrew) an alernate
form of Rebecca.
Rebbeca, Rebecah

Rebecca ☀ **GB** (Hebrew) tied,
bound. Bible: the wife of Isaac.
See also Becca, Becky.
*Rabecca, Reba, Rebbecca,
Rebeca, Rebeccah, Rebeccea,*
*Rebeccka, Rebecha, Rebecka,
Rebeckah, Rebeckia, Rebecky,
Rebekah, Rebeque, Rebi, Reveca,
Riva, Rivka*

Rebekah **GB** (Hebrew) a form of
Rebecca.
*Rebeka, Rebekha, Rebekka,
Rebekkah, Rebekke, Revecca,
Reveka, Revekka, Rifka*

Rebi (Hebrew) a familiar form of
Rebecca.
*Rebbie, Rebe, Rebie, Reby, Ree,
Reebie*

Reece **BG** (Welsh) a form of
Rhys.

Reed **BG** (English) a form of
Reid.

Reena (Greek) peaceful.
(English) a form of Rina.
(Hebrew) a form of Rinah.
Reen, Reenie, Rena, Reyna

Reese **BG** (Welsh) a form of
Reece.

Reet (Estonian) a form of
Margaret.
Reatha, Reta, Retha

Regan **GB** (Irish) a form of
Reagan.
Regane, Reghan

Reganne (Irish) a form of
Reagan.
Raegan, Ragan, Reagan, Regin

Reggie **BG** (English) a familiar
form of Regina.
Reggi, Reggy, Regi, Regia, Regie

Regina (Latin) queen. (English) king's advisor. Geography: the capital of Saskatchewan. See also Gina.
Ragine, Raina, Raine, Rega, Regena, Regennia, Reggie, Regiena, Regine, Reginia, Regis, Reina, Rena

Reginald 🅱🅶 (English) king's advisor.

Regine (Latin) a form of Regina.
Regin

Rei 🅶🅱 (Japanese) polite, well behaved.
Reiko

Reia (Spanish) a form of Reina.

Reid 🅱🅶 (English) redhead.

Reilly 🅱🅶 (Irish) a form of Riley.
Reilee, Reileigh, Reiley, Reili, Reilley, Reily

Reina (Spanish) a short form of Regina. See also Reyna.
Reinah, Reine, Reinette, Reinie, Reinna, Reiny, Reiona, Renia, Rina

Rekha (Hindi) thin line.
Reka, Rekia, Rekiah, Rekiya

Relinda (German) kind-hearted princess.

Remedios (Spanish) remedy.

Remi 🅱🅶 (French) from Rheims, France.
Raymi, Remee, Remie, Remy

Remington 🅱🅶 (English) raven estate.
Remmington

Ren (Japanese) arranger; water lily; lotus.

Rena (Hebrew) song; joy. A familiar form of Irene, Regina, Renata, Sabrina, Serena.
Reena, Rina, Rinna, Rinnah

Renae (French) a form of Renée.
Renay

Renata (French) a form of Renée.
Ranata, Rena, Renada, Renatta, Renita, Rennie, Renyatta, Rinada, Rinata

Rene 🅱🅶 (Greek) a short form of Irene, Renée.
Reen, Reenie, Reney, Rennie

Renee 🅶🅱 (French) a form of René.

Renée (French) born again.
Renae, Renata, Renay, Rene, Renea, Reneigh, Renell, Renelle, Renne

Renita (French) a form of Renata.
Reneeta, Renetta, Renitza

Rennie (English) a familiar form of Renata.
Reni, Renie, Renni

Reseda (Spanish) fragrant mignonette blossom.

Reshawna (American) a combination of the prefix Re + Shawna.
Resaunna, Reshana, Reshaunda,

*Reshawnda, Reshawnna,
Reshonda, Reshonn, Reshonta*

Resi (German) a familiar form of
Theresa.
*Resia, Ressa, Resse, Ressie,
Reza, Rezka, Rezi*

Reta (African) shaken.
Reeta, Retta, Rheta, Rhetta

Reubena (Hebrew) behold a
child.
*Reubina, Reuvena, Rubena,
Rubenia, Rubina, Rubine, Rubyna*

Reva (Latin) revived. (Hebrew)
rain; one-fourth. A form of Reba,
Riva.
Ree, Reeva, Revia, Revida

Reveca, Reveka (Slavic) forms
of Rebecca, Rebekah.
Reve, Revecca, Revekka, Rivka

Rexanne (American) queen.
Rexan, Rexana, Rexann, Rexanna

Reya (Spanish) a form of Reina.

Reyes (Spanish) a form of Reyna.

Reyhan BG (Turkish) sweet-
smelling flower.

Reyna (Greek) peaceful.
(English) a form of Reina.
Reyana, Reyanna, Reyni, Reynna

Reynalda (German) king's
advisor.

Réz BG (Latin, Hungarian)
copper-colored hair.

Reza (Czech) a form of Theresa.
Rezi, Rezka

Rhea (Greek) brook, stream.
Mythology: the mother of Zeus.
*Rheá, Rhéa, Rhealyn, Rheanna,
Rhia, Rhianna*

Rheanna, Rhianna (Greek)
forms of Rhea.
*Rheana, Rheann, Rheanne,
Rhiana, Rhiauna*

Rhett BG (Welsh) a form of Rhys.

Rhian (Welsh) a short form of
Rhiannon.
*Rhianne, Rhyan, Rhyann,
Rhyanne, Rian, Riane, Riann,
Rianne, Riayn*

Rhiannon (Welsh) witch; nymph;
goddess.
*Rheannan, Rheannin, Rheannon,
Rheanon, Rhian, Rhianen,
Rhianna, Rhiannan, Rhiannen,
Rhianon, Rhianwen, Rhinnon,
Rhyanna, Riana, Riannon, Rianon*

Rhoda (Greek) from Rhodes,
Greece.
*Rhode, Rhodeia, Rhodie, Rhody,
Roda, Rodi, Rodie, Rodina*

Rhona (Scottish) powerful,
mighty. (English) king's advisor.
Rhonae, Rhonnie

Rhonda (Welsh) grand.
*Rhondene, Rhondiesha, Ronda,
Ronelle, Ronnette*

Rhys BG (Welsh) enthusiastic;
stream.

Ria (Spanish) river.
Riah

Riana, Rianna (Irish) short
forms of Briana. (Arabic) forms
of Rihana.
Reana, Reanna, Rhianna,
Rhyanna, Riana, Rianah

Rica (Spanish) a short form of
Erica, Frederica, Ricarda. See also
Enrica, Sandrica, Terrica, Ulrica.
Ricca, Rieca, Riecka, Rieka, Rikka,
Riqua, Rycca

Ricarda (Spanish) rich and
powerful ruler.
Rica, Richanda, Richarda, Richi,
Ricki

Ricardo 🅱🅶 (Portuguese,
Spanish) a form of Richard.

Richael (Irish) saint.

Richard 🅱🅶 (English) a form of
Richart (see Boys' Names).

Richelle (German, French) a
form of Ricarda.
Richel, Richela, Richele, Richell,
Richella, Richia

Rickelle (American) a form of
Raquel.
Rickel, Rickela, Rickell

Rickey 🅱🅶 (English) a familiar
form of Richard.

Ricki, Rikki 🅶🅱 (American)
familiar forms of Erica,
Frederica, Ricarda.
Rica, Ricci, Riccy, Rici, Rickee,
Rickia, Rickie, Rickilee, Rickina,
Rickita, Ricky, Ricquie, Riki, Rikia,
Rikita, Rikka, Rikke, Rikkia, Rikkie,
Rikky, Riko

Ricky 🅱🅶 (American) a form of
Ricki.

Rico 🅱🅶 (Spanish) a familiar form
of Richard. (Italian) a short form
of Enrico (see Boys' Names).

Ricquel (American) a form of
Raquel.
Rickquell, Ricquelle, Rikell,
Rikelle

Rida 🅱🅶 (Arabic) favored by God.

Rigel (Spanish) most brilliant star
in the sky.

Rihana (Arabic) sweet basil.
Rhiana, Rhianna, Riana, Rianna

Rika (Swedish) ruler.
Ricka

Rilee (Irish) a form of Riley.
Rielee, Rielle

Riley ☀ 🅱🅶 (Irish) valiant.
Raleigh, Reilly, Rieley, Rielly,
Riély, Rilee, Rileigh, Rilie

Rilla (German) small brook.

Rima (Arabic) white antelope.
Reem, Reema, Reemah, Rema,
Remah, Rhymia, Rim, Ryma

Rimona (Hebrew) pomegranate.
See also Mona.

Rin (Japanese) park. Geography: a
Japanese village.
Rini, Rynn

Rina (English) a short form of names ending in "rina." (Hebrew) a form of Rena, Rinah.
Reena, Rena

Rinah (Hebrew) joyful.
Rina

Río (Spanish) river.

Riona (Irish) saint.

Risa (Latin) laughter.
Reesa, Resa

Risha (Hindi) born during the lunar month of Taurus.
Rishah, Rishay

Rishona (Hebrew) first.
Rishina, Rishon

Rissa (Greek) a short form of Nerissa.
Risa, Rissah, Ryssa, Ryssah

Rita (Sanskrit) brave; honest. (Greek) a short form of Margarita.
Reatha, Reda, Reeta, Reida, Reitha, Rheta, Riet, Ritah, Ritamae, Ritamarie

Ritsa (Greek) a familiar form of Alexandra.
Ritsah, Ritsi, Ritsie, Ritsy

Riva (French) river bank. (Hebrew) a short form of Rebecca. See also Reba, Reva.
Rivalee, Rivi, Rivvy

River **BG** (Latin, French) stream, water.
Rivana, Rivanna, Rivers, Riviane

Rivka (Hebrew) a short form of Rebecca.
Rivca, Rivcah, Rivkah

Riza (Greek) a form of Theresa.
Riesa, Rizus, Rizza

Roanna (American) a form of Rosanna.
Ranna, Roana, Roanda, Roanne

Robbi (English) a familiar form of Roberta.
Robby, Robbye, Robey, Robi, Robia, Roby

Robbie **BG** (English) a form of Robbi.

Robert **BG** (English) famous brilliance.

Roberta (English) a form of Robert.
Roba, Robbi, Robbie, Robena, Robertena, Robertina

Roberto **BG** (Italian, Portuguese, Spanish) a form of Robert.

Robin **GB** (English) robin. A form of Roberta.
Robann, Robbin, Robeen, Roben, Robena, Robian, Robina, Robine, Robinette, Robinia, Robinn, Robinta, Robyn

Robinette (English) a familiar form of Robin.
Robernetta, Robinet, Robinett, Robinita

Robyn GB (English) a form of Robin.
Robbyn, Robbynn, Robyne, Robynn, Robynne

Rochelle GB (French) large stone. (Hebrew) a form of Rachel. See also Shelley.
Reshelle, Roch, Rocheal, Rochealle, Rochel, Rochele, Rochell, Rochella, Rochette, Rockelle, Roshele, Roshell, Roshelle

Rochely (Latin) goddess of the earth.

Rocio (Spanish) dewdrops.
Rocío

Roderica (German) famous ruler.
Rica, Rika, Rodericka, Roderika, Rodreicka, Rodricka, Rodrika

Roderiga (Spanish) notable leader.

Rodnae (English) island clearing.
Rodna, Rodnetta, Rodnicka

Rodneisha (American) a combination of Rodnae + Aisha.
Rodesha, Rodisha, Rodishah, Rodnecia, Rodnesha, Rodneshia, Rodneycia, Rodneysha, Rodnisha

Rodney BG (English) island clearing.

Rogelia (Teutonic) beautiful one.

Rogelio BG (Spanish) famous warrior.

Rohana (Hindi) sandalwood. (American) a combination of Rose + Hannah.
Rochana, Rohena

Rohini (Hindi) woman.

Roja (Spanish) red.

Rolanda (German) a form of Rolando.
Ralna, Rolande, Rolando, Rolaunda, Roleesha, Rolene, Rolinda, Rollande, Rolonda

Rolando BG (German) famous throughout the land.

Rolene (German) a form of Rolanda.
Rolaine, Rolena, Rolleen, Rollene

Roma (Latin) from Rome.
Romai, Rome, Romeise, Romeka, Romelle, Romesha, Rometta, Romia, Romilda, Romilla, Romina, Romini, Romma, Romonia

Romaine (French) from Rome.
Romana, Romanda, Romanelle, Romania, Romanique, Romany, Romayne, Romona, Romy

Romanela (Latin) native of Rome.

Romelia (Hebrew) God's beloved or preferred one.

Romola (Latin) Roman woman.

Rómula (Spanish) possessor of great strength.

Romy GB (French) a familiar form of Romaine. (English) a

familiar form of Rosemary.
Romi, Romie

Rona (Scandinavian) a short form
of Ronalda.
*Rhona, Roana, Ronalda, Ronna,
Ronnae, Ronnay, Ronne, Ronni,
Ronsy*

Ronaele (Greek) the name
Eleanor spelled backwards.
Ronalee, Ronni, Ronnie, Ronny

Ronald BG (Scottish) a form of
Reginald.

Ronda (Welsh) a form of Rhonda.
*Rondai, Rondesia, Rondi, Rondie,
Ronelle, Ronnette, Ronni, Ronnie,
Ronny*

Rondelle (French) short poem.
Rhondelle, Rondel, Ronndelle

Roneisha (American) a
combination of Rhonda + Aisha.
*Roneasha, Ronecia, Ronee,
Roneeka, Roneesha, Roneice,
Ronese, Ronesha, Roneshia,
Ronesia, Ronessa, Ronessia,
Ronichia, Ronicia, Roniesha,
Ronisha, Ronneisha, Ronnesa,
Ronnesha, Ronneshia, Ronni,
Ronnie, Ronniesha, Ronny*

Ronelle (Welsh) a form of
Rhonda, Ronda.
*Ranell, Ranelle, Ronel, Ronella,
Ronielle, Ronnella, Ronnelle*

Ronisha (American) a form of
Roneisha.
*Ronise, Ronnise, Ronnisha,
Ronnishia*

Ronli (Hebrew) joyful.
*Ronia, Ronice, Ronit, Ronlee,
Ronlie, Ronni, Ronnie, Ronny*

Ronnette (Welsh) a familiar form
of Rhonda, Ronda.
*Ronetta, Ronette, Ronit, Ronita,
Ronnetta, Ronni, Ronnie, Ronny*

Ronni (American) a familiar form
of Veronica and names beginning
with "Ron."
*Rone, Ronee, Roni, Ronnee,
Ronney*

Ronnie, Ronny BG (American)
forms of Ronni.

Roquelina (Latin) strong as a
rock.

Rori (Irish) famous brilliance;
famous ruler.
Rorie

Rory BG (Irish) a form of Rori.

Ros, Roz (English) short forms of
Rosalind, Rosalyn.
Rozz, Rozzey, Rozzi, Rozzie, Rozzy

Rosa GB (Italian, Spanish) a form
of Rose. History: Rosa Parks
inspired the American Civil Rights
movement by refusing to give up
her bus seat to a white man in
Montgomery, Alabama. See also
Charo, Roza.

Rosa de Lima (Spanish) a form
of Rosa.

Rosabel (French) beautiful rose.
*Rosabelia, Rosabella, Rosabelle,
Rosebelle*

Rosalba (Latin) white rose.
Rosalva, Roselba

Rosalía (Spanish) a combination of Rosa and Lía.

Rosalie (English) a form of Rosalind.
Rosalea, Rosalee, Rosaleen, Rosaleigh, Rosalene, Rosalia, Rosealee, Rosealie, Roselee, Roseli, Roselia, Roselie, Roseley, Rosely, Rosilee, Rosli, Rozali, Rozália, Rozalie, Rozele

Rosalín, Roselín (Spanish) a combination of Rosa and Linda.

Rosalind (Spanish) fair rose.
Ros, Rosalie, Rosalinda, Rosalinde, Rosalyn, Rosalynd, Rosalynde, Roselind, Roselyn, Rosie, Roz, Rozalind, Rozland

Rosalinda (Spanish) a form of Rosalind.
Rosalina

Rosalyn (Spanish) a form of Rosalind.
Ros, Rosaleen, Rosalin, Rosaline, Rosalyne, Rosalynn, Rosalynne, Rosilyn, Roslin, Roslyn, Roslyne, Roslynn, Roz, Rozalyn, Rozlyn

Rosamond (German) famous guardian.
Rosamund, Rosamunda, Rosemonde, Rozamond

Rosanna, Roseanna (English) combinations of Rose + Anna.
Ranna, Roanna, Rosana, Rosannah, Roseana, Roseannah, Rosehanah, Rosehannah, Rosie, Rossana, Rossanna, Rozana, Rozanna

Rosanne, Roseanne (English) combinations of Rose + Ann.
Roanne, Rosan, Rosann, Roseann, Rose Ann, Rose Anne, Rossann, Rossanne, Rozann, Rozanne

Rosario GB (Filipino, Spanish) rosary.
Rosarah, Rosaria, Rosarie, Rosary, Rosaura

Rose (Latin) rose. See also Chalina, Raisa, Raizel, Roza.
Rada, Rasia, Rasine, Rois, Róise, Rosa, Rosea, Rosella, Roselle, Roses, Rosetta, Rosie, Rosina, Rosita, Rosse

Roselani (Hawaiian) heavenly rose.

Roselyn (Spanish) a form of Rosalind.
Roseleen, Roselene, Roselin, Roseline, Roselyne, Roselynn, Roselynne

Rosemarie (English) a combination of Rose + Marie.
Rosamaria, Rosamarie, Rosemari, Rosemaria, Rose Marie

Rosemary (English) a combination of Rose + Mary.
Romi, Romy

Rosenda (German) excellent lady.

Rosetta (Italian) a form of Rose.
Roseta, Rosette

Roshan (Sanskrit) shining light.

Roshawna (American) a
combination of Rose + Shawna.
*Roshan, Roshana, Roshanda,
Roshani, Roshann, Roshanna,
Roshanta, Roshaun, Roshauna,
Roshaunda, Roshawn,
Roshawnda, Roshawnna,
Roshona, Roshonda, Roshowna,
Roshunda*

Rosie (English) a familiar form of
Rosalind, Rosanna, Rose.
*Rosey, Rosi, Rosio, Rosse, Rosy,
Rozsi, Rozy*

Rosilda (German) horse-riding
warrior.

Rosina (English) a familiar form
of Rose.
*Rosena, Rosenah, Rosene,
Rosheen, Rozena, Rozina*

Rosinda (Teutonic) famous
warrior.

Rosine (Latin) little rose.

Rosita (Spanish) a familiar form
of Rose.
*Roseeta, Roseta, Rozeta, Rozita,
Rozyte*

Roslyn (Scottish) a form of
Rossalyn.
*Roslin, Roslynn, Rosslyn,
Rosslynn*

Rosmarí (Spanish) a combination
of Rosa and María.

Rosmira (German) celebrated
horse-riding warrior.

Ross BG (Latin) rose. (Scottish)
peninsula. (French) red.

Rossalyn (Scottish) cape;
promontory.
*Roslyn, Rosselyn, Rosylin,
Roszaliyn*

Rosura (Latin) golden rose.

Rowan GB (English) tree with
red berries. (Welsh) a form of
Rowena.
Rowana

Rowena (Welsh) fair-haired.
(English) famous friend.
Literature: Ivanhoe's love interest
in Sir Walter Scott's novel
Ivanhoe.
*Ranna, Ronni, Row, Rowan,
Rowe, Roweena, Rowen, Rowina*

Roxana, Roxanna (Persian)
forms of Roxann.
Rocsana, Roxannah

Roxann, Roxanne (Persian)
sunrise. Literature: Roxanne is
the heroine of Edmond Rostand's
play *Cyrano de Bergerac*.
*Rocxann, Roxan, Roxana, Roxane,
Roxanna, Roxianne, Roxy*

Roxy (Persian) a familiar form of
Roxann.
Roxi, Roxie

Royale (English) royal.
*Royal, Royalene, Royalle, Roylee,
Roylene, Ryal, Ryale*

Royanna (English) queenly, royal.
Roya

Royce 🅱🅶 (English) child of Roy.

Roza (Slavic) a form of Rosa.
Roz, Rozalia, Roze, Rozel, Rozele,
Rozell, Rozella, Rozelli, Rozia,
Rozsa, Rozsi, Rozyte, Rozza,
Rozzie

Rozene (Native American) rose
blossom.
Rozena, Rozina, Rozine, Ruzena

Ruana (Hindi) stringed musical
instrument.
Ruan, Ruon

Ruben 🅱🅶 (Hebrew) a form of
Reuben (see Boys' Names).

Rubena (Hebrew) a form of
Reubena.
Rubenia, Rubina, Rubine, Rubinia,
Rubyn, Rubyna

Rubi (French) a form of Ruby.
Ruba, Rubbie, Rubee, Rubí,
Rubia, Rubie

Ruby 🅶🅱 (French) precious stone.
Rubby, Rubetta, Rubette, Rubey,
Rubi, Rubiann, Rubyann, Rubye

Ruchi (Hindi) one who wishes to
please.

Rudecinda (Spanish) a form of
Rosenda.

Rudee (German) famous wolf.
Rudeline, Rudell, Rudella, Rudi,
Rudie, Rudina, Rudy

Rudra (Hindi) seeds of the
rudraksha plant.

Rudy 🅱🅶 (German) a form of
Rudee.

Rue (German) famous. (French)
street. (English) regretful; strong-
scented herbs.
Ru, Ruey

Rufa (Latin) red-haired.

Ruffina (Italian) redhead.
Rufeena, Rufeine, Rufina,
Ruphyna

Rui (Japanese) affectionate.

Rukan (Arabic) steady; confident.

Rula (Latin, English) ruler.

Runa (Norwegian) secret; flowing.
Runna

Ruperta (Spanish) a form of
Roberta.

Rupinder 🅶🅱 (Sanskrit) beautiful.

Ruri (Japanese) emerald.
Ruriko

Rusalka (Czech) wood nymph.
(Russian) mermaid.

Russhell (French) redhead; fox
colored.
Rushell, Rushelle, Russellynn,
Russhelle

Rusti (English) redhead.
Russet, Rustie, Rusty

Rute (Portuguese) a form of Ruth.

Ruth (Hebrew) friendship. Bible: daughter-in-law of Naomi.
Rutha, Ruthalma, Ruthe, Ruthella, Ruthetta, Ruthie, Ruthven

Ruthann (American) a combination of Ruth + Ann.
Ruthan, Ruthanna, Ruthannah, Ruthanne, Ruthina, Ruthine

Ruthie (Hebrew) a familiar form of Ruth.
Ruthey, Ruthi, Ruthy

Rutilda (German) strong because of her fame.

Ruza (Czech) rose.
Ruzena, Ruzenka, Ruzha, Ruzsa

Ryan BG (Irish) little ruler.
Raiann, Raianne, Rhyann, Riana, Riane, Ryana, Ryane, Ryanna, Ryanne, Rye, Ryen, Ryenne

Ryann GB (Irish) a form of Ryan.

Ryba (Czech) fish.

Rylan BG (English) land where rye is grown.

Rylee GB (Irish) valiant.
Rye, Ryelee, Rylea, Ryleigh, Ryley, Rylie, Rylina, Rylyn

Ryleigh, Rylie (Irish) forms of Rylee.
Ryelie, Ryli, Rylleigh, Ryllie

Ryley BG (Irish) a form of Rylee.
Ryeley, Rylly, Ryly

Ryo (Japanese) dragon.
Ryoko

S

S GB (American) an initial used as a first name.

Saarah (Arabic) princess.

Saba (Arabic) morning. (Greek) a form of Sheba.
Sabaah, Sabah, Sabba, Sabbah

Sabana (Latin) from the open plain.

Sabelia (Spanish) a form of Sabina.

Sabi (Arabic) young girl.

Sabina (Latin) History: the Sabine were a tribe in ancient Italy. See also Bina.
Sabeen, Sabena, Sabienne, Sabin, Sabine, Sabinka, Sabinna, Sabiny, Saby, Sabyne, Savina, Sebina, Sebinah

Sabiya (Arabic) morning; eastern wind.
Saba, Sabaya, Sabiyah

Sable (English) sable; sleek.
Sabel, Sabela, Sabella

Sabra (Hebrew) thorny cactus fruit. (Arabic) resting. History: a name for native-born Israelis, who were said to be hard on the outside and soft and sweet on the inside.
Sabera, Sabira, Sabrah, Sabre, Sabrea, Sabreah, Sabree, Sabreea, Sabri, Sabria, Sabriah, Sabriya, Sebra

Sabreena (English) a form of Sabrina.
Sabreen, Sabrena, Sabrene

Sabrina GB (Latin) boundary line. (English) princess. (Hebrew) a familiar form of Sabra. See also Bree, Brina, Rena, Zabrina.
Sabre, Sabreena, Sabrinas, Sabrinah, Sabrine, Sabrinia, Sabrinna, Sabryna, Sebree, Sebrina, Subrina

Sabryna (English) a form of Sabrina.
Sabrynna

Sacha BG (Russian) a form of Sasha.
Sache, Sachia

Sachi (Japanese) blessed; lucky.
Saatchi, Sachie, Sachiko

Sacnite (Mayan) white flower.

Sada (Japanese) chaste. (English) a form of Sadie.
Sadá, Sadah, Sadako

Sade GB (Hebrew) a form of Chadee, Sarah, Shardae, Sharday.
Sáde, Sadé, Sadea, Sadee, Shaday

Sadella (American) a combination of Sade + Ella.
Sadelle, Sydel, Sydell, Sydella, Sydelle

Sadhana (Hindi) devoted.

Sadie (Hebrew) a familiar form of Sarah. See also Sada.
Saddie, Sadee, Sadey, Sadi, Sadiey, Sady, Sadye, Saide, Saidee, Saidey, Saidi, Saidia, Saidie, Saidy, Sayde, Saydee, Seidy

Sadira (Persian) lotus tree. (Arabic) star.
Sadra

Sadiya (Arabic) lucky, fortunate.
Sadi, Sadia, Sadiah, Sadiyah, Sadiyyah, Sadya

Sadzi (Carrier) sunny disposition.

Saffron (English) Botany: a plant with purple or white flowers whose orange stigmas are used as a spice.
Safron

Safiya (Arabic) pure; serene; best friend.
Safa, Safeya, Saffa, Safia, Safiyah

Safo (Greek) she who sees with clarity.

Sagara (Hindi) ocean.

Sage BG (English) wise. Botany: an herb used as a seasoning.
Sagia, Saige, Salvia

Sahara (Arabic) desert; wilderness.
Sahar, Saharah, Sahari, Saheer,
Saher, Sahira, Sahra, Sahrah

Sai (Japanese) talented.
Saiko

Saida (Hebrew) a form of Sarah.
(Arabic) happy; fortunate.
Saidah

Saige (English) a form of Sage.

Saira (Hebrew) a form of Sara.
Sairah, Sairi

Sakaë (Japanese) prosperous.

Sakari (Hindi) sweet.
Sakkara

Saki (Japanese) cloak; rice wine.

Sakti (Hindi) energy, power.

Sakuna (Native American) bird.

Sakura (Japanese) cherry
blossom; wealthy; prosperous.

Sala (Hindi) sala tree. Religion:
the sacred tree under which
Buddha died.

Salaberga (German) she who
defends the sacrifice.

Salali (Cherokee) squirrel.

Salama (Arabic) peaceful. See
also Zulima.

Salbatora (Spanish) savior.

Salena (French) a form of Salina.
Saleana, Saleen, Saleena,
Salene, Salenna, Sallene

Saleta (French) location in the
French Alps where there was a
sighting of the Virgin Mary.

Salima (Arabic) safe and sound;
healthy.
Saleema, Salema, Salim,
Salimah, Salma

Salina (French) solemn, dignified.
Salena, Salin, Salinah, Salinda,
Saline

Salliann (English) a combination
of Sally + Ann.
Sallian, Sallianne, Sallyann,
Sally-Ann, Sallyanne, Sally-Anne

Sally GB (English) princess.
History: Sally Ride, an American
astronaut, became the first U.S.
woman in space.
Sal, Salaid, Sallee, Salletta,
Sallette, Salley, Salli, Sallie

Salome (Hebrew) peaceful.
History: Salome Alexandra was a
ruler of ancient Judea. Bible: the
niece of King Herod.
Saloma, Salomé, Salomey,
Salomi

Salud (Spanish) health.

Salvadora (Spanish) savior.

Salvatora (Italian) savior.

Salvia (Spanish) healthy; saved.
(Latin) a form of Sage.
Sallvia, Salviana, Salviane,
Salvina, Salvine

Sam BG (Aramaic, Hebrew) a
short form of Samantha.

Samala (Hebrew) asked of God.
Samale, Sammala

Samanta (Hebrew) a form of
Samantha.
Samantah, Smanta

Samantha ☀ GB (Aramaic)
listener. (Hebrew) told by God.
*Sam, Samana, Samanath,
Samanatha, Samanitha,
Samanithia, Samanta, Samanth,
Samanthe, Samanthi, Samanthia,
Samatha, Sami, Sammanth,
Sammantha, Semantha,
Simantha, Smantha, Symantha*

Samara (Latin) elm-tree seed.
*Saimara, Samaira, Samar,
Samarah, Samari, Samaria,
Samariah, Samarie, Samarra,
Samarrea, Samary, Samera,
Sameria, Samira, Sammar,
Sammara, Samora*

Samatha (Hebrew) a form of
Samantha.
Sammatha

Sameh (Hebrew) listener.
(Arabic) forgiving.
Samaiya, Samaya

Sami BG (Arabic) praised.
(Hebrew) a short form of
Samantha, Samuela.
*Samia, Samiah, Samiha, Samina,
Sammey, Sammi, Sammie,
Sammijo, Sammy, Sammyjo,
Samya, Samye*

Samira (Arabic) entertaining.
*Samirah, Samire, Samiria,
Samirra, Samyra*

Sammy BG (Arabic, Hebrew) a
form of Sami.

Samone (Hebrew) a form of
Simone.
*Samoan, Samoane, Samon,
Samona, Samoné, Samonia*

Samuel BG (Hebrew) heard God;
asked of God.

Samuela (Hebrew) a form of
Samuel.
*Samala, Samelia, Samella, Sami,
Samielle, Samille, Sammile,
Samuelle*

Samuelle GB (Hebrew) a form
of Samuela.
Samuella

Sana (Arabic) mountaintop;
splendid; brilliant.
*Sanaa, Sanáa, Sanaah, Sane,
Sanah*

Sancia (Spanish) holy, sacred.
*Sanceska, Sancha, Sancharia,
Sanchia, Sancie, Santsia, Sanzia*

Sandeep BG (Punjabi)
enlightened.
Sandip

Sandi (Greek) a familiar form of
Sandra.
*Sandee, Sandia, Sandie, Sandiey,
Sandine, Sanndie*

Sandra (Greek) defender of
mankind. A short form of
Cassandra. History: Sandra Day
O'Connor was the first woman
appointed to the U.S. Supreme
Court. See also Zandra.
*Sahndra, Sandi, Sandira,
Sandrea, Sandria, Sandrica,
Sandy, Sanndra, Saundra*

Sandrea (Greek) a form of
Sandra.
*Sandreea, Sandreia, Sandrell,
Sandria, Sanndria*

Sandrica (Greek) a form of
Sandra. See also Rica.
Sandricka, Sandrika

Sandrine (Greek) a form of
Alexandra.
*Sandreana, Sandrene,
Sandrenna, Sandrianna, Sandrina*

Sandy 𝐆𝐁 (Greek) a familiar
form of Cassandra, Sandra.
Sandya, Sandye

Sanne (Hebrew, Dutch) lily.
Sanea, Saneh, Sanna, Sanneen

Santana 𝐆𝐁 (Spanish) Saint Anne.
*Santa, Santaniata, Santanna,
Santanne, Santena, Santenna,
Shantana*

Santina (Spanish) little saint.
Santinia

Sanura (Swahili) kitten.
Sanora

Sanuye (Moquelumnan) red
clouds at sunset.

Sanya (Sanskrit) born on
Saturday.
Saneiya, Sania, Sanyia

Sanyu 𝐁𝐆 (Luganda) happiness.

Sapata (Native American)
dancing bear.

Sapphira (Hebrew) a form of
Sapphire.
*Safira, Sapheria, Saphira,
Saphyra, Sephira*

Sapphire (Greek) blue gemstone.
*Saffire, Saphire, Saphyre,
Sapphira*

Saqui (Mapuche) preferred one,
chosen one; kind soul.

Sara ☀ 𝐆𝐁 (Hebrew) a form of
Sarah.
Saira, Sarae, Saralee, Sarra, Sera

Sarah ☀ 𝐆𝐁 (Hebrew) princess.
Bible: the wife of Abraham and
mother of Isaac. See also Sadie,
Saida, Sally, Saree, Sharai, Shari,
Zara, Zarita.
*Sahra, Sara, Saraha, Sarahann,
Sarahi, Sarai, Sarann, Saray,
Sarha, Sariah, Sarina, Sarita,
Sarolta, Sarotte, Sarrah, Sasa,
Sayra, Sorcha*

Sarai, Saray (Hebrew) forms of
Sarah.
Saraya

Saralyn (American) a
combination of Sarah + Lynn.
Saralena, Saraly, Saralynn

Saree (Arabic) noble. (Hebrew) a familiar form of Sarah.
Sareeka, Sareka, Sari, Sarika, Sarka, Sarri, Sarrie, Sary

Sariah (Hebrew) forms of Sarah.
Saria, Sarie

Sarila (Turkish) waterfall.

Sarina (Hebrew) a familiar form of Sarah.
Sareen, Sareena, Saren, Sarena, Sarene, Sarenna, Sarin, Sarine, Sarinna, Sarinne

Sarita (Hebrew) a familiar form of Sarah.
Saretta, Sarette, Sarit, Saritia, Saritta

Sarolta (Hungarian) a form of Sarah.

Sarotte (French) a form of Sarah.

Sarrah (Hebrew) a form of Sarah.
Sarra

Sasa (Japanese) assistant. (Hungarian) a form of Sarah, Sasha.

Sasha 🇬🇧 (Russian) defender of mankind. See also Zasha.
Sacha, Sahsha, Sasa, Sascha, Saschae, Sashae, Sashah, Sashai, Sashana, Sashay, Sashea, Sashel, Sashenka, Sashey, Sashi, Sashia, Sashira, Sashsha, Sashya, Sasjara, Sauscha, Sausha, Shasha, Shashi, Shashia

Sasquia (Teutonic) she who carries a knife.

Sass (Irish) Saxon.
Sassie, Sassoon, Sassy

Satara (American) a combination of Sarah + Tara.
Sataria, Satarra, Sateriaa, Saterra, Saterria

Satin (French) smooth, shiny.
Satinder

Satinka (Native American) sacred dancer.

Sato (Japanese) sugar.
Satu

Saturia (Latin) she who has it all.

Saturnina (Spanish) gift of Saturn.

Saul 🅱🅶 (Hebrew) asked for, borrowed.

Saundra (English) a form of Sandra, Sondra.
Saundee, Saundi, Saundie, Saundy

Saura (Hindi) sun worshiper.

Savana, Savanna (Spanish) forms of Savannah.
Saveena, Savhana, Savhanna, Savina, Savine, Savona, Savonna

Savanah (Spanish) a form of Savannah.
Savhannah

Savannah ☀ GB (Spanish)
treeless plain.
*Sahvannah, Savana, Savanah,
Savanha, Savanna, Savannha,
Savauna, Savonnah, Savonne,
Sevan, Sevanah, Sevanh, Sevann,
Sevanna, Svannah*

Saveria (Teutonic) from the new
house.

Savon BG (Spanish) a treeless
plain.

Sawa (Japanese) swamp.
(Moquelumnan) stone.

Sawyer BG (English) wood
worker.
Sawyar, Sawyor

Sayde, Saydee (Hebrew) forms
of Sadie.
Saydi, Saydia, Saydie, Saydy

Sayén (Mapuche) sweet, lovable,
warm; openhearted woman.

Sayo (Japanese) born at night.

Sayra (Hebrew) a form of Sarah.
Sayrah, Sayre, Sayri

Scarlett (English) bright red.
Literature: Scarlett O'Hara is the
heroine of Margaret Mitchell's
novel *Gone with the Wind*.
*Scarlet, Scarlette, Scarlotte,
Skarlette*

Schyler GB (Dutch) sheltering.
*Schuyla, Schuyler, Schuylia,
Schylar*

Scott BG (English) from Scotland.

Scotti (Scottish) from Scotland.
Scota, Scotia, Scottie, Scotty

Sean BG (Irish) a form of John.

Seana, Seanna (Irish) forms of
Sean. See also Shauna, Shawna.
*Seaana, Sean, Seane, Seann,
Seannae, Seannah, Seannalisa,
Seanté, Sianna, Sina*

Sebastian BG (Greek) venerable.
(Latin) revered. (French) a form
of Sebastian.

Sebastiane (Greek, Latin,
French) a form of Sebastian.
*Sebastene, Sebastia, Sebastian,
Sebastiana, Sebastien,
Sebastienne*

Sebastien BG (Greek, Latin,
French) a form of Sebastian.

Seble (Ethiopian) autumn.

Sebrina (English) a form of
Sabrina.
*Sebrena, Sebrenna, Sebria,
Sebriana*

Secilia (Latin) a form of Cecilia.
Saselia, Sasilia, Sesilia, Sileas

Secunda (Latin) second.

Secundina (Latin) family's
second daughter.

Seda (Armenian) forest voices.

Sedna (Eskimo) well-fed.
Mythology: the goddess of sea
animals.

Seelia (English) a form of Sheila.

Seema (Greek) sprout. (Afghan) sky; profile.
Seemah, Sima, Simah

Sefa (Swiss) a familiar form of Josefina.

Séfora (Hebrew) like a small bird.

Segismunda (German) victorious protector.

Segunda (Spanish) second-born.

Seina (Basque) innocent.

Seirra (Irish) a form of Sierra.
Seiara, Seiarra, Seira, Seirria

Seki (Japanese) wonderful.
Seka

Sela (English) a short form of Selena.
Seeley, Selah

Selam (Ethiopian) peaceful.

Selda (German) a short form of Griselda. (Yiddish) a form of Zelda.
Seldah, Selde, Sellda, Selldah

Selena GB (Greek) moon. Mythology: Selene was the goddess of the moon. See also Celena.
Saleena, Sela, Selana, Seleana, Seleena, Selen, Selenah, Selene, Séléné, Selenia, Selenna, Selina, Sena, Syleena, Sylena

Selene (Greek) a form of Selena.
Seleni, Selenie, Seleny

Selia (Latin) a short form of Cecilia.
Seel, Seil, Sela, Silia

Selima (Hebrew) peaceful.
Selema, Selemah, Selimah

Selina (Greek) a form of Celina, Selena.
Selie, Selin, Selinda, Seline, Selinia, Selinka, Sellina, Selyna, Selyne, Selynne, Sylina

Selma (German) divine protector. (Irish) fair, just. (Scandinavian) divinely protected. (Arabic) secure. See also Zelma.
Sellma, Sellmah, Selmah

Selva (Latin) she who was born in the jungle.

Sema (Turkish) heaven; divine omen.
Semaj

Semele (Latin) once.

Seminaris, Semíramis (Assyrian) she who lives harmoniously with the doves.

Sempronia (Spanish) prudent and measured.

Sen BG (Japanese) Mythology: a magical forest elf that lives for thousands of years.

Senalda (Spanish) sign.
Sena, Senda, Senna

Seneca (Iroquois) a tribal name.
Senaka, Seneka, Senequa, Senequae, Senequai, Seneque

Senona (Spanish) lively.

Septima (Latin) seventh.

Sequoia (Cherokee) giant
redwood tree.
*Seqoiyia, Sequoyia, Seqoya,
Sequoi, Sequoiah, Sequora,
Sequoya, Sequoyah, Sikoya*

Serafina (Hebrew) burning;
ardent. Bible: seraphim are an
order of angels.
*Sarafina, Serafine, Seraphe,
Seraphin, Seraphina, Seraphine,
Seraphita, Serapia, Serofina*

Serena (Latin) peaceful. See also
Rena.
*Sarina, Saryna, Seraina, Serana,
Sereen, Sereina, Seren, Serenah,
Serene, Serenea, Serenia,
Serenna, Serina, Serreana,
Serrena, Serrenna*

Serenela (Spanish) a form of
Serena.

Serenity (Latin) peaceful.
*Serenidy, Serenitee, Serenitey,
Sereniti, Serenitiy, Serinity,
Serrennity*

Sergia (Greek) attendant.

Serilda (Greek) armed warrior
woman.

Serina (Latin) a form of Serena.
*Sereena, Serin, Serine, Serreena,
Serrin, Serrina, Seryna*

Servanda (Latin) she who must
be saved and protected.

Servia (Latin) daughter of those
who serve the Lord.

Seth **BG** (Hebrew) appointed.

Sevanda (Latin) she who
deserves to be saved and
guarded.

Severa (Spanish) severe.

Severina (Italian, Portuguese,
Croatian, German, Ancient
Roman) severe.

Sevilla (Spanish) from Seville.
Seville

Shaba (Spanish) rose.
Shabana, Shabina

Shada (Native American) pelican.
*Shadae, Shadea, Shadeana,
Shadee, Shadi, Shadia, Shadiah,
Shadie, Shadiya, Shaida*

Shaday (American) a form of
Sade.
*Shadai, Shadaia, Shadaya,
Shadayna, Shadei, Shadeziah,
Shaiday*

Shadrika (American) a
combination of the prefix Sha +
Rika.
*Shadreeka, Shadreka, Shadrica,
Shadricka, Shadrieka*

Shae **GB** (Irish) a form of Shea.
Shaenel, Shaeya, Shai, Shaia

Shaelee (Irish) a form of Shea.
*Shaeleigh, Shaeley, Shaelie,
Shaely*

Shaelyn (Irish) a form of Shea.
*Shael, Shaelaine, Shaelan,
Shaelanie, Shaelanna, Shaeleen,
Shaelene, Shaelin, Shaeline,
Shaelyne, Shaelynn, Shae-Lynn,
Shaelynne*

Shafira (Swahili) distinguished.
Shaffira

Shahar (Arabic) moonlit.
Shahara

Shahina (Arabic) falcon.
*Shaheen, Shaheena, Shahi,
Shahin*

Shahla (Afghani) beautiful eyes.
Shaila, Shailah, Shalah

Shaianne (Cheyenne) a form of
Cheyenne.
*Shaeen, Shaeine, Shaian,
Shaiana, Shaiandra, Shaiane,
Shaiann, Shaianna*

Shaila (Latin) a form of Sheila.
*Shaela, Shaelea, Shaeyla,
Shailah, Shailee, Shailey, Shaili,
Shailie, Shailla, Shaily, Shailyn,
Shailynn*

Shaina GB (Yiddish) beautiful.
*Shaena, Shainah, Shaine,
Shainna, Shajna, Shanie, Shayna,
Shayndel, Sheina, Sheindel*

Shajuana (American) a
combination of the prefix Sha +
Juanita. See also Shawanna.
*Shajuan, Shajuanda, Shajuanita,
Shajuanna, Shajuanza*

Shaka BG (Hindi) a form of
Shakti. A short form of names
beginning with "Shak. " See also
Chaka.
Shakah, Shakha

Shakarah (American) a combi-
nation of the prefix Sha + Kara.
*Shacara, Shacari, Shaccara,
Shaka, Shakari, Shakkara,
Shikara*

Shakayla (Arabic) a form of
Shakila.
*Shakaela, Shakail, Shakaila,
Shakala*

Shakeena (American) a combi-
nation of the prefix Sha + Keena.
*Shaka, Shakeina, Shakeyna,
Shakina, Shakyna*

Shakeita (American) a combi-
nation of the prefix Sha + Keita.
See also Shaqueita.
*Shaka, Shakeeta, Shakeitha,
Shakeithia, Shaketa, Shaketha,
Shakethia, Shaketia, Shakita,
Shakitra, Sheketa, Shekita,
Shikita, Shikitha*

Shakera (Arabic) a form of
Shakira.
*Chakeria, Shakeira, Shakeirra,
Shakerah, Shakeria, Shakeriah,
Shakeriay, Shakerra, Shakerri,
Shakerria, Shakerya, Shakeryia,
Shakeyra*

Shakia (American) a combination
of the prefix Sha + Kia.
Shakeeia, Shakeeyah, Shakeia,

Shakeya, Shakiya, Shekeia, Shekia, Shekiah, Shikia

Shakila (Arabic) pretty.
Chakila, Shaka, Shakayla, Shakeela, Shakeena, Shakela, Shakelah, Shakilah, Shakyla, Shekila, Shekilla, Shikeela

Shakira (Arabic) thankful.
Shaakira, Shacora, Shaka, Shakeera, Shakeerah, Shakeeria, Shakera, Shakiera, Shakierra, Shakir, Shakirah, Shakirat, Shakirea, Shakirra, Shakora, Shakuria, Shakyra, Shaquira, Shekiera, Shekira, Shikira

Shakti (Hindi) energy, power.
Religion: a form of the Hindu goddess Devi.
Sakti, Shaka, Sita

Shakyra (Arabic) a form of Shakira.
Shakyria

Shalana (American) a combination of the prefix Sha + Lana.
Shalaana, Shalain, Shalaina, Shalaine, Shaland, Shalanda, Shalane, Shalann, Shalaun, Shalauna, Shalayna, Shalayne, Shalaynna, Shallan, Shelan, Shelanda

Shaleah (American) a combination of the prefix Sha + Leah.
Shalea, Shalee, Shaleea, Shalia, Shaliah

Shaleisha (American) a combination of the prefix Sha + Aisha.
Shalesha, Shalesia, Shalicia, Shalisha

Shalena (American) a combination of the prefix Sha + Lena.
Shaleana, Shaleen, Shaleena, Shalen, Shálena, Shalene, Shalené, Shalenna, Shalina, Shalinda, Shaline, Shalini, Shalinna, Shelayna, Shelayne, Shelena

Shalisa (American) a combination of the prefix Sha + Lisa.
Shalesa, Shalese, Shalessa, Shalice, Shalicia, Shaliece, Shalise, Shalisha, Shalishea, Shalisia, Shalissa, Shalisse, Shalyce, Shalys, Shalyse

Shalita (American) a combination of the prefix Sha + Lita.
Shaleta, Shaletta, Shalida, Shalitta

Shalona (American) a combination of the prefix Sha + Lona.
Shalon, Shalone, Shálonna, Shalonne

Shalonda (American) a combination of the prefix Sha + Ondine.
Shalonde, Shalondine, Shalondra, Shalondria

Shalyn (American) a combination of the prefix Sha + Lynn.
Shalin, Shalina, Shalinda, Shaline, Shalyna, Shalynda, Shalyne, Shalynn, Shalynne

Shamara (Arabic) ready for battle.
Shamar, Shamarah, Shamare, Shamarea, Shamaree, Shamari, Shamaria, Shamariah, Shamarra, Shamarri, Shammara, Shamora, Shamori, Shamorra, Shamorria, Shamorriah

Shameka (American) a combination of the prefix Sha + Meka.
Shameaka, Shameakah, Shameca, Shamecca, Shamecha, Shamecia, Shameika, Shameke, Shamekia

Shamika (American) a combination of the prefix Sha + Mika.
Shameeca, Shameeka, Shamica, Shamicia, Shamicka, Shamieka, Shamikia

Shamira (Hebrew) precious stone.
Shamir, Shamiran, Shamiria, Shamyra

Shamiya (American) a combination of the prefix Sha + Mia.
Shamea, Shamia, Shamiah, Shamiyah, Shamyia, Shamyiah, Shamyne

Shana (Hebrew) a form of Shane. (Irish) a form of Jane.
Shaana, Shan, Shanae, Shanda, Shandi, Shane, Shania, Shanna, Shannah, Shauna, Shawna

Shanae (Irish) a form of Shana.
Shanay, Shanea

Shanda (American) a form of Chanda, Shana.
Shandae, Shandah, Shandra, Shannda

Shandi (English) a familiar form of Shana.
Shandee, Shandeigh, Shandey, Shandice, Shandie

Shandra (American) a form of Shanda. See also Chandra.
Shandrea, Shandreka, Shandri, Shandria, Shandriah, Shandrice, Shandrie, Shandry

Shane ☆ (Irish) God is gracious.
Shanea, Shaneah, Shanee, Shanée, Shanie

Shaneisha (American) a combination of the prefix Sha + Aisha.
Shanesha, Shaneshia, Shanessa, Shanisha, Shanissha

Shaneka (American) a form of Shanika.
Shanecka, Shaneeka, Shaneekah, Shaneequa, Shaneeque, Shaneika, Shaneikah, Shanekia, Shanequa, Shaneyka, Shonneka

Shanel, Shanell, Shanelle
(American) forms of Chanel.
*Schanel, Schanell, Shanella,
Shanelly, Shannel, Shannell,
Shannelle, Shenel, Shenela,
Shenell, Shenelle, Shenelly,
Shinelle, Shonelle, Shynelle*

Shaneta (American) a
combination of the prefix Sha +
Neta.
*Seanette, Shaneeta, Shanetha,
Shanethis, Shanetta, Shanette,
Shineta, Shonetta*

Shani (Swahili) a form of Shany.

Shania (American) a form of
Shana.
*Shanasia, Shanaya, Shaniah,
Shaniya, Shanya, Shenia*

Shanice (American) a form of
Janice. See also Chanise.
*Chenise, Shanece, Shaneese,
Shaneice, Shanese, Shanicea,
Shaniece, Shanise, Shanneice,
Shannice, Shanyce, Sheneice*

Shanida (American) a
combination of the prefix Sha +
Ida.
Shaneeda, Shannida

Shanika (American) a
combination of the prefix Sha +
Nika.
*Shaneka, Shanica, Shanicca,
Shanicka, Shanieka, Shanike,
Shanikia, Shanikka, Shanikqua,
Shanikwa, Shaniqua, Shenika,
Shineeca, Shonnika*

Shaniqua (American) a form of
Shanika.
*Shaniqa, Shaniquah, Shanique,
Shaniquia, Shaniquwa,
Shaniqwa, Shenequa, Sheniqua,
Shinequa, Shiniqua*

Shanise (American) a form of
Shanice.
*Shanisa, Shanisha, Shanisia,
Shanissa, Shanisse, Shineese*

Shanita (American) a
combination of the prefix Sha +
Nita.
*Shanitha, Shanitra, Shanitta,
Shinita*

Shanley **GB** (Irish) hero's child.
*Shanlee, Shanleigh, Shanlie,
Shanly*

Shanna (Irish) a form of Shana,
Shannon.
Shanea, Shannah, Shannea

Shannen (Irish) a form of
Shannon.
Shanen, Shanena, Shanene

Shannon **GB** (Irish) small and
wise.
*Shanan, Shanadoah, Shann,
Shanna, Shannan, Shanneen,
Shannen, Shannie, Shannin,
Shannyn, Shanon*

Shanta, Shante (French) forms
of Chantal.
*Shantai, Shantay, Shantaya,
Shantaye, Shanté, Shantea,
Shantee, Shantée, Shanteia*

Shantae GB (French) a form of Chantal.

Shantal (American) a form of Shantel.
Shantall, Shontal

Shantana (American) a form of Santana.
Shantan, Shantanae, Shantanell, Shantanickia, Shantanika, Shantanna

Shantara (American) a combination of the prefix Sha + Tara.
Shantaria, Shantarra, Shantera, Shanteria, Shanterra, Shantira, Shontara, Shuntara

Shanteca (American) a combination of the prefix Sha + Teca.
Shantecca, Shanteka, Shantika, Shantikia

Shantel, Shantell GB (American) song.
Seantelle, Shanntell, Shanta, Shantal, Shantae, Shantale, Shante, Shanteal, Shanteil, Shantele, Shantella, Shantelle, Shantrell, Shantyl, Shantyle, Shauntel, Shauntell, Shauntelle, Shauntrel, Shauntrell, Shauntrella, Shentel, Shentelle, Shontal, Shontalla, Shontalle, Shontel, Shontelle

Shanteria (American) a form of Shantara.
Shanterica, Shanterria, Shanterrie, Shantieria, Shantirea, Shonteria

Shantesa (American) a combination of the prefix Sha + Tess.
Shantese, Shantice, Shantise, Shantisha, Shontecia, Shontessia

Shantia (American) a combination of the prefix Sha + Tia.
Shanteya, Shanti, Shantida, Shantie, Shaunteya, Shauntia, Shontia

Shantille (American) a form of Chantilly.
Shanteil, Shantil, Shantilli, Shantillie, Shantilly, Shantyl, Shantyle

Shantina (American) a combination of the prefix Sha + Tina.
Shanteena, Shontina

Shantora (American) a combination of the prefix Sha + Tory.
Shantoia, Shantori, Shantoria, Shantory, Shantorya, Shantoya, Shanttoria

Shantrice (American) a combination of the prefix Sha + Trice. See also Chantrice.
Shantrece, Shantrecia, Shantreece, Shantreese, Shantrese, Shantress, Shantrezia, Shantricia, Shantriece, Shantris, Shantrisse, Shontrice

Shany (Swahili) marvelous, wonderful.
Shaney, Shannai, Shannea, Shanni, Shannia, Shannie, Shanny, Shanya

Shappa (Native American) red thunder.

Shaquanda (American) a combination of the prefix Sha + Wanda.
Shaquan, Shaquana, Shaquand, Shaquandey, Shaquandra, Shaquandria, Shaquanera, Shaquani, Shaquania, Shaquanna, Shaquanta, Shaquantae, Shaquantay, Shaquante, Shaquantia, Shaquona, Shaquonda, Shaquondra, Shaquondria

Shaqueita, Shaquita (American) forms of Shakeita.
Shaqueta, Shaquetta, Shaquette, Shaquitta, Shequida, Shequita, Shequittia

Shaquila, Shaquilla (American) forms of Shakila.
Shaquail, Shaquia, Shaquil, Shaquilah, Shaquile, Shaquill, Shaquillah, Shaquille, Shaquillia, Shequela, Shequele, Shequila, Shquiyla

Shaquille BG (American) a form of Shaquila.

Shaquira (American) a form of Shakira.
Shaquirah, Shaquire, Shaquirra, Shaqura, Shaqurah, Shaquri

Shara (Hebrew) a short form of Sharon.
Shaara, Sharah, Sharal, Sharala, Sharalee, Sharlyn, Sharlynn, Sharra, Sharrah

Sharai (Hebrew) princess. See also Sharon.
Sharae, Sharaé, Sharah, Sharaiah, Sharay, Sharaya, Sharayah

Sharan (Hindi) protector.
Sharaine, Sharanda, Sharanjeet

Shardae, Sharday (Punjabi) charity. (Yoruba) honored by royalty. (Arabic) runaway. A form of Chardae.
Sade, Shadae, Sharda, Shar-Dae, Shardai, Shar-Day, Sharde, Shardea, Shardee, Shardée, Shardei, Shardeia, Shardey

Sharee (English) a form of Shari.
Shareen, Shareena, Sharine

Shari (French) beloved, dearest. (Hungarian) a form of Sarah. See also Sharita, Sheree, Sherry.
Shara, Share, Sharee, Sharia, Shariah, Sharian, Shariann, Sharianne, Sharie, Sharra, Sharree, Sharri, Sharrie, Sharry, Shary

Sharice (French) a form of Cherice.
Shareese, Sharesse, Sharese, Sharica, Sharicka, Shariece, Sharis, Sharise, Sharish, Shariss, Sharissa, Sharisse, Sharyse

Sharik (African) child of God.

Sharissa (American) a form of
Sharice.
*Sharesa, Sharessia, Sharisa,
Sharisha, Shereeza, Shericia,
Sherisa, Sherissa*

Sharita (French) a familiar form
of Shari. (American) a form of
Charity. See also Sherita.
Shareeta, Sharrita

Sharla (French) a short form of
Sharlene, Sharlotte.

Sharlene (French) little and
strong.
*Scharlane, Scharlene, Shar,
Sharla, Sharlaina, Sharlaine,
Sharlane, Sharlanna, Sharlee,
Sharleen, Sharleine, Sharlena,
Sharleyne, Sharline, Sharlyn,
Sharlyne, Sharlynn, Sharlynne,
Sherlean, Sherleen, Sherlene,
Sherline*

Sharlotte (American) a form of
Charlotte.
*Sharlet, Sharlett, Sharlott,
Sharlotta*

Sharma (American) a short form
of Sharmaine.
Sharmae, Sharme

Sharmaine (American) a form of
Charmaine.
*Sharma, Sharmain, Sharman,
Sharmane, Sharmanta,
Sharmayne, Sharmeen,
Sharmene, Sharmese, Sharmin,
Sharmine, Sharmon, Sharmyn*

Sharna (Hebrew) a form of
Sharon.
*Sharnae, Sharnay, Sharne,
Sharnea, Sharnease, Sharnee,
Sharneese, Sharnell, Sharnelle,
Sharnese, Sharnett, Sharnetta,
Sharnise*

Sharon GB (Hebrew) desert
plain. A form of Sharai.
*Shaaron, Shara, Sharai, Sharan,
Shareen, Sharen, Shari, Sharin,
Sharna, Sharonda, Sharone,
Sharran, Sharren, Sharrin,
Sharron, Sharrona, Sharyn,
Sharyon, Sheren, Sheron, Sherryn*

Sharonda (Hebrew) a form of
Sharon.
Sharronda, Sheronda, Sherrhonda

Sharrona (Hebrew) a form of
Sharon.
*Sharona, Sharone, Sharonia,
Sharonna, Sharony, Sharronne,
Sheron, Sherona, Sheronna,
Sherron, Sherronna, Sherronne,
Shirona*

Shatara (Hindi) umbrella.
(Arabic) good; industrious.
(American) a combination of
Sharon + Tara.
*Shatarea, Shatari, Shataria,
Shatarra, Shataura, Shateira,
Shatera, Shaterah, Shateria,
Shaterra, Shaterri, Shaterria,
Shatherian, Shatierra, Shatiria*

Shatoria (American) a combination of the prefix Sha + Tory.
Shatora, Shatorea, Shatori,

Shatorri, Shatorria, Shatory,
Shatorya, Shatoya

Shaun BG (Hebrew, Irish) God is
gracious.

Shauna (Hebrew) a form of
Shaun. (Irish) a form of Shana.
See also Seana, Shona.
Shaun, Shaunah, Shaunda,
Shaune, Shaunee, Shauneen,
Shaunelle, Shaunette, Shauni,
Shaunice, Shaunicy, Shaunie,
Shaunika, Shaunisha, Shaunna,
Shaunnea, Shaunta, Shaunua,
Shaunya

Shaunda (Irish) a form of
Shauna. See also Shanda,
Shawnda, Shonda.
Shaundal, Shaundala, Shaundel,
Shaundela, Shaundell,
Shaundelle, Shaundra,
Shaundrea, Shaundree,
Shaundria, Shaundrice

Shaunta (Irish) a form of
Shauna. See also Shawnta,
Shonta.
Schunta, Shauntae, Shauntay,
Shaunte, Shauntea, Shauntee,
Shauntée, Shaunteena, Shauntei,
Shauntia, Shauntier, Shauntrel,
Shauntrell, Shauntrella

Shavon GB (American) a form of
Shavonne.
Schavon, Schevon, Shavan,
Shavana, Shavaun, Shavona,
Shavonda, Shavone, Shavonia,
Shivon

Shavonne (American) a combi-
nation of the prefix Sha +
Yvonne. See also Siobhan.
Shavanna, Shavon, Shavondra,
Shavonn, Shavonna, Shavonni,
Shavonnia, Shavonnie,
Shavontae, Shavonte, Shavonté,
Shavoun, Shivaun, Shivawn,
Shivonne, Shyvon, Shyvonne

Shawanna (American) a combi-
nation of the prefix Sha + Wanda.
See also Shajuana, Shawna.
Shawan, Shawana, Shawanda,
Shawante, Shiwani

Shawn BG (Hebrew, Irish) God is
gracious.

Shawna (Hebrew) a form of
Shawn. (Irish) a form of Jane. A
form of Shana, Shauna. See also
Seana, Shona.
Sawna, Shaw, Shawn, Shawnae,
Shawnai, Shawnea, Shawnee,
Shawneen, Shawneena,
Shawnell, Shawnette, Shawnna,
Shawnra, Shawnta, Sheona,
Siân, Siana, Sianna

Shawnda (Irish) a form of
Shawna. See also Shanda,
Shaunda, Shonda.
Shawndal, Shawndala, Shawndan,
Shawndel, Shawndra, Shawndrea,
Shawndree, Shawndreel,
Shawndrell, Shawndria

Shawnee (Irish) a form of
Shawna.
Shawne, Shawneea, Shawney,
Shawni, Shawnie

Shawnika (American) a combination of Shawna + Nika.
Shawnaka, Shawnequa, Shawneika, Shawnicka

Shawnta GB (Irish) a form of Shawna. See also Shaunta, Shonta.
Shawntae, Shawntay, Shawnte, Shawnté, Shawntee, Shawntell, Shawntelle, Shawnteria, Shawntia, Shawntil, Shawntile, Shawntill, Shawntille, Shawntina, Shawntish, Shawntrese, Shawntriece

Shay BG (Irish) a form of Shea.
Shaya, Shayah, Shayda, Shayha, Shayia, Shayla, Shey, Sheye

Shaye (Irish) a form of Shay.

Shayla (Irish) a form of Shay.
Shaylagh, Shaylah, Shaylain, Shaylan, Shaylea, Shayleah, Shaylla, Shaylyn, Sheyla

Shaylee (Irish) a form of Shea.
Shaylei, Shayleigh, Shayley, Shayli, Shaylie, Shayly, Shealy

Shaylyn (Irish) a form of Shea.
Shaylin, Shaylina, Shaylinn, Shaylynn, Shaylynne, Shealyn, Sheylyn

Shayna (Hebrew) beautiful.
Shaynae, Shaynah, Shayne, Shaynee, Shayney, Shayni, Shaynie, Shaynna, Shaynne, Shayny, Sheana, Sheanna

Shayne BG (Hebrew) a form of Shayna.

Shea GB (Irish) fairy palace.
Shae, Shay, Shaylee, Shaylyn, Shealy, Shaelee, Shaelyn, Shealyn, Sheann, Sheannon, Sheanta, Sheaon, Shearra, Sheatara, Sheaunna, Sheavon

Sheba (Hebrew) a short form of Bathsheba. Geography: an ancient country of south Arabia.
Saba, Sabah, Shebah, Sheeba

Sheena (Hebrew) God is gracious. (Irish) a form of Jane.
Sheenagh, Sheenah, Sheenan, Sheeneal, Sheenika, Sheenna, Sheina, Shena, Shiona

Sheila (Latin) blind. (Irish) a form of Cecelia. See also Cheyla, Zelizi.
Seelia, Seila, Selia, Shaila, Sheela, Sheelagh, Sheelah, Sheilagh, Sheilah, Sheileen, Sheiletta, Sheilia, Sheillynn, Sheilya, Shela, Shelagh, Shelah, Shelia, Shiela, Shila, Shilah, Shilea, Shyla

Shelbi, Shelbie (English) forms of Shelby.
Shelbbie, Shellbi, Shellbie

Shelby GB (English) ledge estate.
Chelby, Schelby, Shel, Shelbe, Shelbee, Shelbey, Shelbi, Shelbie, Shelbye, Shellby

Sheldon BG (English) farm on the ledge.
Sheldina, Sheldine, Sheldrina, Sheldyn, Shelton

Shelee (English) a form of Shelley.
Shelee, Sheleen, Shelena, Sheley, Sheli, Shelia, Shelina, Shelinda, Shelita

Shelisa (American) a combination of Shelley + Lisa.
Sheleza, Shelica, Shelicia, Shelise, Shelisse, Sheliza

Shelley, Shelly GB (English) meadow on the ledge. (French) familiar forms of Michelle. See also Rochelle.
Shelee, Shell, Shella, Shellaine, Shellana, Shellany, Shellee, Shellene, Shelli, Shellian, Shelliann, Shellie, Shellina

Shelsea (American) a form of Chelsea.
Shellsea, Shellsey, Shelsey, Shelsie, Shelsy

Shelton BG (English) a form of Sheldon.

Shena (Irish) a form of Sheena.
Shenada, Shenae, Shenah, Shenay, Shenda, Shene, Shenea, Sheneda, Shenee, Sheneena, Shenica, Shenika, Shenina, Sheniqua, Shenita, Shenna, Shennae, Shennah, Shenoa

Shera (Aramaic) light.
Sheera, Sheerah, Sherae, Sherah, Sheralee, Sheralle, Sheralyn, Sheralynn, Sheralynne, Sheray, Sheraya

Sheree (French) beloved, dearest.
Scherie, Sheeree, Shere, Shereé, Sherrelle, Shereen, Shereena

Sherelle (French) a form of Cherelle, Sheryl.
Sherel, Sherell, Sheriel, Sherrel, Sherrell, Sherrelle, Shirelle

Sheri, Sherri (French) forms of Sherry.
Sheria, Sheriah, Sherie, Sherrie

Sherian (American) a combination of Sheri + Ann.
Sherianne, Sherrina

Sherice (French) a form of Cherice.
Scherise, Sherece, Shereece, Sherees, Shereese, Sherese, Shericia, Sherise, Sherisse, Sherrish, Sherryse, Sheryce

Sheridan GB (Irish) wild.
Sherida, Sheridane, Sherideen, Sheriden, Sheridian, Sheridon, Sherridan, Sherridon

Sherika (Punjabi) relative. (Arabic) easterner.
Shereka, Sherica, Shericka, Sherrica, Sherricka, Sherrika

Sherissa (French) a form of Sherry, Sheryl.
Shereeza, Sheresa, Shericia, Sherrish

Sherita (French) a form of Sherry, Sheryl. See also Sharita.
Shereta, Sheretta, Sherette, Sherrita

Sherleen (French, English) a
form of Sheryl, Shirley.
*Sherileen, Sherlene, Sherlin,
Sherlina, Sherline, Sherlyn,
Sherlyne, Sherlynne, Shirlena,
Shirlene, Shirlina, Shirlyn*

Sherry GB (French) beloved,
dearest. A familiar form of Sheryl.
See also Sheree.
*Sherey, Sheri, Sherissa, Sherrey,
Sherri, Sherria, Sherriah, Sherrie,
Sherye, Sheryy*

Sheryl (French) beloved. A familiar
form of Shirley. See also Sherry.
*Sharel, Sharil, Sharilyn, Sharyl,
Sharyll, Sheral, Sherell, Sheriel,
Sheril, Sherill, Sherily, Sherilyn,
Sherissa, Sherita, Sherleen,
Sherral, Sherrelle, Sherril,
Sherrill, Sherryl, Sherylly*

Sherylyn (American) a
combination of Sheryl + Lynn.
See also Cherilyn.
*Sharolin, Sharolyn, Sharyl-Lynn,
Sheralyn, Sherilyn, Sherilynn,
Sherilynne, Sherralyn, Sherralynn,
Sherrilyn, Sherrilynn, Sherrilynne,
Sherrylyn, Sherryn, Sherylanne*

Shevonne (American) a
combination of the prefix She +
Yvonne.
*Shevaun, Shevon, Shevonda,
Shevone*

Sheyenne (Cheyenne) a form of
Cheyenne. See also Shyann,
Shyanne.
Shayhan, Sheyan, Sheyane,

*Sheyann, Sheyanna, Sheyannah,
Sheyanne, Sheyen, Sheyene,
Shiante, Shyanne*

Shianne (Cheyenne) a form of
Cheyenne.
*She, Shian, Shiana, Shianah,
Shianda, Shiane, Shiann,
Shianna, Shiannah, Shiany,
Shieana, Shieann, Shieanne,
Shiena, Shiene, Shienna*

Shifra (Hebrew) beautiful.
Schifra, Shifrah

Shika (Japanese) gentle deer.
Shi, Shikah, Shikha

Shilo (Hebrew) God's gift. Bible: a
sanctuary for the Israelites where
the Ark of the Covenant was kept.
Shiloh

Shina (Japanese) virtuous, good;
wealthy. (Chinese) a form of
China.
Shinae, Shinay, Shine, Shinna

Shino (Japanese) bamboo stalk.

Shiquita (American) a form of
Chiquita.
Shiquata, Shiquitta

Shira (Hebrew) song.
*Shirah, Shiray, Shire, Shiree,
Shiri, Shirit, Shyra*

Shirlene (English) a form of
Shirley.
Shirleen, Shirline, Shirlynn

Shirley (English) bright meadow.
See also Sheryl.
Sherlee, Sherleen, Sherley,

*Sherli, Sherlie, Shir, Shirl, Shirlee,
Shirlie, Shirly, Shirlly, Shurlee,
Shurley*

Shivani (Hindi) life and death.
*Shiva, Shivana, Shivanie,
Shivanna*

Shizu (Japanese) silent.
Shizue, Shizuka, Shizuko, Shizuyo

Shona (Irish) a form of Jane. A
form of Shana, Shauna, Shawna.
*Shiona, Shonagh, Shonah,
Shonalee, Shonda, Shone,
Shonee, Shonette, Shoni, Shonie,
Shonna, Shonnah, Shonta*

Shonda (Irish) a form of Shona.
See also Shanda, Shaunda,
Shawnda.
*Shondalette, Shondalyn, Shondel,
Shondelle, Shondi, Shondia,
Shondie, Shondra, Shondreka,
Shounda*

Shonta (Irish) a form of Shona.
See also Shaunta, Shawnta.
*Shontá, Shontae, Shontai,
Shontalea, Shontasia, Shontavia,
Shontaviea, Shontay, Shontaya,
Shonte, Shonté, Shontedra,
Shontee, Shonteral, Shonti,
Shontol, Shontoy, Shontrail,
Shountáe*

Shoshana (Hebrew) a form of
Susan.
*Shosha, Shoshan, Shoshanah,
Shoshane, Shoshanha, Shoshann,
Shoshanna, Shoshannah,
Shoshauna, Shoshaunah,
Shoshawna, Shoshona,*

*Shoshone, Shoshonee,
Shoshoney, Shoshoni, Shoushan,
Shushana, Sosha, Soshana*

Shu (Chinese) kind, gentle.

Shug (American) a short form of
Sugar.

Shula (Arabic) flaming, bright.
Shulah

Shulamith (Hebrew) peaceful.
See also Sula.
Shulamit, Sulamith

Shunta (Irish) a form of Shonta.
*Shuntae, Shunté, Shuntel,
Shuntell, Shuntelle, Shuntia*

Shura (Russian) a form of
Alexandra.
*Schura, Shurah, Shuree, Shureen,
Shurelle, Shuritta, Shurka,
Shurlana*

Shyann, Shyanne (Cheyenne)
forms of Cheyenne. See also
Sheyenne.
*Shyan, Shyana, Shyandra,
Shyane, Shynee, Shyanna,
Shyannah, Shye, Shyene,
Shyenna, Shyenne*

Shyla **GB** (English) a form of
Sheila.
*Shya, Shyah, Shylah, Shylan,
Shylayah, Shylana, Shylane,
Shyle, Shyleah, Shylee, Shyley,
Shyli, Shylia, Shylie, Shylo,
Shyloe, Shyloh, Shylon, Shylyn*

Shyra (Hebrew) a form of Shira.
Shyrae, Shyrah, Shyrai, Shyrie, Shyro

Sianna (Irish) a form of Seana.
Sian, Siana, Sianae, Sianai, Sianey, Siannah, Sianne, Sianni, Sianny, Siany

Siara (Irish) a form of Sierra.
Siarah, Siarra, Siarrah, Sieara

Sibeta (Moquelumnan) finding a fish under a rock.

Sibila (Greek) she who prophesizes.

Sibley (English) sibling; friendly.
(Greek) a form of Sybil.
Sybley

Sidney GB (French) a form of Sydney.
Sidne, Sidnee, Sidnei, Sidneya, Sidni, Sidnie, Sidny, Sidnye

Sidonia (Hebrew) enticing.
Sydania, Syndonia

Sidonie (French) from Saint-Denis, France. See also Sydney.
Sedona, Sidaine, Sidanni, Sidelle, Sidoine, Sidona, Sidonae, Sidonia, Sidony

Sidra (Latin) star child.
Sidrah, Sidras

Sienna (American) a form of Ciana.
Seini, Siena

Siera (Irish) a form of Sierra.
Sierah, Sieria

Sierra ☀ GB (Irish) black.
(Spanish) saw toothed.
Geography: any rugged range of mountains that, when viewed from a distance, has a jagged profile. See also Ciara.
Seara, Searria, Seera, Seirra, Siara, Siearra, Siera, Sierrah, Sierre, Sierrea, Sierriah, Syerra

Sigfreda (German) victorious peace. See also Freda.
Sigfreida, Sigfrida, Sigfrieda, Sigfryda

Sigmunda (German) victorious protector.
Sigmonda

Signe (Latin) sign, signal.
(Scandinavian) a short form of Sigourney.
Sig, Signa, Signy, Singna, Singne

Sigourney (English) victorious conquerer.
Signe, Sigournee, Sigourny

Sigrid (Scandinavian) victorious counselor.
Siegrid, Siegrida, Sigritt

Sihu (Native American) flower; bush.

Siko (African) crying baby.

Silas BG (Latin) a short form of Silvan (see Boys' Names).

Silvana (Latin) a form of Sylvana.
Silvaine, Silvanna, Silviane

Silveria (Spanish) she who was born in the jungle.

Silvia (Latin) a form of Sylvia.
Silivia, Silva, Silvya

Silvina (Spanish) a form of
Silvana.

Simcha BG (Hebrew) joyful.

Simon BG (Hebrew) he heard.
Bible: one of the Twelve
Disciples.

Simone GB (Hebrew, French) a
form of Simon.
*Samone, Siminie, Simmi, Simmie,
Simmona, Simmone, Simoane,
Simona, Simonetta, Simonette,
Simonia, Simonina, Simonne,
Somone, Symone*

Simran GB (Sikh) absorbed in
God.
Simren, Simrin, Simrun

Sina (Irish) a form of Seana.
*Seena, Sinai, Sinaia, Sinan,
Sinay*

Sinclaire (French) prayer.
Sinclair

Sinclética (Greek) she who is
invited.

Sindy (American) a form of Cindy.
*Sinda, Sindal, Sindee, Sindi,
Sindia, Sindie, Sinnedy, Synda,
Syndal, Syndee, Syndey, Syndi,
Syndia, Syndie, Syndy*

Sinead (Irish) a form of Jane.
Seonaid, Sine, Sinéad

Sinforosa (Latin) full of
misfortunes.

Sintiques (Greek) she who
arrives on a special occasion.

Siobhan GB (Irish) a form of
Joan. See also Shavonne.
*Shibahn, Shibani, Shibhan,
Shioban, Shobana, Shobha,
Shobhana, Siobahn, Siobhana,
Siobhann, Siobhon, Siovaun,
Siovhan*

Sira (Latin) she who comes from
Syria.

Sirena (Greek) enchanter.
Mythology: Sirens were sea
nymphs whose singing enchanted
sailors and made them crash
their ships into nearby rocks.
*Sireena, Sirene, Sirine, Syrena,
Syrenia, Syrenna, Syrina*

Siria (Persian) brilliant as the
sun.

Sisika (Native American)
songbird.

Sissy (American) a familiar form
of Cecelia.
Sisi, Sisie, Sissey, Sissie

Sita (Hindi) a form of Shakti.
Sitah, Sitarah, Sitha, Sithara

Siti (Swahili) respected woman.

Skye GB (Arabic) water giver.
(Dutch) a short form of Skyler.
Geography: an island in the
Hebrides, Scotland.
*Ski, Skie, Skii, Skky, Sky, Skya,
Skyy*

Skylar BG (Dutch) a form of Skyler.
Skyela, Skyelar, Skyla, Skylair, Skyylar

Skyler BG (Dutch) sheltering.
Skila, Skilah, Skye, Skyeler, Skyelur, Skyla, Skylar, Skylee, Skylena, Skyli, Skylia, Skylie, Skylin, Skyllar, Skylor, Skylyn, Skylynn, Skylyr, Skyra

Sloane (Irish) warrior.
Sloan, Sloanne

Socorro (Spanish) helper.

Sofia ☀ GB (Greek) a form of Sophia. See also Zofia, Zsofia.
Sofeea, Sofeeia, Soffi, Sofi, Soficita, Sofie, Sofija, Sofiya, Sofka, Sofya

Sofía (Greek) a form of Sofia.

Sol (Latin) she who possesses brightness.

Solada (Tai) listener.

Solana (Spanish) sunshine.
Solande, Solanna, Soleil, Solena, Soley, Solina, Solinda

Solange (French) dignified.

Soledad (Spanish) solitary.
Sole, Soleda

Soledada (Spanish) solitary.

Solenne (French) solemn, dignified.
Solaine, Solene, Soléne, Solenna, Solina, Soline, Solonez, Souline, Soulle

Solita (Latin) solitary.

Solomon BG (Hebrew) peaceful.

Soma (Hindi) lunar.

Sommer (English) summer; summoner. (Arabic) black. See also Summer.
Somara, Somer, Sommar, Sommara, Sommers

Somoche (Mapuche) distinguished woman, woman of her word.

Sondra (Greek) defender of mankind.
Saundra, Sondre, Sonndra, Sonndre

Sonia (Russian, Slavic) a form of Sonya.
Sonica, Sonida, Sonita, Sonna, Sonni, Sonnia, Sonnie, Sonny

Sonja (Scandinavian) a form of Sonya.
Sonjae, Sonjia

Sonny BG (Russian, Slavic) a form of Sonia.

Sonora (Spanish) pleasant sounding.

Sonya GB (Greek) wise. (Russian, Slavic) a form of Sophia.
Sonia, Sonja, Sonnya, Sonyae, Sunya

Sook (Korean) pure.

Sopheary (Cambodian) beautiful girl.

Sophia ☆ GB (Greek) wise. See
also Sonya, Zofia.
Sofia, Sophie

Sophie GB (Greek) a familiar
form of Sophia. See also Zocha.
Sophey, Sophi, Sophy

Sophronia (Greek) wise;
sensible.
Soffrona, Sofronia

Sora (Native American) chirping
songbird.

Soraya (Persian) princess.
Suraya

Sorrel GB (French) reddish
brown. Botany: a plant whose
leaves are used as salad greens.

Sorya (Spanish) she who is
eloquent.

Soso (Native American) tree
squirrel dining on pine nuts;
chubby-cheeked baby.

Souzan (Persian) burning fire.
Sousan, Souzanne

Spencer BG (English) dispenser
of provisions.
Spenser

Speranza (Italian) a form of
Esperanza.
Speranca

Spica (Latin) star's name.

Spring (English) springtime.
Spryng

Stacey, Stacy GB (Greek)
resurrection. (Irish) a short form
of Anastasia, Eustacia, Natasha.
*Stace, Stacee, Staceyan,
Staceyann, Staicy, Stasey, Stasya,
Stayce, Staycee, Staci, Steacy*

Staci, Stacie (Greek) forms of
Stacey.
Stacci, Stacia, Stayci

Stacia (English) a short form of
Anastasia.
Stasia, Staysha

Stanley BG (English) stony
meadow.

Starla (English) a form of Starr.
Starrla

Starleen (English) a form of Starr.
*Starleena, Starlena, Starlene,
Starlin, Starlyn, Starlynn, Starrlen*

Starley (English) a familiar form
of Starr.
Starle, Starlee, Staly

Starling BG (English) bird.

Starr GB (English) star.
*Star, Staria, Starisha, Starla,
Starleen, Starlet, Starlette,
Starley, Starlight, Starre, Starri,
Starria, Starrika, Starrsha,
Starsha, Starshanna, Startish*

Stasya (Greek) a familiar form of
Anastasia. (Russian) a form of
Stacey.
*Stasa, Stasha, Stashia, Stasia,
Stasja, Staska*

Stefani, Steffani (Greek) forms of Stephanie.
Stafani, Stefanni, Steffane, Steffanee, Stefini, Stefoni

Stefanía (Greek) a form of Stefanie.

Stefanie (Greek) a form of Stephanie.
Stafanie, Staffany, Stefane, Stefanee, Stefaney, Stefania, Stefanié, Stefanija, Stefannie, Stefcia, Stefenie, Steffanie, Steffi, Stefinie, Stefka

Stefany, Steffany (Greek) forms of Stephanie.
Stefanny, Stefanya, Steffaney

Steffi (Greek) a familiar form of Stefanie, Stephanie.
Stefa, Stefcia, Steffee, Steffie, Steffy, Stefi, Stefka, Stefy, Stepha, Stephi, Stephie, Stephy

Stella GB (Latin) star. (French) a familiar form of Estelle.
Steile, Stellina

Stepania (Russian) a form of Stephanie.
Stepa, Stepahny, Stepanida, Stepanie, Stepanyda, Stepfanie, Stephana

Stephane BG (Greek) a form of Stephanie.

Stephani (Greek) a form of Stephanie.
Stephania, Stephanni

Stephanie ☀ GB (Greek) a form of Stephen. See also Estefani, Estephanie, Panya, Stevie, Zephania.
Stamatios, Stefani, Stefanie, Stefany, Steffie, Stepania, Stephaija, Stephaine, Stephanas, Stephane, Stephanee, Stephani, Stephanida, Stéphanie, Stephanine, Stephann, Stephannie, Stephany, Stephene, Stephenie, Stephianie, Stephney, Stesha, Steshka, Stevanee

Stephany GB (Greek) a form of Stephanie.
Stephaney, Stephanye

Stephen BG (Greek) crowned.

Stephene (Greek) a form of Stephanie.
Stephina, Stephine, Stephyne

Stephenie (Greek) a form of Stephanie.
Stephena, Stephenee, Stepheney, Stepheni, Stephenny, Stepheny, Stephine, Stephinie

Stephney (Greek) a form of Stephanie.
Stephne, Stephni, Stephnie, Stephny

Sterling BG (English) valuable; silver penny.

Stetson BG (Danish) stepchild.

Steven BG (Greek) a form of Stephen.

Stevie GB (Greek) a familiar
form of Stephanie.
*Steva, Stevana, Stevanee, Stevee,
Stevena, Stevey, Stevi, Stevy,
Stevye*

Stewart BG (English) a form of
Stuart.

Stina (German) a short form of
Christina.
Steena, Stena, Stine, Stinna

Stockard (English) stockyard.

Storm BG (English) a short form
of Stormy.

Stormie (English) a form of Stormy.
Stormee, Stormi, Stormii

Stormy GB (English) impetuous
by nature.
*Storm, Storme, Stormey, Stormie,
Stormm*

Stuart BG (English) caretaker,
steward.

Suchin (Tai) beautiful thought.

Sue (Hebrew) a short form of
Susan, Susanna.

Sueann, Sueanna (American)
combinations of Sue + Ann, Sue
+ Anna.
*Suann, Suanna, Suannah,
Suanne, Sueanne*

Suela (Spanish) consolation.
Suelita

Sugar (American) sweet as sugar.
Shug

Sugi (Japanese) cedar tree.

Suke (Hawaiian) a form of Susan.

Sukey (Hawaiian) a familiar form
of Susan.
Suka, Sukee, Suki, Sukie, Suky

Sukhdeep GB (Sikh) light of
peace and bliss.
Sukhdip

Suki (Japanese) loved one.
(Moquelumnan) eagle-eyed.
Sukie

Sula (Icelandic) large sea bird.
(Greek, Hebrew) a short form of
Shulamith, Ursula.

Suletu (Moquelumnan) soaring
bird.

Sulamita (Hebrew) gentle,
peaceful woman.

Sulia (Latin) a form of Julia.
Suliana

Sulwen (Welsh) bright as the sun.

Sumalee (Tai) beautiful flower.

Sumati (Hindi) unity.

Sumaya (American) a combination of Sue + Maya.
Sumayah, Sumayya, Sumayyah

Sumi (Japanese) elegant, refined.
Sumiko

Summer GB (English)
summertime. See also Sommer.
Sumer, Summar, Summerann,
Summerbreeze, Summerhaze,
Summerine, Summerlee,
Summerlin, Summerlyn,
Summerlynn, Summers, Sumrah,
Summyr, Sumyr

Sun (Korean) obedient.
Suncance, Sundee, Sundeep,
Sundi, Sundip, Sundrenea, Santa,
Sunya

Sun-Hi (Korean) good; joyful.

Sunee (Tai) good.
Suni

Suni (Zuni) native; member of
our tribe.
Sunita, Sunitha, Suniti, Sunne,
Sunni, Sunnie, Sunnilei

Sunki (Hopi) swift.
Sunkia

Sunny BG (English) bright,
cheerful.
Sunni, Sunnie

Sunshine (English) sunshine.
Sunshyn, Sunshyne

Surata (Pakistani) blessed joy.

Suri (Todas) pointy nose.
Suree, Surena, Surenia

Surya (Sanskrit) Mythology: a sun
god.
Suria, Suriya, Surra

Susammi (French) a
combination of Susan + Aimee.
Suzami, Suzamie, Suzamy

Susan GB (Hebrew) lily. See also
Shoshana, Sukey, Zsa Zsa, Zusa.
Sawsan, Siusan, Sosan, Sosana,
Sue, Suesan, Sueva, Suisan,
Suke, Susana, Susann, Susanna,
Suse, Susen, Susette, Susie,
Suson, Suzan, Suzanna,
Suzannah, Suzanne, Suzette

Susana GB (Hebrew) a form of
Susan.
Susanah, Susane

Susanita (Spanish) a form of
Susana.

Susanna, Susannah (Hebrew)
forms of Susan. See also Xuxa,
Zanna, Zsuzsanna.
Sonel, Sosana, Sue, Suesanna,
Susana, Susanah, Susanka,
Susette, Susie, Suzanna

Suse (Hawaiian) a form of Susan.

Susette (French) a familiar form
of Susan, Susanna.
Susetta

Susie, Suzie (American) familiar
forms of Susan, Susanna.
Suse, Susey, Susi, Sussi, Sussy,
Susy, Suze, Suzi, Suzy, Suzzie

Suzanna, Suzannah (Hebrew)
forms of Susan.
Suzana, Suzenna, Suzzanna

Suzanne GB (English) a form of Susan.
Susanne, Suszanne, Suzane, Suzann, Suzzane, Suzzann, Suzzanne

Suzette (French) a form of Susan.
Suzetta, Suzzette

Suzu (Japanese) little bell.
Suzue, Suzuko

Suzuki (Japanese) bell tree.

Svetlana (Russian) bright light.
Sveta, Svetochka

Syá (Chinese) summer.

Sybella (English) a form of Sybil.
Sebila, Sibbella, Sibeal, Sibel, Sibell, Sibella, Sibelle, Sibilla, Sibylla, Sybel, Sybelle, Sybila, Sybilla

Sybil (Greek) prophet. Mythology: sibyls were oracles who relayed the messages of the gods. See also Cybele, Sibley.
Sib, Sibbel, Sibbie, Sibbill, Sibby, Sibeal, Sibel, Sibyl, Sibylle, Sibylline, Sybella, Sybille, Syble

Sydnee GB (French) a form of Sydney.
Sydne, Sydnea, Sydnei

Sydney ☆ GB (French) from Saint-Denis, France. See also Sidonie.
Cidney, Cydney, Sidney, Sy, Syd, Sydel, Sydelle, Sydna, Sydnee, Sydni, Sydnie, Sydny, Sydnye, Syndona, Syndonah

Sydni, Sydnie (French) forms of Sydney.

Syed BG (Arabic) happy.

Sying BG (Chinese) star.

Sylvana (Latin) forest.
Sylva, Sylvaine, Sylvanah, Sylvania, Sylvanna, Sylvie, Sylvina, Sylvinnia, Sylvonah, Sylvonia, Sylvonna

Sylvia (Latin) forest. Literature: Sylvia Plath was a well-known American poet. See also Silvia, Xylia.
Sylvette, Sylvie, Sylwia

Sylvianne (American) a combination of Sylvia + Anne.
Sylvian

Sylvie (Latin) a familiar form of Sylvia.
Silvi, Silvie, Silvy, Sylvi

Symone (Hebrew) a form of Simone.
Symmeon, Symmone, Symona, Symoné, Symonne

Symphony (Greek) symphony, harmonious sound.
Symfoni, Symphanie, Symphany, Symphanée, Symphoni, Symphoni

Syreeta (Hindi) good traditions. (Arabic) companion.
Syretta, Syrrita

T

T BG (American) an initial used as a first name.

Tabatha GB (Greek, Aramaic) a form of Tabitha.
Tabathe, Tabathia, Tabbatha

Tabby (English) a familiar form of Tabitha.
Tabbi

Tabetha (Greek, Aramaic) a form of Tabitha.

Tabia (Swahili) talented.
Tabea

Tabina (Arabic) follower of Muhammad.

Tabitha (Greek, Aramaic) gazelle.
Tabatha, Tabbee, Tabbetha, Tabbey, Tabbi, Tabbie, Tabbitha, Tabby, Tabetha, Tabiatha, Tabita, Tabithia, Tabotha, Tabtha, Tabytha

Tabora (Arabic) plays a small drum.

Tabytha (Greek, Aramaic) a form of Tabitha.
Tabbytha

Tacey (English) a familiar form of Tacita.
Tace, Tacee, Taci, Tacy, Tacye

Taci (Zuni) washtub. (English) a form of Tacey.
Tacia, Taciana, Tacie

Tacita (Latin) silent.
Tacey

Tadita (Omaha) runner.
Tadeta, Tadra

Taelor (English) a form of Taylor.
Taelar, Taeler, Taellor, Taelore, Taelyr

Taesha (Latin) a form of Tisha. (American) a combination of the prefix Ta + Aisha.
Tadasha, Taeshayla, Taeshia, Taheisha, Tahisha, Taiesha, Taisha, Taishae, Teasha, Teashia, Teisha, Tesha

Taffy GB (Welsh) beloved.
Taffia, Taffine, Taffye, Tafia, Tafisa, Tafoya

Tahira (Arabic) virginal, pure.
Taheera, Taheerah, Tahera, Tahere, Taheria, Taherri, Tahiara, Tahirah, Tahireh

Tahlia (Greek, Hebrew) a form of Talia.
Tahleah, Tahleia

Tailor (English) a form of Taylor.
Tailar, Tailer, Taillor, Tailyr

Taima GB (Native American) clash of thunder.
Taimi, Taimia, Taimy

Taipa (Moquelumnan) flying quail.

Tais (Greek) she who is beautiful.

Taite (English) cheerful.
Tate, Tayte, Tayten

Taja (Hindi) crown.
Taiajára, Taija, Tajae, Tajah, Tahai, Tehya, Teja, Tejah, Tejal

Taka (Japanese) honored.

Takala (Hopi) corn tassel.

Takara (Japanese) treasure.
Takarah, Takaria, Takarra, Takra

Takayla (American) a combination of the prefix Ta + Kayla.
Takayler, Takeyli

Takeisha (American) a combination of the prefix Ta + Keisha.
Takecia, Takesha, Takeshia, Takesia, Takisha, Takishea, Takishia, Tekeesha, Tekeisha, Tekeshi, Tekeysia, Tekisha, Tikesha, Tikisha, Tokesia, Tykeisha

Takenya (Hebrew) animal horn. (Moquelumnan) falcon. (American) a combination of the prefix Ta + Kenya.
Takenia, Takenja

Takeria (American) a form of Takira.
Takera, Takeri, Takerian, Takerra, Takerria, Takierria, Takoria

Taki (Japanese) waterfall.
Tiki

Takia (Arabic) worshiper.
Takeia, Takeiyah, Takeya, Takeyah, Takhiya, Takiah, Takija, Takiya, Takiyah, Takkia, Takya, Takyah, Takyia, Taqiyya, Taquaia, Taquaya, Taquiia, Tekeiya, Tekeiyah, Tekeyia, Tekiya, Tekiyah, Tikia, Tykeia, Tykia

Takila (American) a form of Tequila.
Takayla, Takeila, Takela, Takelia, Takella, Takeyla, Takiela, Takilah, Takilla, Takilya, Takyla, Takylia, Tatakyla, Tehilla, Tekeila, Tekela, Tekelia, Tekilaa, Tekilia, Tekilla, Tekilyah, Tekla

Takira (American) a combination of the prefix Ta + Kira.
Takara, Takarra, Takeara, Takeera, Takeira, Takeirah, Takera, Takiara, Takiera, Takierah, Takierra, Takirah, Takiria, Takirra, Takora, Takyra, Takyrra, Taquera, Taquira, Tekeria, Tikara, Tikira, Tykera

Tala (Native American) stalking wolf.

Talasi (Hopi) corn tassel.
Talasea, Talasia

Taleah (American) a form of Talia.
Talaya, Talayah, Talayia, Talea, Taleana, Taleea, Taleéi, Talei, Taleia, Taleiya, Tylea, Tyleah, Tylee

Taleisha (American) a combination of Talia + Aisha.
Taileisha, Taleise, Talesha, Talicia, Taliesha, Talisa, Talisha, Talysha, Telisha, Tilisha, Tyleasha, Tyleisha, Tylicia, Tylisha, Tylishia

Talena (American) a combination of the prefix Ta + Lena.
Talayna, Talihna, Taline, Tallenia, Talná, Tilena, Tilene, Tylena

Talesha (American) a form of Taleisha.
Taleesha, Talesa, Talese, Taleshia, Talesia, Tallese, Tallesia, Tylesha, Tyleshia, Tylesia

Talia (Greek) blooming. (Hebrew) dew from heaven. (Latin, French) birthday. A short form of Natalie. See also Thalia.
Tahlia, Taleah, Taliah, Taliatha, Taliea, Taliyah, Talley, Tallia, Tallya, Talya, Tylia

Talía (Greek) a form of Talia.

Talina (American) a combination of Talia + Lina.
Talin, Talinda, Taline, Tallyn, Talyn, Talynn, Tylina, Tyline

Talisa (English) a form of Tallis.
Talisha, Talishia, Talisia, Talissa, Talysa, Talysha, Talysia, Talyssa

Talitha (Arabic) young girl.
Taleetha, Taletha, Talethia, Taliatha, Talita, Talithia, Taliya, Telita, Tiletha

Taliyah (Greek) a form of Talia.
Taleya, Taleyah, Talieya, Talliyah, Talya, Talyah, Talyia

Talley (French) a familiar form of Talia.
Tali, Talle, Tallie, Tally, Taly, Talye

Tallis (French, English) forest.
Talice, Talisa, Talise, Tallys

Tallulah (Choctaw) leaping water.
Tallou, Talula

Talon 🅱🅶 (French, English) claw, nail.

Tam 🅱🅶 (Vietnamese) heart.

Tama (Japanese) jewel.
Tamaa, Tamah, Tamaiah, Tamala, Tema

Tamaka (Japanese) bracelet.
Tamaki, Tamako, Timaka

Tamar 🅶🅱 (Hebrew) a short form of Tamara. (Russian) History: a twelfth-century Georgian queen. (Hebrew) a short form of Tamara.
Tamer, Tamor, Tamour

Tamara (Hebrew) palm tree. See also Tammy.
Tamar, Tamará, Tamarae, Tamarah, Tamaria, Tamarin, Tamarla, Tamarra, Tamarria, Tamarrian, Tamarsha, Tamary, Tamera, Tamira, Tamma, Tammara, Tamora, Tamoya, Tamra, Tamura, Tamyra, Temara, Temarian, Thama, Thamar, Thamara, Thamarra, Timara, Tomara, Tymara

Tamassa (Hebrew) a form of
Thomasina.
*Tamasin, Tamasine, Tamsen,
Tamsin, Tamzen, Tamzin*

Tamaya (Quechua) in the center.

Tameka (Aramaic) twin.
*Tameca, Tamecia, Tamecka,
Tameeka, Tamekia, Tamiecka,
Tamieka, Temeka, Timeeka,
Timeka, Tomeka, Tomekia,
Trameika, Tymeka, Tymmeeka,
Tymmeka*

Tamera (Hebrew) a form of
Tamara.
*Tamer, Tamerai, Tameran,
Tameria, Tamerra, Tammera,
Thamer, Timera*

Tamesha (American) a
combination of the prefix Ta +
Mesha.
*Tameesha, Tameisha, Tameshia,
Tameshkia, Tameshya, Tamisha,
Tamishia, Tamnesha, Temisha,
Timesha, Timisha, Tomesha,
Tomiese, Tomise, Tomisha,
Tramesha, Tramisha, Tymesha*

Tamika (Japanese) a form of
Tamiko.
*Tamica, Tamieka, Tamikah,
Tamikia, Tamikka, Tammika,
Tamyka, Timika, Timikia, Tomika,
Tymika, Tymmicka*

Tamiko (Japanese) child of the
people.
*Tami, Tamika, Tamike, Tamiqua,
Tamiyo, Tammiko*

Tamila (American) a combination
of the prefix Ta + Mila.
*Tamala, Tamela, Tamelia, Tamilla,
Tamille, Tamillia, Tamilya*

Tamira (Hebrew) a form of
Tamara.
*Tamir, Tamirae, Tamirah, Tamiria,
Tamirra, Tamyra, Tamyria,
Tamyrra*

Tammi, Tammie (English) forms
of Tammy.
*Tameia, Tami, Tamia, Tamiah,
Tamie, Tamijo, Tamiya*

Tammy **GB** (English) twin.
(Hebrew) a familiar form of
Tamara.
*Tamilyn, Tamlyn, Tammee,
Tammey, Tammi, Tammie, Tamy,
Tamya*

Tamra (Hebrew) a short form of
Tamara.
Tammra, Tamrah

Tamsin (English) a short form of
Thomasina.

Tana (Slavic) a short form of
Tanya.
*Taina, Tanae, Tanaeah, Tanah,
Tanairi, Tanairy, Tanalia, Tanara,
Tanavia, Tanaya, Tanaz, Tanna,
Tannah*

Tandy (English) team.
*Tanda, Tandalaya, Tandi, Tandie,
Tandis, Tandra, Tandrea, Tandria*

Taneisha (American) a combination of the prefix Ta + Nesha.
Tahniesha, Taineshia, Tanasha, Tanashia, Tanaysia, Tanniecia, Tanniesha, Tantashea

Tanesha GB (American) a combination of the prefix Ta + Nesha.
Taneshea, Taneshia, Taneshya, Tanesia, Tanesian, Tanessa, Tanessia, Taniesha, Tannesha, Tanneshia, Tantashea

Taneya (Russian, Slavic) a form of Tanya.
Tanea, Taneah, Tanee, Taneé, Taneia

Tangia (American) a combination of the prefix Ta + Angela.
Tangela, Tangi, Tangie, Tanja, Tanji, Tanjia, Tanjie

Tani GB (Japanese) valley. (Slavic) stand of glory. A familiar form of Tania.
Tahnee, Tahni, Tahnie, Tanee, Taney, Tanie, Tany

Tania (Russian, Slavic) fairy queen.
Taneea, Tani, Taniah, Tanija, Tanika, Tanis, Taniya, Tannia, Tannis, Tanniya, Tannya, Tarnia

Taniel (American) a combination of Tania + Danielle.
Taniele, Tanielle, Teniel, Teniele, Tenielle

Tanika (American) a form of Tania.
Tanikka, Tanikqua, Taniqua, Tanique, Tannica, Tianeka, Tianika

Tanis GB (Slavic) a form of Tania, Tanya.
Tanas, Tanese, Taniese, Tanise, Tanisia, Tanka, Tenice, Tenise, Tenyse, Tiannis, Tonise, Trance, Tranise, Tynice, Tyniece, Tyniese, Tynise

Tanisha (American) a combination of the prefix Ta + Nisha.
Tahniscia, Tahnisha, Tanasha, Tanashea, Tanicha, Taniesha, Tanish, Tanishah, Tanishia, Tanitia, Tannicia, Tannisha, Tenisha, Tenishka, Tinisha, Tonisha, Tonnisha, Tynisha

Tanissa (American) a combination of the prefix Tania + Nissa.
Tanesa, Tanisa, Tannesa, Tannisa, Tennessa, Tranissa

Tanita (American) a combination of the prefix Ta + Nita.
Taneta, Tanetta, Tanitra, Tanitta, Teneta, Tenetta, Tenita, Tenitta, Tyneta, Tynetta, Tynette, Tynita, Tynitra, Tynitta

Tanith (Phoenician) Mythology: Tanit is the goddess of love.
Tanitha

Tanner BG (English) leather worker, tanner.
Tannor

Tannis (Slavic) a form of Tania, Tanya.
Tannese, Tanniece, Tanniese, Tannis, Tannise, Tannus, Tannyce, Tiannis

Tansy (Greek) immortal. (Latin) tenacious, persistent.
Tancy, Tansee, Tansey, Tanshay, Tanzey

Tanya (Russian, Slavic) fairy queen.
Tahnee, Tahnya, Tana, Tanaya, Taneya, Tania, Tanis, Taniya, Tanka, Tannis, Tannya, Tanoya, Tany, Tanyia, Taunya, Tawnya, Thanya

Tao (Chinese, Vietnamese) peach.

Tara GB (Aramaic) throw; carry. (Irish) rocky hill. (Arabic) a measurement.
Taira, Tairra, Taraea, Tarah, Taráh, Tarai, Taralee, Tarali, Tarasa, Tarasha, Taraya, Tarha, Tari, Tarra, Taryn, Tayra, Tehra

Taraneh (Persian) melody.

Taree (Japanese) arching branch.
Tarea, Tareya, Tari, Taria

Tari (Irish) a familiar form of Tara.
Taria, Tarika, Tarila, Tarilyn, Tarin, Tarina, Tarita

Tarissa (American) a combination of Tara + Rissa.
Taris, Tarisa, Tarise, Tarisha

Tarra (Irish) a form of Tara.
Tarrah

Tarsicia (Greek) valiant.

Tarsilia (Greek) basket weaver.

Taryn GB (Irish) a form of Tara.
Taran, Tareen, Tareena, Taren, Tarene, Tarin, Tarina, Tarren, Tarrena, Tarrin, Tarrina, Tarron, Tarryn, Taryna

Tasarla (Gypsy) dawn.

Tasha GB (Greek) born on Christmas day. (Russian) a short form of Natasha. See also Tashi, Tosha.
Tacha, Tachiana, Tahsha, Tasenka, Tashae, Tashana, Tashay, Tashe, Tashee, Tasheka, Tashka, Tasia, Taska, Taysha, Thasha, Tiaisha, Tysha

Tashana (American) a combination of the prefix Ta + Shana.
Tashan, Tashanda, Tashani, Tashanika, Tashanna, Tashiana, Tashianna, Tashina, Tishana, Tishani, Tishanna, Tishanne, Toshanna, Toshanti, Tyshana

Tashara (American) a combination of the prefix Ta + Shara.
Tashar, Tasharah, Tasharia, Tasharna, Tasharra, Tashera, Tasherey, Tasheri, Tasherra, Tashira, Tashirah

Tashawna (American) a combination of the prefix Ta + Shawna.
Tashauna, Tashauni, Tashaunie, Tashaunna, Tashawanna, Tashawn, Tashawnda, Tashawnna, Tashawnnia, Tashonda, Tashondra, Tiashauna, Tishawn, Tishunda, Tishunta, Toshauna, Toshawna, Tyshauna, Tyshawna

Tasheena (American) a combination of the prefix Ta + Sheena.
Tasheana, Tasheeana, Tasheeni, Tashena, Tashenna, Tashennia, Tasheona, Tashina, Tisheena, Tosheena, Tysheana, Tysheena, Tyshyna

Tashelle (American) a combination of the prefix Ta + Shelley.
Tachell, Tashell, Techell, Techelle, Teshell, Teshelle, Tochell, Tochelle, Toshelle, Tychell, Tychelle, Tyshell, Tyshelle

Tashi (Hausa) a bird in flight. (Slavic) a form of Tasha.
Tashia, Tashie, Tashika, Tashima, Tashiya

Tasia (Slavic) a familiar form of Tasha.
Tachia, Tashea, Tasiya, Tassi, Tassia, Tassiana, Tassie, Tasya

Tassos (Greek) a form of Theresa.

Tata (Russian) a familiar form of Tatiana.
Tatia

Tate BG (English) a short form of Tatum. A form of Taite, Tata.

Tatiana (Slavic) fairy queen. See also Tanya, Tiana.
Tata, Tatania, Tatanya, Tateana, Tati, Tatia, Tatianna, Tatie, Tatihana, Tatiyana, Tatjana, Tatyana, Tiatiana

Tatianna (Slavic) a form of Tatiana.
Taitiann, Taitianna, Tateanna, Tateonna, Tationna

Tatiyana (Slavic) a form of Tatiana.
Tateyana, Tatiayana, Tatiyanna, Tatiyona, Tatiyonna

Tatum GB (English) cheerful.
Tate, Tatumn

Tatyana (Slavic) a form of Tatiana.
Tatyanah, Tatyani, Tatyanna, Tatyannah, Tatyona, Tatyonna

Taura (Latin) bull. Astrology: Taurus is a sign of the zodiac.
Taurae, Tauria, Taurina

Tauri (English) a form of Tory.
Taure, Taurie, Taury

Tavia (Latin) a short form of Octavia. See also Tawia.
Taiva, Tauvia, Tava, Tavah, Tavita

Tavie (Scottish) twin.
Tavey, Tavi

Tawanna (American) a combination of the prefix Ta + Wanda.
Taiwana, Taiwanna, Taquana, Taquanna, Tawan, Tawana, Tawanda, Tawanne, Tequana, Tequanna, Tequawna, Tewanna, Tewauna, Tiquana, Tiwanna, Tiwena, Towanda, Towanna, Tywania, Tywanna

Tawia (African) born after twins. (Polish) a form of Tavia.

Tawni (English) a form of Tawny.
Tauni, Taunia, Tawnia, Tawnie, Tawnnie, Tiawni

Tawny (Gypsy) little one. (English) brownish yellow, tan.
Tahnee, Tany, Tauna, Tauné, Taunisha, Tawnee, Tawnesha, Tawney, Tawni, Tawnyell, Tiawna

Tawnya (American) a combination of Tawny + Tonya.
Tawna

Taya, Taye (English) short forms of Taylor.
Tay, Tayah, Tayana, Tayiah, Tayna, Tayra, Taysha, Taysia, Tayva, Tayvonne, Teya, Teyanna, Teyona, Teyuna, Tiaya, Tiya, Tiyah, Tiyana, Tye

Tayla (English) a short form of Taylor.
Taylah, Tayleah, Taylee, Tayleigh, Taylie, Teila

Taylar (English) a form of Taylor.
Talar, Tayla, Taylah, Taylare, Tayllar

Tayler 🄶🄱 (English) a form of Taylor.
Tayller

Taylor ✹ 🄶🄱 (English) tailor.
Taelor, Tailor, Taiylor, Talor, Talora, Taya, Taye, Tayla, Taylar, Tayler, Tayllor, Tayllore, Tayloir, Taylorann, Taylore, Taylorr, Taylour, Taylur, Teylor

Tazu (Japanese) stork; longevity.
Taz, Tazi, Tazia

Tea (Spanish) a short form of Dorothy.

Teagan 🄶🄱 (Welsh) beautiful, attractive.
Taegen, Teage, Teagen, Teaghan, Teaghanne, Teaghen, Teagin, Teague, Teegan, Teeghan, Tegan, Tegwen, Teigan, Tejan, Tiegan, Tigan, Tijan, Tijana

Teaira (Latin) a form of Tiara.
Teairra, Teairre, Teairria, Teara, Tearah, Teareya, Teari, Tearia, Teariea, Tearra, Tearria

Teal (English) river duck; blue green.
Teala, Teale, Tealia, Tealisha

Teanna (American) a combination of the prefix Te + Anna. A form of Tiana.
Tean, Teana, Teanah, Teann, Teannah, Teanne, Teaunna, Teena, Teuana

Teca (Hungarian) a form of Theresa.
Techa, Teka, Tica, Tika

Tecla (Greek) God's fame.
Tekla, Theckla

Teddi (Greek) a familiar form of Theodora.
Tedde, Teddey, Teddie, Teddy, Tedi, Tediah, Tedy

Tedra (Greek) a short form of Theodora.
Teddra, Teddreya, Tedera, Teedra, Teidra

Tegan GB (Welsh) a form of Teagan.
Tega, Tegen, Teggan, Teghan, Tegin, Tegyn, Teigen

Telisha (American) a form of Taleisha.
Teleesha, Teleisia, Telesa, Telesha, Teleshia, Telesia, Telicia, Telisa, Telishia, Telisia, Telissa, Telisse, Tellisa, Tellisha, Telsa, Telysa

Telma (Spanish) will.

Telmao (Greek) loving with her fellow people.

Temira (Hebrew) tall.
Temora, Timora

Temis (Greek) she who establishes order and justice.

Tempest GB (French) stormy.
Tempesta, Tempeste, Tempestt, Tempist, Tempistt, Tempress, Tempteste

Tenesha, Tenisha (American) combinations of the prefix Te + Niesha.
Tenecia, Teneesha, Teneisha, Teneshia, Tenesia, Tenessa, Teneusa, Teniesha, Tenishia

Tennille (American) a combination of the prefix Te + Nellie.
Taniel, Tanille, Teneal, Teneil, Teneille, Teniel, Tenille, Tenneal, Tenneill, Tenneille, Tennia, Tennie, Tennielle, Tennile, Tineal, Tiniel, Tonielle, Tonille

Teodelina, Teodolinda (German) she who is loving with the people in her village; she loves her village.

Teodequilda (German) warrior of her village.

Teodomira (Spanish) an important woman in the village.

Teodora (Czech) a form of Theodora.
Teadora

Teofania, Teofanía (Greek) manifestation of God.

Teofila, Teófila (Greek) friend of God, loved by God.

Teolinda (German) a form of Teodelina.

Teona, Teonna (Greek) forms of Tiana, Tianna.
Teon, Teoni, Teonia, Teonie, Teonney, Teonnia, Teonnie

Tequila (Spanish) a kind of liquor. See also Takila.
Taquela, Taquella, Taquila, Taquilla, Tequilia, Tequilla, Tiquila, Tiquilia

Tera, Terra GB (Latin) earth. (Japanese) swift arrow. (American) forms of Tara.
Terah, Terai, Teria, Terrae, Terrah, Terria, Tierra

Teralyn (American) a combination of Terri + Lynn.
Taralyn, Teralyn, Teralynn, Terralin, Terralyn

Tercera (Spanish) third-born.

Terence BG (Latin) a form of Terrence (see Boys' Names).

Teresa (Greek) a form of Theresa. See also Tressa.
Taresa, Taressa, Tarissa, Terasa, Tercza, Tereasa, Tereatha, Terese, Teresea, Teresha, Teresia, Teresina, Teresita, Tereska, Tereson, Teressa, Teretha, Tereza, Terezia, Terezie, Terezilya, Terezinha, Terezka, Terezsa, Terisa, Terisha, Teriza, Terrasa, Terresa, Terresha, Terresia, Terressa, Terrosina, Tersa, Tersea, Teruska, Terza, Teté, Tyresa, Tyresia

Terese (Greek) a form of Teresa.
Tarese, Taress, Taris, Tarise, Tereece, Tereese, Teress, Terez, Teris, Terrise

Teresinha (Portuguese) a form of Theresa.

Teri GB (Greek) reaper. A familiar form of Theresa.
Terie

Terpsícore (Greek) she who enjoys dancing.

Terrance BG (Latin) a form of Terrence (see Boys' Names).

Terrell BG (Greek) a form of Terrelle.

Terrelle (Greek) a form of Theresa.
Tarrell, Teral, Terall, Terel, Terell, Teriel, Terral, Terrall, Terrell, Terrella, Terriel, Terriell, Terrielle, Terrill, Terryelle, Terryl, Terryll, Terrylle, Teryl, Tyrell, Tyrelle

Terrene (Latin) smooth.
Tareena, Tarena, Teran, Teranee, Tereena, Terena, Terencia, Terene, Terenia, Terentia, Terina, Terran, Terren, Terrena, Terrin, Terrina, Terron, Terrosina, Terryn, Terun, Teryn, Teryna, Terynn, Tyreen, Tyrene

Terri GB (Greek) reaper. A familiar form of Theresa.
Terree, Terria, Terrie

Terriann (American) a combination of Terri + Ann.
Teran, Terian, Teriann, Terianne, Teriyan, Terria, Terrian, Terrianne, Terryann

Terrianna (American) a combination of Terri + Anna.
Teriana, Terianna, Terriana, Terriauna, Terrina, Terriona, Terrionna, Terriyana, Terriyanna, Terryana, Terryauna, Tyrina

Terrica (American) a combination of Terri + Erica. See also Rica.
Tereka, Terica, Tericka, Terika, Terreka, Terricka, Terrika, Tyrica, Tyricka, Tyrika, Tyrikka, Tyronica

Terry 🄱🄶 (Greek) a short form of Theresa.
Tere, Teree, Terelle, Terene, Teri, Terie, Terrey, Terri, Terrie, Terrye, Tery

Terry-Lynn (American) a combination of Terry + Lynn.
Terelyn, Terelynn, Terri-Lynn, Terrilynn, Terrylynn

Tertia (Latin) third.
Tercia, Tercina, Tercine, Terecena, Tersia, Terza

Tesira (Greek) founder.

Tess 🄶🄱 (Greek) a short form of Quintessa, Theresa.
Tes, Tese

Tessa 🄶🄱 (Greek) reaper.
Tesa, Tesah, Tesha, Tesia, Tessah, Tessia, Tezia

Tessie (Greek) a familiar form of Theresa.
Tesi, Tessey, Tessi, Tessy, Tezi

Tetis (Greek) wet nurse; nursemaid.

Tetsu (Japanese) strong as iron.

Tetty (English) a familiar form of Elizabeth.

Tevin 🄱🄶 (American) a combination of the prefix Te + Kevin.

Tevy (Cambodian) angel.
Teva

Teylor (English) a form of Taylor.
Teighlor, Teylar

Thaddea (Greek) courageous. (Latin) praiser.
Thada, Thadda

Thalassa (Greek) sea, ocean.

Thalia (Greek) a form of Talia. Mythology: the Muse of comedy.
Thaleia, Thalie, Thalya

Thana (Arabic) happy occasion.
Thaina, Thania, Thanie

Thanh (Vietnamese) bright blue. (Punjabi) good place.
Thantra, Thanya

Thao (Vietnamese) respectful of parents.

Thea (Greek) goddess. A short form of Althea.
Theo

Thelma (Greek) willful.
Thelmalina

Thema (African) queen.

Theodora (Greek) a form of
Theodore. See also Dora,
Dorothy, Feodora.
Taedra, Teddi, Tedra, Teodora,
Teodory, Teodosia, Theda,
Thedorsha, Thedrica, Theo,
Theodore, Theodoria, Theodorian,
Theodosia, Theodra

Theodore **BG** (Greek) gift of God.

Theone (Greek) a form of
Theodore.
Theondra, Theoni, Theonie

Theophania (Greek) God's
appearance. See also Tiffany.
Theo, Theophanie

Theophila (Greek) loved by God.
Theo

Theresa **GB** (Greek) reaper. See
also Resi, Reza, Riza, Tassos,
Teca, Terrelle, Tracey, Tracy,
Zilya.
Teresa, Teri, Terri, Terry, Tersea,
Tess, Tessa, Tessie, Theresia,
Theresina, Theresita, Theressa,
Thereza, Therisa, Therissie,
Thersa, Thersea, Tresha, Tressa,
Trice

Therese (Greek) a form of
Theresa.
Terese, Thérése, Theresia,
Theressa, Therra, Therressa,
Thersa

Theta (Greek) Linguistics: a letter
in the Greek alphabet.

Thetis (Greek) disposed.
Mythology: the mother of
Achilles.

Thi (Vietnamese) poem.
Thia, Thy, Thya

Thirza (Hebrew) pleasant.
Therza, Thirsa, Thirzah, Thursa,
Thurza, Thyrza, Tirshka, Tirza

Thomas **BG** (Greek, Aramaic)
twin.

Thomasina (Hebrew) twin. See
also Tamassa.
Tamsin, Thomasa, Thomasia,
Thomasin, Thomasine,
Thomazine, Thomencia,
Thomethia, Thomisha, Thomsina,
Toma, Tomasa, Tomasina,
Tomasine, Tomina, Tommie,
Tommina

Thora (Scandinavian) thunder.
Thordia, Thordis, Thorri, Thyra,
Tyra

Thuy (Vietnamese) gentle.

Tia (Greek) princess. (Spanish)
aunt.
Téa, Teah, Teeya, Teia, Ti,
Tiakeisha, Tialeigh, Tiamarie,
Tianda, Tiandria, Tiante, Tiia, Tiye,
Tyja

Tiana, Tianna (Greek) princess.
(Latin) short forms of Tatiana.
Teana, Teanna, Tiahna, Tianah,
Tiane, Tianea, Tianee, Tiani,
Tiann, Tiannah, Tianne, Tianni,
Tiaon, Tiauna, Tiena, Tiona,
Tionna, Tiyana

Tiara (Latin) crowned.
*Teair, Teaira, Teara, Téare, Tearia,
Tearria, Teearia, Teira, Teirra,
Tiaira, Tiare, Tiarea, Tiareah, Tiari,
Tiaria, Tiarra, Tiera, Tierra, Tyara*

Tiarra GB (Latin) a form of Tiara.
Tiairra, Tiarrah, Tyarra

Tiauna (Greek) a form of Tiana.
Tiaunah, Tiaunia, Tiaunna

Tiberia (Latin) Geography: the
Tiber River in Italy.
Tib, Tibbie, Tibby

Tiburcia (Spanish) born in the
place of pleasures.

Tichina (American) a
combination of the prefix Ti +
China.
Tichian, Tichin, Tichinia

Ticiana (Latin) valiant defender.

Tida (Tai) daughter.

Tiera, Tierra (Latin) forms of
Tiara.
*Tieara, Tiéra, Tierah, Tierre,
Tierrea, Tierria*

Tierney GB (Irish) noble.
*Tieranae, Tierani, Tieranie,
Tieranni, Tierany, Tiernan,
Tiernee, Tierny*

Tiff (Latin) a short form of Tiffani,
Tiffanie, Tiffany.

Tiffani, Tiffanie (Latin) forms of
Tiffany.
*Tephanie, Tifanee, Tifani, Tifanie,
Tiff, Tiffanee, Tiffayne, Tiffeni,
Tiffenie, Tiffennie, Tiffiani,
Tiffianie, Tiffine, Tiffini, Tiffinie,
Tiffni, Tiffy, Tiffynie, Tifni*

Tiffany GB (Latin) trinity. (Greek)
a short form of Theophania. See
also Tyfany.
*Taffanay, Taffany, Tifaney, Tifany,
Tiff, Tiffaney, Tiffani, Tiffanie,
Tiffanny, Tiffeney, Tiffiany,
Tiffiney, Tiffiny, Tiffnay, Tiffney,
Tiffny, Tiffy, Tiphanie, Triffany*

Tiffy (Latin) a familiar form
of Tiffani, Tiffany.
Tiffey, Tiffi, Tiffie

Tijuana (Spanish) Geography: a
border town in Mexico.
*Tajuana, Tajuanna, Thejuana,
Tiajuana, Tiajuanna, Tiawanna*

Tilda (German) a short form of
Matilda.
Tilde, Tildie, Tildy, Tylda, Tyldy

Tillie (German) a familiar form of
Matilda.
Tilia, Tilley, Tilli, Tillia, Tilly, Tillye

Timi (English) a familiar form of
Timothea.
Timia, Timie, Timmi, Timmie

Timotea (Greek) she who honors
and praises God.

Timothea (English) honoring
God.
Thea, Timi

Timothy BG (Greek) honoring
God.

Tina **GB** (Spanish, American) a short form of Augustine, Martina, Christina, Valentina.
Teanna, Teena, Teina, Tena, Tenae, Tinai, Tine, Tinea, Tinia, Tiniah, Tinna, Tinnia, Tyna, Tynka

Tinble (English) sound bells make.
Tynble

Tinesha (American) a combination of the prefix Ti + Niesha.
Timnesha, Tinecia, Tineisha, Tinesa, Tineshia, Tinessa, Tinisha, Tinsia

Tinisha (American) a form of Tenisha.
Tiniesha, Tinieshia, Tinishia, Tinishya

Tiona, Tionna (American) forms of Tiana.
Teona, Teonna, Tionda, Tiondra, Tiondre, Tioné, Tionette, Tioni, Tionia, Tionie, Tionja, Tionnah, Tionne, Tionya, Tyonna

Tiphanie (Latin) a form of Tiffany.
Tiphanee, Tiphani, Tiphany

Tiponya (Native American) great horned owl.
Tipper

Tipper (Irish) water pourer. (Native American) a short form of Tiponya.

Tira (Hindi) arrow.
Tirah, Tirea, Tirena

Tirtha (Hindi) ford.

Tirza (Hebrew) pleasant.
Thersa, Thirza, Tierza, Tirsa, Tirzah, Tirzha, Tyrzah

Tisa (Swahili) ninth-born.
Tisah, Tysa, Tyssa

Tish (Latin) a short form of Tisha.

Tisha **GB** (Latin) joy. A short form of Leticia.
Taesha, Tesha, Teisha, Tiesha, Tieshia, Tish, Tishal, Tishia, Tysha, Tyshia

Tita (Greek) giant. (Spanish) a short form of names ending in "tita. "

Titania (Greek) giant. Mythology: the Titans were a race of giants.
Tania, Teata, Titanna, Titanya, Titiana, Tiziana, Tytan, Tytania, Tytiana

Titiana (Greek) a form of Titania.
Titianay, Titiania, Titianna, Titiayana, Titionia, Titiyana, Titiyanna, Tityana

Tivona (Hebrew) nature lover.

Tiwa (Zuni) onion.

Tiyana (Greek) a form of Tiana.
Tiyan, Tiyani, Tiyania, Tiyanna, Tiyonna

Tobi **GB** (Hebrew) God is good.
Tobe, Tobee, Tobey, Tobie, Tobit, Toby, Tobye, Tova, Tovah, Tove, Tovi, Tybi, Tybie

Toby **BG** (Hebrew) a form of Tobi.

Tocarra (American) a combination of the prefix To + Cara.
Tocara, Toccara

Todd BG (English) fox.

Toinette (French) a short form of Antoinette.
Toinetta, Tola, Tonetta, Tonette, Toni, Toniette, Twanette

Toki (Japanese) hopeful.
Toko, Tokoya, Tokyo

Tola (Polish) a form of Toinette.
Tolsia

Tomi GB (Japanese) rich.
Tomie, Tomiju

Tommie BG (Hebrew) a short form of Thomasina.
Tomme, Tommi, Tommia, Tommy

Tommy BG (Hebrew) a form of Tommie.

Tomo (Japanese) intelligent.
Tomoko

Tonesha (American) a combination of the prefix To + Niesha.
Toneisha, Toneisheia, Tonesha, Tonesia, Toniece, Tonisha, Tonneshia

Toni GB (Greek) flourishing. (Latin) praiseworthy.
Tonee, Toney, Tonia, Tonie, Toniee, Tonni, Tonnie, Tony, Tonye

Tonia (Latin, Slavic) a form of Toni, Tonya.
Tonea, Toniah, Toniea, Tonja, Tonje, Tonna, Tonni, Tonnia, Tonnie, Tonnja

Tonisha (American) a form of Toneisha.
Toniesha, Tonisa, Tonise, Tonisia, Tonnisha

Tony BG (Greek, Latin) a form of Toni.

Tonya (Slavic) fairy queen.
Tonia, Tonnya, Tonyea, Tonyetta, Tonyia

Topaz (Latin) golden yellow gem.

Topsy (English) on top. Literature: a slave in Harriet Beecher Stowe's novel *Uncle Tom's Cabin*.
Toppsy, Topsey, Topsie

Tora (Japanese) tiger.

Tori GB (Japanese) bird. (English) a form of Tory.
Toria, Toriana, Torie, Torri, Torrie, Torrita

Toria (English) a form of Tori, Tory.
Toriah, Torria

Toriana (English) a form of Tori.
Torian, Toriane, Toriann, Torianna, Torianne, Toriauna, Torin, Torina, Torine, Torinne, Torion, Torionna, Torionne, Toriyanna, Torrina

Toribia (Latin) she who moves on to another life.

Torie, Torrie (English) forms of Tori.
Tore, Toree, Torei, Torre, Torree

Torilyn (English) a combination of Tori + Lynn.
Torilynn, Torrilyn, Torrilynn

Torri (English) a form of Tori.

Tory GB (English) victorious.
(Latin) a short form of Victoria.
Tauri, Torey, Tori, Torrey, Torreya,
Torry, Torrye, Torya, Torye, Toya

Tosca (Latin) native of Toscana,
Italy.

Toscana (Latin) she who was
born in Etruria, Tuscany.

Tosha (Punjabi) armaments.
(Polish) a familiar form of
Antonia. (Russian) a form of
Tasha.
Toshea, Toshia, Toshiea, Toshke,
Tosia, Toska

Toshi (Japanese) mirror image.
Toshie, Toshiko, Toshikyo

Toski (Hopi) squashed bug.

Totsi (Hopi) moccasins.

Tottie (English) a familiar form of
Charlotte.
Tota, Totti, Totty

Tovah (Hebrew) good.
Tova, Tovia

Toya (Spanish) a form of Tory.
Toia, Toyanika, Toyanna, Toyea,
Toylea, Toyleah, Toylenn, Toylin,
Toylyn

Tracey GB (Greek) a familiar
form of Theresa. (Latin) warrior.
Trace, Tracee, Tracell, Traci,
Tracie, Tracy, Traice, Trasey,
Treesy

Traci, Tracie GB (Latin) forms of
Tracey.
Tracia, Tracilee, Tracilyn,
Tracilynn, Tracina, Traeci

Tracy GB (Greek) a familiar form
of Theresa. (Latin) warrior.
Treacy

Tralena (Latin) a combination of
Tracy + Lena.
Traleen, Tralene, Tralin, Tralinda,
Tralyn, Tralynn, Tralynne

Tranesha (American) a combi-
nation of the prefix Tra + Niesha.
Traneice, Traneis, Traneise,
Traneisha, Tranese, Traneshia,
Tranice, Traniece, Traniesha,
Tranisha, Tranishia

Tranquila (Spanish) calm, tranquil.

Tránsito (Latin) she who moves
on to another life.

Trashawn BG (American) a
combination of the prefix Tra +
Shawn.
Trashan, Trashana, Trashauna,
Trashon, Trayshauna

Trava (Czech) spring grasses.

Travis BG (English) a form of
Travers (see Boys' Names).

Travon BG (American) a form of
Trevon.

Treasure (Latin) treasure, wealth;
valuable.
Treasa, Treasur, Treasuré,
Treasury

Trella (Spanish) a familiar form of Estelle.

Tremaine BG (Scottish) house of stone.

Trent BG (Latin) torrent, rapid stream. (French) thirty. Geography: a city in northern Italy.

Tresha (Greek) a form of Theresa.
Trescha, Trescia, Tréshana, Treshia

Tressa (Greek) a short form of Theresa. See also Teresa.
Treaser, Tresa, Tresca, Trese, Treska, Tressia, Tressie, Trez, Treza, Trisa

Trevina (Irish) prudent. (Welsh) homestead.
Treva, Trevanna, Trevena, Trevenia, Treveon, Trevia, Treviana, Trevien, Trevin, Trevona

Trevon BG (Irish) a form of Trevona.

Trevona (Irish) a form of Trevina.
Trevion, Trevon, Trevonia, Trevonna, Trevonne, Trevonye

Trevor BG (Irish) prudent. (Welsh) homestead.

Triana (Latin) third. (Greek) a form of Trina.
Tria, Triann, Trianna, Trianne

Trice (Greek) a short form of Theresa.
Treece

Tricia (Latin) a form of Trisha.
Trica, Tricha, Trichelle, Tricina, Trickia

Trilby (English) soft hat.
Tribi, Trilbie, Trillby

Trina GB (Greek) pure.
Treena, Treina, Trenna, Triana, Trinia, Trinchen, Trind, Trinda, Trine, Trinette, Trini, Trinica, Trinice, Triniece, Trinika, Trinique, Trinisa, Tryna

Trini (Greek) a form of Trina.
Trinia, Trinie

Trinidad (Latin) three people in one God.

Trinity ✵ GB (Latin) triad. Religion: the Father, the Son, and the Holy Spirit.
Trinita, Trinite, Trinitee, Triniti, Trinnette, Trinty

Tripaileo (Mapuche) explosion of flames, explosive bomb; explosive, impulsive, passionate, and vehement woman.

Trish (Latin) a short form of Beatrice, Trisha.
Trishell, Trishelle

Trisha (Latin) noblewoman. (Hindi) thirsty. See also Tricia.
Treasha, Trish, Trishann, Trishanna, Trishanne, Trishara, Trishia, Trishna, Trissha, Trycia

Trissa (Latin) a familiar form of Patricia.
Trisa, Trisanne, Trisia, Trisina, Trissi, Trissie, Trissy, Tryssa

Trista (Latin) a short form of Tristen.
Trisatal, Tristess, Tristia, Trysta, Trystia

Tristan BG (Latin) bold.
Trista, Tristane, Tristanni, Tristany, Tristen, Tristian, Tristiana, Tristin, Triston, Trystan, Trystyn

Tristana (Latin) she who carries sadness with her.

Tristen BG (Latin) a form of Tristan.
Tristene, Trysten

Tristin BG (Latin) a form of Tristan.
Tristina, Tristine, Tristinye, Tristn, Trystin

Triston BG (Latin) a form of Tristan.
Tristony

Trystyn (Latin) a form of Tristan.

Trixie (American) a familiar form of Beatrice.
Tris, Trissie, Trissina, Trix, Trixi, Trixy

Troy BG (Irish) foot soldier.

Troya (Irish) a form of Troy.
Troi, Troia, Troiana, Troiya

Trudel (Dutch) a form of Trudy.

Trudy (German) a familiar form of Gertrude.
Truda, Trude, Trudel, Trudessa, Trudey, Trudi, Trudie

Trycia (Latin) a form of Trisha.

Tryna (Greek) a form of Trina.
Tryane, Tryanna, Trynee

Tryne (Dutch) pure.
Trine

Tsigana (Hungarian) a form of Zigana.
Tsigane, Tzigana, Tzigane

Tu BG (Chinese) jade.

Tucker BG (English) fuller, tucker of cloth.

Tuesday (English) born on the third day of the week.
Tuesdae, Tuesdea, Tuesdee, Tuesdey, Tusdai

Tula (Hindi) born in the lunar month of Capricorn.
Tulah, Tulla, Tullah, Tuula

Tullia (Irish) peaceful, quiet.
Tulia, Tulliah

Tulsi (Hindi) basil, a sacred Hindi herb.
Tulsia

Turner BG (Latin) lathe worker; wood worker.

Turquoise (French) blue-green semi-precious stone.
Turkois, Turkoise, Turkoys, Turkoyse

Tusa (Zuni) prairie dog.

Tusnelda (German) she who fights giants.

Tuyen (Vietnamese) angel.

Tuyet (Vietnamese) snow.

Twyla (English) woven of double thread.
Twila, Twilla

Ty 🅱🅶 (English) a short form of Tyler, Tyson.

Tyanna (American) a combination of the prefix Ty + Anna.
Tya, Tyana, Tyann, Tyannah, Tyanne, Tyannia

Tyeisha (American) a form of Tyesha.
Tyeesha, Tyeishia, Tyieshia, Tyisha, Tyishea, Tyishia

Tyesha (American) a combination of Ty + Aisha.
Tyasha, Tyashia, Tyasia, Tyasiah, Tyeisha, Tyeshia, Tyeyshia, Tyisha

Tyfany (American) a short form of Tiffany.
Tyfani, Tyfanny, Tyffani, Tyffanni, Tyffany, Tyffini, Typhanie, Typhany

Tykeisha (American) a form of Takeisha.
Tkeesha, Tykeisa, Tykeishia, Tykesha, Tykeshia, Tykeysha, Tykeza, Tykisha

Tykera (American) a form of Takira.
Tykeira, Tykeirah, Tykereiah, Tykeria, Tykeriah, Tykerria, Tykiera, Tykierra, Tykira, Tykiria, Tykirra

Tyler 🅱🅶 (English) tailor.
Tyller, Tylor

Tylor 🅱🅶 (English) a form of Tyler.

Tyna (Czech) a short form of Kristina.
Tynae, Tynea, Tynia

Tyne (English) river.
Tine, Tyna, Tynelle, Tynessa, Tynetta

Tynesha (American) a combination of Ty + Niesha.
Tynaise, Tynece, Tyneicia, Tynesa, Tynesha, Tyneshia, Tynessia, Tyniesha, Tynisha, Tyseisha

Tynisha (American) a form of Tynesha.
Tyneisha, Tyneisia, Tynisa, Tynise, Tynishi

Tyra 🅶🅱 (Scandinavian) battler. Mythology: Tyr was the god of war. A form of Thora. (Hindi) a form of Tira.
Tyraa, Tyrah, Tyran, Tyree, Tyria

Tyree 🅱🅶 (Scandinavian) a form of Tyra.

Tyrell 🅱🅶 (Greek) a form of Terrelle.

Tyshanna (American) a combination of Ty + Shawna.
Tyshana, Tyshanae, Tyshane, Tyshaun, Tyshaunda, Tyshawn, Tyshawna, Tyshawnah, Tyshawnda, Tyshawnna, Tysheann, Tysheanna, Tyshonia, Tyshonna, Tyshonya

Tyson 🅱🅶 (French) child of Ty.

Tytiana (Greek) a form of Titania.
*Tytana, Tytanna, Tyteana,
Tyteanna, Tytianna, Tytianni,
Tytionna, Tytiyana, Tytiyanna,
Tytyana, Tytyauna*

U

U (Korean) gentle.

Ubaldina (Teutonic) audacious,
daring; intelligent.

Udele (English) prosperous.
Uda, Udella, Udelle, Yudelle

Ula (Irish) sea jewel.
(Scandinavian) wealthy.
(Spanish) a short form of Eulalia.
Uli, Ulla

Ulani (Polynesian) cheerful.
Ulana, Ulane

Ulima (Arabic) astute; wise.
Ullima

Ulla (German, Swedish) willful.
(Latin) a short form of Ursula.
Ulli

Ulrica (German) wolf ruler; ruler
of all. See also Rica.
*Ulka, Ullrica, Ullricka, Ullrika,
Ulrika, Ulrike*

Ultima (Latin) last, endmost,
farthest.

Ululani (Hawaiian) heavenly
inspiration.

Ulva (German) wolf.

Uma (Hindi) mother. Religion:
another name for the Hindu
goddess Devi.

Umay (Turkish) hopeful.
Umai

Umbelina (Latin) she who gives
protective shade.

Umeko (Japanese) plum-blossom
child; patient.
Ume, Umeyo

Una (Latin) one; united. (Hopi)
good memory. (Irish) a form of
Agnes. See also Oona.
Unna, Uny

Undine (Latin) little wave.
Mythology: the undines were
water spirits. See also Ondine.
Undeen, Undene

Unice (English) a form of Eunice.

Unika GB (American) a form of
Unique.
*Unica, Unicka, Unik, Unikqua,
Unikue*

Unique GB (Latin) only one.
Unika, Uniqia, Uniqua, Uniquia

Unity (English) unity.
Uinita, Unita, Unitee

Unn (Norwegian) she who is
loved.

Unna (German) woman.

Urania (Greek) heavenly.
Mythology: the Muse of astronomy.
Urainia, Uranie, Uraniya, Uranya

Urbana (Latin) city dweller.
Urbanah, Urbanna

Uriel BG (Hebrew) God is my light.

Urika (Omaha) useful to everyone.
Ureka

Urit (Hebrew) bright.
Urice

Urraca (German) magpie.

Ursa (Greek) a short form of Ursula. (Latin) a form of Orsa.
Ursey, Ursi, Ursie, Ursy

Ursina (Latin) little bear.

Ursula (Greek) little bear. See also Sula, Ulla, Vorsila.
Irsaline, Ursa, Ursala, Ursel, Ursela, Ursella, Ursely, Ursilla, Ursillane, Ursola, Ursule, Ursulina, Ursuline, Urszula, Urszuli, Urzula

Úrsula (Portuguese) a form of Ursula.

Usha (Hindi) sunrise.

Ushi (Chinese) ox. Astrology: a sign of the Chinese zodiac.

Uta (German) rich. (Japanese) poem.
Utako

Utina (Native American) woman of my country.
Utahna, Utona, Utonna

V GB (American) an initial used as a first name.

Vail BG (English) valley.
Vale, Vayle

Val BG (Latin) a short form of Valentina, Valerie.

Vala (German) singled out.
Valla

Valarie (Latin) a form of Valerie.
Valarae, Valaree, Valarey, Valari, Valaria, Vallarie

Valburga (German) she who defends on the battlefield.

Valda (German) famous ruler.
Valida, Velda

Valdrada (German) she who gives advice.

Valencia (Spanish) strong. Geography: a region in eastern Spain.
Valecia, Valence, Valenica, Valentia, Valenzia

Valene (Latin) a short form of Valentina.
Valaine, Valean, Valeda, Valeen, Valen, Valena, Valeney, Valien, Valina, Valine, Vallan, Vallen

Valentina (Latin) strong. History: Valentina Tereshkova, a Soviet cosmonaut, was the first woman in space. See also Tina, Valene, Valli.
Val, Valantina, Vale, Valenteen, Valentena, Valentijn, Valentin, Valentine, Valiaka, Valtina, Valyn, Valynn

Valera (Russian) a form of Valerie. See also Lera.

Valeria (Latin) a form of Valerie.
Valaria, Valeriana, Valeriane, Veleria

Valéria (Hungarian, Portuguese) a form of Valerie.

Valerie GB (Latin) strong.
Vairy, Val, Valarie, Vale, Valera, Valeree, Valeri, Valeria, Valérie, Valery, Valka, Valleree, Valleri, Vallerie, Valli, Vallirie, Valora, Valorie, Valry, Valya, Velerie, Waleria

Valery (Latin) a form of Valerie.
Valerye, Vallary, Vallery

Valeska (Slavic) glorious ruler.
Valesca, Valese, Valeshia, Valeshka, Valezka, Valisha

Valli (Latin) a familiar form of Valentina, Valerie. Botany: a plant native to India.
Vallie, Vally

Valma (Finnish) loyal defender.

Valonia (Latin) shadow valley.
Vallon, Valona

Valora (Latin) a form of Valerie.
Valoria, Valorya, Velora

Valorie (Latin) a form of Valerie.
Vallori, Vallory, Valori, Valory

Vance BG (English) thresher.

Vanda GB (German) a form of Wanda.
Vandana, Vandella, Vandetta, Vandi, Vannda

Vanesa (Greek) a form of Vanessa.
Vanesha, Vaneshah, Vanesia, Vanisa

Vanessa ☆ GB (Greek) butterfly. Literature: a name invented by Jonathan Swift as a nickname for Esther Vanhomrigh. See also Nessie.
Van, Vanassa, Vanesa, Vaneshia, Vanesse, Vanessia, Vanessica, Vanetta, Vaneza, Vaniece, Vaniessa, Vanija, Vanika, Vanissa, Vanita, Vanna, Vannesa, Vannessa, Vanni, Vannie, Vanny, Varnessa, Venessa

Vanetta (English) a form of Vanessa.
Vaneta, Vanita, Vanneta, Vannetta, Vannita, Venetta

Vania, Vanya (Russian) familiar forms of Anna.
Vanija, Vanina, Vaniya, Vanja, Vanka, Vannia

Vanity (English) vain.
Vaniti, Vanitty

Vanna (Cambodian) golden.
(Greek) a short form of Vanessa.
*Vana, Vanae, Vanelly, Vannah,
Vannalee, Vannaleigh, Vannie,
Vanny*

Vannesa, Vannessa (Greek)
forms of Vanessa.
Vannesha, Vanneza

Vanora (Welsh) white wave.
Vannora

Vantrice (American) a combi-
nation of the prefix Van + Trice.
*Vantrece, Vantricia, Vantrisa,
Vantrissa*

Varda (Hebrew) rose.
*Vadit, Vardia, Vardice, Vardina,
Vardis, Vardit*

Varinia (Ancient Roman, Spanish)
versatile.

Varvara (Slavic) a form of Barbara.
*Vara, Varenka, Varina, Varinka,
Varya, Varyusha, Vava, Vavka*

Vashti (Persian) lovely. Bible: the
wife of Ahasuerus, king of Persia.
Vashtee, Vashtie, Vashty

Vaughn 🅱️🅶 (Welsh) small.

Veanna (American) a combination of the prefix Ve + Anna.
Veeana, Veena, Veenaya, Veeona

Veda (Sanskrit) sacred lore;
knowledge. Religion: the Vedas
are the sacred writings of
Hinduism.
*Vedad, Vedis, Veeda, Veida,
Veleda, Vida*

Vedette (Italian) sentry; scout.
(French) movie star.
Vedetta

Vega (Arabic) falling star.

Velda (German) a form of Valda.

Velika (Slavic) great, wondrous.

Velma (German) a familiar form
of Vilhelmina.
Valma, Vellma, Vilma, Vilna

Velvet (English) velvety.

Venancia (Latin) hunter; she
likes to hunt deer.

Venecia (Italian) from Venice,
Italy.
*Vanecia, Vanetia, Veneise,
Venesa, Venesha, Venesher,
Venesse, Venessia, Venetia,
Venette, Venezia, Venice, Venicia,
Veniece, Veniesa, Venise,
Venisha, Venishia, Venita, Venitia,
Venize, Vennesa, Vennice,
Vennisa, Vennise, Vonitia, Vonizia*

Venessa (Latin) a form of Vanessa.
*Veneese, Venesa, Venese,
Veneshia, Venesia, Venisa,
Venissa, Vennessa*

Ventana (Spanish) window.

Ventura (Spanish) good fortune.

Venus (Latin) love. Mythology: the
goddess of love and beauty.
Venis, Venusa, Venusina, Vinny

Vera (Latin) true. (Slavic) faith. A short form of Elvera, Veronica. See also Verena, Wera.
Vara, Veera, Veira, Veradis, Verasha, Vere, Verka, Verla, Viera, Vira

Verbena (Latin) sacred plants.
Verbeena, Verbina

Verda (Latin) young, fresh.
Verdi, Verdie, Viridiana, Viridis

Verdad (Spanish) truthful.

Veredigna (Latin) she who has earned great honors for her dignity.

Verena (Latin) truthful. A familiar form of Vera, Verna.
Verene, Verenis, Vereniz, Verina, Verine, Verinka, Veroshka, Verunka, Verusya, Virna

Verenice (Latin) a form of Veronica.
Verenis, Verenise, Vereniz

Verity (Latin) truthful.
Verita, Veritie

Verlene (Latin) a combination of Veronica + Lena.
Verleen, Verlena, Verlin, Verlina, Verlinda, Verline, Verlyn

Verna (Latin) springtime. (French) a familiar form of Laverne. See also Verena, Wera.
Verasha, Verla, Verne, Vernetia, Vernetta, Vernette, Vernia, Vernice, Vernita, Verusya, Viera, Virida, Virna, Virnell

Vernice (Latin) a form of Bernice, Verna.
Vernese, Vernesha, Verneshia, Vernessa, Vernica, Vernicca, Verniece, Vernika, Vernique, Vernis, Vernise, Vernisha, Vernisheia, Vernissia

Veronica (Latin) true image. See also Ronni, Weronika.
Varonica, Vera, Veranique, Verenice, Verhonica, Verinica, Verohnica, Veron, Verona, Verone, Veronic, Véronic, Veronice, Veronika, Veronique, Véronique, Veronne, Veronnica, Veruszhka, Vironica, Vron, Vronica

Verónica (Spanish) a form of Veronica.

Verônica (Portuguese) a form of Veronica.

Veronika (Latin) a form of Veronica.
Varonika, Veronick, Véronick, Veronik, Veronike, Veronka, Veronkia, Veruka

Veronique, Véronique (French) forms of Veronica.

Vespera (Latin) evening star.

Vesta (Latin) keeper of the house. Mythology: the goddess of the home.
Vessy, Vest, Vesteria

Veta (Slavic) a familiar form of Elizabeth.
Veeta, Vita

Vi (Latin, French) a short form of
Viola, Violet.
Vye

Vianca (Spanish) a form of
Bianca.
Vianeca, Vianica

Vianey (American) a familiar
form of Vianna.
Vianney, Viany

Vianna (American) a combination
of Vi + Anna.
Viana, Vianey, Viann, Vianne

Vica (Hungarian) a form of Eve.

Vicente 🅱🅶 (Spanish) a form of
Vincent.

Vicki, Vickie (Latin) familiar
forms of Victoria.
*Vic, Vicci, Vicke, Vickee, Vickiana,
Vickilyn, Vickki, Vicky, Vika, Viki,
Vikie, Vikki, Vikky*

Vicky 🇬🇧 (Latin) a familiar form
of Victoria.
Viccy, Vickey, Viky, Vikkey, Vikky

Victoria ☀ 🇬🇧 (Latin) victorious.
See also Tory, Wicktoria, Wisia.
*Vicki, Vicky, Victoire, Victoriana,
Victorianna, Victorie, Victorina,
Victorine, Victoriya, Victorria,
Victorriah, Victory, Victorya,
Viktoria, Vitoria, Vyctoria*

Vida (Sanskrit) a form of Veda.
(Hebrew) a short form of Davida.
Vidamarie

Vidonia (Portuguese) branch of a
vine.
Vedonia, Vidonya

Vienna (Latin) Geography: the
capital of Austria.
*Veena, Vena, Venna, Vienette,
Vienne, Vina*

Viktoria (Latin) a form of
Victoria.
*Viktorie, Viktorija, Viktorina,
Viktorine, Viktorka*

Vilhelmina (German) a form of
Wilhelmina.
Velma, Vilhelmine, Vilma

Villette (French) small town.
Vietta

Vilma (German) a short form of
Vilhemina.

Vina (Hindi) Religion: a musical
instrument played by the Hindu
goddess of wisdom. (Spanish)
vineyard. (Hebrew) a short form
of Davina. (English) a short form
of Alvina. See also Lavina.
*Veena, Vena, Viña, Vinesha,
Vinessa, Vinia, Viniece, Vinique,
Vinisha, Viñita, Vinna, Vinni,
Vinnie, Vinny, Vinora, Vyna*

Vincent 🅱🅶 (Latin) victor,
conqueror.

Vincentia (Latin) a form of
Vincent.
*Vicenta, Vincenta, Vincentena,
Vincentina, Vincentine, Vincenza,
Vincy, Vinnie*

Viñita (Spanish) a form of Vina.
*Viñeet, Viñeeta, Viñetta, Viñette,
Viñitha, Viñta, Viñti, Viñtia,
Vyñetta, Vyñette*

Viola (Latin) violet; stringed
instrument in the violin family.
Literature: the heroine of
Shakespeare's play *Twelfth Night*.
*Vi, Violaine, Violanta, Violante,
Viole, Violeine*

Violet (French) Botany: a plant
with purplish blue flowers.
*Vi, Violeta, Violette, Vyolet,
Vyoletta, Vyolette*

Violeta (French) a form of Violet.
Violetta

Virgilia (Latin) rod bearer, staff
bearer.
Virgillia

Virginia (Latin) pure, virginal.
Literature: Virginia Woolf was a
well-known British writer. See
also Gina, Ginger, Ginny, Jinny.
*Verginia, Verginya, Virge, Virgen,
Virgenia, Virgenya, Virgie,
Virgine, Virginie, Virginië,
Virginio, Virginnia, Virgy, Virjeana*

Virginie (French) a form of
Virginia.

Viridiana (Latin) a form of
Viridis.

Viridis (Latin) green.
Virdis, Virida, Viridia, Viridiana

Virtudes (Latin) blessed spirit.

Virtue (Latin) virtuous.

Visitación (Latin) refers to the
Virgin Mary visiting Saint Isabel,
who was her cousin.

Vita (Latin) life.
*Veeta, Veta, Vitaliana, Vitalina,
Vitel, Vitella, Vitia, Vitka, Vitke*

Vitalia (Latin) she who is full of
life.

Vitoria (Spanish) a form of
Victoria.
Vittoria

Vitória (Portuguese) a form of
Victoria.

Viv (Latin) a short form of Vivian.

Viva (Latin) a short form of Aviva,
Vivian.
Vica, Vivan, Vivva

Viveca (Scandinavian) a form of
Vivian.
*Viv, Vivecca, Vivecka, Viveka,
Vivica, Vivieca, Vyveca*

Vivian GB (Latin) full of life.
*Vevay, Vevey, Viv, Viva, Viveca,
Vivee, Vivi, Vivia, Viviana,
Viviane, Viviann, Vivianne, Vivie,
Vivien, Vivienne, Vivina, Vivion,
Vivyan, Vivyann, Vivyanne,
Vyvyan, Vyvyann, Vyvyanne*

Viviana (Latin) a form of Vivian.
Viv, Vivianna, Vivyana, Vyvyana

Vondra (Czech) loving woman.
Vonda, Vondrea

Voneisha (American) a combination of Yvonne + Aisha.
Voneishia, Vonesha, Voneshia

Vonna (French) a form of Yvonne.
Vona

Vonny (French) a familiar form of Yvonne.
Vonney, Vonni, Vonnie

Vontricia (American) a combination of Yvonne + Tricia.
Vontrece, Vontrese, Vontrice, Vontriece

Vorsila (Greek) a form of Ursula.
Vorsilla, Vorsula, Vorsulla, Vorsyla

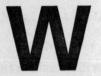

W BG (American) an initial used as a first name.

Wadd (Arabic) beloved.

Waheeda (Arabic) one and only.

Wainani (Hawaiian) beautiful water.

Wakana (Japanese) plant.

Wakanda (Dakota) magical power.
Wakenda

Wakeisha (American) a combination of the prefix Wa + Keisha.
Wakeishia, Wakesha, Wakeshia, Wakesia

Walad (Arabic) newborn.
Waladah, Walidah

Walda (German) powerful; famous.
Waldina, Waldine, Walida, Wallda, Welda

Waleria (Polish) a form of Valerie.
Wala

Walker BG (English) cloth; walker.
Wallker

Wallis (English) from Wales.
Wallie, Walliss, Wally, Wallys

Wanda (German) wanderer. See also Wendy.
Vanda, Wahnda, Wandah, Wandely, Wandie, Wandis, Wandja, Wandzia, Wannda, Wonda, Wonnda

Wandie (German) a familiar form of Wanda.
Wandi, Wandy

Waneta (Native American) charger. See also Juanita.
Waneeta, Wanita, Wanite, Wanneta, Waunita, Wonita, Wonnita, Wynita

Wanetta (English) pale face.
Wanette, Wannetta, Wannette

Wanika (Hawaiian) a form of Juanita.
Wanicka

Wanya BG (Russian) a form of Vania.

Warda (German) guardian.
Wardah, Wardeh, Wardena,
Wardenia, Wardia, Wardine

Washi (Japanese) eagle.

Wattan (Japanese) homeland.

Wauna (Moquelumnan) snow
geese honking.
Waunakee

Wava (Slavic) a form of Barbara.

Waverly **GB** (English) quaking
aspen-tree meadow.
Waverley, Waverli, Wavierlee

Wayna (Quechua) young.

Waynesha (American) a
combination of Waynette +
Niesha.
Wayneesha, Wayneisha, Waynie,
Waynisha

Waynette (English) wagon
maker.
Waynel, Waynelle, Waynetta,
Waynlyn

Weeko (Dakota) pretty girl.

Wehilani (Hawaiian) heavenly
adornment.

Wenda (Welsh) a form of Wendy.
Wendaine, Wendayne

Wendelle (English) wanderer.
Wendaline, Wendall, Wendalyn,
Wendeline, Wendella,
Wendelline, Wendelly

Wendi (Welsh) a form of Wendy.
Wendie

Wendy (Welsh) white; light
skinned. A familiar form of
Gwendolyn, Wanda.
Wenda, Wende, Wendee,
Wendey, Wendi, Wendye,
Wuendy

Wera (Polish) a form of Vera. See
also Verna.
Wiera, Wiercia, Wierka

Weronika (Polish) a form of
Veronica.
Weronikra

Wesisa (Musoga) foolish.

Weslee (English) western
meadow.
Weslea, Wesleigh, Weslene,
Wesley, Wesli, Weslia, Weslie,
Weslyn

Wesley **BG** (English) a form of
Weslee.

Weston **BG** (English) western
town.

Whitley **GB** (English) white field.
Whitely, Whitlee, Whitleigh,
Whitlie, Whittley

Whitney **GB** (English) white
island.
Whiteney, Whitne, Whitné,
Whitnee, Whitneigh, Whitnie,
Whitny, Whitnye, Whytne,
Whytney, Witney

Whitnie (English) a form of
Whitney.
Whitani, Whitnei, Whitni,
Whytni, Whytnie

Whittney (English) a form of
Whitney.
*Whittaney, Whittanie, Whittany,
Whitteny, Whittnay, Whittnee,
Whittney, Whittni, Whittnie*

Whoopi (English) happy; excited.
Whoopie, Whoopy

Wicktoria (Polish) a form of
Victoria.
Wicktorja, Wiktoria, Wiktorja

Wilda (German) untamed.
(English) willow.
Willda, Wylda

Wileen (English) a short form of
Wilhelmina.
Wilene, Willeen, Willene

Wilhelmina (German) a form of
Wilhelm (see Boys' Names). See
also Billie, Guillerma, Helma,
Minka, Minna, Minnie.
*Vilhelmina, Wileen, Wilhelmine,
Willa, Willamina, Willamine,
Willemina, Willette, Williamina,
Willie, Willmina, Willmine,
Wilma, Wimina*

Wilikinia (Hawaiian) a form of
Virginia.

Willa (German) a short form of
Wilhelmina.
Willabella, Willette, Williabelle

Willette (English) a familiar form
of Wilhelmina, Willa.
*Wiletta, Wilette, Willetta,
Williette*

William 🅱🅖 (English) a form of
Wilhelm (see Boys' Names).

Willie 🅱🅖 (English) a familiar
form of Wilhelmina.
*Willi, Willina, Willisha, Willishia,
Willy*

Willow (English) willow tree.
Willough

Wilma (German) a short form of
Wilhelmina.
*Williemae, Wilmanie, Wilmayra,
Wilmetta, Wilmette, Wilmina,
Wilmyne, Wylma*

Wilona (English) desired.
Willona, Willone, Wilone

Wilson 🅱🅖 (English) child of Will.

Win 🅱🅖 (German) a short form of
Winifred. See also Edwina.
Wyn

Winda (Swahili) hunter.

Windy (English) windy.
*Windee, Windey, Windi, Windie,
Wyndee, Wyndy*

Winema (Moquelumnan) woman
chief.

Winifred (German) peaceful
friend. (Welsh) a form of
Guinevere. See also Freddi, Una,
Winnie.
*Win, Winafred, Winefred,
Winefride, Winfreda, Winfrieda,
Winiefrida, Winifrid, Winifryd,
Winnafred, Winnefred,
Winniefred, Winnifred, Winnifrid,
Wynafred, Wynifred, Wynnifred*

Winna (African) friend.
Winnah

Winnie (English) a familiar form
of Edwina, Gwyneth, Winnifred,
Winona, Wynne. History: Winnie
Mandela kept the anti-apartheid
movement alive in South Africa
while her then-husband, Nelson
Mandela, was imprisoned.
Literature: the lovable bear in A.
A. Milne's children's story
Winnie-the-Pooh.
*Wina, Winne, Winney, Winni,
Winny, Wynnie*

Winola (German) charming
friend.
Wynola

Winona (Lakota) oldest daughter.
*Wanona, Wenona, Wenonah,
Winnie, Winonah, Wynonna*

Winter GB (English) winter.
Wintr, Wynter

Wira (Polish) a form of Elvira.
Wiria, Wirke

Wisia (Polish) a form of Victoria.
Wicia, Wikta

Wren (English) wren, songbird.

Wyanet (Native American)
legendary beauty.
Wyaneta, Wyanita, Wynette

Wyatt BG (French) little warrior.

Wynne (Welsh) white, light
skinned. A short form of
Blodwyn, Guinivere, Gwyneth.
Winnie, Wyn, Wynn

Wynonna (Lakota) a form of
Winona.
Wynnona, Wynona

Wynter (English) a form of
Winter.
Wynteria

Wyoming (Native American)
Geography: a western U.S. state.
Wy, Wye, Wyoh, Wyomia

Xandra (Greek) a form of Zandra.
(Spanish) a short form of
Alexandra.
Xander, Xandrea, Xandria

Xanthe (Greek) yellow, blond. See
also Zanthe.
*Xanne, Xantha, Xanthia,
Xanthippe*

Xanthippe (Greek) a form of
Xanthe. History: Socrates's wife.
Xantippie

Xavier BG (Arabic) bright.
(Basque) owner of the new
house.

Xaviera (Arabic, Basque) a form
of Xavier. See also Javiera,
Zaviera.
Xavia, Xaviére, Xavyera, Xiveria

Xela (Quiché) my mountain
home.

Xena (Greek) a form of Xenia.

Xenia (Greek) hospitable. See also Zena, Zina.
Xeenia, Xena, Xenea, Xenya, Xinia

Xiang (Chinese) fragrant.

Xiomara (Teutonic) glorious forest.
Xiomaris, Xiomayra

Xiu Mei (Chinese) beautiful plum.

Xochitl (Aztec) place of many flowers.
Xochil, Xochilt, Xochilth, Xochiti

Xuan (Vietnamese) spring.

Xuxa (Portuguese) a familiar form of Susanna.

Xylia (Greek) a form of Sylvia.
Xylina, Xylona

Yachne (Hebrew) hospitable.

Yadira GB (Hebrew) friend.
Yadirah, Yadirha, Yadyra

Yael GB (Hebrew) strength of God. See also Jael.
Yaeli, Yaella, Yeala

Yaffa (Hebrew) beautiful. See also Jaffa.
Yafeal, Yaffit, Yafit

Yahaira (Hebrew) a form of Yakira.
Yahara, Yahayra, Yahira

Yaíza (Guanche) rainbow.

Yajaira (Hebrew) a form of Yakira.
Yahaira, Yajara, Yajayra, Yajhaira

Yakira (Hebrew) precious; dear.
Yahaira, Yajaira

Yalanda (Greek) a form of Yolanda.
Yalando, Yalonda, Ylana, Ylanda

Yalena (Greek, Russian) a form of Helen. See also Lena, Yelena.

Yaletha (American) a form of Oletha.
Yelitsa

Yamary (American) a combination of the prefix Ya + Mary.
Yamairy, Yamarie, Yamaris, Yamayra

Yamelia (American) a form of Amelia.
Yameily, Yamelya, Yamelys

Yamila (Arabic) a form of Jamila.
Yamela, Yamely, Yamil, Yamile, Yamilet, Yamiley, Yamilla, Yamille

Yaminah (Arabic) right, proper.
Yamina, Yamini, Yemina, Yeminah, Yemini

Yamka (Hopi) blossom.

Yamuna (Hindi) sacred river.

Yan **BG** (Russian) a form of John.

Yana (Slavic) a form of Jana.
*Yanae, Yanah, Yanay, Yanaye,
Yanesi, Yanet, Yaneth, Yaney,
Yani, Yanik, Yanina, Yanis,
Yanisha, Yanitza, Yanixia, Yanna,
Yannah, Yanni, Yannica, Yannick,
Yannina*

Yanaba (Navajo) brave.

Yanamaría (Slavic) bitter grace.

Yaneli (American) a combination
of the prefix Ya + Nellie.
*Yanela, Yanelis, Yaneliz, Yanelle,
Yanelli, Yanely, Yanelys*

Yanet (American) a form of Janet.
*Yanete, Yaneth, Yanethe, Yanette,
Yannet, Yanneth, Yannette*

Yáng (Chinese) sun.

Yara (Tupi) she is a lady.

Yareli (American) a form of Oralee.
Yarely, Yaresly

Yarina (Slavic) a form of Irene.
Yaryna

Yaritza (American) a combination
of Yana + Ritsa.
Yaritsa, Yarítsa

Yarkona (Hebrew) green.

Yarmilla (Slavic) market trader.

Yashira (Afghan) humble; takes it
easy. (Arabic) wealthy.

Yasmeen (Persian) a form of
Yasmin.
Yasemeen, Yasemin, Yasmeena,

*Yasmen, Yasmene, Yasmeni,
Yasmenne, Yassmeen, Yassmen*

Yasmin, Yasmine (Persian)
jasmine flower.
*Yashmine, Yasiman, Yasimine,
Yasma, Yasmain, Yasmaine,
Yasmina, Yasminda, Yasmon,
Yasmyn, Yazmin, Yesmean,
Yesmeen, Yesmin, Yesmina,
Yesmine, Yesmyn*

Yasmín (Persian) a form of
Yasmin.

Yasu (Japanese) resting, calm.
Yasuko, Yasuyo

Yazmin (Persian) a form of
Yasmin.
*Yazmeen, Yazmen, Yazmene,
Yazmina, Yazmine, Yazmyn,
Yazmyne, Yazzmien, Yazzmine,
Yazzmine, Yazzmyn*

Yecenia (Arabic) a form of
Yesenia.

Yehudit (Hebrew) a form of
Judith.
Yudit, Yudita, Yuta

Yei (Japanese) flourishing.

Yeira (Hebrew) light.

Yekaterina (Russian) a form of
Katherine.

Yelena (Russian) a form of
Helen, Jelena. See also Lena,
Yalena.
*Yeleana, Yelen, Yelenna, Yelenne,
Yelina, Ylena, Ylenia, Ylenna*

Yelisabeta (Russian) a form of Elizabeth.
Yelizaveta

Yemena (Arabic) from Yemen.
Yemina

Yen (Chinese) yearning; desirous.
Yeni, Yenih, Yenny

Yenay (Chino) she who loves.

Yenene (Native American) shaman.

Yenifer (Welsh) a form of Jennifer.
Yenefer, Yennifer

Yeo (Korean) mild.
Yee

Yepa (Native American) snow girl.

Yeruti (Guarani) turtledove.

Yesenia (Arabic) flower.
Yasenya, Yecenia, Yesinia, Yesnia, Yessenia

Yesica (Hebrew) a form of Jessica.
Yesika, Yesiko

Yésica (Hebrew) a form of Yesica.

Yessenia (Arabic) a form of Yesenia.
Yessena, Yessenya, Yissenia

Yessica (Hebrew) a form of Jessica.
Yessika, Yesyka

Yetta (English) a short form of Henrietta.
Yette, Yitta, Yitty

Yeva (Ukrainian) a form of Eve.

Yiesha (Arabic, Swahili) a form of Aisha.
Yiasha

Yín (Chinese) silver.

Ynez (Spanish) a form of Agnes. See also Inez.
Ynes, Ynesita

Yoanna (Hebrew) a form of Joanna.
Yoana, Yohana, Yohanka, Yohanna, Yohannah

Yocasta (Greek) violet.

Yocelin, Yocelyn (Latin) forms of Jocelyn.
Yoceline, Yocelyne, Yuceli

Yoconda (Italian) happy and jovial.

Yoi (Japanese) born in the evening.

Yoki (Hopi) bluebird.
Yokie

Yoko (Japanese) good girl.
Yo

Yolanda (Greek) violet flower. See also Iolanthe, Jolanda, Olinda.
Yalanda, Yolie, Yolaine, Yolana, Yoland, Yolande, Yolane, Yolanna, Yolantha, Yolanthe, Yolette, Yolonda, Yorlanda, Youlanda, Yulanda, Yulonda

Yole, Yone (Greek) beautiful as a violet.

Yolie (Greek) a familiar form of Yolanda.
Yola, Yoley, Yoli, Yoly

Yoluta (Native American) summer flower.

Yomara (American) a combination of Yolanda + Tamara.
Yomaira, Yomarie, Yomira

Yon (Burmese) rabbit. (Korean) lotus blossom.
Yona, Yonna

Yoné (Japanese) wealth; rice.

Yonina (Hebrew) a form of Jonina.
Yona, Yonah

Yonita (Hebrew) a form of Jonita.
Yonat, Yonati, Yonit

Yoomee (Coos) star.
Yoome

Yordana (Basque) descendant. See also Jordana.

Yori (Japanese) reliable.
Yoriko, Yoriyo

Yoselin GB (Latin) a form of Jocelyn.
Yoseline, Yoselyn, Yosselin, Yosseline, Yosselyn

Yosepha (Hebrew) a form of Josephine.
Yosefa, Yosifa, Yuseffa

Yoshi (Japanese) good; respectful.
Yoshie, Yoshiko, Yoshiyo

Yovela (Hebrew) joyful heart; rejoicer.

Ysabel (Spanish) a form of Isabel.
Ysabell, Ysabella, Ysabelle, Ysbel, Ysbella, Ysobel

Ysanne (American) a combination of Ysabel + Ann.
Ysande, Ysann, Ysanna

Yseult (German) ice rule. (Irish) fair; light skinned. (Welsh) a form of Isolde.
Yseulte, Ysolt

Yuana (Spanish) a form of Juana.
Yuan, Yuanna

Yudelle (English) a form of Udele.
Yudela, Yudell, Yudella

Yudita (Russian) a form of Judith.
Yudit, Yudith, Yuditt

Yuki BG (Japanese) snow.
Yukie, Yukiko, Yukiyo

Yulene (Basque) a form of Julia.
Yuleen

Yulia (Russian) a form of Julia.
Yula, Yulenka, Yulinka, Yulka, Yulya

Yuliana (Spanish) a form of Juliana.
Yulenia, Yuliani

Yuri GB (Japanese) lily.
Yuree, Yuriko, Yuriyo

Yvanna (Slavic) a form of Ivana.
Yvan, Yvana, Yvannia

Yvette (French) a familiar form of Yvonne. See also Evette, Ivette.
Yavette, Yevett, Yevette, Yevetta, Yvet, Yveta, Yvett, Yvetta

Yvonne GB (French) young archer. (Scandinavian) yew wood; bow wood. See also Evonne, Ivonne, Vonna, Vonny, Yvette.
Yavanda, Yavanna, Yavanne, Yavonda, Yavonna, Yavonne, Yveline, Yvon, Yvone, Yvonna, Yvonnah, Yvonnia, Yvonnie, Yvonny

Z

Z BG (American) an initial used as a first name.

Zaba (Hebrew) she who offers a sacrifice to God.

Zabrina (American) a form of Sabrina.
Zabreena, Zabrinia, Zabrinna, Zabryna

Zachariah BG (Hebrew) God remembered.

Zacharie BG (Hebrew) God remembered.
Zacari, Zacceaus, Zacchaea, Zachary, Zachoia, Zackaria, Zackeisha, Zackeria, Zakaria, Zakaya, Zakeshia, Zakiah, Zakiria, Zakiya, Zakiyah, Zechari

Zachary BG (Hebrew) a form of Zacharie.
Zackery, Zakary

Zada (Arabic) fortunate, prosperous.
Zaida, Zayda, Zayeda

Zafina (Arabic) victorious.

Zafirah (Arabic) successful; victorious.

Zahar (Hebrew) daybreak; dawn.
Zahara, Zaharra, Zahera, Zahira, Zahirah, Zeeherah

Zahavah (Hebrew) golden.
Zachava, Zachavah, Zechava, Zechavah, Zehava, Zehavi, Zehavit, Zeheva, Zehuva

Zahra (Swahili) flower. (Arabic) white.
Zahara, Zahraa, Zahrah, Zahreh, Zahria

Zaira (Hebrew) a form of Zara.
Zaire, Zairea, Zirrea

Zakia BG (Swahili) smart. (Arabic) chaste.
Zakea, Zakeia, Zakiah, Zakiya

Zakira (Hebrew) a form of Zacharie.
Zaakira, Zakiera, Zakierra, Zakir, Zakirah, Zakiria, Zakiriya, Zykarah, Zykera, Zykeria, Zykerria, Zykira, Zykuria

Zakiya (Arabic) a form of Zakia.
Zakeya, Zakeyia, Zakiyaa, Zakiyah, Zakiyya, Zakiyyah, Zakkiyya, Zakkiyyah, Zakkyyah

Zalika (Swahili) born to royalty.
Zuleika

Zaltana (Native American) high
mountain.

Zana **GB** (Spanish) a form of
Zanna.

Zandra (Greek) a form of Sandra.
*Zahndra, Zandrea, Zandria, Zandy,
Zanndra, Zondra*

Zane **BG** (English) a form of
John.

Zaneta (Spanish) a form of Jane.
Zanita, Zanitra

Zanna (Spanish) a form of Jane.
(English) a short form of
Susanna.
*Zaina, Zainah, Zainna, Zana,
Zanae, Zanah, Zanella, Zanette,
Zannah, Zannette, Zannia, Zannie*

Zanthe (Greek) a form of Xanthe.
Zanth, Zantha

Zara (Hebrew) a form of Sarah,
Zora.
*Zaira, Zarah, Zarea, Zaree,
Zareea, Zareen, Zareena, Zareh,
Zareya, Zari, Zaria, Zariya, Zarria*

Zarifa (Arabic) successful.

Zarina (Slavic) empress.

Zarita (Spanish) a form of Sarah.

Zasha (Russian) a form of Sasha.
Zascha, Zashenka, Zashka, Zasho

Zaviera (Spanish) a form of
Xaviera.
Zavera, Zavirah

Zawati (Swahili) gift.

Zayit **BG** (Hebrew) olive.

Zaynah (Arabic) beautiful.
Zayn, Zayna

Zea (Latin) grain.

Zechariah **BG** (Hebrew) a form
of Zachariah.

Zelda (Yiddish) gray haired.
(German) a short form of
Griselda. See also Selda.
Zelde, Zella, Zellda

Zelene (English) sunshine.
Zeleen, Zelena, Zeline

Zelia (Spanish) sunshine.
Zele, Zelene, Zelie, Zélie, Zelina

Zelizi (Basque) a form of Sheila.

Zelma (German) a form of Selma.

Zelmira (Arabic) brilliant one.

Zemirah (Hebrew) song of joy.

Zena (Greek) a form of Xenia.
(Ethiopian) news. (Persian)
woman. See also Zina.
*Zanae, Zanah, Zeena, Zeenat,
Zeenet, Zeenia, Zeenya, Zein,
Zeina, Zenah, Zenana, Zenea,
Zenia, Zenna, Zennah, Zennia,
Zenya*

Zenadia (Greek) she who is
dedicated to God.

Zenaida (Greek) white-winged dove.
Zenaide, Zenaïde, Zenayda, Zenochka

Zenda GB (Persian) sacred; feminine.

Zenobia (Greek) sign, symbol. History: a queen who ruled the city of Palmyra in ancient Syria.
Zeba, Zeeba, Zenobie, Zenovia

Zephania, Zephanie (Greek) forms of Stephanie.
Zepania, Zephanas, Zephany

Zephyr BG (Greek) west wind.
Zefiryn, Zephra, Zephria, Zephyer, Zephyrine

Zera (Hebrew) seeds.
Zerah, Zeriah

Zerdali (Turkish) wild apricot.

Zerlina (Latin, Spanish) beautiful dawn. Music: a character in Mozart's opera *Don Giovanni*.
Zerla, Zerlinda

Zerrin (Turkish) golden.
Zerren

Zeta (English) rose. Linguistics: a letter in the Greek alphabet.
Zayit, Zetana, Zetta

Zetta (Portuguese) rose.

Zhana (Slavic) a form of Zhane.
Zhanay, Zhanaya, Zhaniah, Zhanna

Zhane GB (Slavic) a form of Jane.
Zhanae, Zhané, Zhanea, Zhanee, Zhaney, Zhani

Zhen (Chinese) chaste.

Zia GB (Latin) grain. (Arabic) light.
Zea

Zidanelia (Greek) she who is God's judge; bluish lotus flower.

Zigana (Hungarian) gypsy girl. See also Tsigana.
Zigane

Zihna (Hopi) one who spins tops.

Zilla (Hebrew) shadow.
Zila, Zillah, Zylla

Zilpah (Hebrew) dignified. Bible: Jacob's wife.
Zilpha, Zylpha

Zilya (Russian) a form of Theresa.

Zimra (Hebrew) song of praise.
Zamora, Zemira, Zemora, Zimria

Zina (African) secret spirit. (English) hospitable. (Greek) a form of Zena.
Zinah, Zine

Zinnia (Latin) Botany: a plant with beautiful, rayed, colorful flowers.
Zinia, Zinny, Zinnya, Zinya

Zipporah (Hebrew) bird. Bible: Moses' wife.
Zipora, Ziporah, Zipporia, Ziproh

Zita (Spanish) rose. (Arabic)
mistress. A short form of names
ending in "sita" or "zita."
Zeeta, Zyta, Zytka

Ziva (Hebrew) bright; radiant.
Zeeva, Ziv, Zivanka, Zivi, Zivit

Zizi (Hungarian) a familiar form
of Elizabeth.
Zsi Zsi

Zobeida (Arabic) pleasant as
cream.

Zocha (Polish) a form of Sophie.

Zoe ☆ GB (Greek) life.
*Zoé, Zoë, Zoee, Zoelie, Zoeline,
Zoelle, Zoey, Zoi, Zoie, Zowe,
Zowey, Zowie, Zoya*

Zoey GB (Greek) a form of Zoe.
Zooey

Zofia (Slavic) a form of Sophia.
See also Sofia.
Zofka, Zsofia

Zohar Bg (Hebrew) shining,
brilliant.
Zoheret

Zohra (Hebrew) blossom.

Zohreh (Persian) happy.
Zahreh, Zohrah

Zola (Italian) piece of earth.
Zoela, Zoila

Zona (Latin) belt, sash.
Zonia

Zondra (Greek) a form of Zandra.
Zohndra

Zora (Slavic) aurora; dawn. See
also Zara.
*Zorah, Zorana, Zoreen, Zoreena,
Zorna, Zorra, Zorrah, Zorya*

Zoraida (Arabic) she who is
eloquent.

Zorina (Slavic) golden.
*Zorana, Zori, Zorie, Zorine, Zorna,
Zory*

Zoya (Slavic) a form of Zoe.
*Zoia, Zoyara, Zoyechka, Zoyenka,
Zoyya*

Zsa Zsa (Hungarian) a familiar
form of Susan.
Zhazha

Zsofia (Hungarian) a form of
Sofia.
Zofia, Zsofi, Zsofika

Zsuzsanna (Hungarian) a form
of Susanna.
*Zsuska, Zsuzsa, Zsuzsi, Zsuzsika,
Zsuzska*

Zudora (Sanskrit) laborer.

Zuleica (Arabic) beautiful and
plump.

Zuleika (Arabic) brilliant.
*Zeleeka, Zul, Zulay, Zulekha,
Zuleyka*

Zulima (Arabic) a form of
Salama.
*Zuleima, Zulema, Zulemah,
Zulimah*

Zulma (Arabic) healthy and
vigorous woman.

Zulmara (Spanish) a form of
Zulma.

Zurafa (Arabic) lovely.
Ziraf, Zuruf

Zuri (Basque) white; light skinned.
(Swahili) beautiful.
Zuria, Zurie, Zurisha, Zury

Zurina, Zurine (Basque) white.

Zurisaday (Arabic) over the
earth.

Zusa (Czech, Polish) a form of
Susan.
*Zuzana, Zuzanka, Zuzia, Zuzka,
Zuzu*

Zuwena (Swahili) good.
Zwena

Zyanya (Zapotec) always.

Zytka (Polish) rose.

Boys

A

'Aziz (Arabic) strong.

A GB (American) an initial used as a first name.

Aakash (Hindi) a form of Akash.

Aaliyah GB (Hebrew) a form of Aliya (see Girls' Names).

Aaron ☀ BG (Hebrew) enlightened. (Arabic) messenger. Bible: the brother of Moses and the first high priest. See also Ron.
Aahron, Aaran, Aaren, Aareon, Aarin, Aaronn, Aarron, Aarronn, Aaryn, Aarynn, Aeron, Aharon, Ahran, Ahren, Aranne, Arek, Aren, Ari, Arin, Aron, Aronek, Aronne, Aronos, Arran, Arron

Aaronjames (American) a combination of Aaron + James.
Aaron James, Aaron-James

Aarronn (Hebrew) enlightened. (Arabic) messenger.
Aarynn

Abad (Hebrew) unique man.

Aban (Persian) Mythology: a figure associated with water and the arts.

Abasi (Swahili) stern.
Abasee, Abasey, Abasie, Abasy

Abban (Latin) white.
Abben, Abbin, Abbine, Abbon

Abbas (Arabic) lion.

Abbey GB (Hebrew) a familiar form of Abe.
Abbee, Abbie, Abby, Abey, Aby

Abbie GB (Hebrew) a form of Abbey.

Abbigail GB (Hebrew) a form of Abigail (see Girls' Names).

Abbott (Hebrew) father; abbot.
Ab, Abba, Abbah, Abbán, Abbé, Abboid Abbot, Abot, Abott

Abbud (Arabic) devoted.

Abby GB (Hebrew) a form of Abbey.

Abdi (African) my servant.

Abdías (Hebrew) God's servant.

Abdirahman (Arabic) a form of Abdulrahman.
Abdirehman

Abdón (Hebrew) servant of God; the very helpful man.

Abdul (Arabic) servant.
Abdal, Abdeel, Abdel, Abdoul, Abdual, Abdull, Abul

Abdulaziz (Arabic) servant of the Mighty.
Abdelazim, Abdelaziz, Abdulazaz, Abdulazeez

Abdullah (Arabic) servant of Allah.
Abdala, Abdalah, Abdalla, Abdallah, Abdela, Abduala, Abdualla, Abduallah, Abdula,

*Abdulah, Abdulahi, Abdulha,
Abdulla, Abdullahi*

Abdulmalik (Arabic) servant of
the Master.

Abdulrahman (Arabic) servant of
the Merciful.
*Abdelrahim, Abdelrahman,
Abdirahman, Abdolrahem,
Abdularahman, Abdurrahman,
Abdurram*

Abe (Hebrew) a short form of
Abel, Abraham.
Abb, Abbe

Abel BG (Hebrew) breath.
(Assyrian) meadow. (German) a
short form of Abelard. Bible:
Adam and Eve's second son.
*Abe, Abele, Abell, Able, Adal,
Avel*

Abelard (German) noble;
resolute.
*Ab, Abalard, Abel, Abelarde,
Abelardo, Abelhard, Abilard,
Adalard, Adelard*

Abercio (Greek) first son.

Abernethy (Scottish) river's
beginning.
Abernathie, Abernethi

Abi (Turkish) older brother.
Abee, Abbi

Abiah (Hebrew) God is my father.
*Abia, Abiel, Abija, Abijah, Abisha,
Abishai, Aviya, Aviyah*

Abidan (Hebrew) father of
judgment.
*Abiden, Abidin, Abidon, Abydan,
Abyden, Abydin, Abydon, Abydyn*

Abie (Hebrew) a familiar form of
Abraham.

Abiel (Hebrew) a form of Abiah.

Abir (Hebrew) strong.
Abyr

Abisha (Hebrew) gift of God.
*Abijah, Abishai, Abishal, Abysha,
Abyshah*

Abner (Hebrew) father of light.
Bible: the commander of Saul's
army.
Ab, Avner, Ebner

Abo (Hebrew) father.

Abraham (Hebrew) father of
many nations. Bible: the first
Hebrew patriarch. See also
Avram, Bram, Ibrahim.
*Abarran, Abe, Aberham, Abey,
Abhiram, Abie, Abrahaim,
Abrahame, Abrahamo, Abrahan,
Abrahán, Abraheem, Abrahem,
Abrahim, Abrahm, Abram,
Abramo, Abrán, Abrao, Arram,
Avram*

Abrahan (Spanish) a form of
Abraham.
Abrahin, Abrahon

Abram (Hebrew) a short form of
Abraham. See also Bram.
Abrama, Abramo, Abrams, Avram

Absalom (Hebrew) father of peace. Bible: the rebellious third son of King David. See also Avshalom, Axel.
Absalaam, Absalon, Abselon, Absolam, Absolom, Absolum

Absalón (Hebrew) a form of Absalom.

Abundancio (Latin) rich, affluent.

Abundio (Latin) he who has a lot of property.

Acab (Hebrew) uncle.

Acacio (Greek) is not evil and is honorable.

Acañir (Mapuche) liberated fox.

Acapana (Quechua) lightning; small hurricane.

Acar (Turkish) bright.

Ace (Latin) unity.
Acer, Acey, Acie

Achachic (Aymara) ancestor; grandfather.

Achic (Quechua) luminous; resplendent.

Achilles (Greek) Mythology: a hero of the Trojan War. Literature: the hero of Homer's epic poem *Iliad*.
Achil, Achill, Achille, Achillea, Achilleus, Achillios, Achyl, Achyll, Achylle, Achylleus Akil, Akili, Akilles

Acisclo (Latin) a pick used to work on rocks.

Ackerley (English) meadow of oak trees.
Accerlee, Accerleigh, Accerley, Ackerlea, Ackerlee, Ackerleigh, Ackerli, Ackerlie, Ackersley, Acklea, Ackleigh, Ackley, Acklie, Akerlea, Akerlee, Akerleigh, Akerley, Akerli, Akerlie, Akerly

Acklee (English) a short form of Ackerley.
Ackli, Ackly

Aconcauac (Quechua) stone sentinel.

Acton (English) oak-tree settlement.
Actan, Acten, Actin, Actun, Actyn

Acursio (Latin) he who heads towards God.

Adahy (Cherokee) in the woods.
Adahi

Adair GB (Scottish) oak-tree ford.
Adaire, Adare, Adayr, Adayre, Addair, Addaire, Addar, Addare, Addayr, Addyre

Adalbaro (Greek) combatant of nobility.

Adalberto (Germanic) belonging to nobility.

Adalgiso, Adalvino (Greek) lance of nobility.

Adalrico (Greek) noble chief of his lineage.

Adam ☆ BG (Phoenician) man;
mankind. (Hebrew) earth; man
of the red earth. Bible: the first
man created by God. See also
Adamson, Addison, Damek,
Keddy, Macadam.
*Ad, Adama, Adamec, Adamo,
Adão, Adas, Addam, Addams,
Addis, Addy, Adem, Adham,
Adhamh, Adim, Adné, Adok,
Adomas, Adym*

Adamec (Czech) a form of Adam.
*Adamek, Adamik, Adamka,
Adamko, Adamok*

Adamson (Hebrew) son of Adam.
Adams, Adamsson, Addamson

Adan (Irish) a form of Aidan.
Aden, Adian, Adin, Adun

Adán (Hebrew) a form of Adam.

Adar (Syrian) ruler; prince.
(Hebrew) noble; exalted.
Addar

Adarius (American) a
combination of Adam + Darius.
*Adareus, Adarias, Adarrius,
Adarro, Adarruis, Adaruis,
Adauris*

Adaucto (Latin) increase.

Addel (German) a short form of
Adelard.
Adell

Addison BG (English) son of
Adam.
Addis, Addisen, Addisun,

*Addoson, Addyson, Adison,
Adisson, Adyson*

Addy (Hebrew) a familiar form of
Adam, Adlai. (German) a familiar
form of Adelard.
Addey, Addi, Addie, Ade, Adi

Ade (Yoruba) royal.

Adelard (German) noble;
courageous.
*Adal, Adalar, Adalard, Adalarde,
Addy, Adel, Adél, Adelar,
Adelarde, Adelhard*

Adelardo, Adelino (Greek)
daring prince.

Adelfo (Greek) male friend.

Adelio (Germanic) father of the
noble prince.

Adelmaro (Greek) distinguished
because of his lineage.

Adelmo (Germanic) noble
protector.

Adelric (German) noble ruler.
*Adalric, Adelrich, Adelrick,
Adelrik, Adelryc, Adelryck,
Adelryk*

**Ademar, Ademaro, Adhemar,
Adimar** (German) he whose
battles have made him
distinguished; celebrated and
famous combatant.

Aden (Arabic) Geography: a
region in southern Yemen.
(Irish) a form of Aidan, Aiden.

Adham (Arabic) black.

Adhelmar (Greek) ennobled by his battles.

Adiel (Hebrew) he was adorned by God.

Adil (Arabic) just; wise.
Adeel, Adeele, Adill, Adyl, Adyll

Adin (Hebrew) pleasant.
Addin, Addyn, Adyn

Adir (Hebrew) majestic; noble.
Adeer

Adirán (Latin) from the Adriatic Sea.

Aditya (Hindi) sun.

Adiv (Hebrew) pleasant; gentle.
Adeev, Adev

Adlai (Hebrew) my ornament.
Ad, Addlai, Addlay, Addy, Adlay, Adley

Adler (German) eagle.
Ad, Addlar, Addler, Adlar

Adli (Turkish) just; wise.
Adlea, Adlee, Adleigh, Adlie, Adly

Admon (Hebrew) peony.

Adnan (Arabic) pleasant.
Adnaan, Adnane

Adney (English) noble's island.
Adnee, Adni, Adnie, Adny

Adolf (German) noble wolf.
History: Adolf Hitler's German army was defeated in World War II. See also Dolf.
Ad, Addof, Addoff, Adof, Adolfo, Adolfus, Adolph

Adolfo (Spanish) a form of Adolf.
Addofo, Adolffo, Adolpho, Andolffo, Andolfo, Andolpho

Adolph (German) a form of Adolf.
Adolphe, Adolpho, Adolphus, Adulphus

Adolphus (French) a form of Adolf.
Adolphius

Adom (Akan) help from God.

Adon (Hebrew) Lord. (Greek) a short form of Adonis.

Adonai (Hebrew) my Lord.

Adonías (Hebrew) God is my Lord.

Adonis (Greek) highly attractive. Mythology: the attractive youth loved by Aphrodite.
Adon, Adonise, Adonnis, Adonys, Adonyse

Adri (Indo-Pakistani) rock.
Adree, Adrey, Adrie, Adry

Adrian ☆ BG (Greek) rich. (Latin) dark. (Swedish) a short form of Hadrian.
Adarian, Ade, Adorjan, Adrain, Adreian, Adreyan, Adri, Adriaan, Adriane, Adriann, Adrianne, Adriano, Adrianus, Adriean, Adrien, Adrik, Adrin, Adrion, Adrionn, Adrionne, Adron, Adryan, Adryn, Adryon

Adrián (Latin) a form of Adrian.

Adriana, Adrianna **GB** (Italian) forms of Adrienne.

Adriano (Italian) a form of Adrian.
Adrianno

Adriel (Hebrew) member of God's flock.
Adrial, Adriall, Adriell, Adryel, Adryell

Adrien **BG** (French) a form of Adrian.
Adriene, Adrienne, Adryen

Adrienne **GB** (French) a form of Adrien.

Adrik (Russian) a form of Adrian.
Adric

Adulfo (Germanic) of noble heritage.

Adwin (Ghanian) creative.
Adwyn

Aeneas (Greek) praised. (Scottish) a form of Angus. Literature: the Trojan hero of Vergil's epic poem *Aeneid*. See also Eneas.

Afram (African) Geography: a river in Ghana, Africa.

Afton **GB** (English) from Afton, England.
Affton, Aftan, Aften, Aftin, Aftyn

Agamemnon (Greek) resolute. Mythology: the king of Mycenae who led the Greeks in the Trojan War.

Agamenón (Greek) he who moves slowly down the path.

Agapito (Hebrew) beloved one.

Agar (Hebrew) he who escaped.

Agatón (Greek) victor; good.

Agenor (Greek) strong man.

Ageo (Hebrew) having a festive character.

Agesislao (Greek) leader of villages.

Agila (Teutonic) he who possesses combat support.

Agnelo (Latin) reference to the lamb of God.

Agni (Hindi) Religion: the Hindu fire god.

Agostine (Italian) a form of Augustine.
Agostyne

Agostiño (Latin) a form of Augusto.

Agrippa (Latin) born feet first. History: the commander of the Roman fleet that defeated Mark Antony and Cleopatra at Actium.
Agripa, Agripah, Agrippah, Agrypa, Agrypah, Agryppa, Agryppah

Agu (Ibo) leopard.

Agús (Spanish) a form of Agustín.

Agusteen (Latin) a form of Augustine.
Agustyne

Agustin (Latin) a form of Augustine.
Agostino, Agoston, Aguistin, Agustein, Agusteyne, Agustine, Agustis, Agusto, Agustus, Agustyn

Agustín (Latin) a form of Augustin.

Ahab (Hebrew) father's brother. Literature: the captain of the Pequod in Herman Melville's novel *Moby-Dick.*

Ahanu (Native American) laughter.

Ahdik (Native American) caribou; reindeer.
Ahdic, Ahdick, Ahdyc, Ahdyck, Ahdyk

Ahearn (Scottish) lord of the horses. (English) heron.
Ahearne, Aherin, Ahern, Aherne, Aheron, Aheryn, Hearn

Ahir (Turkish) last.

Ahkeem (Hebrew) a form of Akeem.
Ahkiem, Ahkyem, Ahkyeme

Ahmad (Arabic) most highly praised. See also Muhammad.
Achmad, Achmed, Ahamad, Ahamada, Ahamed, Ahmaad, Ahmaud, Amad, Amahd, Amed

Ahmed BG (Swahili) praiseworthy.

Ahsan (Arabic) charitable.

Aidan ✦ BG (Irish) fiery.
Adan, Aden, Aiden, Aidun, Aydan, Ayden, Aydin

Aidano (Teutonic) he who distinguishes himself.

Aiden ✦ BG (Irish) a form of Aidan.
Aden, Aidon, Aidwin, Aidwyn, Aidyn

Aiken (English) made of oak.
Aicken, Aikin, Ayken, Aykin

Ailwan (English) noble friends.
Ailwen, Ailwin

Aimery (French) a form of Emery.
Aime, Aimeree, Aimerey, Aimeri, Aimeric, Aimerie, Amerey, Aymeric, Aymery

Aimon (French) house. (Irish) a form of Eamon.

Aindrea (Irish) a form of Andrew.
Aindreas

Ainsley GB (Scottish) my own meadow.
Ainslea, Ainslee, Ainslei, Ainsleigh, Ainsli, Ainslie, Ainsly, Ansley, Aynslee, Aynsley, Aynslie

Aizik (Russian) a form of Isaac.

Aja GB (Punjabi) a form of Ajay.

Ajala (Yoruba) potter.
Ajalah

Ajay (Punjabi) victorious;
undefeatable. (American) a
combination of the initials A. + J.
*Aj, Aja, Ajae, Ajai, Ajaye, Ajaz,
Ajé, Ajee, Ajit*

Ajit (Sanskrit) unconquerable.
Ajeet, Ajith

Akar (Turkish) flowing stream.
Akara, Akare

Akash (Hindi) sky.
Aakash, Akasha, Akshay

Akbar (Arabic) great.
Akbara, Akbare

Akecheta (Sioux) warrior.
Akechetah

Akeem, Akim (Hebrew) short
forms of Joachim.
*Achim, Achym, Ackeem, Ackim,
Ackime, Ackym, Ackyme
Ahkieme, Akeam, Akee, Akiem,
Akima, Akym, Arkeem*

Akemi (Japanese) dawn.
Akemee, Akemie, Akemy

Akil (Arabic) intelligent. (Greek)
a form of Achilles.
*Ahkeel, Akeel, Akeil, Akeyla,
Akhil, Akiel, Akila, Akilah, Akile,
Akili, Akyl, Akyle*

Akins (Yoruba) brave.
Akin, Akyn, Akyns

Akira GB (Japanese) intelligent.
*Akihito, Akio, Akirah, Akiyo,
Akyra, Akyrah*

Akiva (Hebrew) a form of Jacob.
Akiba, Kiva

Aklea (English) a short form of
Ackerley.
*Aklee, Akleigh, Akley, Akli, Aklie,
Akly*

Akmal (Arabic) perfect.
Ackmal

Akram (Arabic) most generous.

Aksel (Norwegian) father of
peace.
Aksell

Akshat (Sanskrit) uninjurable.

Akshay (American) a form of
Akash.
Akshaj, Akshaya

Akule (Native American) he looks
up.
Akul

Akyo (Japanese) bright.

Al (Irish) a short form of Alan,
Albert, Alexander.

Aladdin (Arabic) height of faith.
Literature: the hero of a story in
the *Arabian Nights*.
*Ala, Alaa, Alaaddin, Aladan,
Aladdan, Aladden, Aladdyn,
Aladean, Aladen, Aladin, Aladino,
Aladyn*

Alain (French) a form of Alan.
*Alaen, Alaine, Alainn, Alayn,
Alein, Aleine, Aleyn, Aleyne,
Allain, Allayn*

Alaire (French) joyful.
Alayr, Alayre

Alam (Arabic) universe.
Alame

Alan ☒☒ (Irish) handsome;
peaceful.
*Ailan, Ailin, Al, Alaan, Alain, Alair,
Aland, Alande, Alando, Alane,
Alani, Alann, Alano, Alanson,
Alante, Alao, Allan, Allen, Alon,
Alun, Alune, Alyn, Alyne*

Alardo (Greek) courageous
prince.

Alaric (German) ruler of all. See
also Ulrich.
*Alarich, Alarick, Alarico, Alarik,
Alaryc, Alaryck, Alaryk Aleric,
Allaric, Allarick, Alric, Alrick, Alrik*

Alastair (Scottish) a form of
Alexander.
*Alaisdair, Alaistair, Alaister,
Alasdair, Alasteir, Alaster,
Alastor, Aleister, Alester, Alistair,
Allaistar, Allastair, Allaster,
Allastir, Allysdair, Alystair*

Alba (Latin) town on the white hill.

Alban (Latin) from Alba, Italy.
*Albain, Albany, Albean, Albein,
Alby, Auban, Auben*

Albano (Germanic) belonging to
the house of Alba.

Alberic (German) smart; wise
ruler.
*Alberich, Alberick, Alberyc,
Alberyck, Alberyk*

Albern (German) noble;
courageous.
Alberne, Alburn, Alburne

Albert ☒☒ (German, French)
noble and bright. See also **Elbert,
Ulbrecht.**
*Adelbert, Ailbert, Al, Albertik,
Alberto, Alberts, Albertus, Albie,
Albrecht, Albret, Alby, Albyrt,
Albyrte, Alvertos, Aubert*

Alberto (Italian) a form of Albert.
Albertino, Berto

Albie, Alby (German, French)
familiar forms of Albert.
Albee, Albey, Albi

Albin (Latin) a form of Alvin.
*Alben, Albeno, Albinek, Albino,
Albins, Albinson, Albun, Alby,
Albyn, Auben*

Albion (Latin) white cliffs.
Geography: a reference to the
white cliffs in Dover, England.
Albon, Albyon, Allbion, Allbyon

Alcandor (Greek) manly; strong.

Alceo (Greek) man of great
strength and vigor.

Alcibiades (Greek) generous
and violent.

Alcibíades (Greek) strong and
valiant man.

Alcides (Greek) strong and
vigorous.

Alcott (English) old cottage.
*Alcot, Alkot, Alkott, Allcot,
Allcott, Allkot, Allkott*

Alcuino (Teutonic) friend of
sacred places, friend of the
temple.

Aldair (German, English) a form
of Alder.
Aldahir, Aldayr

Aldano, Aldino (Celtic) noble;
experienced man.

Alden BG (English) old; wise
protector.
*Aldan, Aldean, Aldin, Aldous,
Aldyn, Elden*

Alder (German, English) alder
tree.
Aldair, Aldar, Aldare, Aldyr

Alderidge (English) alder ridge.
Alderige, Aldrydge, Aldryge

Aldise (English) old house.
(German) a form of Aldous.
Aldiss, Aldys

Aldo (Italian) old; elder.
(German) a short form of
Aldous.
Alda

Aldous (German) a form of
Alden.
*Aldis, Aldo, Aldon, Aldos, Aldus,
Elden*

Aldred (English) old; wise
counselor.
Alldred, Eldred

Aldrich (English) wise.
*Aldric, Aldrick, Aldridge, Aldrige,
Aldritch, Aldryc, Aldryck Aldryk,
Alldric, Alldrich, Alldrick,
Alldridge, Eldridge*

Aldwin (English) old friend.
*Aldwan, Aldwen, Aldwon,
Aldwyn, Edlwin*

Alec, Alek BG (Greek) short
forms of Alexander.
Aleck, Aleik, Alekko, Aleko, Elek

Aleczander (Greek) a form of
Alexander.
*Alecander, Aleckxander,
Alecsander, Alecxander*

Alejandra GB (Spanish) a form
of Alexandra.

Alejandrino (Greek) he is the
protector and defender of men.

Alejandro ✵ BG (Spanish) a
form of Alexander.

Alejándro (Spanish) a form of
Alexander.
*Alejándra, Aléjo, Alexjandro,
Alexjándro*

Alejo (Greek) he who protects
and defends.

Aleksandar, Aleksander
(Greek) forms of Alexander.
*Aleksandor, Aleksandr,
Aleksandras, Aleksandur*

Aleksei (Russian) a short form of
Alexander.
*Aleks, Aleksey, Aleksi, Aleksis,
Aleksy, Alexei, Alexey*

Alekzander, Alexzander
(Greek) forms of Alexander.
Alekxander, Alekxzander,
Alexkzandr, Alexzandr, Alexzandyr

Alem (Arabic) wise.

Aleric (German) a form of Alaric.
Alerick, Alerik, Alleric, Allerick,
Alleryc, Alleryck, Alleryk

Aleron (Latin) winged.
Aleronn

Alesio (Italian) a form of Alejo.

Alessandro 🄱🄶 (Italian) a form
of Alexander.
Alessand, Alessander,
Alessandre, Allessandro

Alex ☀ 🄱🄶 (Greek) a short form
of Alexander.
Alax, Alexx, Allax, Allex, Allyx,
Allyxx, Alyx, Elek

Alexa 🄶🄱 (Greek) a short form of
Alexandra.

Alexander ☀ 🄱🄶 (Greek)
defender of mankind. History:
Alexander the Great was the
conqueror of the civilized world.
See also Alastair, Alistair, Iskander,
Jando, Leks, Lex, Lexus,
Macallister, Oleksandr, Olés,
Sander, Sándor, Sandro, Sandy,
Sasha, Xan, Xander, Zander, Zindel.
Al, Alec, Alecsandar, Alejándro,
Alek, Alekos, Aleksandar,
Aleksander, Aleksei, Alekzander,
Alessandro, Alex, Alexandar,
Alexandor, Alexandr, Alexandre,
Alexandro, Alexandros, Alexi,

Alexis, Alexxander, Alexzander,
Alic, Alick, Alisander, Alixander

Alexandra 🄶🄱 (Greek) defender
of humankind.

Alexandre 🄱🄶 (French) a form
of Alexander.

Alexandria 🄶🄱 (Greek) a form
of Alexandra.

Alexandro (Greek) a form of
Alexander.
Alexandras, Alexandros,
Alexandru

Alexe 🄶🄱 (Russian) a form of
Alexi. (Greek) a form of Alex.

Alexi 🄶🄱 (Russian) a form of
Aleksei. (Greek) a short form of
Alexander.
Alexe, Alexee, Alexey, Alexie,
Alexio, Alexy, Alezio

Alexie 🄶🄱 (Russian, Greek) a
form of Alexi.

Alexis 🄶🄱 (Greek) a short form
of Alexander.
Alexei, Alexes, Alexey, Alexios,
Alexius, Alexiz, Alexsis, Alexsus,
Alexus, Alexys

Alexsander (Greek) a form of
Alexander.

Alexus 🄶🄱 (Greek) a form of
Alexis.

Aleydis (Teutonic) born into a
noble family.

Alfie BG (English) a familiar form of Alfred.
Alfy

Alfio (Greek) he who has a white complexion.

Alfonso (Italian, Spanish) a form of Alphonse.
Affonso, Alfons, Alfonse, Alfonsus, Alfonza, Alfonzo, Alfonzus

Alford (English) old river ford.
Allford

Alfred (English) elf counselor; wise counselor. See also Fred.
Ailfrid, Ailfryd, Alf, Alfeo, Alfie, Alfredo, Alfredus, Alfrid, Alfried, Alfryd, Alured

Alfredo (Italian, Spanish) a form of Alfred.
Alfrido

Alger (German) noble spearman. (English) a short form of Algernon. See also Elger.
Aelfar, Algar, Algor, Allgar

Algernon (English) bearded, wearing a moustache.
Aelgernon, Algenon, Alger, Algie, Algin, Algon

Algie (English) a familiar form of Algernon.
Algee, Algia, Algy

Algis (German) spear.
Algiss

Algiso (Greek) lance of nobility.

Ali BG (Arabic) greatest. (Swahili) exalted.
Aly

Alí (Arabic) a form of Ali.

Alic (Greek) a short form of Alexander.
Alick, Aliek, Alik, Aliko, Alyc, Alyck, Alyk, Alyko

Alice GB (Greek) truthful. (German) noble.

Alicia GB (English) a form of Alice.

Alijah (Hebrew) a form of Elijah.

Alim (Arabic) scholar. (Arabic) a form of Alem.
Alym

Alipio (Greek) he who is not affected by suffering.

Alisander (Greek) a form of Alexander.
Alisandre, Alisaunder, Alissander, Alissandre, Alsandair, Alsandare, Alsander

Alisha GB (Greek) truthful. (German) noble. (English) a form of Alicia.

Alison, Allison GB (English) Alice's son.
Allisan, Allisen, Allisun, Allisyn, Allysan, Allysen, Allysin, Allyson, Allysun, Allysyn

Alissa GB (Greek) a form of Alice.

Alistair (English) a form of Alexander.
Alisdair, Alistaire, Alistar, Alister, Allistair, Allistar, Allister, Allistir, Alstair, Alystayr, Alystyre

Alix GB (Greek) a short form of Alex.
Alixx, Allix, Allixx, Allyx, Allyxx

Alixander (Greek) a form of Alexander.
Alixandre, Alixandru, Alixsander, Alixxander, Alixxzander, Alixzander, Alyxxander, Alyxxsander, Alyxxzander, Alyxzander

Allambee (Australian) quiet place.
Alambee, Alambey, Alambi, Alambie, Alamby, Allambey, Allambi, Allambie, Allamby

Allan BG (Irish) a form of Alan.
Allane, Allayne

Allante, Allanté (Spanish) forms of Alan.

Allard (English) noble, brave.
Alard, Ellard

Allen BG (Irish) a form of Alan.
Alen, Allene, Alley, Alleyn, Alleyne, Allie, Allin, Alline, Allon, Allyn, Allyne

Allie GB (Irish) a form of Allen.

Alma GB (Arabic) learned. (Latin) soul.

Almeric (German) powerful ruler.
Almauric, Amaurick, Amaurik, Amauryc, Amauryck, Amauryk, Americk, Amerik, Ameryc, Ameryck, Ameryk

Almon (Hebrew) widower.
Alman, Almen, Almin, Almyn

Alois (German) a short form of Aloysius.
Aloys

Aloisio (Spanish) a form of Louis.

Alok (Sanskrit) victorious cry.

Alon (Hebrew) oak.
Alonn

Alondra GB (Spanish) a form of Alexandra.

Alonso, Alonzo (Spanish) forms of Alphonse.
Alano, Alanzo, Alon, Alonz, Alonza, Alonze, Allonza, Allonzo, Elonzo, Lon, Lonnie, Lonso, Lonzo

Aloysius (German) a form of Louis.
Alaois, Alois, Aloisius, Aloisio

Alphonse (German) noble and eager.
Alf, Alfie, Alfonso, Alonzo, Alphons, Alphonsa, Alphonso, Alphonsus, Alphonza, Alphonzus, Fonzie

Alphonso (Italian) a form of Alphonse.
Alphanso, Alphonzo, Fonso

Alpin (Irish) attractive.
Alpine, Alpyn, Alpyne

Alroy (Spanish) king.
Alroi

Alston (English) noble's
settlement.
*Allston, Alstan, Alsten, Alstin,
Alstun, Alstyn*

Altair (Greek) star. (Arabic)
flying.
Altayr, Altayre

Alterio (Greek) like a starry night.

Altman (German) old man.
Altmann, Altmen, Atman

Alton (English) old town.
Alten

Alucio (Latin) he is lucid and
illustrious.

Alula (Latin) winged; swift.

Alva BG (Hebrew) sublime.
Alvah

Alvan (German) a form of Alvin.
Alvand, Alvun

Alvar (English) army of elves.
Alvara

Alvaro (Spanish) just; wise.

Alvern (Latin) spring.
Alverne, Elvern

Alvero (Germanic) completely
prudent.

Alvin (Latin) white; light skinned.
(German) friend to all; noble
friend; friend of elves. See also
Albin, Elvin.
*Aloin, Aluin, Aluino, Alvan, Alven,
Alvie, Alvino, Alvon, Alvy, Alvyn,
Alwin, Elwin*

Alvis (Scandinavian) all-knowing.

Alwin (German) a form of Alvin.
*Ailwyn, Alwan, Alwen, Alwon,
Alwun, Alwyn, Alwynn, Aylwin*

Alyssa GB (Greek) rational.
Botany: alyssum is a flowering
herb.

Amadeo (Italian) a form of
Amadeus.

Amadeus (Latin) loves God.
Music: Wolfgang Amadeus Mozart
was a famous eighteenth-century
Austrian composer.
*Amad, Amadeaus, Amadée,
Amadeo, Amadei, Amadio,
Amadis, Amado, Amador,
Amadou, Amando, Amedeo,
Amodaos*

Amal GB (Hebrew) worker.
(Arabic) hopeful.
Amahl

Amalio (Greek) a man who is
carefree.

Aman (Hebrew) magnificent one.

Amancio (Latin) he who loves
God.

Amanda GB (Latin) lovable.

Amandeep BG (Punjabi) light of
peace.
*Amandip, Amanjit, Amanjot,
Amanpreet*

Amando (French) a form of
Amadeus.
*Amand, Amandio, Amaniel,
Amato*

Amani (Arabic) believer.
(Yoruba) strength; builder.
Amanee

Amar (Punjabi) immortal.
(Arabic) builder.
Amare, Amaree, Amari, Amario,
Amaris, Amarjit, Amaro,
Amarpreet, Amarri, Ammar,
Ammer

Amaranto (Greek) he who does
not slow down.

Amaruquispe (Quechua) free,
like the sacred Amaru.

Amarutopac (Quechua) glorious,
majestic Amaru.

Amaruyupanqui (Quechua) he
who honors Amaru; memorable
Amaru.

Amato (French) loved.
Amat, Amatto

Ambar 𝐆𝐁 (Sanskrit) sky.

Amber 𝐆𝐁 (French) amber.

Ambrois (French) a form of
Ambrose.

Ambrose (Greek) immortal.
Ambie, Ambrogio, Ambroise,
Ambroisius, Ambros, Ambrosi,
Ambrosio, Ambrosios, Ambrosius,
Ambrossye, Ambrosye, Ambrotos,
Ambroz Ambrus, Amby

Ameen (Hebrew, Arabic, Hindi) a
form of Amin.

Ameer (Hebrew) a form of Amir.
Ameir, Amer, Amere

Amelio (Teutonic) very hard
worker, energetic.

Americ (French) a form of
Emery.

Américo (Germanic) prince in
action.

Amerigo (Teutonic) industrious.
History: Amerigo Vespucci was
the Italian explorer for whom
America is named.
Americo, Americus, Amerygo

Amérigo (Italian) a form of
Amerigo.

Ames (French) friend.
Amess

Ami (Hebrew) builder.

Amicus (English, Latin) beloved
friend.
Amic, Amick, Amicko, Amico,
Amik, Amiko, Amyc, Amyck,
Amycko, Amyk, Amyko

Amiel (Hebrew) God of my
people.
Amiell, Ammiel, Amyel, Amyell

Amílcar (Punic) he who governs
the city.

Amin (Hebrew, Arabic)
trustworthy; honest. (Hindi)
faithful.
Amen, Amine, Ammen, Ammin,
Ammyn, Amyn, Amynn

Amín (Arabic) a form of Amin.

Amintor (Greek) protector.

Amir **GB** (Hebrew) proclaimed.
(Punjabi) wealthy; king's
minister. (Arabic) prince.
*Aamer, Aamir, Ameer, Amire,
Amiri, Amyr*

Amish (Sanskrit) honest.

Amit (Punjabi) unfriendly.
(Arabic) highly praised.
Amita, Amitan, Amreet

Ammon (Egyptian) hidden.
Mythology: the ancient god
associated with reproduction.
Amman

Amol (Hindi) priceless, valuable.
Amul

Amoldo (Spanish) power of an
eagle.

Amon (Hebrew) trustworthy;
faithful.
Amun

Amón (Hebrew) a form of Amon.

Amory (German) a form of Emory.
*Ameree, Ameri, Amerie, Amery,
Ammeree, Ammerey, Ammeri,
Ammerie, Ammery, Ammoree,
Ammorey, Ammori, Ammorie,
Ammory, Amor, Amoree, Amorey,
Amori, Amorie*

Amos (Hebrew) burdened,
troubled. Bible: an Old Testament
prophet.
Amose, Amous

Amós (Hebrew) a form of Amos.

Ampelio (Greek) he who makes
wine from his own grapes.

Ampelo (Greek) son of a satyr and
a nymph, who died while trying to
pick grapes from a grapevine.

Amram (Hebrew) mighty nation.
Amarien, Amran, Amren, Amryn

Amrit **BG** (Sanskrit) nectar.
(Punjabi, Arabic) a form of Amit.
Amryt

Amritpal (Sikh) protector of the
Lord's nectar.

Amuillan (Mapuche) movement
from the altar; he who warmly
serves others.

Amy **GB** (Latin) beloved.

An **BG** (Chinese, Vietnamese)
peaceful.
Ana

Anacario (Greek) not without
grace.

Anacleto (Greek) he who was
called upon.

Anaías (Hebrew) Lord answers.

Anand (Hindi) blissful.
Ananda, Anant, Ananth

Ananías (Hebrew) he who has
the grace of God.

Anastasius (Greek) resurrection.
*Anas, Anastacio, Anastacios,
Anastagio, Anastas, Anastase,
Anastasi, Anastasio, Anastasios,
Anastatius, Anastice, Anastisis,
Anaztáz, Athanasius*

Anatole (Greek) east.
*Anatol, Anatoley, Anatoli,
Anatolie, Anatolijus, Anatolio,
Anatolis, Anatoliy, Anatoly,
Anitoly, Antoly*

Anbesa (Spanish) a Saracen
governor of Spain.

Anca (Quechua) eagle; black
eagle.

Ancasmayu (Quechua) blue like
the river.

Ancaspoma, Ancaspuma
(Quechua) bluish puma.

Ancavil (Mapuche) identical
mythological being.

Ancavilo (Mapuche) snake's
body; a body that is half snake.

Anchali (Taos) painter.
*Anchalee, Anchaley, Anchalie,
Anchaly*

Ancuguiyca (Quechua) having
sacred resistance.

Anders (Swedish) a form of
Andrew.
Andar, Ander

Anderson 🅱🄶 (Swedish) son of
Andrew.
Andersen

Andonios (Greek) a form of
Anthony.
Andoni, Andonis, Andonny

Andor (Hungarian) a form of
Andrew.

András (Hungarian) a form of
Andrew.
*Andraes, Andri, Andris, Andrius,
Andriy, Aundras, Aundreas*

Andre, André 🅱🄶 (French)
forms of Andrew.
*Andra, Andrae, Andrecito,
Andree, Andrei, Aundre, Aundré*

Andrea 🄶🄱 (Greek) a form of
Andrew.
Andrean, Andreani, Andrian

Andreas 🅱🄶 (Greek) a form of
Andrew.
Andres, Andries

Andrei (Bulgarian, Romanian,
Russian) a form of Andrew.
*Andreian, Andrej, Andrey,
Andreyan, Andrie, Aundrei*

Andreo (Greek) manly.

Andres 🅱🄶 (Spanish) a form of
Andrew.
Andras, Andrés, Andrez

Andrew ☆ 🅱🄶 (Greek) strong;
manly; courageous. Bible: one of
the Twelve Apostles. See also
Bandi, Drew, Endre, Evangelos,
Kendrew, Ondro.
*Aindrea, Anders, Andery,
Andonis, Andor, András, Andre,
André, Andrea, Andreas, Andrei,
Andres, Andrews, Andru, Andrue,
Andrus, Andy, Anker, Anndra,
Antal, Audrew*

Androcles (Greek) man covered
with glory.

Andrónico (German) victorious
man.

Andros (Polish) sea. Mythology:
the god of the sea.
Andris, Andrius, Andrus

Andrzej (Polish) a form of
Andrew.

Andy BG (Greek) a short form of
Andrew.
*Ande, Andee, Andey, Andi, Andie,
Andino, Andis, Andje*

Aneurin (Welsh) honorable; gold.
See also Nye.
Aneirin

Anfernee (Greek) a form of
Anthony.
*Anferney, Anfernie, Anferny,
Anfranee, Anfrene, Anfrenee,
Anpherne*

Anfión (Greek) mythological son
of Antiope and Jupiter.

Anfonee (Greek) a form of
Anthony.
Anfoney, Anfoni, Anfonie, Anfony

Angel ☆ BG (Greek) angel.
(Latin) messenger. See also
Gotzon.
*Ange, Angell, Angelo, Angie,
Angy, Anjel, Anjell*

Ángel (Greek) a form of Angel.

Angela GB (Greek) angel;
messenger.

Angelina GB (Russian) forms of
Angela.

Angeline (Russian) forms of
Angela.

Angelino (Latin) messenger.

Angelo (Italian) a form of Angel.
*Angeleo, Angelito, Angello,
Angelos, Angelous, Angiolo,
Anglo, Anjello, Anjelo*

Angilberto (Teutonic) he who
shines with the power of God. A
combination of Ángel and
Alberto.

Angus (Scottish) exceptional;
outstanding. Mythology: Angus Og
was the Celtic god of youth, love,
and beauty. See also Ennis, Gus.
Aeneas, Aonghas

Anh (Vietnamese) peace; safety.

Aniano (Greek) he who is sad
and upset.

Anías (Hebrew) God answers.

Anibal (Phoenician) a form of
Hannibal.

Aníbal (Punic) he who has the
grace of God.

Anicet, Aniceto (Greek)
invincible man of great strength.

Anik GB (Czech) a form of Anica
(see Girls' Names).

Anil (Hindi) wind god.
*Aneal, Aneel, Anel, Aniel,
Aniello, Anielo, Anyl, Anyll*

Anisha GB (English) a form of
Agnes (see Girls' Names).

Anita GB (Spanish) a form of Anna.

Anka GB (Turkish) phoenix.

Anker (Danish) a form of Andrew.
Ankor, Ankur

Anna GB (Greek) a form of Annas.

Annan (Scottish) brook. (Swahili) fourth-born son.
Annen, Annin, Annon, Annun, Annyn

Annas (Greek) gift from God.
Anis, Anish, Anna, Annais

Anne GB (English) gracious.

Anno (German) a familiar form of Johann.
Ano

Anoki (Native American) actor.
Anokee, Anokey, Anokie, Anoky

Anoop (Sikh) beauty.

Ansaldo (German) he who represents God; God is with him.

Ansel (French) follower of a nobleman.
Ancell, Ansa, Anselino, Ansell, Ansellus, Anselyno, Ansyl

Anselm (German) divine protector. See also Elmo.
Anse, Anselme, Anselmi, Anselmo

Ansis (Latvian) a form of Janis.

Ansley GB (Scottish) a form of Ainsley.
Anslea, Anslee, Ansleigh, Ansli, Anslie, Ansly, Ansy

Anson (German) divine. (English) Anne's son.
Ansan, Ansen, Ansin, Ansun, Ansyn

Anta, Antay (Quechua) copper, copperish.

Antal (Hungarian) a form of Anthony.
Antek, Anti, Antos

Antares (Greek) giant, red star. Astronomy: the brightest star in the constellation Scorpio.
Antar, Antario, Antarious, Antarius, Antarr, Antarus

Antauaya (Quechua) copper-colored meadow; copper-colored grass.

Antavas (Lithuanian) a form of Anthony.
Antae, Antaeus, Antavious, Antavius, Ante, Anteo

Antelmo (Germanic) protector of the homeland.

Antenor (Greek) he who is a fighter.

Anthany (Latin, Greek) a form of Anthony.
Antanas, Antanee, Antanie, Antenee, Anthan, Antheny, Anthine, Anthney

Anthonie (Latin, Greek) a form of Anthony.
Anthone, Anthonee, Anthoni, Anthonia

Anthony ☆ **BG** (Latin) praiseworthy. (Greek) flourishing. See also Tony.
Anathony, Andonios, Andor, András, Anothony, Antal, Antavas, Anfernee, Anthany, Anthawn, Anthey, Anthian, Anthino, Anthone, Anthoney, Anthonie, Anthonio, Anthonu, Anthonysha, Anthoy, Anthyoine, Anthyonny, Antione, Antjuan, Antoine, Anton, Antonio, Antony, Antwan, Antwon

Antígono (Greek) he who stands out amongst all of his fellow men.

Antilaf (Mapuche) happy day, joyous day.

Antininan (Quechua) copperish like fire.

Antioco (Greek) he who commands the chariot in the fight against the enemy.

Antione **BG** (French) a form of Anthony.
Antion, Antionio, Antionne, Antiono

Antipan (Mapuche) sunny branch of a clear brown color.

Antipas (Greek) he is the enemy of all, in opposition to everyone.

Antivil (Mapuche) sunny snake.

Antjuan (Spanish) a form of Anthony.
Antajuan, Anthjuan, Antuan, Antuane

Antoan (Vietnamese) safe, secure.

Antoine (French) a form of Anthony.
Anntoin, Anthoine, Antoiné, Antoinne, Atoine

Antolín (Greek) flourishing, beautiful like a flower.

Anton (Slavic) a form of Anthony.
Anthon, Antone, Antonn, Antonne, Antons, Antos

Antón (Spanish) a form of Antonio.

Antonia **GB** (Greek) flourishing. (Latin) praiseworthy.

Antonio ☆ **BG** (Italian) a form of Anthony. See also Tino, Tonio.
Anthonio, Antinio, Antoinio, Antoino, Antonello, Antoneo, Antonin, Antonín, Antonino, Antonnio, Antonios, Antonius, Antonyia, Antonyio, Antonyo

Antony (Latin) a form of Anthony.
Antin, Antini, Antius, Antonee, Antoney, Antoni, Antonie, Antonin, Antonios, Antonius, Antonyia, Antonyio, Antonyo, Anty

Antti (Finnish) manly.
Anthey, Anthi, Anthie, Anthy, Anti, Antty

Antu (Indigenous) salt.

Antwan (Arabic) a form of
Anthony.
*Antaw, Antawan, Antawn,
Anthawn, Antowan, Antowaun,
Antowine, Antowne, Antowyn,
Antuwan, Antwain, Antwaina,
Antwaine, Antwainn, Antwaion,
Antwane, Antwann, Antwanne,
Antwarn, Antwaun, Antwen,
Antwian, Antwine, Antwuan,
Antwun, Antwyné*

Antwon (Arabic) a form of
Anthony.
*Antown, Antuwon, Antwion,
Antwione, Antwoan, Antwoin,
Antwoine, Antwone, Antwonn,
Antwonne, Antwoun, Antwyon,
Antwyone, Antyon, Antyonne,
Antywon*

Anwar (Arabic) luminous.
Anour, Anouar, Anwi

Anyaypoma, Anyaypuma
(Quechua) he who roars and
becomes angry like the puma.

Aparicio (Latin) he who refers to
the appearances of the Virgin in
different stages.

Apeles (Greek) he who is in a
sacred place.

Apiatan (Kiowa) wooden lance.

Apo, Apu (Quechua) chief, Lord
God; he who moves forward.

Apólito (Latin) dedicated to the
god Apollo.

Apollo (Greek) manly. Mythology:
the god of prophecy, healing,
music, poetry, and light. See also
Polo.
*Apolinar, Apolinario, Apollos,
Apolo, Apolonio, Appollo, Appolo,
Appolonio*

Apolodoro (Griego) skill of
Apollo.

April 🆖 (Latin) opening.

Apucachi (Quechua) lord of salt,
salty.

Apucatequil, Apucatiquil
(Quechua) god of lightning.

Apumaita (Quechua) where are
you, master?

Apurimac (Quechua) eloquent
master.

Apuyurac (Quechua) white chief.

Aquila (Latin, Spanish) eagle.
*Acquilla, Aquil, Aquilas, Aquileo,
Aquiles, Aquilino, Aquill, Aquilla,
Aquille, Aquillino, Aquyl, Aquyla,
Aquyll, Aquylla*

Arafat (Arabic) mountain of
recognition. History: Yasir Arafat
led Al Fatah, an Arab guerilla
group, and the Palestine
Liberation Organization,
advocating an independent
Palestinian state.

Araldo (Spanish) a form of
Harold.
Aralodo, Aralt, Aroldo, Arry

Aram (Syrian) high, exalted.
*Ara, Aramia, Arem, Arim, Arra,
Arram, Arum, Arym*

Aramis (French) Literature: one of
the title characters in Alexandre
Dumas's novel *The Three
Musketeers*.
Airamis, Aramith, Aramys

Aran (Tai) forest. (Danish) a form
of Aren. (Hebrew, Scottish) a
form of Arran.
Arane

Arcángel (Greek) prince of all
angels.

Archer (English) bowman.
Archar, Archie, Archor

Archibald (German) bold. See
also Arkady.
*Arch, Archaimbaud, Archambault,
Archibaldes, Archibaldo,
Archibold, Archie, Archybald,
Archybalde, Archybaldes,
Archybauld, Archybaulde*

Archie (German, English) a
familiar form of Archer, Archibald.
*Arche, Archee, Archey, Archi,
Archy*

Ardal (Irish) a form of Arnold.
Ardale, Ardall

Ardell (Latin) eager; industrious.
Ardel

Arden **GB** (Latin) ardent; fiery.
*Ard, Ardan, Ardene, Ardent,
Ardian, Ardie, Ardin, Ardint, Ardn,
Arduino, Ardyn, Ardynt*

Ardley (English) ardent meadow.
*Ardlea, Ardlee, Ardleigh, Ardli,
Ardlie, Ardly*

Ardon (Hebrew) bronzed.
Ardun

Areli **GB** (American) a form of
Oralee (see Girls' names).

Aren (Danish) eagle; ruler.
(Hebrew, Arabic) a form of
Aaron.

Aretas (Arabic) metal forger.

Aretino (Greek, Italian)
victorious.
Aretin, Aretine, Artyn, Artyno

Argenis (Greek) he who has a
great whiteness.

Argentino, Argento (Latin)
shines like silver.

Argimiro (Greek) careful;
vigilant.

Argus (Danish) watchful, vigilant.
Agos, Arguss

Argyle (Irish) from Ireland.
Argile, Argiles, Argyles

Ari **GB** (Hebrew) a short form of
Ariel. (Greek) a short form of
Aristotle.
*Aree, Arey, Arias, Arie, Arieh,
Arih, Arij, Ario, Arri, Ary, Arye*

Aria (Hebrew) a form of Ariel.

Arian (Greek) a form of Arion.
Ariann, Arrian, Aryan

Ariana GB (Greek) a form of Arian.

Ariane GB (Greek) a form of Arian.

Arianne GB (Greek) a form of Arian.

Aric (German) a form of Richard. (Scandinavian) a form of Eric.
Aaric, Aarick Aarik Arec, Areck, Arich, Arick, Ariek, Arik, Arrek, Arric, Arrick, Arrik, Aryc, Aryck, Aryk

Ariel GB (Hebrew) lion of God. Bible: another name for Jerusalem. Literature: the name of a sprite in the Shakespearean play *The Tempest*.
Airal, Airel, Arel, Areli, Ari, Ariele, Ariell, Arielle, Ariya, Ariyel, Arrial, Arriel, Aryel, Aryell, Aryl, Aryll, Arylle

Aries (Latin) ram. Astrology: the first sign of the zodiac.
Arees, Ares, Arie, Ariez, Aryes

Arif (Arabic) knowledgeable.
Areef, Aryf

Arion (Greek) enchanted. (Hebrew) melodious.
Arian, Arien, Ario, Arione, Aryon

Aristarco (Greek) best of the princes.

Aristeo (Greek) outstanding one.

Aristides (Greek) son of the best.
Aris, Aristede, Aristedes,

Aristeed, Aristide, Aristides, Aristidis, Arystides, Arystydes

Arístides (Greek) a form of Aristides.

Aristóbulo (Greek) greatest and best counselor; he who gives very good advice.

Aristofanes (Greek) best, the optimum.

Aristóteles (Greek) best; the most renowned; the most optimistic; he who has noble intentions.

Aristotle (Greek) best; wise. History: a third-century B.C. philosopher who tutored Alexander the Great.
Ari, Aris, Aristito, Aristo, Aristokles, Aristotal, Aristotel, Aristotelis, Aristotol, Aristott, Aristotyl, Arystotle

Arjun (Hindi) white; milk colored.
Arjen, Arjin, Arju, Arjuna, Arjune

Arkady (Russian) a form of Archibald.
Arcadio, Arkadee, Arkadey, Arkadi, Arkadie, Arkadij, Arkadiy

Arkin (Norwegian) son of the eternal king.
Aricin, Arkeen, Arkyn

Arledge (English) lake with the hares.
Arlege, Arlidge, Arlledge, Arllege

Arlen (Irish) pledge.
Arlan, Arland, Arlend, Arlin, Arlinn, Arlon, Arlyn, Arlynn

Arley (English) a short form of Harley.
Arleigh, Arlie, Arly

Arlo (Spanish) barberry. (English) fortified hill. A form of Harlow. (German) a form of Charles.
Arlow

Arman (Persian) desire, goal.
Armaan, Armahn, Armaine

Armand (Latin, German) a form of Herman. See also Mandek.
Armad, Arman, Armanda, Armando, Armands, Armanno, Armaude, Armenta, Armond

Armando (Spanish) a form of Armand.
Armondo

Armani 🅱🅶 (Hungarian) sly. (Hebrew) a form of Armon.
Arman, Armanee, Armaney, Armanie, Armann, Armany Armoni, Armonie, Armonio, Armonni, Armony

Armentario (Greek) herder of livestock.

Armon (Hebrew) high fortress, stronghold.
Armani, Armen, Armin, Armino, Armonn, Armons, Armyn

Armstrong (English) strong arm. History: astronaut Neil Armstrong was the commander of Apollo 11 and the first person to walk on the moon.
Armstron, Armstronge

Arnaud (French) a form of Arnold.
Arnaude, Arnauld, Arnault, Arnoll

Arne (German) a form of Arnold.
Arna, Arnay, Arnel, Arnele, Arnell, Arnelle

Arnette (English) little eagle.
Arnat, Arnatt, Arnet, Arnett, Arnetta, Arnot, Arnott

Arnie (German) a familiar form of Arnold.
Arnee, Arney, Arni, Arnny, Arny

Arno (German) a short form of Arnold. (Czech) a short form of Ernest.
Arnou, Arnoux

Arnold (German) eagle ruler.
Ardal, Arnald, Arnaldo, Arnaud, Arndt, Arne, Arnhold, Arnie, Arno, Arnol, Arnoldas, Arnolde, Arnoldo, Arnoll, Arnolt, Arnoud, Arnulfo, Arnyld

Arnon (Hebrew) rushing river.
Arnan, Arnen, Arnin, Arnyn

Arnulfo (German) a form of Arnold.

Aron, Arron 🅱🅶 (Hebrew) forms of Aaron. (Danish) forms of Aren.
Arrion

Aroon (Tai) dawn.
Aroone

Arquelao (Greek) governor of his village.

Arquimedes (Greek) he who has profound thoughts.

Arquímedes (Greek) deep thinker.

Arquipo (Greek) horse breaker.

Arran (Scottish) island dweller. Geography: an island off the west coast of Scotland. (Hebrew) a form of Aaron.
Aeran, Arren, Arrin, Arryn, Aryn

Arrigo (Italian) a form of Harry.
Alrigo, Arrighetto

Arrio (Spanish) warlike.
Ario, Arrow, Arryo, Aryo

Arsenio (Greek) masculine; virile. History: Saint Arsenius was a teacher in the Roman Empire.
Arsen, Arsène, Arseneo, Arsenius, Arseny, Arsenyo, Arsinio, Arsinyo, Arsynio, Arsynyo

Arsha (Persian) venerable.
Arshah

Art (English) a short form of Arthur.

Artemus (Greek) gift of Artemis. Mythology: Artemis was the goddess of the hunt and the moon.
Artemas, Artemio, Artemis, Artimas, Artimis, Artimus

Arthur ☼Ⓖ (Irish) noble; lofty hill. (Scottish) bear. (English) rock. (Icelandic) follower of Thor. See also Turi.
Art, Artair, Artek, Arth, Arther,
Arthor, Arthyr, Artie, Artor, Arturo, Artus, Aurthar, Aurther, Aurthur

Artie (English) a familiar form of Arthur.
Arte, Artee, Artian, Artis, Arty, Atty

Arturo (Italian) a form of Arthur.
Arthuro, Artur

Arun (Cambodian, Hindi) sun.
Aruns

Arundel (English) eagle valley.

Arve (Norwegian) heir, inheritor.

Arvel (Welsh) wept over.
Arval, Arvell, Arvelle, Arvil, Arvol, Arvyn

Arvid (Hebrew) wanderer. (Norwegian) eagle tree. See also Ravid.
Arv, Arvad, Arve, Arvie, Arvind, Arvinder, Arvyd, Arvydas

Arvin (German) friend of the people; friend of the army.
Arv, Arvan, Arven, Arvie, Arvind, Arvinder, Arvon, Arvy, Arvyn, Arwan, Arwen, Arwin, Arwon, Arwyn

Arya (Hebrew) a form of Aria.

Aryeh (Hebrew) lion.

Asa ⒷⒼ (Hebrew) physician, healer. (Yoruba) falcon.
Asaa, Asah, Ase

Asád (Arabic) lion.
Asaad, Asad, Asid, Assad, Azad

Asadel (Arabic) prosperous.
Asadour, Asadul, Asadyl, Asael

Asaf (Hebrew) one chosen by God.

Ascensión (Spanish) mystical name that alludes to the ascension of Jesus Christ to heaven.

Ascot (English) eastern cottage; style of necktie. Geography: a village near London and the site of the Royal Ascot horseraces.
Ascott

Asdrúbal (Punic) he who is protected by God.

Asgard (Scandinavian) court of the gods.

Ash (Hebrew) ash tree.
Ashby

Ashanti GB (Swahili) from a tribe in West Africa.
Ashan, Ashani, Ashante, Ashantee, Ashaunte

Ashburn (English) from the ash-tree stream.
Ashbern, Ashberne, Ashbirn, Ashbirne, Ashborn, Ashborne, Ashbourn, Ashbourne, Ashburne, Ashbyrn, Ashbyrne

Ashby (Scandinavian) ash-tree farm. (Hebrew) a form of Ash.
Ashbee, Ashbey, Ashbi, Ashbie

Asher (Hebrew) happy; blessed.
Ashar, Ashir, Ashor, Ashur, Ashyr

Ashford (English) ash-tree ford.
Ash, Ashforde, Ashtin

Ashlee GB (English) a form of Ashley.

Ashleigh GB (English) a form of Ashley.

Ashley GB (English) ash-tree meadow.
Ash, Asheley, Ashelie, Ashely, Ashlan, Ashlea, Ashlen, Ashli, Ashlie, Ashlin, Ashling, Ashlinn, Ashlone, Ashly, Ashlynn, Aslan

Ashlyn GB (English) a form of Ashley.

Ashon (Swahili) seventh-born son.

Ashraf (Arabic) most honorable.

Ashton ☆ BG (English) ash-tree settlement.
Ashtan, Ashten, Ashtian, Ashtin, Ashtion, Ashtonn, Ashtown, Ashtun

Ashtyn GB (English) a form of Ashton.

Ashur (Swahili) Mythology: the principal Assyrian deity.

Ashwani (Hindi) first. Religion: the first of the twenty-seven galaxies revolving around the moon.
Ashwan

Ashwin (Hindi) star.
Ashwen, Ashwon, Ashwyn

Asiel (Hebrew) created by God.
Asyel

Asif (Arabic) forgiveness.

Asker (Turkish) soldier.

Aspen GB (English) aspen tree.

Asterio (Greek) mythical figure
that was thrown into the sea
because of his escape from Zeus.

Astley (Greek) starry field.
*Asterlea, Asterlee, Asterleigh,
Asterley, Asterli, Asterlie, Asterly,
Astlea, Astlee, Astleigh, Astli,
Astlie, Astly*

Asto, Astu (Quechua) bird of the
Andes.

Astolfo (Greek) he who helps
with his lance.

Aston (English) eastern town.
*Astan, Asten, Astin, Astown,
Astyn*

Astuguaraca (Quechua) he who
hunts astus with a sling.

Aswad (Arabic) dark skinned,
black.
Aswald

Ata (Fante) twin.
Atah

Atahualpa (Quechua) bird of
fortune.

Atanasio (Greek) immortal.

Atau (Quechua) fortunate.

Atauaipa (Quechua) bird of
fortune; creator of fortune.

Atauanca (Quechua) fortunate
eagle.

Atauchi (Quechua) he who
makes us good fortunes.

Atek (Polish) a form of Tanek.

Atenodoro (Greek) gift of
wisdom.

Athan (Greek) immortal.
*Athen, Athens, Athin, Athon,
Athons, Athyn, Athyns*

Atherton (English) town by a
spring.
Atharton, Athorton

Athol (Scottish) from Ireland.
*Affol, Athal, Athel, Athil,
Atholton, Athyl*

Atid (Tai) sun.
Atyd

Atif (Arabic) caring.
Ateef, Atef, Atyf

Atila (Gothic) a form of Attila.

Atilano (Spanish) a form of Atila.

Atkins (English) from the home
of the relatives.
Atkin, Atkyn, Atkyns

Atlas (Greek) lifted; carried.
Mythology: Atlas was forced by
Zeus to carry the heavens on his
shoulders as a punishment for
his share of the war of the Titans.

Atley (English) meadow.
Atlea, Atlee, Atleigh, Atli, Atlie,
Atly, Attlea, Attlee, Attleigh
Attley, Attli, Attlie, Attly

Atoc, Atuc (Quechua) sly as a
fox; wolf.

Atocuaman (Quechua) he who
possesses the strength of a falcon
and the shrewdness of a fox.

Atticus (Latin) from Attica, a
region outside Athens.

Attila (Gothic) little father.
History: the Hun leader who
invaded the Roman Empire.
Atalik, Atila, Atilio, Atilla, Atiya,
Attal, Attilah, Attilio, Attyla,
Attylah

Atwater (English) at the water's
edge.
Attwater

Atwell (English) at the well.
Attwel, Atwel

Atwood (English) at the forest.
Attwood

Atworth (English) at the
farmstead.
Attworth

Auberon (German) a form of
Oberon.
Auberron, Aubrey

Auberto (French) a form of
Alberto.

Aubree GB (German, French) a
form of Aubrey.

Aubrey GB (German) noble;
bearlike. (French) a familiar
form of Auberon.
Aubary, Aube, Aubery, Aubie,
Aubré, Aubreii, Aubri, Aubry,
Aubury

Aubrie GB (German, French) a
form of Aubrey.

Auburn (Latin) reddish brown.
Abern, Aberne, Abirn, Abirne,
Aburn, Aburne, Abyrn, Abyrne,
Aubern, Auberne, Aubin, Aubirn,
Aubirne, Aubun, Auburne,
Aubyrn, Aubyrne

Auden (English) old friend.
Audan, Audin, Audyn

Audie (German) noble; strong.
(English) a familiar form of
Edward.
Audee, Audey Audi, Audiel,
Audley, Audy

Audomaro (Greek) famous
because of his riches.

Audon (French) old; rich.
Audelon

Audra GB (English) a form of
Audrey.

Audrey GB (English) noble
strength.
Audre, Audrea, Audri, Audrius,
Audry

Audric (English) wise ruler.
Audrick, Audrik, Audryc, Audryck,
Audryk

Audun (Scandinavian) deserted, desolate.

Augie (Latin) a familiar form of August.
Auggie, Augy

August B G (Latin) a short form of Augustine, Augustus.
Agosto, Augie, Auguste, Augusto

Augustín (Spanish) a form of Augustine.

Augustine B G (Latin) majestic. Religion: Saint Augustine was the first archbishop of Canterbury. See also Austin, Gus, Tino.
Agustin, August, Augusteen, Augustein, Augusteyn, Augusteyne Augustin, Augustinas, Augustino, Augustyn, Augustyne Austen, Austin, Auston, Austyn

Augusto (Latin) a form of August.

Augustus (Latin) majestic; venerable. History: an honorary title given to the first Roman emperor, Octavius Caesar.
Agustas, Agustys, August

Aukai (Hawaiian) seafarer.
Aukay

Aundre (Greek) a form of Andre.
Aundrae, Aundray, Aundrea, Aundrey, Aundry

Auqui (Quechua) master; prince.

Auquipuma (Quechua) a prince who is as strong as a puma.

Auquitupac (Quechua) glorious prince.

Auquiyupanqui (Quechua) he who honors his masters.

Aurek (Polish) golden haired.
Aurec

Aurelia (Latin) gold.

Aurelio (Latin) a short form of Aurelius.
Aurel, Aurele, Aureli, Aurellio

Aurelius (Latin) golden. History: Marcus Aurelius was a second-century A.D. philosopher and emperor of Rome.
Arelian, Areliano, Aurèle, Aureliano, Aurelien, Aurélien, Aurelio, Aurelyus, Aurey, Auriel, Aury

Aurick (German) protecting ruler.
Auric, Aurik, Auryc, Auryck, Auryk

Austen, Auston, Austyn B G (Latin) short forms of Augustine.
Austan, Austun, Austyne

Austin ☀ B G (Latin) a short form of Augustine.
Astin, Austine, Oistin, Ostin

Austín (Spanish) a form of Augustín.

Autumn G B (Latin) autumn.

Auxilio (Latin) he who saves, who brings help.

Avel (Greek) breath.
Avell

Avelino (Latin) he who was born in Avella, Italy.

Avent (French) born during Advent.
Advent, Aventin, Aventino, Aventyno

Averill (French) born in April.
Ave, Averal, Averall, Averel, Averell, Averiel, Averil, Averyl, Averyll, Avrel, Avrell, Avrill, Avryll

Avery BG (English) a form of Aubrey.
Avary, Aveary, Avere, Averee, Averey, Averi, Averie, Avrey, Avry

Avi (Hebrew) God is my father.
Avian, Avidan, Avidor, Avie, Aviel, Avion, Avy

Avito (Latin) he who is from the grandfather.

Aviv (Hebrew) youth; springtime.

Avneet GB (Hebrew) a form of Avner.

Avner (Hebrew) a form of Abner.
Avniel

Avram (Hebrew) a form of Abraham, Abram.
Arram, Avraam, Avraham, Avrahom, Avrohom, Avrom, Avrum

Avshalom (Hebrew) father of peace. See also Absalom.
Avsalom

Awan (Native American) somebody.

Axel (Latin) axe. (German) small oak tree; source of life. (Scandinavian) a form of Absalom.
Aksel, Ax, Axe, Axell, Axil, Axill, Axl, Axle, Axyle

Ayar (Quechua) wild quinoa.

Ayden (Irish) a form of Aidan.
Aydean

Aydin (Turkish) intelligent.

Ayers (English) heir to a fortune.

Ayinde (Yoruba) we gave praise and he came.

Aylmer (English) a form of Elmer.
Aillmer, Ailmer, Allmer, Ayllmer

Aymil (Greek) a form of Emil.
Aimil, Aimyl

Aymon (French) a form of Raymond.
Aiman, Aimen, Aimin, Aimyn

Ayo (Yoruba) happiness.

Azad (Turkish) free.

Azanías (Hebrew) God hears him.

Azarias (Hebrew) Lord sustains me; divine salvation; God is my soul.

Azarías (Hebrew) Lord sustains and guides me.

Azariel (Hebrew) he who has control over the waters.

Azeem (Arabic) a form of Azim.
Aseem, Asim

Azi (Nigerian) youth.

Azim (Arabic) defender.
Azeem

Aziz (Arabic) strong.

Azizi (Swahili) precious.

Azriel (Hebrew) God is my aid.

Azuriah (Hebrew) aided by God.
Azaria, Azariah, Azuria

B

B 🆖 (American) an initial used as a first name.

Baal (Chaldean) he who dominates a territory; owner and lord.

Baco (Greek) he who creates disturbances.

Baden (German) bather.
Baeden, Bayden, Baydon

Bahir (Arabic) brilliant, dazzling.

Bahram (Persian) ancient king.

Bailee 🆖 (French) a form of Bailey.

Bailey 🆖 (French) bailiff, steward.
Bail, Bailie, Bailio, Baillie, Baily, Bailye, Baley, Bayley

Bain (Irish) a short form of Bainbridge.
Baine, Bayne, Baynn

Bainbridge (Irish) fair bridge.
Bain, Baynbridge, Bayne, Baynebridge

Baird (Irish) traveling minstrel, bard; poet.
Bairde, Bard

Bakari (Swahili) noble promise.
Bacari, Baccari, Bakarie

Baker (English) baker. See also Baxter.
Bakir, Bakory, Bakr

Bal (Sanskrit) child born with lots of hair.

Balasi (Basque) flat footed.

Balbino (Latin) he who mumbles, who speaks in a stammering manner.

Balbo (Latin) stammerer.
Bailby, Balbi, Ballbo

Baldemar (German) bold; famous.
Baldemer, Baldomero, Baumar, Baumer

Balder (Scandinavian) bald. Mythology: the Norse god of light, summer, purity, and innocence.
Baldier, Baldur, Baudier

Baldovín (Spanish) a form of Balduino.

Baldric (German) brave ruler.
Baldrick, Baudric

Balduino (Germanic) valiant friend.

Baldwin (German) bold friend.
Bald, Baldovino, Balduin, Baldwinn, Baldwyn, Baldwynn, Balldwin, Baudoin

Balfour (Scottish) pastureland.
Balfor, Balfore

Balin (Hindi) mighty soldier.
Bali, Baylen, Baylin, Baylon, Valin

Ballard (German) brave; strong.
Balard

Balraj (Hindi) strongest.

Baltazar (Greek) a form of Balthasar.
Baltasar

Balthasar (Greek) God save the king. Bible: one of the three wise men who bore gifts for the infant Jesus.
Badassare, Baldassare, Baltazar, Balthasaar, Balthazar, Balthazzar, Baltsaros, Belshazar, Belshazzar, Boldizsár

Bancroft (English) bean field.
Ban, Bancrofft, Bank, Bankroft, Banky, Binky

Bandi BG (Hungarian) a form of Andrew.
Bandit

Bane (Hawaiian) a form of Bartholomew.

Banner (Scottish, English) flag bearer.
Bannor, Banny

Banning (Irish) small and fair.
Bannie, Banny

Barak (Hebrew) lightning bolt. Bible: the valiant warrior who helped Deborah.
Barrak

Baran (Russian) ram.
Baren

Barasa (Kikuyu) meeting place.

Barclay (Scottish, English) birch-tree meadow.
Bar, Barcley, Barklay, Barkley, Barklie, Barrclay, Berkeley

Bard (Irish) a form of Baird.
Bar, Barde, Bardia, Bardiya, Barr

Bardolf (German) bright wolf.
Bardo, Bardolph, Bardou, Bardoul, Bardulf, Bardulph

Bardrick (Teutonic) axe ruler.
Bardric, Bardrik

Baris (Turkish) peaceful.

Barker (English) lumberjack; advertiser at a carnival.

Barlow (English) bare hillside.
Barlowe, Barrlow, Barrlowe

Barnabas (Greek, Hebrew, Aramaic, Latin) son of the missionary. Bible: Christian apostle and companion of Paul on his first missionary journey.
Bane, Barna, Barnaba, Barnabus, Barnaby, Barnebas, Barnebus, Barney

Barnaby (English) a form of
Barnabas.
*Barnabe, Barnabé, Barnabee,
Barnabey, Barnabi, Barnabie,
Bernabé, Burnaby*

Barnard (French) a form of
Bernard.
*Barn, Barnard, Barnhard,
Barnhardo*

Barnes (English) bear; son of
Barnett.

Barnett (English) nobleman;
leader.
*Barn, Barnet, Barney, Baronet,
Baronett, Barrie, Barron, Barry*

Barney (English) a familiar form
of Barnabas, Barnett.
Barnie, Barny

Barnum (German) barn; storage
place. (English) baron's home.
Barnham

Baron (German, English)
nobleman, baron.
*Baaron, Barion, Baronie, Barrin,
Barrion, Barron, Baryn, Bayron,
Berron*

Barrett 🅱🅶 (German) strong as a
bear.
*Bar, Baret, Barrat, Barret,
Barretta, Barrette, Barry, Berrett,
Berrit*

Barric (English) grain farm.
*Barrick, Beric, Berric, Berrick,
Berrik*

Barrington (English) fenced
town. Geography: a town in
England.

Barry 🅱🅶 (Welsh) son of Harry.
(Irish) spear, marksman.
(French) gate, fence.
Baris, Barri, Barrie, Barris, Bary

Bart (Hebrew) a short form of
Bartholomew, Barton.
Barrt, Bartel, Bartie, Barty

Bartholomew (Hebrew) son of
Talmaí. Bible: one of the Twelve
Apostles. See also Jerney, Parlan,
Parthalán.
*Balta, Bane, Bart, Bartek, Barth,
Barthel, Barthelemy, Barthélemy,
Barthélmy, Bartho, Bartholo,
Bartholomaus, Bartholome,
Bartholomeo, Bartholomeus,
Bartholomieu, Bartimous, Bartlet,
Barto, Bartolome, Bartolomé,
Bartolomeo, Bartolomeô,
Bartolommeo, Bartome, Bartz,
Bat*

Bartlet (English) a form of
Bartholomew.
Bartlett, Bartley

Barto (Spanish) a form of
Bartholomew.
*Bardo, Bardol, Bartol, Bartoli,
Bartolo, Bartos*

Barton (English) barley town;
Bart's town.
Barrton, Bart

Bartram (English) a form of
Bertram.
Barthram

Baruc (Hebrew) he who is
blessed by God.

Baruch (Hebrew) blessed.
Boruch

Basam (Arabic) smiling.
Basem, Basim, Bassam

Basil (Greek, Latin) royal, kingly.
Religion: a saint and founder of
monasteries. Botany: an herb
often used in cooking. See also
Vasilis, Wasili.
*Bas, Basal, Base, Baseal, Basel,
Basle, Basile, Basilio, Basilios,
Basilius, Bassel, Bazek, Bazel,
Bazil, Bazyli*

Basir (Turkish) intelligent,
discerning.
*Bashar, Basheer, Bashir, Bashiyr,
Bechir, Bhasheer*

Bassett (English) little person.
Basett, Basit, Basset, Bassit

Bastien (German) a short form of
Sebastian.
Baste, Bastiaan, Bastian, Bastion

Bat (English) a short form of
Bartholomew.

Baudilio (Teutonic) he who is
brave and valiant.

Baul (Gypsy) snail.

Bautista (Greek) he who
baptizes.

Bavol (Gypsy) wind; air.

Baxter (English) a form of Baker.
Bax, Baxie, Baxty, Baxy

Bay (Vietnamese) seventh son.
(French) chestnut brown color;
evergreen tree. (English) howler.

Bayard (English) reddish brown
hair.
*Baiardo, Bay, Bayardo, Bayerd,
Bayrd*

Baylee GB (French) a form of
Bayley.

Bayley GB (French) a form of
Bailey.
Bayleigh, Baylie, Bayly

Beacan (Irish) small.
Beacán, Becan

Beacher (English) beech trees.
*Beach, Beachy, Beech, Beecher,
Beechy*

Beagan (Irish) small.
Beagen, Beagin

Beale (French) a form of Beau.
Beal, Beall, Bealle, Beals

Beaman (English) beekeeper.
*Beamann, Beamen, Beeman,
Beman*

Beamer (English) trumpet player.

Beasley (English) field of peas.

Beatriz GB (Latin) a form of
Beatrice (see Girls' Names).

Beattie (Latin) blessed; happy; bringer of joy.
Beatie, Beatty, Beaty

Beau 🆖 (French) handsome.
Beale, Beaux, Bo

Beaufort (French) beautiful fort.

Beaumont (French) beautiful mountain.

Beauregard (French) handsome; beautiful; well regarded.

Beaver (English) beaver.
Beav, Beavo, Beve, Bevo

Bebe 🆖 (Spanish) baby.

Beck (English, Scandinavian) brook.
Beckett

Beda (Teutonic) he who orders and provides for.

Bede (English) prayer. Religion: the patron saint of lectors.

Bela 🆖 (Czech) white. (Hungarian) bright.
Béla, Belaal, Belal, Belall, Belay, Bellal

Belarmino (Germanic) having beautiful armor.

Belden (French, English) pretty valley.
Beldin, Beldon, Bellden, Belldon

Belen 🆖🅱 (Greek) arrow.

Belisario (Greek) he who shoots arrows skillfully.

Bell (French) handsome. (English) bell ringer.

Bellamy (French) beautiful friend.
Belamy, Bell, Bellamey, Bellamie

Bello (African) helper or promoter of Islam.

Belmiro (Portuguese) good-looking; attractive.

Bem (Tiv) peace.
Behm

Ben (Hebrew) a short form of Benjamin.
Behn, Benio, Benn, Benne, Benno

Ben Zion (Hebrew) son of Zion.
Benson, Benzi

Ben-ami (Hebrew) son of my people.
Baram, Barami

Benedict (Latin) blessed. See also Venedictos, Venya.
Benci, Bendick, Bendict, Bendino, Bendix, Bendrick, Benedetto, Benedick, Benedicto, Benedictus, Benedikt, Bengt, Benito, Benoit

Benedikt (German, Slavic) a form of Benedict.
Bendek, Bendik, Benedek, Benedik

Bengt (Scandinavian) a form of Benedict.
Beng, Benke, Bent

Beniam (Ethiopian) a form of Benjamin.
Beneyam, Beniamin, Beniamino

Benicio (Latin) riding friend.

Benigno (Latin) prodigal son; he who does good deeds.

Benildo (Teutonic) fights against bears.

Benito (Italian) a form of Benedict. History: Benito Mussolini led Italy during World War II.
Benedo, Benino, Benno, Beno, Betto, Beto

Benjamen (Hebrew) a form of Benjamin.
Benejamen, Benjermen, Benjjmen

Benjamin ✹ BG (Hebrew) son of my right hand. See also Peniamina, Veniamin.
Behnjamin, Bejamin, Bemjiman, Ben, Benejaminas, Bengamin, Beniam, Benja, Benjahmin, Benjaim, Benjam, Benjamaim, Benjaman, Benjamen, Benjamine, Benjaminn, Benjamino, Benjamon, Benjamyn, Benjamynn, Benjemin, Benjermain, Benjermin, Benji, Benjie, Benjiman, Benjy, Benkamin, Bennjamin, Benny, Benyamin, Benyamino, Binyamin, Mincho

Benjamín (Hebrew) a form of Benjamin.

Benjiman (Hebrew) a form of Benjamin.
Benjimen, Benjimin, Benjimon, Benjmain

Benjiro (Japanese) enjoys peace.

Bennett BG (Latin) little blessed one.
Benet, Benett, Bennet, Benette, Bennete, Bennette

Benny (Hebrew) a familiar form of Benjamin.
Bennie

Beno (Hebrew) son. (Mwera) band member.

Benoit (French) a form of Benedict.
Benott

Benoni (Hebrew) son of my sorrow. Bible: Ben-oni was the son of Jacob and Rachel.
Ben-Oni

Benson (Hebrew) son of Ben. A short form of Ben Zion.
Bensan, Bensen, Benssen, Bensson

Bentley (English) moor; coarse grass meadow.
Bent, Bentlea, Bentlee, Bentlie, Lee

Benton (English) Ben's town; town on the moors.
Bent

Benzi (Hebrew) a familiar form of Ben Zion.

Beppe (Italian) a form of Joseph.
Beppy

Ber (English) boundary. (Yiddish) bear.

Berardo (Germanic) a form of Bernard.

Beredei (Russian) a form of Hubert.
Berdry, Berdy, Beredej, Beredy

Berenguer (Teutonic) bear that is prepared for battle.

Berg (German) mountain.
Berdj, Berge, Bergh, Berje

Bergen (German, Scandinavian) hill dweller.
Bergin, Birgin

Berger (French) shepherd.

Bergren (Scandinavian) mountain stream.
Berg

Berk (Turkish) solid, rugged.

Berkeley (English) a form of Barclay.
Berk, Berkely, Berkie, Berkley, Berklie, Berkly, Berky

Berl (German) a form of Burl.
Berle, Berlie, Berlin, Berlyn

Berlyn (German) boundary line. See also Burl.
Berlin, Burlin

Bern (German) a short form of Bernard.
Berne

Bernadette 🇬🇧 (French) a form of Bernadine (see Girls' Names).

Bernal (German) strong as a bear.
Bernald, Bernaldo, Bernel, Bernhald, Bernhold, Bernold

Bernaldino (German) strong bear.

Bernard (German) brave as a bear. See also Bjorn.
Barnard, Bear, Bearnard, Benek, Ber, Berend, Bern, Bernabé, Bernadas, Bernardel, Bernardin, Bernardo, Bernardus, Bernardyn, Bernarr, Bernat, Bernek, Bernal, Bernel, Bernerd, Berngards, Bernhard, Bernhards, Bernhardt, Bernie, Bjorn, Burnard

Bernardo (Spanish) a form of Bernard.
Barnardino, Barnardo, Barnhardo, Benardo, Bernardino, Bernhardo, Berno, Burnardo, Nardo

Bernie (German) a familiar form of Bernard.
Berney, Berni, Berny, Birney, Birnie, Birny, Burney

Berry (English) berry; grape.
Berrie

Bersh (Gypsy) one year.

Bert (German, English) bright, shining. A short form of Berthold, Berton, Bertram, Bertrand, Egbert, Filbert.
Bertie, Bertus, Birt, Burt

Berthold (German) bright; illustrious; brilliant ruler.
Bert, Berthoud, Bertold, Bertolde

Bertie (English) a familiar form of Bert, Egbert.
Berty, Birt, Birtie, Birty

Bertín (Spanish) distinguished friend.
Berti

Berto (Spanish) a short form of Alberto.

Bertoldo (Germanic) splendid boss.

Berton (English) bright settlement; fortified town.
Bert

Bertram (German) bright; illustrious. (English) bright raven. See also Bartram.
Beltran, Beltrán, Beltrano, Bert, Berton, Bertrae, Bertraim, Bertraum, Bertron

Bertrand (German) bright shield.
Bert, Bertran, Bertrando, Bertranno

Bertulfo (Teutonic) warrior who shines.

Berwyn (Welsh) white head.
Berwin, Berwynn, Berwynne

Besarión (Greek) walker.

Betsabé (Hebrew) oath of God.

Bevan (Welsh) son of Evan.
Beavan, Beaven, Beavin, Bev, Beve, Beven, Bevin, Bevo, Bevon

Beverly 🅖🅑 (English) beaver meadow.
Beverlea, Beverleigh, Beverley, Beverlie

Bevis (French) from Beauvais, France; bull.
Beauvais, Bevys

Bhagwandas (Hindi) servant of God.

Bianca 🅖🅑 (Italian) white.

Bibiano (Spanish) small man.

Bickford (English) axe-man's ford.

Bienvenido (Filipino) welcome.

Bijan (Persian) ancient hero.
Bihjan, Bijann, Bijhan, Bijhon, Bijon

Bilal (Arabic) chosen.
Bila, Bilaal, Bilale, Bile, Bilel, Billaal, Billal

Bill (German) a short form of William.
Bil, Billee, Billijo, Billye, Byll, Will

Billie 🅖🅑 (German) a form of Billy.

Billy 🅑🅖 (German) a familiar form of Bill, William.
Bille, Billey, Billie, Billy, Bily, Willie

Binah (Hebrew) understanding; wise.
Bina

Bing (German) kettle-shaped hollow.

Binh (Vietnamese) peaceful.

Binkentios (Greek) a form of Vincent.

Binky (English) a familiar form of Bancroft, Vincent.
Bink, Binkentios, Binkie

Birch (English) white; shining; birch tree.
Birk, Burch

Birger (Norwegian) rescued.

Birkey (English) island with birch trees.
Birk, Birkie, Birky

Birkitt (English) birch-tree coast.
Birk, Birket, Birkit, Burket, Burkett, Burkitt

Birley (English) meadow with the cow barn.
Birlee, Birlie, Birly

Birney (English) island with a brook.
Birne, Birnie, Birny, Burney, Burnie, Burny

Birtle (English) hill with birds.

Bishop (Greek) overseer. (English) bishop.
Bish, Bishup

Bjorn (Scandinavian) a form of Bernard.
Bjarne

Blackburn (Scottish) black brook.

Blade (English) knife, sword.
Bladen, Bladon, Bladyn, Blae, Blaed, Blayde

Bladimir (Russian) a form of Vladimir.
Bladimer

Bladimiro (Slavic) prince of peace.

Blaine BG (Irish) thin, lean. (English) river source.
Blain, Blane, Blayne

Blair BG (Irish) plain, field. (Welsh) place.
Blaire, Blare, Blayr, Blayre

Blaise, Blaize BG (French) forms of Blaze.
Ballas, Balyse, Blais, Blaisot, Blas, Blase, Blasi, Blasien, Blasius, Blass, Blaz, Blaze, Blayz, Blayze, Blayzz

Blake ☀ BG (English) attractive; dark.
Blaik, Blaike, Blakely, Blakeman, Blakey, Blayke

Blakely BG (English) dark meadow.
Blakelee, Blakeleigh, Blakeley, Blakelie, Blakelin, Blakelyn, Blakeny, Blakley, Blakney

Blanca GB (Italian) a form of Bianca.

Blanco (Spanish) light skinned; white; blond.

Blandino (Latin) he who is flattered.

Blane (Irish) a form of Blaine.
Blaney, Blanne

Blasco (Latin) of a pale color.

Blayne (Irish) a form of Blaine.
Blayn, Blayney

Blaze (Latin) stammerer. (English) flame; trail mark made on a tree.
Balázs, Biaggio, Biagio, Blaise, Blaize, Blazen, Blazer

Bliss GB (English) blissful; joyful.

Bly (Native American) high.

Blythe GB (English) carefree; merry, joyful.
Blithe, Blyth

Bo BG (English) a form of Beau, Beauregard. (German) a form of Bogart.
Boe

Boaz (Hebrew) swift; strong.
Bo, Boas, Booz, Bos, Boz

Bob (English) a short form of Robert.
Bobb, Bobby, Bobek, Rob

Bobbi, Bobbie GB (English) a form of Bobby.

Bobby BG (English) a familiar form of Bob, Robert.
Bobbey, Bobbie, Bobbye, Boby

Bobek (Czech) a form of Bob, Robert.

Bobi (English) a form of Bobby.

Boden (Scandinavian) sheltered. (French) messenger, herald.
Bodie, Bodin, Bodine, Bodyne, Boe

Bodie (Scandinavian) a familiar form of Boden.
Boddie, Bode, Bodee, Bodey, Bodhi, Bodi, Boedee, Boedi, Boedy

Bodil (Norwegian) mighty ruler.

Bodua (Akan) animal's tail.

Boecio (Greek) he who helps; the defender, who goes into battle ready.

Bogart (German) strong as a bow. (Irish, Welsh) bog, marshland.
Bo, Bogey, Bogie, Bogy

Bohdan (Ukrainian) a form of Donald.
Bogdan, Bogdashka, Bogdon, Bohden, Bohdon

Boleslao (Slavic) most glorious of the glorious.

Bonaro (Italian, Spanish) friend.
Boña, Bonar

Bonaventure (Italian) good luck.

Bond (English) tiller of the soil.
Bondie, Bondon, Bonds, Bondy

Boniface (Latin) do-gooder.
Bonifacio, Bonifacius, Bonifacy

Booker (English) bookmaker;
book lover; Bible lover.
Bookie, Books, Booky

Boone (Latin, French) good.
History: Daniel Boone was an
American pioneer.
Bon, Bone, Bonne, Boonie, Boony

Booth (English) hut.
(Scandinavian) temporary
dwelling.
Boot, Boote, Boothe

Borak (Arabic) lightning.
Mythology: the horse that carried
Muhammad to seventh heaven.

Borden (French) cottage. (English)
valley of the boar; boar's den.
Bord, Bordie, Bordy

Boreas (Greek) north wind.

Borg (Scandinavian) castle.

Boris (Slavic) battler, warrior.
Religion: the patron saint of
Moscow, princes, and Russia.
*Boriss, Borja, Borris, Borya,
Boryenka, Borys*

Borka (Russian) fighter.
Borkinka

Boseda (Tiv) born on Saturday.

Bosley (English) grove of trees.

Botan (Japanese) blossom, bud.

Bourey (Cambodian) country.

Bourne (Latin, French) boundary.
(English) brook, stream.

Boutros (Arabic) a form of Peter.

Bowen (Welsh) son of Owen.
Bow, Bowe, Bowie

Bowie (Irish) yellow haired.
History: James Bowie was an
American-born Mexican colonist
who died during the defense of
the Alamo.
Bow, Bowen

Boyce (French) woods, forest.
Boice, Boise, Boy, Boycey, Boycie

Boyd (Scottish) yellow haired.
Boid, Boyde

Brad 🅱🅶 (English) a short form of
Bradford, Bradley.
Bradd, Brade

Bradburn (English) broad stream.

Braden 🅱🅶 (English) broad valley.
*Bradan, Bradden, Bradeon,
Bradin, Bradine, Bradyn, Braeden,
Braiden, Brayden, Bredan, Bredon*

Bradford (English) broad river
crossing.
Brad, Braddford, Ford

Bradlee (English) a form of
Bradley.
Bradlea, Bradleigh, Bradlie

Bradley 🅱🅶 (English) broad
meadow.
*Brad, Braddly, Bradlay, Bradlee,
Bradly, Bradlyn, Bradney*

Bradly (English) a form of Bradley.

Bradon (English) broad hill.
Braedon, Braidon, Braydon

Bradshaw (English) broad forest.

Brady **BG** (Irish) spirited. (English) broad island.
Bradey, Bradi, Bradie, Bradye, Braidy

Bradyn (English) a form of Braden.
Bradynne, Breidyn

Braedan (English) a form of Braeden.

Braeden, Braiden **BG** (English) forms of Braden.
Braedin, Braedyn, Braidyn

Braedon (English) a form of Bradon.
Breadon

Bragi (Scandinavian) poet. Mythology: the god of poetry, eloquence, and song.
Brage

Braham (Hindi) creator.
Braheem, Braheim, Brahiem, Brahima, Brahm

Brainard (English) bold raven; prince.
Brainerd

Bram (Scottish) bramble, brushwood. (Hebrew) a short form of Abraham, Abram.
Brame, Bramm, Bramdon

Bramwell (English) bramble spring.
Brammel, Brammell, Bramwel, Bramwyll

Branch (Latin) paw; claw; tree branch.

Brand (English) firebrand; sword. A short form of Brandon.
Brandall, Brande, Brandel, Brandell, Brander, Brandley, Brandol, Brandt, Brandy, Brann

Brandan **BG** (English) a form of Brandon.

Brandeis (Czech) dweller on a burned clearing.
Brandis

Branden (English) beacon valley.
Brandden, Brandene, Brandin, Brandine, Brandyn, Breandan

Brandi **GB** (Dutch, English) a form of Brandy.

Brandon ✮ **BG** (English) beacon hill.
Bran, Brand, Branddon, Brandone, Brandonn, Brandyn, Branndan, Branndon, Brannon, Breandon, Brendon

Brandt (English) a form of Brant.

Brandy **GB** (Dutch) brandy. (English) a familiar form of Brand.
Branddy, Brandey, Brandi, Brandie

Brandyn (English) a form of Branden, Brandon.
Brandynn

Brannon (Irish) a form of Brandon.
Branen, Brannan, Brannen, Branon

Branson (English) son of Brandon, Brant. A form of Bronson.
Bransen, Bransin, Brantson

Brant (English) proud.
Brandt, Brannt, Brante, Brantley, Branton

Brantley 🅱🅶 (English) a form of Brant.
Brantlie, Brantly, Brentlee, Brentley, Brently

Braulio (Italian) a form of Brawley.
Brauli, Brauliuo

Brawley (English) meadow on the hillside.
Braulio, Brawlee, Brawly

Braxton 🅱🅶 (English) Brock's town.
Brax, Braxdon, Braxston, Braxten, Braxtin, Braxxton

Brayan (Irish, Scottish) a form of Brian.
Brayn, Brayon

Brayden 🅱🅶 (English) a form of Braden.
Braydan, Braydn, Bradyn, Breydan, Breyden, Brydan, Bryden

Braydon 🅱🅶 (English) a form of Bradon.
Braydoon, Brydon, Breydon

Breana, Breanna 🅶🅱 (Irish) forms of Briana.

Breann, Breanne 🅶🅱 (Irish) short forms of Briana.

Breck 🅱🅶 (Irish) freckled.
Brec, Breckan, Brecken, Breckie, Breckin, Breckke, Breckyn, Brek, Brexton

Brede (Scandinavian) iceberg, glacier.

Brencis (Latvian) a form of Lawrence.
Brence

Brenda 🅶🅱 (Irish) little raven. (English) sword.

Brendan 🅱🅶 (Irish) little raven. (English) sword.
Breandan, Bren, Brenden, Brendis, Brendon, Brendyn, Brenn, Brennan, Brennen, Brenndan, Brenyan, Bryn

Brenden 🅱🅶 (Irish) a form of Brendan.
Bren, Brendene, Brendin, Brendine, Brennden

Brendon (English) a form of Brandon. (Irish, English) a form of Brendan.
Brenndon

Brenna 🅶🅱 (English, Irish) a form of Brennan.

Brennan, Brennen 🅱🅶 (English, Irish) forms of Brendan.
Bren, Brenan, Brenen, Brenin, Brenn, Brennann, Brenner,

Brennin, Brennon, Brennor, Brennyn, Brenon

Brent (English) a short form of Brenton.
Brendt, Brente, Brentson, Brentt

Brenton BG (English) steep hill.
Brent, Brentan, Brenten, Brentin, Brentten, Brentton, Brentyn

Breogán (Spanish) indicative of family or origin.

Breon BG (Irish, Scottish) a form of Brian.

Bret, Brett BG (Scottish) from Great Britain. See also Britton.
Bhrett, Braten, Braton, Brayton, Bretin, Bretley, Bretlin, Breton, Brettan, Brette, Bretten, Bretton, Brit, Britt

Brewster (English) brewer.
Brew, Brewer, Bruwster

Breyon (Irish, Scottish) a form of Brian.
Breyan

Brian ☆ BG (Irish, Scottish) strong; virtuous; honorable. History: Brian Boru was an eleventh-century Irish king and national hero. See also Palaina.
Brayan, Breyon, Briann, Briano, Briant, Briante, Briaun, Briayan, Brien, Brience, Brient, Brin, Briny, Brion, Bryan, Bryen

Briana GB (Irish, Scottish) a form of Brian.

Brianna GB (Irish, Scottish) a form of Brian.

Brianne GB (Irish, Scottish) a form of Brian.

Briar (French) heather.
Brier, Brierly, Bryar, Bryer, Bryor

Brice BG (Welsh) alert; ambitious. (English) son of Rice.
Bricen, Briceton, Bryce

Bricio (Celtic) represents strength.

Brick (English) bridge.
Bricker, Bricklen, Brickman, Brik

Bridger (English) bridge builder.
Bridd, Bridge, Bridgeley, Bridgely

Bridget GB (Irish) strong.

Brielle GB (French) a form of Brie (see Girls' Names).

Brigham (English) covered bridge. (French) troops, brigade.
Brig, Brigg, Briggs, Brighton

Brighton (English) bright town.
Breighton, Bright, Brightin, Bryton

Brion (Irish, Scottish) a form of Brian.
Brieon, Brione, Brionn, Brionne

Brit, Britt (Scottish) forms of Bret, Brett. See also Britton.
Brit, Brityce

Britany, Brittany GB (English) from Britain.

Britney, Brittney, Brittny GB (English) forms of Britany.

Britton (Scottish) from Great Britain. See also Bret, Brett, Brit, Britt.
Britain, Briten, Britian, Britin, Briton, Brittain, Brittan, Britten, Brittian, Brittin, Britton

Brock 🅱🅶 (English) badger.
Broc, Brocke, Brockett, Brockie, Brockley, Brockton, Brocky, Brok, Broque

Brod (English) a short form of Broderick.
Brode, Broden

Broderick (Welsh) son of the famous ruler. (English) broad ridge. See also Roderick.
Brod, Broddie, Brodderick, Brodderrick, Broddy, Broderic, Broderrick, Brodrick

Brodie 🅱🅶 (Irish) a form of Brody.
Brodi, Broedi

Brodrick (Welsh, English) a form of Broderick.
Broddrick, Brodric, Brodryck

Brody 🅱🅶 (Irish) ditch; canal builder.
Brodee, Broden, Brodey, Brodie, Broedy

Brogan (Irish) a heavy work shoe.
Brogen, Broghan, Broghen

Bromley (English) brushwood meadow.

Bron (Afrikaans) source.

Bronislaw (Polish) weapon of glory.

Bronson (English) son of Brown.
Bransen, Bransin, Branson, Bron, Bronnie, Bronnson, Bronny, Bronsan, Bronsen, Bronsin, Bronsonn, Bronsson, Bronsun, Bronsyn, Brunson

Bronwyn 🅶🅱 (Welsh) white breasted.

Brook 🅶🅱 (English) brook, stream.
Brooker, Brookin

Brooke 🅶🅱 (English) a form of Brook.

Brooklyn, Brooklynn 🅶🅱 (American) combinations of Brook + Lynn.

Brooks 🅱🅶 (English) son of Brook.
Brookes, Broox

Brown (English) brown; bear.

Bruce 🅱🅶 (French) brushwood thicket; woods.
Brucey, Brucy, Brue, Bruis

Bruno (German, Italian) brown haired; brown skinned.
Brunon, Bruns

Bryan ☀ (Irish) a form of Brian.
Brayan, Bryann, Bryant, Bryen

Bryana, Bryanna 🅶🅱 (Irish) forms of Bryan.

Bryanne (Irish) a form of Bryan.

Bryant (Irish) a form of Bryan.
Bryent

Bryce **BG** (Welsh) a form of
Brice.
Brycen, Bryceton, Bryson, Bryston

Bryden **BG** (English) a form of
Brayden.

Brylee **GB** (American) a
combination of the letter B +
Riley.

Brynn **GB** (German) a form of
Bryon.

Bryon (German) cottage.
(English) bear.
*Bryeon, Bryn, Bryne, Brynne,
Bryone*

Bryson **BG** (Welsh) child of
Brice.

Bryton **Bg** (English) a form of
Brighton.
*Brayten, Brayton, Breyton,
Bryeton, Brytan, Bryten, Brytin,
Brytten, Brytton*

Bubba (German) a boy.
Babba, Babe, Bebba

Buck (German, English) male
deer.
*Buckie, Buckley, Buckner, Bucko,
Bucky*

Buckley (English) deer meadow.
Bucklea, Bucklee

Buckminster (English) preacher.

Bud (English) herald, messenger.
Budd, Buddy

Buddy (American) a familiar form
of Bud.
Budde, Buddey, Buddie

Buell (German) hill dweller.
(English) bull.

Buenaventura (Latin) he who
predicts happiness.

Buford (English) ford near the
castle.
Burford

Burcardo (Germanic) daring
protector; the defender of the
fortress.

Burgess (English) town dweller;
shopkeeper.
*Burg, Burges, Burgh, Burgiss,
Burr*

Burian (Ukrainian) lives near
weeds.

Burke (German, French) fortress,
castle.
*Berk, Berke, Birk, Bourke, Burk,
Burkley*

Burl (English) cup bearer; wine
servant; knot in a tree. (German)
a short form of Berlyn.
Berl, Burley, Burlie, Byrle

Burleigh (English) meadow with
knotted tree trunks.
*Burlee, Burley, Burlie, Byrleigh,
Byrlee*

Burne (English) brook.
*Beirne, Burn, Burnell, Burnett,
Burney, Byrn, Byrne*

Burney (English) island with a brook. A familiar form of Rayburn.

Burr (Swedish) youth. (English) prickly plant.

Burris (English) town dweller.

Burt (English) a form of Bert. A short form of Burton.
Burrt, Burtt, Burty

Burton (English) fortified town.
Berton, Burt

Busby (Scottish) village in the thicket; tall military hat made of fur.
Busbee, Buzby, Buzz

Buster (American) hitter, puncher.

Butch (American) a short form of Butcher.

Butcher (English) butcher.
Butch

Buzz (Scottish) a short form of Busby.
Buzzy

Byford (English) by the ford.

Byram (English) cattle yard.

Byrd (English) birdlike.
Bird, Birdie, Byrdie

Byrne (English) a form of Burne.
Byrn, Byrnes

Byron (French) cottage. (English) barn.
Beyren, Beyron, Biren, Biron, Buiron, Byram, Byran, Byrann, Byren, Byrom, Byrone

C BG (American) an initial used as a first name.

Cable (French, English) rope maker.
Cabell

Cachayauri (Quechua) hard as a shard of copper; sharp as a spine or needle.

Cadao (Vietnamese) folksong.

Cadby (English) warrior's settlement.

Caddock (Welsh) eager for war.

Cade BG (Welsh) a short form of Cadell.
Cady

Cadell (Welsh) battler.
Cade, Cadel, Cedell

Caden BG (American) a form of Kadin.
Cadan, Caddon, Cadian, Cadien, Cadin, Cadon, Cadyn, Caeden, Caedon, Caid, Caiden, Cayden

Cadmus (Greek) from the east. Mythology: a Phoenician prince who founded Thebes and introduced writing to the Greeks.

Caelan (Scottish) a form of Nicholas.
Cael, Caelon, Caelyn, Cailan, Cailean, Caillan, Cailun, Cailyn,

Calan, Calen, Caleon, Caley,
Calin, Callan, Callon, Callyn,
Calon, Calyn, Caylan, Cayley

Caesar (Latin) long-haired.
History: a title for Roman
emperors. See also Kaiser, Kesar,
Sarito.
Caesarae, Caesear, Caeser,
Caezar, Caseare, Ceasar, Cesar,
Ceseare, Cezar, Cézar, Czar,
Seasar

Cahil (Turkish) young, naive.

Cai (Welsh) a form of Gaius.
Caio, Caius, Caw

Caifas (Assyrian) man of little
energy.

Cain (Hebrew) spear; gatherer.
Bible: Adam and Eve's oldest son.
See also Kabil, Kane, Kayne.
Cainaen, Cainan, Caine, Cainen,
Caineth, Cayn, Cayne

Caín (Hebrew) a form of Cain.

Cairn (Welsh) landmark made of
a mound of stones.
Cairne, Carn, Carne

Cairo (Arabic) Geography: the
capital of Egypt.
Kairo

Caitlin GB (Irish) pure.

Caiya (Quechua) close, nearby;
unique.

Calder (Welsh, English) brook,
stream.

Caldwell (English) cold well.

Cale (Hebrew) a short form of
Caleb.

Caleb ⭐ BG (Hebrew) dog;
faithful. (Arabic) bold, brave.
Bible: one of the twelve spies sent
by Moses. See also Kaleb, Kayleb.
Caeleb, Calab, Calabe, Cale,
Caley, Calib, Calieb, Callob,
Calob, Calyb, Cayleb, Caylebb,
Caylib, Caylob

Caleigh GB (Irish) a form of
Caley.

Calen, Calin (Scottish) forms of
Caelan.
Caelen, Caelin, Caellin, Cailen,
Cailin, Caillin, Calean, Callen,
Caylin

Calepodio (Greek) he who has
beautiful feet.

Caley (Irish) a familiar form of
Caleb.
Calee, Caleigh

Calfumil (Mapuche) glazed
ceramic tile; brilliant blue.

Calhoun (Irish) narrow woods.
(Scottish) warrior.
Colhoun, Colhoune, Colquhoun

Calígula (Latin) he who wears
sandals.

Calimaco (Greek) excellent
fighter.

Calímaco (Greek) good fighter.

Calimerio (Greek) he who ushers in a beautiful day.

Calinico (Greek) he who secures a beautiful victory.

Calistenes (Greek) beautiful and strong.

Calisto, Calixto (Greek) best and the most beautiful.

Calistrato (Greek) he who commands a great army.

Calístrato (Greek) chief of a great army.

Callahan (Irish) descendant of Ceallachen.
Calahan, Callaghan

Callum 🅱🅶 (Irish) dove.
Callam, Calum, Calym

Calogero (Greek) wise one; the beautiful man; he who is going to age well.

Calvert (English) calf herder.
Cal, Calbert, Calvirt

Calvin (Latin) bald. See also Kalvin, Vinny.
Cal, Calv, Calvien, Calvon, Calvyn

Calvino (Latin) bald.

Calvucura (Mapuche) blue stone.

Cam 🅱🅶 (Gypsy) beloved. (Scottish) a short form of Cameron. (Latin, French, Scottish) a short form of Campbell.
Camm, Cammie, Cammy, Camy

Camaron (Scottish) a form of Cameron.
Camar, Camari, Camaran, Camaren

Camden 🅱🅶 (Scottish) winding valley.
Kamden

Cameron ☀ 🅱🅶 (Scottish) crooked nose. See also Kameron.
Cam, Camaron, Cameran, Cameren, Camerin, Cameroun, Camerron, Camerson, Camerun, Cameryn, Camiren, Camiron, Cammeron, Camron

Camille 🅶🅱 (French) young ceremonial attendant.
Camile

Camilo (Latin) child born to freedom; noble.
Camiel, Camillo, Camillus

Campbell (Latin, French) beautiful field. (Scottish) crooked mouth.
Cam, Camp, Campy

Camron 🅱🅶 (Scottish) a short form of Cameron.
Camren, Cammrin, Cammron, Camran, Camreon, Camrin, Camryn, Camrynn

Canaan (French) a form of Cannon. History: an ancient region between the Jordan River and the Mediterranean.
Canan, Canen, Caynan

Cancio (Latin) founder of the city of Anzio.

Candice GB (Greek) a form of Candace (see Girls' Names).

Candide (Latin) pure; sincere.
Candid, Candido, Candonino

Cándido (Latin) a form of Candide.

Cannon (French) church official; large gun. See also Kannon.
Canaan, Cannan, Cannen, Cannin, Canning, Canon

Canute (Latin) white haired. (Scandinavian) knot. History: a Danish king who became king of England after 1016. See also Knute.
Cnut, Cnute

Canuto (Latin) wise man with abundant white hair.

Capac, Capah (Quechua) Lord; rich in kindness; great, powerful, just, correct.

Capacuari (Quechua) kind-hearted master and untamable like the vicuna.

Capaquiupanqui (Quechua) he who honors his master; memorable master.

Cappi (Gypsy) good fortune.

Caquia (Quechua) thunder; bolt of lightning.

Car (Irish) a short form of Carney.

Carey BG (Greek) pure. (Welsh) castle; rocky island. See also Karey.
Care, Caree, Cari, Carre, Carree, Carrie, Cary

Carim (Arabic) generous.

Carina GB (Italian) dear little one. (Swedish) a form of Karen. (Greek) a familiar form of Cora (see Girls' Names).

Carl BG (German, English) a short form of Carlton. A form of Charles. See also Carroll, Kale, Kalle, Karl, Karlen, Karol.
Carle, Carles, Carless, Carlis, Carll, Carlo, Carlos, Carlson, Carlston, Carlus, Carolos

Carlee GB (English) a form of Carly.

Carley GB (English) a familiar form of Carlin.

Carli GB (English) a form of Carly.

Carlie GB (English) a familiar form of Carlin.

Carlin BG (Irish) little champion.
Carlan, Carlen, Carley, Carlie, Carling, Carlino, Carly

Carlisle (English) Carl's island.
Carlyle, Carlysle

Carlito (Spanish) a familiar form of Carlos.
Carlitos

Carlo (Italian) a form of Carl, Charles.
Carolo

Carlomagno (Spanish) Charles the great.

Carlos ☀ **BG** (Spanish) a form of Carl, Charles.
Carlito

Carlton **BG** (English) Carl's town.
Carl, Carleton, Carllton, Carlston, Carltonn, Carltton, Charlton

Carly **GB** (English) a familiar form of Carlin.

Carmel (Hebrew) vineyard, garden. See also Carmine.
Carmello, Carmelo, Karmel

Carmen **GB** (Latin) a form of Carmine.

Carmichael (Scottish) follower of Michael.

Carmine (Latin) song; crimson. (Italian) a form of Carmel.
Carmain, Carmaine, Carman, Carmen, Carmon

Carnelius (Greek, Latin) a form of Cornelius.
Carnealius, Carneilius, Carnellius, Carnilious

Carnell (English) defender of the castle. (French) a form of Cornell.

Carney (Irish) victorious. (Scottish) fighter. See also Kearney.
Car, Carny, Karney

Carol **GB** (Irish, German) a form of Carroll.

Carolina **GB** (Italian) a form of Caroline.

Caroline **GB** (French) little and strong.

Carolyn **GB** (English) a form of Caroline.

Carpo (Greek) valuable fruit.

Carr (Scandinavian) marsh. See also Kerr.
Karr

Carrick (Irish) rock.
Carooq, Carricko

Carrie **GB** (Greek, Welsh) a form of Carey.

Carrington (Welsh) rocky town.

Carroll (Irish) champion. (German) a form of Carl.
Carel, Carell, Cariel, Cariell, Carol, Carole, Carolo, Carols, Carollan, Carolus, Carrol, Cary, Caryl

Carson **BG** (English) son of Carr.
Carsen, Carsino, Carrson, Karson

Carsten (Greek) a form of Karsten.
Carston

Carter ☀ **BG** (English) cart driver.
Cart

Cartwright (English) cart builder.

Caruamayu (Quechua) yellow river.

Carvell (French, English) village on the marsh.
Carvel, Carvelle, Carvellius

Carver (English) wood-carver; sculptor.

Cary (Welsh) a form of Carey. (German, Irish) a form of Carroll.
Carray, Carry

Casandro (Greek) hero's brother.

Case (Irish) a short form of Casey. (English) a short form of Casimir.

Casey BG (Irish) brave.
Case, Casie, Casy, Cayse, Caysey, Kacey, Kasey

Cash (Latin) vain. (Slavic) a short form of Casimir.
Cashe

Casiano (Latin) he who is equipped with a helmet.

Casildo (Arabic) youth that carries the lance.

Casimir (Slavic) peacemaker.
Cachi, Cas, Case, Cash, Cashemere, Cashi, Cashmeire, Cashmere, Casimere, Casimire, Casimiro, Castimer, Kasimir, Kazio

Casiodoro (Greek) gift from a friend.

Casper (Persian) treasurer. (German) imperial. See also Gaspar, Jasper, Kasper.
Caspar, Cass

Cass BG (Irish, Persian) a short form of Casper, Cassidy.

Cassandra GB (Greek) helper.

Cassidy GB (Irish) clever; curly haired.
Casidy, Cass, Cassady, Cassie, Kassidy

Cassie (Irish) a familiar form of Cassidy.
Casi, Casie, Casio, Cassey, Cassy, Casy

Cassius (Latin, French) box; protective cover.
Cassia, Cassio, Cazzie

Casta (Spanish) pure.

Castle (Latin) castle.
Cassle, Castel

Casto (Greek) pure, honest, clean.

Castor (Greek) beaver. Astrology: one of the twins in the constellation Gemini. Mythology: one of the patron saints of mariners.
Caster, Caston

Cástor (Greek) a form of Castor.

Cataldo (Greek) outstanding in war.

Catari (Aymara) serpent.

Catequil, Catiquil, Catuilla (Quechua) ray of light.

Cater (English) caterer.

Catherine GB (Greek) pure. (English) a form of Katherine.

Cato (Latin) knowledgeable, wise.
Caton

Catón (Latin) a form of Cato.
Caton, Catón

Catricura (Mapuche) cut stone.

Catulo (Latin) puppy; soft.

Cátulo (Spanish) a form of Catulo.

Cauac (Quechua) sentinel; he who guards.

Cauachi (Quechua) he who makes us attentive, vigilant.

Cauana (Quechua) he who is in a place where all can be seen.

Cautaro (Araucanian) daring and enterprising.

Cavan (Irish) handsome. See also Kevin.
Caven, Cavin, Cavan, Cawoun

Cayden (American) a form of Caden.
Cayde, Caydin

Cayetano (Latin) he who is from Gaeta, an ancient city in the Lacio region.

Caylan (Scottish) a form of Caelan.
Caylans, Caylen, Caylon

Cayo (Latin) happy and fun.

Cayua (Quechua) he who follows, follower; faithful.

Cazzie (American) a familiar form of Cassius.
Caz, Cazz, Cazzy

Ceasar (Latin) a form of Caesar.
Ceaser

Cecil 🅱🅶 (Latin) blind.
Cece, Cecile, Cecilio, Cecilius, Cecill, Celio, Siseal

Cedric (English) battle chieftain. See also Kedrick, Rick.
Cad, Caddaric, Ced, Cederic, Cedrec, Cédric, Cedrick, Cedryche, Sedric

Cedrick (English) a form of Cedric.
Ceddrick, Cederick, Cederrick, Cedirick, Cedrik

Cedro (Spanish) strong gift.

Ceejay (American) a combination of the initials C. + J.
Cejay, C.J.

Ceferino (Greek) he who caresses like the wind.

Celedonio (Latin) he is like the swallow.

Celestino (Latin) resident of the celestial reign.

Celine 🅶🅱 (Greek) a form of Celena (see Girls' Names).

Celso (Latin) tall, elevated; noble.

Cemal (Arabic) attractive.

Cencio (Italian) a form of Vicente.

Cenobio (Latin) he who rejects the strangers; God gives him protection and good health.

Cephas (Latin) small rock. Bible: the term used by Jesus to describe Peter.
Cepheus, Cephus

Cerdic (Welsh) beloved.
Caradoc, Caradog, Ceredig, Ceretic

Cerek (Polish) lordly. (Greek) a form of Cyril.

Cesar BG (Spanish) a form of Caesar.
Casar, César, Cesare, Cesareo, Cesario, Cesaro, Cessar

Cesáreo (Latin) relating to Caesar.

Cesarión (Latin) Caesar's follower.

Cestmir (Czech) fortress.

Cezar (Slavic) a form of Caesar.
Cézar, Cezary, Cezek, Chezrae, Sezar

Chace (French) a form of Chase.
Chayce

Chad BG (English) warrior. A short form of Chadwick. Geography: a country in north-central Africa.
Ceadd, Chaad, Chadd, Chaddie, Chaddy, Chade, Chadleigh, Chadler, Chadley, Chadlin, Chadlyn, Chadmen, Chado, Chadron, Chady

Chadrick (German) mighty warrior.
Chaddrick, Chaderic, Chaderick, Chadrack, Chadric

Chadwick (English) warrior's town.
Chad, Chaddwick, Chadvic, Chadwyck

Chago (Spanish) a form of Jacob.
Chango, Chanti

Chaicu (Aymara) he who has great strength in order to fling stones, is skillful with the sling.

Chaim (Hebrew) life. See also Hyman.
Chai, Chaimek, Haim, Khaim

Chaise (French) a form of Chase.
Chais, Chaisen, Chaison

Chal (Gypsy) boy; son.
Chalie, Chalin

Chale (Spanish) strong and youthful.

Chalmers (Scottish) son of the lord.
Chalmer, Chalmr, Chamar, Chamarr

Chalten (Tehuelchean) bluish.

Cham (Vietnamese) hard worker.
Chams

Chambi, Champi (Aymara) halberd, lance; he who brings good news.

Chambigüiyca, Champigüiyca
(Aymara) beam of sunlight; sent
from the gods.

Chan 🅑🅖 (Sanskrit) shining.
(English) a form of Chauncey.
(Spanish) a form of Juan.
Chann, Chano, Chayo

Chanan (Hebrew) cloud.

Chance 🅑🅖 (English) a short
form of Chancellor, Chauncey.
*Chanc, Chancee, Chancey,
Chancie, Chancy, Chanse, Chansy,
Chants, Chantz, Chanze, Chanz,
Chaynce*

Chancellor (English) record
keeper.
*Chance, Chancelar, Chancelen,
Chanceleor, Chanceler,
Chanceller, Chancelor, Chanselor,
Chanslor*

Chander (Hindi) moon.
*Chand, Chandan, Chandany,
Chandara, Chandon*

Chandler 🅑🅖 (English) candle
maker.
*Chandelar, Chandlan, Chandlar,
Chandlier, Chandlor, Chandlyr*

Chane (Swahili) dependable.

Chaney (French) oak.
*Chayne, Cheaney, Cheney, Cheyn,
Cheyne, Cheyney*

Chankrisna (Cambodian) sweet
smelling tree.

Channing (English) wise.
(French) canon; church official.
Chane, Chann

Chanse (English) a form of
Chance.
Chans, Chansey

Chantal 🅖🅑 (French) song.

Chante 🅑🅖 (French) singer.
*Chant, Chantha, Chanthar,
Chantra, Chantry, Shantae*

Chantel 🅖🅑 (French) a form of
Chantal.

Chapman (English) merchant.
Chap, Chappie, Chappy

Charity 🅖🅑 (Latin) charity,
kindness.

Charles ☀ 🅑🅖 (German) farmer.
(English) strong and manly. See
also Carl, Searlas, Tearlach,
Xarles.
*Arlo, Chareles, Charels, Charlese,
Carlo, Carlos, Charl, Charle,
Charlen, Charlie, Charlot, Charlz,
Charlzell, Chaz, Chick, Chip,
Chuck*

Charlie 🅑🅖 (German, English) a
familiar form of Charles.
*Charle, Charlee, Charley, Charli,
Charly*

Charlton (English) a form of
Carlton.
*Charlesten, Charleston,
Charleton, Charlotin*

Charro (Spanish) cowboy.

Chase ☀ BG (French) hunter.
Chace, Chaise, Chasen, Chason,
Chass, Chasse, Chastan, Chasten,
Chastin, Chastinn, Chaston,
Chasyn, Chayse

Chaska (Sioux) first-born son.

Chauar (Quechua) fiber, rope.

Chauncey BG (English)
chancellor; church official.
Chan, Chance, Chancey, Chaunce,
Chauncei, Chauncy, Chaunecy,
Chaunesy, Chaunszi

Chaupi (Quechua) he who is in
the middle of everything.

Chavez (Hispanic) a surname
used as a first name.
Chavaz, Chaves, Chaveze,
Chavies, Chavis, Chavius, Chevez,
Cheveze, Cheviez, Chevious,
Chevis, Chivass, Chivez

Chayse (French) a form of Chase.
Chaysea, Chaysen, Chayson,
Chaysten

Chayton (Lakota) falcon.

Chaz BG (English) a familiar form
of Charles.
Chas, Chasz, Chaze, Chazwick,
Chazy, Chazz, Chez

Che (Spanish) God will add or
multiply.

Ché (Spanish) a familiar form
of José. History: Ernesto "Che"
Guevara was a revolutionary who
fought at Fidel Castro's side in
Cuba.
Chay

Checha (Spanish) a familiar form
of Jacob.

Cheche (Spanish) a familiar form
of Joseph.

Chelsea GB (English) seaport.

Chelsey GB (English) a form of
Chelsea.

Chelsie GB (English) a form of
Chelsea.

Chen (Chinese) great, tremendous.

Chencho (Spanish) a familiar
form of Lawrence.

Chepe (Spanish) a familiar form
of Joseph.
Cepito

Cherokee GB (Cherokee) people
of a different speech.
Cherrakee

Chesmu (Native American) gritty.

Chester (English) a short form of
Rochester.
Ches, Cheslav, Cheston, Chet

Chet (English) a short form of
Chester.
Chett, Chette

Cheung (Chinese) good luck.

Chevalier (French) horseman, knight.
Chev, Chevy

Chevy (French) a familiar form of Chevalier. Geography: Chevy Chase is a town in Maryland. Culture: a short form of Chevrolet, an American automobile company.
Chev, Chevey, Chevi, Chevie, Chevvy, Chewy

Cheyenne 🅖🅑 (Cheyenne) a tribal name.
Chayann, Chayanne, Cheyeenne, Cheyene, Chyenne, Shayan

Chi 🅑🅖 (Chinese) younger generation. (Nigerian) personal guardian angel.

Chican (Quechua) unique, different from the rest.

Chick (English) a familiar form of Charles.
Chic, Chickie, Chicky

Chico (Spanish) boy.

Chik (Gypsy) earth.

Chike (Ibo) God's power.

Chiko (Japanese) arrow; pledge.

Chilo (Spanish) a familiar form of Francisco.

Chilton (English) farm by the spring.
Chil, Chill, Chillton, Chilt

Chim (Vietnamese) bird.

China 🅖🅑 (Chinese) fine porcelain. Geography: a country in eastern Asia.

Chincolef (Mapuche) swift squad; rapid.

Chinua (Ibo) God's blessing.
Chino, Chinou

Chioke (Ibo) gift of God.

Chip (English) a familiar form of Charles.
Chipman, Chipper

Chiram (Hebrew) exalted; noble.

Chloe 🅖🅑 (Greek) blooming, verdant.

Choque, Chuqui (Quechua) lance; dancer.

Chorche (Aragonese) a form of George.

Chris 🅑🅖 (Greek) a short form of Christian, Christopher. See also Kris.
Chriss, Christ, Chrys, Cris, Crist

Christa 🅖🅑 (Greek) a form of Christian.

Christain 🅑🅖 (Greek) a form of Christian.
Christai, Christan, Christane, Christaun, Christein

Christen 🅖🅑 (Greek) a form of Christian.

Christian ☆ 🅑🅖 (Greek) follower of Christ; anointed. See also Jaan, Kerstan, Khristian, Kit,

Krister, Kristian, Krystian.
Chretien, Chris, Christa, Christain,
Christé, Christen, Christensen,
Christiaan, Christiana, Christiane,
Christiann, Christianna,
Christianno, Christiano,
Christianos, Christien, Christin,
Christino, Christion, Christon,
Christos, Christyan, Christyon,
Chritian, Chrystian, Cristian,
Crystek

Christie GB (Greek) a short form of Christina, Christine.

Christien (Greek) a form of Christian.
Christienne, Christinne, Chrystien

Christin GB (Greek) a form of Christian.

Christina GB (Greek) Christian; anointed.

Christine GB (French, English) a form of Christina.

Christofer (Greek) a form of Christopher.
Christafer, Christafur, Christefor,
Christerfer, Christifer, Christoffer,
Christofher, Christofper,
Chrystofer

Christoff (Russian) a form of Christopher.
Chrisof, Christif, Christof, Cristofe

Christophe BG (French) a form of Christopher.
Christoph

Christopher ☆ BG (Greek) Christ-bearer. Religion: the patron saint of travelers. See also Cristopher, Kester, Kit, Kristopher, Risto, Stoffel, Tobal, Topher.
Chris, Chrisopherson, Christapher,
Christepher, Christerpher,
Christhoper, Christipher,
Christobal, Christofer, Christoff,
Christoforo, Christoher,
Christopehr, Christoper,
Christophe, Christopherr,
Christophor, Christophoros,
Christophr, Christophre,
Christophyer, Christophyr,
Christorpher, Christos, Christovao,
Christpher, Christphere,
Christphor, Christpor, Christrpher,
Chrystopher, Cristobal

Christophoros (Greek) a form of Christopher.
Christoforo, Christoforos,
Christophor, Christophorus,
Christphor, Cristoforo, Cristopher

Christos (Greek) a form of Christopher. See also Khristos.

Christy GB (English) a short form of Christina, Christine.

Chucho (Hebrew) a familiar form of Jesus.

Chuck (American) a familiar form of Charles.
Chuckey, Chuckie, Chucky

Chui (Swahili) leopard.

Chul (Korean) firm.

Chuma (Ibo) having many beads, wealthy. (Swahili) iron.

Chuminga (Spanish) a familiar form of Dominic.
Chumin

Chumo (Spanish) a familiar form of Thomas.

Chun 🅱🅶 (Chinese) spring.

Chung (Chinese) intelligent.
Chungo, Chuong

Chuquigüaman (Quechua) dancing falcon; golden falcon.

Chuquigüiyca (Quechua) sacred dance.

Chuquilla (Quechua) ray of light; golden light.

Churchill (English) church on the hill. History: Sir Winston Churchill served as British prime minister and won a Nobel Prize for literature.

Chuscu (Quechua) fourth son.

Chuya (Quechua) clear as water, pure.

Cian (Irish) ancient.
Céin, Cianán, Kian

Ciara 🅶🅱 (Irish) black.

Cibrao (Latin) inhabitant of Cyprus.

Cicero (Latin) chickpea. History: a famous Roman orator, philosopher, and statesman.
Cicerón

Cid (Spanish) lord. History: title for Rodrigo Díaz de Vivar, an eleventh-century Spanish soldier and national hero.
Cyd

Cidro (Spanish) strong gift.

Cindy 🅶🅱 (Greek) moon. (Latin) a familiar form of Cynthia.

Ciqala (Dakota) little.

Ciríaco (Greek) he who belongs to the Lord.

Cirineo (Greek) native of Cyrene (present-day Libya).

Cirrillo (Italian) a form of Cyril.
Cirilio, Cirillo, Cirilo, Ciro

Cisco (Spanish) a short form of Francisco.

Ciset (Spanish) a form of Narciso.

Citino (Latin) quick to act.

Claire 🅶🅱 (French) a form of Clara.

Clancy (Irish) redheaded fighter.
Clancey, Claney

Clara 🅶🅱 (Latin) clear; bright.

Clare 🅶🅱 (Latin) a short form of Clarence.
Clair, Clarey, Clary

Clarence 🅱🅶 (Latin) clear; victorious.
Clarance, Clare, Clarrance, Clarrence, Clearence

Clarissa **GB** (Greek) brilliant.
(Italian) a form of Clara.

Clark **BG** (French) cleric; scholar.
Clarke, Clerc, Clerk

Claro (Latin) he who is clean and
transparent.

Claude **BG** (Latin, French) lame.
*Claud, Claudan, Claudel, Claudell,
Claudey, Claudi, Claudian,
Claudianus, Claudie, Claudien,
Claudin, Claudio, Claudis,
Claudius, Claudy*

Claudie **GB** (Latin, French) a
form of Claude.

Claudino (Latin) he who belongs
to the ancient Roman family
Claudios.

Claudio **BG** (Italian) a form of
Claude.

Claus (German) a short form of
Nicholas. See also Klaus.
Claas, Claes, Clause

Clay (English) clay pit. A short
form of Clayborne, Clayton.
Klay

Clayborne (English) brook near
the clay pit.
*Claibern, Claiborn, Claiborne,
Claibrone, Clay, Claybon,
Clayborn, Claybourn, Claybourne,
Clayburn, Clebourn*

Clayton **BG** (English) town built
on clay.
*Clay, Clayten, Cleighton, Cleyton,
Clyton, Klayton*

Cleandro (Greek) glorious man.

Cleary (Irish) learned.

Cleavon (English) cliff.
*Clavin, Clavion, Clavon, Clavone,
Clayvon, Claywon, Clévon,
Clevonn, Clyvon*

Clem (Latin) a short form of
Clement.
Cleme, Clemmy, Clim

Clement (Latin) merciful. Bible: a
coworker of Paul. See also
Klement, Menz.
*Clem, Clemens, Clément,
Clemente, Clementius, Clemmons*

Clemente (Italian, Spanish) a
form of Clement.
Clemento, Clemenza

Cleofas (Greek) he is the glory of
his father.

Cleon (Greek) famous.
Kleon

Cleto (Greek) he was chosen to
fight.

Cletus (Greek) illustrious.
History: a Roman pope and
martyr.
*Cleatus, Cledis, Cleotis, Clete,
Cletis*

Cleveland (English) land of cliffs.
*Cleaveland, Cleavland, Cleavon,
Cleve, Clevelend, Clevelynn,
Clevey, Clevie, Clevon*

Cliff (English) a short form of Clifford, Clifton.
Clif, Clift, Clive, Clyff, Clyph, Kliff

Clifford (English) cliff at the river crossing.
Cliff, Cliford, Clyfford, Klifford

Clifton BG (English) cliff town.
Cliff, Cliffton, Clift, Cliften, Clyfton

Climaco (Greek) he who climbs the ladder.

Clímaco (Greek) he who ascends.

Clímene (Greek) famous, celebrated.

Clint (English) a short form of Clinton.
Klint

Clinton (English) hill town.
Clenten, Clint, Clinten, Clintion, Clintton, Clynton, Klinton

Clive (English) a form of Cliff.
Cleve, Clivans, Clivens, Clyve, Klyve

Clodio (German) glorious.

Clodoaldo (Teutonic) prince that is the chosen and illustrious captain.

Clodomiro (Germanic) he of illustrious fame.

Clodulfo (Germanic) glory.

Clorindo (Greek) he who is like the grass.

Clotario (Gothic) a form of Lotario.

Clove (Spanish) nail.

Clovis (German) famous soldier. See also Louis.

Cluny (Irish) meadow.

Clyde (Welsh) warm. (Scottish) Geography: a river in Scotland.
Cly, Clywd, Klyde

Coby (Hebrew) a familiar form of Jacob.
Cob, Cobby, Cobe, Cobey, Cobi, Cobia, Cobie

Cochise (Apache) hardwood. History: a famous Chiricahua Apache leader.

Coco GB (French) a familiar form of Jacques.
Coko, Koko

Codey BG (English) a form of Cody.
Coday

Codi BG (English) a form of Cody.

Codie BG (English) a form of Cody.
Coadi, Codea

Cody ☀ BG (English) cushion. History: William "Buffalo Bill" Cody was an American frontier scout who toured America and Europe with his Wild West show. See also Kody.
Coady, Coddy, Code, Codee,

Codell, Codey, Codi, Codiak,
Codie, Coedy

Coffie (Ewe) born on Friday.

Coique (Quechua) silver.

Coiquiyoc (Quechua) he who is
rich with silver.

Cola (Italian) a familiar form of
Nicholas, Nicola.
Colas

Colar (French) a form of
Nicholas.

Colbert (English) famous
seafarer.
Cole, Colt, Colvert, Culbert

Colby BG (English) dark; dark
haired.
Colbey, Colbi, Colbie, Colbin,
Colebee, Coleby, Collby, Kolby

Cole ☆ BG (Latin) cabbage
farmer. (English) a short form of
Coleman.
Colet, Coley, Colie, Kole

Coleman BG (Latin) cabbage
farmer. (English) coal miner.
Cole, Colemann, Colm, Colman,
Koleman

Colin ☆ BG (Irish) young cub.
(Greek) a short form of Nicholas.
Cailean, Colan, Cole, Colen,
Coleon, Colinn, Collin, Colyn,
Kolin

Colla, Culla (Quechua) from the
village Colla; eminent, excellent.

Collacapac, Cullacapac
(Quechua) Lord Colla, eminent
and kind-hearted lord.

Collana, Cullana (Quechua)
best; he who excels.

Collatupac, Cullatupac
(Quechua) glorious, majestic
Colla; royal eminence.

Colley (English) black haired;
swarthy.
Colee, Collie, Collis

Collier (English) miner.
Colier, Collayer, Collie, Collyer,
Colyer

Collin BG (Scottish) a form of
Colin, Collins.
Collan, Collen, Collian, Collon,
Collyn

Collins (Greek) son of Colin.
(Irish) holly.
Collin, Collis

Colon (Latin) he has the beauty of
a dove.

Colson (Greek, English) son of
Nicholas.
Colsen, Coulson

Colt BG (English) young horse;
frisky. A short form of Colter,
Colton.
Colte

Colten (English) a form of Colton.

Colter (English) herd of colts.
Colt

Colton 🅱🅶 (English) coal town.
*Colt, Coltan, Colten, Coltin, Coltinn,
Coltn, Coltrane, Colttan, Coltton,
Coltun, Coltyn, Coltyne, Kolton*

Columba (Latin) dove.
*Coim, Colum, Columbia,
Columbus*

Colwyn (Welsh) Geography: a
river in Wales.
Colwin, Colwinn

Coman (Arabic) noble. (Irish)
bent.
Comán

Coñalef (Mapuche) swift youngster;
rapid, agile; well meaning.

Conall (Irish) high, mighty.
*Conal, Connal, Connel, Connell,
Connelly, Connolly*

Conan (Irish) praised; exalted.
(Scottish) wise.
*Conant, Conary, Connen, Connie,
Connon, Connor, Conon*

Conary (Irish) a form of Conan.
Conaire

Coni (Quechua) warm.

Coniraya (Quechua) heat from
the sun; he who has heat from
the sun.

Conlan (Irish) hero.
Conlen, Conley, Conlin, Conlyn

Conner 🅱🅶 (Irish) a form of
Connor.
*Connar, Connary, Conneer,
Connery, Konner*

Connie 🅶🅱 (English, Irish) a
familiar form of Conan, Conrad,
Constantine, Conway.
Con, Conn, Conney, Conny

Connor ☀ 🅱🅶 (Scottish) wise.
(Irish) a form of Conan.
*Conner, Connoer, Connory,
Connyr, Conor, Konner, Konnor*

Cono (Mapuche) ringdove.

Conor 🅱🅶 (Irish) a form of
Connor.
Conar, Coner, Conour, Konner

Conrad (German) brave
counselor.
*Connie, Conrade, Conrado,
Corrado, Konrad*

Conroy (Irish) wise.
Conry, Roy

Constancio (Latin) perseverant
one.

Constant (Latin) a short form of
Constantine.

Constantine (Latin) firm,
constant. History: Constantine the
Great was the Roman emperor
who adopted the Christian faith.
See also Dinos, Konstantin,
Stancio.
*Connie, Constadine, Constandine,
Constandios, Constanstine,
Constant, Constantin,
Constantino, Constantinos,
Constantios, Costa*

Contardo (Teutonic) he who is
daring and valiant.

Conun-Huenu (Mapuche) entrance to the sky; elevated hill.

Conway (Irish) hound of the plain.
Connie, Conwy

Cook (English) cook.
Cooke

Cooper BG (English) barrel maker. See also Keiffer.
Coop, Couper

Corbett (Latin) raven.
Corbbitt, Corbet, Corbette, Corbit, Corbitt

Corbin BG (Latin) raven.
Corban, Corben, Corbey, Corbie, Corbon, Corby, Corbyn, Korbin

Corcoran (Irish) ruddy.

Cordaro (Spanish) a form of Cordero.
Coradaro, Cordairo, Cordara, Cordarel, Cordarell, Cordarelle, Cordareo, Cordarin, Cordario, Cordarion, Cordarious, Cordarius, Cordarrel, Cordarrell, Cordarris, Cordarrius, Cordarro, Cordarrol, Cordarus, Cordarryl, Cordaryal, Corddarro, Corrdarl

Cordell (French) rope maker.
Cord, Cordae, Cordale, Corday, Cordeal, Cordeil, Cordel, Cordele, Cordelle, Cordie, Cordy, Kordell

Cordero (Spanish) little lamb.
Cordaro, Cordeal, Cordeara, Cordearo, Cordeiro, Cordelro, Corder, Cordera, Corderall, Corderias, Corderious, Corderral, Corderro, Corderryn, Corderun, Corderus, Cordiaro, Cordierre, Cordy, Corrderio

Corey BG (Irish) hollow. See also Korey, Kory.
Core, Coreaa, Coree, Cori, Corian, Corie, Corio, Correy, Corria, Corrie, Corry, Corrye, Cory

Cori GB (Irish) a form of Corey.

Coriguaman (Quechua) golden falcon.

Coriñaui (Quechua) he who has eyes that are the color and beauty of gold.

Coripoma (Quechua) golden puma.

Cormac (Irish) raven's son. History: a third-century king of Ireland who was a great lawmaker.
Cormack, Cormick

Cornelius BG (Greek) cornel tree. (Latin) horn colored. See also Kornel, Kornelius, Nelek.
Carnelius, Conny, Cornealous, Corneili, Corneilius, Corneilus, Corneliaus, Cornelious, Cornelias, Cornelis, Corneliu, Cornell, Cornellious, Cornellis, Cornellius, Cornelous, Corneluis, Cornelus, Corney, Cornie, Cornielius, Corniellus, Corny, Cournelius, Cournelyous, Nelius, Nellie

Cornell (French) a form of Cornelius.
Carnell, Cornall, Corneil, Cornel, Cornelio, Corney, Cornie, Corny, Nellie

Cornwallis (English) from Cornwall.

Corona (Latin) crown.

Corrado (Italian) a form of Conrad.
Carrado

Corrigan (Irish) spearman.
Carrigan, Carrigen, Corrigon, Corrigun, Korrigan

Corrin (Irish) spear carrier.
Corin, Corion

Corry (Latin) a form of Corey.

Cort (German) bold. (Scandinavian) short. (English) a short form of Courtney.
Corte, Cortie, Corty, Kort

Cortez (Spanish) conqueror. History: Hernando Cortés was a Spanish conquistador who conquered Aztec Mexico.
Cartez, Cortes, Cortis, Cortize, Courtes, Courtez, Curtez, Kortez

Cortney GB (English) a form of Courtney.

Corwin (English) heart's companion; heart's delight.
Corwinn, Corwyn, Corwynn, Corwynne

Cory BG (Latin) a form of Corey. (French) a familiar form of Cornell. (Greek) a short form of Corydon.
Corye

Corydon (Greek) helmet, crest.
Coridon, Corradino, Cory, Coryden, Coryell

Cosgrove (Irish) victor, champion.

Cosimus (Italian) a form of Cosme.

Cosme (Greek) a form of Cosmo.

Cosmo (Greek) orderly; harmonious; universe.
Cos, Cosimo, Cosme, Cosmé, Cozmo, Kosmo

Costa (Greek) a short form of Constantine.
Costandinos, Costantinos, Costas, Costes

Coty BG (French) slope, hillside.
Cote, Cotee, Cotey, Coti, Cotie, Cotty, Cotye

Courtland (English) court's land.
Court, Courtlan, Courtlana, Courtlandt, Courtlin, Courtlind, Courtlon, Courtlyn, Kourtland

Courtney GB (English) court.
Cort, Cortnay, Cortne, Cortney, Court, Courten, Courtenay, Courteney, Courtnay, Courtnee, Curt, Kortney

Cowan (Irish) hillside hollow.
Coe, Coven, Covin, Cowen, Cowey, Cowie

Coy (English) woods.
Coye, Coyie, Coyt

Coyahue (Mapuche) meeting place for speaking and debating.

Coyle (Irish) leader in battle.

Coyne (French) modest.
Coyan

Craddock (Welsh) love.
Caradoc, Caradog

Craig BG (Irish, Scottish) crag; steep rock.
Crag, Craige, Craigen, Craigery, Craigh, Craigon, Creag, Creg, Cregan, Cregg, Creig, Creigh, Criag, Kraig

Crandall (English) crane's valley.
Cran, Crandal, Crandel, Crandell, Crendal

Crawford (English) ford where crows fly.
Craw, Crow, Ford

Creed (Latin) belief.
Creedon

Creighton (English) town near the rocks.
Cray, Crayton, Creighm, Creight, Creighto, Crichton

Crepin (French) a form of Crispin.

Crescencio (Latin) he who constantly increases his virtue.

Crescente (Latin) growing.

Cripín, Cripo (Latin) having curly hair.

Crisanto (Greek) golden flower.

Crisipo (Greek) golden horse.

Crisoforo (Greek) he who wears gold.

Crisóforo (Greek) he who gives advice that has value; his word is valuable.

Crisologo (Greek) he who says words that are like gold.

Crisólogo (Greek) he who gives advice that is as good as gold.

Crisostomo (Greek) mouth of gold.

Crisóstomo (Greek) he who gives valuable advice.

Crispin (Latin) curly haired.
Crepin, Cris, Crispian, Crispien, Crispino, Crispo, Krispin

Cristal GB (Latin) a form of Crystal.

Cristian BG (Greek) a form of Christian.
Crétien, Cristean, Cristhian, Cristiano, Cristien, Cristino, Cristle, Criston, Cristos, Cristy, Cristyan, Crystek, Crystian

Cristián (Latin) Christian, he who follows Christ.

Cristo (Greek) because of the Messiah.

Cristobal (Greek) a form of Christopher.
Cristóbal, Cristoval, Cristovao

Cristoforo (Italian) a form of Christopher.
Cristofor

Cristopher (Greek) a form of Christopher.
Cristaph, Cristhofer, Cristifer, Cristofer, Cristoph, Cristophe, Crystapher, Crystifer

Cristovo (Greek) Christ's servant.

Crofton (Irish) town with cottages.

Cromwell (English) crooked spring, winding spring.

Crosby (Scandinavian) shrine of the cross.
Crosbey, Crosbie, Cross

Crosley (English) meadow of the cross.
Cross

Crowther (English) fiddler.

Cruz BG (Portuguese, Spanish) cross.
Cruze, Kruz

Crystal GB (Latin) clear, brilliant glass.

Crystek (Polish) a form of Christian.

Cuarto (Spanish) born fourth.

Cuasimodo (Latin) he who is child-like.

Cuirpuma (Quechua) golden puma.

Cuiycui (Quechua) silver.

Cullen BG (Irish) handsome.
Cull, Cullan, Cullie, Cullin

Culley (Irish) woods.
Cullie, Cully

Culver (English) dove.
Colver, Cull, Cullie, Cully

Cuminao (Mapuche) crimson glow, the sun's last twinkle.

Cumya (Quechua) thunder, thundering; luminous.

Cunac (Quechua) he who counsels; counselor.

Cuñi (Quechua) warm.

Cunibaldo (Greek) of noble birth.

Cuniberto (Teutonic) he who stands apart from the other noble gentlemen because of his heritage.

Cuñiraya (Quechua) heat from the sun; he who has heat from the sun.

Cunningham (Irish) village of the milk pail.

Cuntur (Quechua) condor.

Cunturcanqui, Cunturchaua (Quechua) he who has all the virtues of a condor.

Cunturi (Aymara) representative of the gods; sent from the ancestral spirits.

Cunturpoma, Cunturpuma (Quechua) powerful as the puma and the condor.

Cunturuari (Quechua) untamable and savage like the vicuna and the condor.

Cunturumi (Quechua) strong as the stone and the condor.

Curamil (Mapuche) brilliant stone of gold and silver.

Curi (Quechua) golden.

Curiguaman (Quechua) golden falcon.

Curileo (Mapuche) black river.

Curiman (Mapuche) black condor.

Curiñaui (Quechua) he who has eyes that are the color and beauty of gold.

Curipan (Mapuche) leafy stinging nettle; furious puma.

Curran BG (Irish) hero.
Curan, Curon, Curr, Curren, Currey, Curri, Currie, Currin, Curry

Currito (Spanish) a form of Curtis.
Curcio

Curro (Spanish) polite or courteous.

Curt (Latin) a short form of Courtney, Curtis. See also Kurt.

Curtis BG (Latin) enclosure. (French) courteous. See also Kurtis.
Curio, Currito, Curt, Curtice, Curtiss, Curtus

Cusi (Quechua) happy, fortunate, prosperous man who is always lucky in all that he does.

Cusiguaman (Quechua) happy falcon.

Cusiguaypa (Quechua) happy rooster; creator of joyous things.

Cusiñaui (Quechua) smiling, with happy eyes.

Cusipoma, Cusipuma (Quechua) happy puma.

Cusirimachi (Quechua) he who fills us with happy words.

Cusiyupanqui (Quechua) honored and fortunate.

Custodio (Latin) guardian spirit, guardian angel.

Cuthbert (English) brilliant.

Cutler (English) knife maker.
Cut, Cuttie, Cutty

Cutmano (Anglo Saxon) man who is famous.

Cuycusi (Quechua) he who moves happily.

Cuyquiyuc (Quechua) he who is rich with silver.

D

Cuyuc (Quechua) he who moves; restless.

Cuyuchi (Quechua) he who makes us move.

Cy (Persian) a short form of Cyrus.

Cyle (Irish) a form of Kyle.

Cynthia 🇬🇧 (Greek) moon.

Cyprian (Latin) from the island of Cyprus.
Ciprian, Cipriano, Ciprien, Cyprien

Cyrano (Greek) from Cyrene, an ancient city in North Africa. Literature: *Cyrano de Bergerac* is a play by Edmond Rostand about a great guardsman and poet whose large nose prevented him from pursuing the woman he loved.

Cyril (Greek) lordly. See also Kiril.
Cerek, Cerel, Ceril, Ciril, Cirillo, Cirrillo, Cyra, Cyrel, Cyrell, Cyrelle, Cyrill, Cyrille, Cyrillus, Syrell, Syril

Cyrus (Persian) sun. Historical: Cyrus the Great was a king in ancient Persia. See also Kir.
Ciro, Cy, Cyress, Cyris, Cyriss, Cyruss, Syris, Syrus

D 🅱🇬 (American) an initial used as a first name.

D'andre 🅱🇬 (French) a form of Deandre.

Dabi (Basque) a form of David.

Dabir (Arabic) tutor.

Dacey 🇬🇧 (Latin) from Dacia, an area now in Romania. (Irish) southerner.
Dace, Dache, Dacian, Dacias, Dacio, Dacy, Daicey, Daicy

Dada (Yoruba) curly haired.
Dadi

Daegel (English) from Daegel, England.

Daelen (English) a form of Dale.
Daelan, Daelin, Daelon, Daelyn, Daelyne

Daemon (Greek) a form of Damian. (Greek, Latin) a form of Damon.
Daemean, Daemeon, Daemien, Daemin, Daemion, Daemyen

Daequan (American) a form of Daquan.
Daequane, Daequon, Daequone, Daeqwan

Daeshawn (American) a combination of the prefix Da + Shawn.
Daesean, Daeshaun, Daeshon, Daeshun, Daisean, Daishaun, Daishawn, Daishon, Daishoun

Daevon (American) a form of Davon.
Daevion, Daevohn, Daevonne, Daevonte, Daevontey

Dafydd (Welsh) a form of David.
Dafyd

Dag (Scandinavian) day; bright.
Daeg, Daegan, Dagen, Dagny, Deegan

Dagan (Hebrew) corn; grain.
Daegan, Daegon, Dagen, Dageon, Dagon

Dagoberto (Germanic) he who shines like the sun.

Dagwood (English) shining forest.

Dai **GB** (Japanese) big.

Daimian (Greek) a form of Damian.
Daiman, Daimean, Daimen, Daimeon, Daimeyon, Daimien, Daimin, Daimion, Daimyan

Daimon (Greek, Latin) a form of Damon.
Daimone

Daiquan (American) a form of Dajuan.
Daekwaun, Daekwon, Daiqone,

Daiqua, Daiquane, Daiquawn, Daiquon, Daiqwan, Daiqwon

Daivon (American) a form of Davon.
Daivain, Daivion, Daivonn, Daivonte, Daiwan

Dajon (American) a form of Dajuan.
Dajean, Dajiawn, Dajin, Dajion, Dajn, Dajohn, Dajonae

Dajuan (American) a combination of the prefix Da + Juan. See also Dejuan.
Daejon, Daejuan, Daiquan, Dajon, Da Jon, Da-Juan, Dajwan, Dajwoun, Dakuan, Dakwan, Dawan, Dawaun, Dawawn, Dawon, Dawoyan, Dijuan, Diuan, Dujuan, D'Juan, D'juan, Dwaun

Dakarai (Shona) happy.
Dakairi, Dakar, Dakaraia, Dakari, Dakarri

Dakoda (Dakota) a form of Dakota.
Dacoda, Dacodah, Dakodah, Dakodas

Dakota **BG** (Dakota) friend; partner; tribal name.
Dac, Dack, Dackota, Dacota, DaCota, Dak, Dakcota, Dakkota, Dakoata, Dakoda, Dakotah, Dakotha, Dakotta, Dekota

Dakotah **BG** (Dakota) a form of Dakota.
Dakottah

Daksh (Hindi) efficient.

Dalal (Sanskrit) broker.

Dalbert (English) bright, shining. See also Delbert.

Dale B️G (English) dale, valley.
Dael, Daelen, Dal, Dalen, Daley, Dalibor, Dallan, Dallin, Dallyn, Daly, Dayl, Dayle

Dalen (English) a form of Dale.
Dailin, Dalaan, Dalan, Dalane, Daleon, Dalian, Dalibor, Dalione, Dallan, Dalon, Daylan, Daylen, Daylin, Daylon

Daley (Irish) assembly. (English) a familiar form of Dale.
Daily, Daly, Dawley

Dallan (English) a form of Dale.
Dallen, Dallon

Dallas B️G (Scottish) valley of the water; resting place. Geography: a town in Scotland; a city in Texas.
Dal, Dalieass, Dall, Dalles, Dallis, Dalys, Dellis

Dallen B️G (English) a form of Dallan.

Dallin, Dallyn B️G (English) pride's people.
Dalin, Dalyn

Dalmacio (Latin) native of Dalmatia, the western part of the Balkans.

Dalmazio (Italian) a form of Dalmacio.

Dalmiro (Germanic) illustrious one because of his heritage.

Dalston (English) Daegel's place.
Dalis, Dallon

Dalton B️G (English) town in the valley.
Dal, Dalaton, Dallton, Dalt, Daltan, Dalten, Daltin, Daltyn, Daulton, Delton

Dalvin (English) a form of Delvin.
Dalven, Dalvon, Dalvyn

Dalziel (Scottish) small field.

Damar (American) a short form of Damarcus, Damario.
Damare, Damari, Damarre, Damauri

Damarcus (American) a combination of the prefix Da + Marcus.
Damacus, Damar, Damarco, Damarcue, Damarick, Damark, Damarkco, Damarkis, Damarko, Damarkus, Damarques, Damarquez, Damarquis, Damarrco

Damario (Greek) gentle. (American) a combination of the prefix Da + Mario.
Damar, Damarea, Damareus, Damaria, Damarie, Damarino, Damarion, Damarious, Damaris, Damarius, Damarrea, Damarrion, Damarrious, Damarrius, Damaryo, Dameris, Damerius

Damaris G️B (Greek, American) a form of Damario.

Damaso (Greek) skillful horse breaker.

Dámaso (Greek) skillful tamer.

Damek (Slavic) a form of Adam.
Damick, Damicke

Dameon (Greek) a form of
Damian.
Damein, Dameion, Dameone

Dametrius (Greek) a form of
Demetrius.
*Dametri, Dametries, Dametrious,
Damitri, Damitric, Damitrie,
Damitrious, Damitrius*

Damian BG (Greek) tamer;
soother.
*Daemon, Daimian, Damaiaon,
Damaian, Damaien, Damain,
Damaine, Damaion, Damani,
Damanni, Damaun, Damayon,
Dame, Damean, Dameon,
Damián, Damiane, Damiann,
Damiano, Damianos, Damien,
Damion, Damiyan, Damján,
Damyan, Daymian, Dema,
Demyan*

Damien BG (Greek) a form of
Damian. Religion: Father Damien
ministered to the leper colony on
the Hawaiian island Molokai.
*Daemien, Daimien, Damie,
Damienne, Damyen*

Damion (Greek) a form of
Damian.
*Damieon, Damiion, Damin,
Damine, Damionne, Damiyon,
Dammion, Damyon*

Damocles (Greek) gives glory to
his village.

Damon BG (Greek) constant,
loyal. (Latin) spirit, demon.
*Daemen, Daemon, Daemond,
Daimon, Daman, Damen,
Damond, Damone, Damoni,
Damonn, Damonni, Damonta,
Damontae, Damonte, Damontez,
Damontis, Damyn, Daymon,
Daymond*

Dan BG (Vietnamese) yes.
(Hebrew) a short form of Daniel.
Dahn, Danh, Danne

Dana GB (Scandinavian) from
Denmark.
Dain, Daina, Dayna

Dandin (Hindi) holy man.

Dandré (French) a combination
of the prefix De + André.
*D'André, Dandrae, D'andrea,
Dandras, Dandray, Dandre,
Dondrea*

Dane BG (English) from
Denmark. See also Halden.
*Dain, Daine, Danie, Dayne,
Dhane*

Danek (Polish) a form of Daniel.

Danforth (English) a form of
Daniel.

Danial (Hebrew) a form of
Daniel.
*Danal, Daneal, Danieal, Daniyal,
Dannial*

Danick, Dannick (Slavic)
familiar forms of Daniel.
*Danek, Danieko, Danik, Danika,
Danyck*

Daniel ☀ B☖ (Hebrew) God is
my judge. Bible: a Hebrew
prophet. See also Danno,
Kanaiela.
*Dacso, Dainel, Dan, Daneel,
Daneil, Danek, Danel, Danforth,
Danial, Danick, Dániel, Daniël,
Daniele, Danielius, Daniell,
Daniels, Danielson, Danilo,
Daniyel, Dan'l, Dannel, Dannick,
Danniel, Dannil, Danno, Danny,
Dano, Danukas, Dany, Danyel,
Danyell, Daoud, Dasco, Dayne,
Deniel, Doneal, Doniel, Donois,
Dusan, Nelo*

Daniele (Hebrew) a form of
Daniel.
Danile, Danniele

Danielle G☖ (Hebrew, French) a
form of Daniel

Danika G☖ (Slavic) a form of
Danick.

Danilo (Slavic) a form of Daniel.
*Danielo, Danil, Danila, Danilka,
Danylo*

Danior (Gypsy) born with teeth.

Danladi (Hausa) born on Sunday.

Danno (Hebrew) a familiar form
of Daniel. (Japanese) gathering
in the meadow.
Dannon, Dano

Dannon (American) a form of
Danno.
*Daenan, Daenen, Dainon,
Danaan, Danen, Danon*

Danny, Dany B☖ (Hebrew)
familiar forms of Daniel.
*Daney, Dani, Dannee, Danney,
Danni, Dannie, Dannye*

Dano (Czech) a form of Daniel.
Danko, Danno

Dante, Danté B☖ (Latin) lasting,
enduring.
*Danatay, Danaté, Dant, Dantae,
Dantay, Dantee, Dauntay,
Dauntaye, Daunté, Dauntrae,
Deante, Dontae, Donté*

Dantel (Latin) enduring.

Dantrell (American) a combi-
nation of Dante + Darell.
*Dantrel, Dantrey, Dantril,
Dantyrell, Dontrell*

Danyel G☖ (Hebrew) a form of
Daniel.
*Danya, Danyal, Danyale, Danyele,
Danyell, Danyiel, Danyl, Danyle,
Danylets, Danylo, Donyell*

Daoud (Arabic) a form of David.
Daudi, Daudy, Dauod, Dawud

Daquan (American) a combi-
nation of the prefix Da + Quan.
*Daequan, Daqon, Daquain,
Daquaine, Da'quan, Daquandre,
Daquandrey, Daquane, Daquann,
Daquantae, Daquante, Daquarius,
Daquaun, Daquawn, Daquin,
Daquon, Daquone, Daquwon,*

*Daqwain, Daqwan, Daqwane,
Daqwann, Daqwon, Daqwone,
Dayquan, Dequain, Dequan,
Dequann, Dequaun*

Dar (Hebrew) pearl.

Dara **GB** (Cambodian) stars.

Daran (Irish) a form of Darren.
*Darann, Darawn, Darian, Darran,
Dayran, Deran*

Darby **GB** (Irish) free. (English)
deer park.
*Dar, Darb, Darbee, Darbey,
Darbie, Derby*

Darcy **GB** (Irish) dark. (French)
from Arcy, France.
*Dar, Daray, D'Aray, Darce,
Darcee, Darcel, Darcey, Darcio,
D'Arcy, Darsey, Darsy*

Dardo (Greek) astute and skillful.

Dareh (Persian) wealthy.

Darell (English) a form of Darrell.
*Darall, Daralle, Dareal, Darel,
Darelle, Darral, Darrall*

Daren (Hausa) born at night.
(Irish, English) a form of Darren.
Dare, Dayren, Dheren

Darian, Darrian **BG** (Irish)
forms of Darren.
Daryan

Darick (German) a form of
Derek.
*Darek, Daric, Darico, Darieck,
Dariek, Darik, Daryk*

Darien, Darrien **BG** (Irish)
forms of Darren.

Darin **BG** (Irish) a form of Darren.
*Daryn, Darynn, Dayrin, Dearin,
Dharin*

Dario (Spanish) affluent.

Darío (Spanish) a form of Dario.

Darion, Darrion **BG** (Irish)
forms of Darren.
Daryeon, Daryon

Darius **BG** (Greek) wealthy.
*Dairus, Dare, Darieus, Darioush,
Dariuse, Dariush, Dariuss,
Dariusz, Darrius*

Darnell **BG** (English) hidden place.
*Dar, Darn, Darnall, Darneal,
Darneil, Darnel, Darnelle,
Darnyell, Darnyll*

Daron **BG** (Irish) a form of Darren.
*Daeron, Dairon, Darone, Daronn,
Darroun, Dayron, Dearon, Dharon,
Diron*

Darrell **BG** (French) darling,
beloved; grove of oak trees.
*Dare, Darel, Darell, Darral, Darrel,
Darrill, Darrol, Darryl, Derrell*

Darren **BG** (Irish) great.
(English) small; rocky hill.
*Daran, Dare, Daren, Darian,
Darien, Darin, Darion, Daron,
Darran, Darrian, Darrien,
Darrience, Darrin, Darrion,
Darron, Darryn, Darun, Daryn,
Dearron, Deren, Dereon, Derren,
Derron*

Darrick (German) a form of Derek.
Darrec, Darrek, Darric, Darrik, Darryk

Darrin (Irish) a form of Darren.

Darrion 🅱🅶 (Irish) a form of Darren.
Dairean, Dairion, Darian, Darien, Darion, Darrian, Darrien, Darrione, Darriyun, Derrian, Derrion

Darrius (Greek) a form of Darius.
Darreus, Darrias, Darrious, Darris, Darriuss, Darrus, Darryus, Derrious, Derris, Derrius

Darron (Irish) a form of Darren.
Darriun, Darroun

Darryl 🅱🅶 (French) darling, beloved; grove of oak trees. A form of Darrell.
Dahrll, Darryle, Darryll, Daryl, Daryle, Daryll, Derryl

Darshan (Hindi) god; godlike. Religion: another name for the Hindu god Shiva.
Darshaun, Darshon

Darton (English) deer town.
Dartel, Dartrel

Darwin (English) dear friend. History: Charles Darwin was the British naturalist who established the theory of evolution.
Darvin, Darvon, Darwyn, Derwin, Derwynn, Durwin

Daryl 🅱🅶 (French) a form of Darryl.
Darel, Daril, Darl, Darly, Daryell, Daryle, Daryll, Darylle, Daroyl

Dasan (Pomo) leader of the bird clan.
Dassan

Dashawn 🅱🅶 (American) a combination of the prefix Da + Shawn.
Dasean, Dashan, Dashane, Dashante, Dashaun, Dashaunte, Dashean, Dashon, Dashonnie, Dashonte, Dashuan, Dashun, Dashwan, Dayshawn

Dativo (Latin) term from Roman law, which is applied to educators.

Dato (Latin) a form of Donato.

Dauid (Swahili) a form of David.

Daulton (English) a form of Dalton.

Davante (American) a form of Davonte.
Davanta, Davantay, Davinte

Davaris (American) a combination of Dave + Darius.
Davario, Davarious, Davarius, Davarrius, Davarus

Dave 🅱🅶 (Hebrew) a short form of David, Davis.

Davey (Hebrew) a familiar form of David.
Davee, Davi, Davie, Davy

David ☀ BG (Hebrew) beloved.
Bible: the second king of Israel.
See also Dov, Havika, Kawika,
Taaveti, Taffy, Tevel.
*Dabi, Daevid, Dafydd, Dai, Daivid,
Daoud, Dauid, Dav, Dave, Daved,
Daveed, Daven, Davey, Davidde,
Davide, Davidek, Davido, Davon,
Davoud, Davyd, Dawid, Dawit,
Dawud, Dayvid, Dodya, Dov*

Davin BG (Scandinavian) brilliant
Finn.
*Daevin, Davion, Davon, Davyn,
Dawan, Dawin, Dawine, Dayvon,
Deavan, Deaven*

Davion BG (American) a form of
Davin.
*Davione, Davionne, Daviyon,
Davyon, Deaveon*

Davis BG (Welsh) son of David.
Dave, Davidson, Davies, Davison

Davon BG (American) a form of
Davin.
*Daevon, Daivon, Davon, Davone,
Davonn, Davonne, Deavon,
Deavone, Devon*

Davonte BG (American) a combi-
nation of Davon + the suffix Te.
*Davante, Davonnte, Davonta,
Davontae, Davontah, Davontai,
Davontay, Davontaye, Davontea,
Davontee, Davonti*

Dawan (American) a form of
Davin.
*Dawann, Dawante, Dawaun,
Dawayne, Dawon, Dawone,
Dawoon, Dawyne, Dawyun*

Dawit (Ethiopian) a form of
David.

Dawn GB (English) sunrise, dawn.

Dawson BG (English) son of
David.
Dawsyn

Dax (French, English) water.

Day (English) a form of Daniel.

Daylon (American) a form of
Dillon.
*Daylan, Daylen, Daylin, Daylun,
Daylyn*

Daymian (Greek) a form of
Damian.
*Daymayne, Daymen, Daymeon,
Daymiane, Daymien, Daymin,
Dayminn, Daymion, Daymn*

Dayne (Scandinavian) a form of
Dane.
Dayn

Dayquan (American) a form of
Daquan.
*Dayquain, Dayquawane, Dayquin,
Dayqwan*

Dayshawn (American) a form of
Dashawn.
*Daysean, Daysen, Dayshaun,
Dayshon, Dayson*

Dayton BG (English) day town;
bright, sunny town.
*Daeton, Daiton, Daythan,
Daython, Daytona, Daytonn,
Deyton*

Dayvon (American) a form of Davin.
Dayven, Dayveon, Dayvin, Dayvion, Dayvonn

De 🅱🅶 (Chinese) virtuous.

Deacon (Greek) one who serves.
Deke

Dean 🅱🅶 (French) leader. (English) valley. See also Dino.
Deane, Deen, Dene, Deyn, Deyne

Deana 🅶🅱 (Latin) divine. (English) valley.

Deandre 🅱🅶 (French) a combination of the prefix De + André.
D'andre, D'andré, D'André, D'andrea, Deandra, Deandrae, Déandre, Deandré, De André, Deandrea, De Andrea, Deandres, Deandrey, Deaundera, Deaundra, Deaundray, Deaundre, De Aundre, Deaundrey, Deaundry, Deondre, Diandre, Dondre

Deangelo (Italian) a combination of the prefix De + Angelo.
Dang, Dangelo, D'Angelo, Danglo, Deaengelo, Deangelio, Deangello, Déangelo, De Angelo, Deangilio, Deangleo, Deanglo, Deangulo, Diangelo, Di'angelo

Deanna 🅶🅱 (Latin) a form of Deana, Diana.

Deante (Latin) a form of Dante.
Deanta, Deantai, Deantay, Deanté, De Anté, Deanteé,

Deaunta, Diantae, Diante, Diantey

Deanthony (Italian) a combination of the prefix De + Anthony.
D'anthony, Danton, Dianthony

Dearborn (English) deer brook.
Dearbourn, Dearburne, Deaurburn, Deerborn

Deborah 🅶🅱 (Hebrew) bee.

Decarlos (Spanish) a combination of the prefix De + Carlos.
Dacarlos, Decarlo, Di'carlos

Decha (Tai) strong.

Decimus (Latin) tenth.

Decio (Latin) tenth.

Declan (Irish) man of prayer. Religion: Saint Declan was a fifth-century Irish bishop.
Deklan

Decoroso (Latin) he is well; he is practical.

Dédalo (Greek) industrious and skillful artisan.

Dedrick (German) ruler of the people. See also Derek, Theodoric.
Deadrick, Deddrick, Dederick, Dedrek, Dedreko, Dedric, Dedrix, Dedrrick, Deedrick, Diedrich, Diedrick, Dietrich, Detrick

Deems (English) judge's child.

Deicola (Latin) he who cultivates a relationship with God.

Deion **BG** (Greek) a form of Dion.
Deione, Deionta, Deionte

Deja **GB** (French) a form of Déja (see Girls' Names).

Dejuan (American) a combination of the prefix De + Juan. See also Dajuan.
Dejan, Dejon, Dejuane, Dejun, Dewan, Dewaun, Dewon, Dijaun, Djuan, D'Juan, Dujuan, Dujuane, D'Won

Dekel (Hebrew, Arabic) palm tree, date tree.

Dekota (Dakota) a form of Dakota.
Decoda, Dekoda, Dekodda, Dekotes

Del (English) a short form of Delbert, Delvin, Delwin.

Delaney **GB** (Irish) descendant of the challenger.
Delaine, Delainey, Delainy, Delan, Delane, Delanny, Delany

Delano (French) nut tree. (Irish) dark.
Delanio, Delayno, Dellano

Delbert (English) bright as day. See also Dalbert.
Bert, Del, Dilbert

Delfín (Greek) playful one with a graceful and beautiful form.

Delfino (Latin) dolphin.
Delfine

Déli (Chinese) virtuous.

Dell (English) small valley. A short form of Udell.

Delling (Scandinavian) scintillating.

Delmar (Latin) sea.
Dalmar, Dalmer, Delmare, Delmario, Delmarr, Delmer, Delmor, Delmore

Delon (American) a form of Dillon.
Deloin, Delone, Deloni, Delonne

Delphine **GB** (Greek) from Delphi, Greece.

Delroy (French) belonging to the king. See also Elroy, Leroy.
Delray, Delree, Delroi

Delshawn (American) a combination of Del + Shawn.
Delsean, Delshon, Delsin, Delson

Delsin (Native American) he is so.
Delsy

Delton (English) a form of Dalton.
Delten, Deltyn

Delvin (English) proud friend; friend from the valley.
Dalvin, Del, Delavan, Delvian, Delvon, Delvyn, Delwin

Delwin (English) a form of Delvin.
Dalwin, Dalwyn, Del, Dellwin, Dellwyn, Delwyn, Delwynn

Deman (Dutch) man.

Demarco (Italian) a combination of the prefix De + Marco.
Damarco, Demarcco, Demarceo, Demarcio, Demarkco, Demarkeo, Demarko, Demarquo, D'Marco

Demarcus (American) a combination of the prefix De + Marcus.
Damarcius, Damarcus, Demarces, Demarcis, Demarcius, Demarcos, Demarcuse, Demarkes, Demarkis, Demarkos, Demarkus, Demarqus, D'Marcus

Demario (Italian) a combination of the prefix De + Mario.
Demarea, Demaree, Demareo, Demari, Demaria, Demariea, Demarion, Demarreio, Demariez, Demarious, Demaris, Demariuz, Demarrio, Demerio, Demerrio

Demarius (American) a combination of the prefix De + Marius.

Demarquis (American) a combination of the prefix De + Marquis.
Demarques, Demarquez, Demarqui

Dembe (Luganda) peaceful.
Damba

Demetri, Demitri (Greek) short forms of Demetrius.
Dametri, Damitré, Demeter, Demetre, Demetrea, Demetriel, Demitre, Demitrie, Domotor

Demetria GB (Greek) cover of the earth.

Demetris (Greek) a short form of Demetrius.
Demeatric, Demeatrice, Demeatris, Demetres, Demetress, Demetric, Demetrice, Demetrick, Demetrics, Demetricus, Demetrik, Demitrez, Demitries, Demitris

Demetrius BG (Greek) lover of the earth. Mythology: a follower of Demeter, the goddess of the harvest. See also Dimitri, Mimis, Mitsos.
Dametrius, Demeitrius, Demeterious, Demetreus, Demetri, Demetrias, Demetrio, Demetrios, Demetrious, Demetris, Demetriu, Demetrium, Demetrois, Demetruis, Demetrus, Demitirus, Demitri, Demitrias, Demitriu, Demitrius, Demitrus, Demtrius, Demtrus, Dimitri, Dimitrios, Dimitrius, Dmetrius, Dymek

Demian (Greek) he who emerged from the village.

Demián (Spanish) a form of Demian.

Demichael (American) a combination of the prefix De + Michael.
Dumichael

Demócrito (Greek) chosen by the villagers to be judge; the arbiter of the village.

Demond (Irish) a short form of Desmond.
Demonde, Demonds, Demone, Dumonde

Demont (French) mountain.
Démont, Demonta, Demontae, Demontay, Demontaz, Demonte, Demontez, Demontre

Demorris (American) a combination of the prefix De + Morris.
Demoris, DeMorris, Demorus

Demos (Greek) people.
Demas, Demosthenes

Demóstenes (Greek) strength of the village.

Demothi (Native American) talks while walking.

Dempsey (Irish) proud.
Demp, Demps, Dempsie, Dempsy

Dempster (English) one who judges.
Demster

Denby (Scandinavian) Geography: a Danish village.
Danby, Den, Denbey, Denney, Dennie, Denny

Denham (English) village in the valley.

Denholm (Scottish) Geography: a town in Scotland.

Denis **BG** (Greek) a form of Dennis.
Deniz

Denise **GB** (Greek) a form of Denis.

Denley (English) meadow; valley.
Denlie, Denly

Denman (English) man from the valley.

Dennis **BG** (Greek) Mythology: a follower of Dionysus, the god of wine. See also Dion, Nicho.
Den, Dénes, Denies, Denis, Deniz, Dennes, Dennet, Dennez, Denny, Dennys, Denya, Denys, Deon, Dinis

Dennison (English) son of Dennis. See also Dyson, Tennyson.
Den, Denison, Denisson, Dennyson

Denny (Greek) a familiar form of Dennis.
Den, Denney, Dennie, Deny

Denton (English) happy home.
Dent, Denten, Dentin

Denver **BG** (English) green valley. Geography: the capital of Colorado.

Denzel **BG** (Cornish) a form of Denzell.
Danzel, Dennzel, Denzal, Denzale, Denzall, Denzell, Denzelle, Denzle, Denzsel

Denzell (Cornish) Geography: a location in Cornwall, England.
Dennzil, Dennzyl, Denzel, Denzial, Denziel, Denzil, Denzill, Denzyel, Denzyl, Donzell

Deodato (Latin) he who serves
God.

Deon B G (Greek) a form of
Dennis. See also Dion.
Deion, Deone, Deonn, Deonno

Deondre (French) a form of
Deandre.
*Deiondray, Deiondre, Deondra,
Deondrae, Deondray, Deondré,
Deondrea, Deondree, Deondrei,
Deondrey, Diondra, Diondrae,
Diondre, Diondrey*

Deontae (American) a
combination of the prefix De +
Dontae.
*Deonta, Deontai, Deontay,
Deontaye, Deonte, Deonté,
Deontea, Deonteya, Deonteye,
Deontia, Dionte*

Deonte, Deonté B G (American)
forms of Deontae.
*D'Ante, Deante, Deontée,
Deontie*

Deontre (American) a form of
Deontae.
*Deontrae, Deontrais, Deontray,
Deontrea, Deontrey, Deontrez,
Deontreze, Deontrus*

Dequan (American) a
combination of the prefix De +
Quan.
*Dequain, Dequane, Dequann,
Dequante, Dequantez, Dequantis,
Dequaun, Dequavius, Dequawn,
Dequian, Dequin, Dequine,
Dequinn, Dequion, Dequoin,*

*Dequon, Dequwan, Deqwon,
Deqwone*

Dereck, Derick (German) forms
of Derek.
*Derekk, Dericka, Derico, Deriek,
Derique, Deryck, Deryk, Deryke,
Detrek*

Derek B G (German) a short form
of Theodoric. See also Dedrick,
Dirk.
*Darek, Darick, Darrick, Derak,
Dereck, Derecke, Derele, Deric,
Derick, Derik, Derk, Derke,
Derrek, Derrick, Deryek*

Deric, Derik (German) forms of
Derek.
Deriek, Derikk

Dermot (Irish) free from envy.
(English) free. (Hebrew) a short
form of Jeremiah. See also
Kermit.
*Der, Dermod, Dermott, Diarmid,
Diarmuid*

Deron (Hebrew) bird; freedom.
(American) a combination of the
prefix De + Ron.
*Daaron, Daron, Da-Ron, Darone,
Darron, Dayron, Dereon, Deronn,
Deronne, Derrin, Derrion, Derron,
Derronn, Derronne, Derryn, Diron,
Duron, Durron, Dyron*

Deror (Hebrew) lover of freedom.
Derori, Derorie

Derrek (German) a form of
Derek.
Derrec, Derreck

Derrell (French) a form of Darrell.
Derel, Derele, Derell, Derelle, Derrel, Dérrell, Derriel, Derril, Derrill, Deryl, Deryll

Derren (Irish, English) a form of Darren.
Deren, Derran, Derraun, Derreon, Derrian, Derrien, Derrin, Derrion, Derron, Derryn, Deryan, Deryn, Deryon

Derrick BG (German) ruler of the people. A form of Derek.
Derric, Derrik, Derryck, Derryk

Derry BG (Irish) redhead. Geography: a city in Northern Ireland.
Darrie, Darry, Derri, Derrie, Derrye, Dery

Derryl (French) a form of Darryl.
Deryl, Deryll

Derward (English) deer keeper.

Derwin (English) a form of Darwin.
Derwyn

Desean (American) a combination of the prefix De + Sean.
Dasean, D'Sean, Dusean

Deshane (American) a combination of the prefix De + Shane.
Deshan, Deshayne

Deshaun (American) a combination of the prefix De + Shaun.
Deshan, Deshane, Deshann, Deshaon, Deshaune, D'shaun, D'Shaun, Dushaun

Deshawn BG (American) a combination of the prefix De + Shawn.
Dashaun, Dashawn, Deshauwn, Deshawan, Deshawon, Deshon, D'shawn, D'Shawn, Dushan, Dushawn

Deshea (American) a combination of the prefix De + Shea.
Deshay

Déshì (Chinese) virtuous.

Deshon (American) a form of Deshawn.
Deshondre, Deshone, Deshonn, Deshonte, Deshun, Deshunn

Desiderato (Latin) he who is desired.

Desiderio (Spanish) desired.

Desiderius (German) a form of Desiderio.

Desmond (Irish) from south Munster.
Demond, Des, Desi, Desimon, Desman, Desmand, Desmane, Desmen, Desmine, Desmon, Desmound, Desmund, Desmyn, Dezmon, Dezmond

Destin BG (French) destiny, fate.
Destan, Desten, Destine, Deston, Destry, Destyn

Destiny GB (French) fate.

Destry (American) a form of
Destin.
Destrey, Destrie

Detrick (German) a form of
Dedrick.
*Detrek, Detric, Detrich, Detrik,
Detrix*

Devan 🅱🅶 (Irish) a form of
Devin.
*Devaan, Devain, Devane, Devann,
Devean, Devun, Diwan*

Devante (American) a
combination of Devan + the
suffix Te.
*Devanta, Devantae, Devantay,
Devanté, Devantée, Devantez,
Devanty, Devaughntae,
Devaughnte, Devaunte,
Deventae, Deventay, Devente,
Divante*

Devaughn (American) a form of
Devin.
Devaugh, Devaun

Devayne (American) a form of
Dewayne.
*Devain, Devaine, Devan, Devane,
Devayn, Devein, Deveion*

Deven 🅱🅶 (Hindi) for God.
(Irish) a form of Devin.
*Deaven, Deiven, Devein, Devenn,
Devven, Diven*

Deverell (English) riverbank.

Devin ☆ 🅱🅶 (Irish) poet.
*Deavin, Deivin, Dev, Devan,
Devaughn, Deven, Devlyn, Devon,
Devvin, Devy, Devyn, Dyvon*

Devine (Latin) divine. (Irish) ox.
*Davon, Devinn, Devon, Devyn,
Devyne, Dewine*

Devlin (Irish) brave, fierce.
*Dev, Devlan, Devland, Devlen,
Devlon, Devlyn*

Devon 🅱🅶 (Irish) a form of
Devin.
*Deavon, Deivon, Deivone,
Deivonne, Deveon, Deveone,
Devion, Devoen, Devohn,
Devonae, Devone, Devoni,
Devonio, Devonn, Devonne,
Devontaine, Devvon, Devvonne,
Dewon, Dewone, Divon, Diwon*

Devonta 🅱🅶 (American) a
combination of Devon + the
suffix Ta.
*Deveonta, Devonnta, Devonntae,
Devontae, Devontai, Devontay,
Devontaye*

Devonte 🅱🅶 (American) a
combination of Devon + the
suffix Te.
*Deveonte, Devionte, Devonté,
Devontea, Devontee, Devonti,
Devontia, Devontre*

Devyn 🅱🅶 (Irish) a form of Devin.
Devyin, Devynn, Devynne

Dewayne (Irish) a form of
Dwayne. (American) a
combination of the prefix De +
Wayne.
*Deuwayne, Devayne, Dewain,
Dewaine, Dewan, Dewane,
Dewaun, Dewaune, Dewayen,
Dewean, Dewon, Dewune*

Dewei (Chinese) highly virtuous.

Dewey (Welsh) prized.
Dew, Dewi, Dewie

DeWitt (Flemish) blond.
Dewitt, Dwight, Wit

Dexter (Latin) dexterous, adroit.
(English) fabric dyer.
Daxter, Decca, Deck, Decka,
Dekka, Dex, Dextar, Dextor,
Dextrel, Dextron

Dezmon, Dezmond (Irish) forms
of Desmond.
Dezman, Dezmand, Dezmen,
Dezmin

Diamond **GB** (English) brilliant
gem; bright guardian.
Diaman, Diamanta, Diamante,
Diamend, Diamenn, Diamont,
Diamonta, Diamonte, Diamund,
Dimond, Dimonta, Dimontae,
Dimonte

Diana **GB** (Latin) divine.
Mythology: the goddess of the
hunt, the moon, and fertility.

Dick (German) a short form of
Frederick, Richard.
Dic, Dicken, Dickens, Dickie,
Dickon, Dicky, Dik

Dickran (Armenian) History: an
ancient Armenian king.
Dicran, Dikran

Dickson (English) son of Dick.
Dickenson, Dickerson, Dikerson,
Diksan

Diderot (Spanish) a form of
Desiderio.

Didi (Hebrew) a familiar form of
Jedidiah, Yedidyah.

Didier (French) desired, longed
for.

Didimo (Greek) twin brother.

Dídimo (Greek) identical twin
brother.

Diedrich (German) a form of
Dedrick, Dietrich.
Didrich, Didrick, Didrik, Diederick

Diego ☆ (Spanish) a form of
Jacob, James.
Iago, Diaz, Jago

Dietbald (German) a form of
Theobald.
Dietbalt, Dietbolt

Dieter (German) army of the
people.
Deiter

Dietrich (German) a form of
Dedrick.
Deitrich, Deitrick, Deke, Diedrich,
Dietrick, Dierck, Dieter, Dieterich,
Dieterick, Dietz

Digby (Irish) ditch town; dike
town.

Dillan **BG** (Irish) a form of Dillon.
Dilan, Dillian, Dilun, Dilyan

Dillon BG (Irish) loyal, faithful.
See also Dylan.
*Daylon, Delon, Dil, Dill, Dillan,
Dillen, Dillie, Dillin, Dillion, Dilly,
Dillyn, Dilon, Dilyn, Dilynn*

Dilwyn (Welsh) shady place.
Dillwyn

Dima (Russian) a familiar form of
Vladimir.
Dimka

Dimas (Greek) loyal comrade;
exemplary companion.

Dimitri BG (Russian) a form of
Demetrius.
*Dimetra, Dimetri, Dimetric,
Dimetrie, Dimitr, Dimitric,
Dimitrie, Dimitrik, Dimitris,
Dimitry, Dimmy, Dmitri, Dymitr,
Dymitry*

Dimitrios (Greek) a form of
Demetrius.
*Dhimitrios, Dimitrius, Dimos,
Dmitrios*

Dimitrius (Greek) a form of
Demetrius.
*Dimetrius, Dimitricus, Dimitrius,
Dimetrus, Dmitrius*

Dingbang (Chinese) protector of
the country.

Dinh (Vietnamese) calm, peaceful.
Din

Dinís (Greek) devoted to
Dionysus.

Dino (German) little sword.
(Italian) a form of Dean.
Deano

Dinos (Greek) a familiar form of
Constantine, Konstantin.

Dinsmore (Irish) fortified hill.
Dinnie, Dinny, Dinse

Diodoro (Greek) Mythology: the
grandson of Hercules who
brought to submission many
villages.

Diogenes (Greek) honest.
History: an ancient philosopher
who searched with a lantern in
daylight for an honest man.
Diogenese

Diógenes (Greek) a form of
Diogenes.

Diómedes (Greek) he who trusts
in God's protection.

Dion BG (Greek) a short form of
Dennis, Dionysus.
*Deion, Deon, Dio, Dione, Dionigi,
Dionis, Dionn, Dionne, Diontae,
Dionte, Diontray*

Dionisio (Greek) a form of
Dionysus.

Dionte (American) a form of
Deontae.
*Diante, Dionta, Diontae, Diontay,
Diontaye, Dionté, Diontea*

Dionysus (Greek) celebration.
Mythology: the god of wine.
Dion, Dionesios, Dionicio,

Dionisio, Dionisios, Dionusios, Dionysios, Dionysius, Dunixi

Dioscoro (Latin) he who is of the Lord.

Dióscoro (Greek) a form of Dioscoro.

Diquan (American) a combination of the prefix Di + Quan.
Diqawan, Diqawn, Diquane

Dirk (German) a short form of Derek, Theodoric.
Derk, Dirck, Dirke, Durc, Durk, Dyrk

Dixon (English) son of Dick.
Dickson, Dix

Dmitri (Russian) a form of Dimitri.
Dmetriy, Dmitiri, Dmitri, Dmitrik, Dmitriy

Doane (English) low, rolling hills.
Doan

Dob (English) a familiar form of Robert.
Dobie

Dobry (Polish) good.

Doherty (Irish) harmful.
Docherty, Dougherty, Douherty

Dolan (Irish) dark haired.
Dolin, Dolyn

Dolf, Dolph (German) short forms of Adolf, Adolph, Rudolf, Rudolph.
Dolfe, Dolfi, Dolphe, Dolphus

Dolores **GB** (Spanish) sorrowful.

Dom (Latin) a short form of Dominic.
Dome, Domó

Domenic **Bg** (Latin) an alternate form of Dominic.
Domanick, Domenick

Domenico (Italian) a form of Dominic.
Domenic, Domicio, Dominico, Menico

Domiciano (Spanish) a form of Domicio.

Domicio (Italian) a form of Domenico.

Domingo (Spanish) born on Sunday. See also Mingo.
Demingo, Domingos

Dominic ☀ **Bg** (Latin) belonging to the Lord. See also Chuminga.
Deco, Demenico, Dom, Domanic, Domeka, Domenic, Domenico, Domini, Dominie, Dominik, Dominique, Dominitric, Dominy, Domminic, Domnenique, Domokos, Domonic, Nick

Dominick **Bg** (Latin) a form of Dominic.
Domiku, Domineck, Dominick, Dominicke, Dominiek, Dominik, Dominnick, Dominyck, Domminick, Dommonick, Domnick, Domokos, Domonick, Donek, Dumin

Dominik (Latin) a form of Dominic.
Domenik, Dominiko, Dominyk, Domonik

Dominique 🇬🇧 (French) a form of Dominic.
Domeniq, Domeniqu, Domenique, Domenque, Dominiqu, Dominque, Dominiqueia, Domnenique, Domnique, Domoniqu, Domonique, Domunique

Dominque 🇧🇬 (French) a form of Dominique.

Domokos (Hungarian) a form of Dominic.
Dedo, Dome, Domek, Domok, Domonkos

Domonique 🇬🇧 (French) a form of Dominique.

Don 🇧🇬 (Scottish) a short form of Donald. See also Kona.
Donn

Donahue (Irish) dark warrior.
Donohoe, Donohue

Donal (Irish) a form of Donald.

Donald (Scottish) world leader; proud ruler. See also Bohdan, Tauno.
Don, Donal, Dónal, Donaldo, Donall, Donalt, Donát, Donaugh, Donnie

Donardo (Celtic) he who governs boldly.

Donatien (French) gift.
Donathan, Donathon

Donato (Italian) gift.
Dodek, Donatello, Donati, Donatien, Donatus

Donavan (Irish) a form of Donovan.
Donaven, Donavin, Donavon, Donavyn

Dondre (French) a form of Deandre.
Dondra, Dondrae, Dondray, Dondré, Dondrea

Dong (Vietnamese) easterner.
Duong

Donkor (Akan) humble.

Donnell 🇧🇬 (Irish) brave; dark.
Doneal, Donel, Donele, Donell, Donelle, Doniel, Donielle, Donnel, Donnele, Donnelle, Donnelly, Donniel, Donyel, Donyell

Donnelly (Irish) a form of Donnell.
Donelly, Donlee, Donley

Donnie, Donny 🇧🇬 (Irish) familiar forms of Donald.

Donovan (Irish) dark warrior.
Dohnovan, Donavan, Donevan, Donevon, Donivan, Donnivan, Donnovan, Donnoven, Donoven, Donovin, Donovon, Donvan

Dontae, Donté (American) forms of Dante.
Donta, Dontai, Dontao, Dontate, Dontavious, Dontavius, Dontay, Dontaye, Dontea, Dontee, Dontez

Donte BG (Latin) a form of Donata (see Girls' Names).

Dontrell BG (American) a form of Dantrell.
Dontral, Dontrall, Dontray, Dontre, Dontreal, Dontrel, Dontrelle, Dontriel, Dontriell

Donzell (Cornish) a form of Denzell.
Donzeil, Donzel, Donzelle, Donzello

Dooley (Irish) dark hero.
Dooly

Dor (Hebrew) generation.

Doran (Greek, Hebrew) gift. (Irish) stranger; exile.
Dore, Dorin, Dorran, Doron, Dorren, Dory

Dorian BG (Greek) from Doris, Greece. See also Isidore.
Dore, Dorey, Dorie, Dorien, Dorin, Dorion, Dorján, Doron, Dorrian, Dorrien, Dorrin, Dorrion, Dorron, Dorryen, Dory

Doroteo (Greek) gift of God.

Dorrell (Scottish) king's door-keeper. See also Durell.
Dorrel, Dorrelle

Dositeo (Greek) God's possession.

Dotan (Hebrew) law.
Dothan

Doug (Scottish) a short form of Dougal, Douglas.
Dougie, Dougy, Dugey, Dugie, Dugy

Dougal (Scottish) dark stranger. See also Doyle.
Doug, Dougall, Dugal, Dugald, Dugall, Dughall

Douglas BG (Scottish) dark river, dark stream. See also Koukalaka.
Doug, Douglass, Dougles, Dugaid, Dughlas

Dov (Yiddish) bear. (Hebrew) a familiar form of David.
Dovid, Dovidas, Dowid

Dovev (Hebrew) whisper.

Dow (Irish) dark haired.

Doyle (Irish) a form of Dougal.
Doy, Doyal, Doyel

Drago (Italian) a form of Drake.

Drake BG (English) dragon; owner of the inn with the dragon trademark.
Drago

Draper (English) fabric maker.
Dray, Draypr

Draven BG (American) a combination of the letter D + Raven.
Dravian, Dravin, Dravion, Dravon, Dravone, Dravyn, Drayven, Drevon

Dreng (Norwegian) hired hand; brave.

Dreshawn (American) a combination of Drew + Shawn.
Dreshaun, Dreshon, Dreshown

Drevon (American) a form of Draven.
Drevan, Drevaun, Dreven, Drevin, Drevion, Drevone

Drew B̄Ḡ (Welsh) wise. (English) a short form of Andrew.
Drewe, Dru

Dru (English) a form of Drew.
Druan, Drud, Drue, Drugi, Drui

Drummond (Scottish) druid's mountain.
Drummund, Drumond, Drumund

Drury (French) loving. Geography: Drury Lane is a street in London's theater district.

Dryden (English) dry valley.
Dry

Duane B̄Ḡ (Irish) a form of Dwayne.
Deune, Duain, Duaine, Duana

Duardo (Spanish) prosperous guardian.

Duarte (Portuguese) rich guard. See also Edward.

Duc (Vietnamese) moral.
Duoc, Duy

Dudd (English) a short form of Dudley.
Dud, Dudde, Duddy

Dudley (English) common field.
Dudd, Dudly

Duer (Scottish) heroic.

Duff (Scottish) dark.
Duffey, Duffie, Duffy

Dugan (Irish) dark.
Doogan, Dougan, Douggan, Duggan

Duilio (Latin) ready to fight.

Duke (French) leader; duke.
Dukey, Dukie, Duky

Dukker (Gypsy) fortuneteller.

Dulani (Nguni) cutting.

Dulcidio (Latin) sweet.

Dumaka (Ibo) helping hand.

Duman (Turkish) misty, smoky.

Duncan (Scottish) brown warrior. Literature: King Duncan was Macbeth's victim in Shakespeare's play *Macbeth*.
Dunc, Dunn

Dunham (Scottish) brown.

Dunixi (Basque) a form of Dionysus.

Dunley (English) hilly meadow.

Dunlop (Scottish) muddy hill.

Dunmore (Scottish) fortress on the hill.

Dunn (Scottish) a short form of Duncan.
Dun, Dune, Dunne

Dunstan (English) brownstone fortress.
Dun, Dunston

Dunton (English) hill town.

Dur (Hebrew) stacked up. (English) a short form of Durwin.

Durand (Latin) a form of Durant.

Durant (Latin) enduring.
Duran, Durance, Durand, Durante, Durontae, Durrant

Durell (Scottish, English) king's doorkeeper. See also Dorrell.
Durel, Durial, Durreil, Durrell, Durrelle

Durko (Czech) a form of George.

Durriken (Gypsy) fortuneteller.

Durril (Gypsy) gooseberry.
Durrel, Durrell

Durward (English) gatekeeper.
Dur, Ward

Durwin (English) a form of Darwin.

Dushawn (American) a combination of the prefix Du + Shawn.
Dusan, Dusean, Dushan, Dushane, Dushaun, Dushon, Dushun

Dustin BG (German) valiant fighter. (English) brown rock quarry.
Dust, Dustain, Dustan, Dusten, Dustie, Dustine, Dustion, Duston, Dusty, Dustyn, Dustynn

Dusty BG (English) a familiar form of Dustin.

Dustyn (English) a form of Dustin.

Dutch (Dutch) from the Netherlands; from Germany.

Duval (French) a combination of the prefix Du + Val.
Duvall, Duveuil

Dwaun (American) a form of Dajuan.
Dwan, Dwaunn, Dwawn, Dwon, Dwuann

Dwayne BG (Irish) dark. See also Dewayne.
Dawayne, Dawyne, Duane, Duwain, Duwan, Duwane, Duwayn, Duwayne, Dwain, Dwaine, Dwan, Dwane, Dwyane, Dywan, Dywane, Dywayne, Dywone

Dwight (English) a form of DeWitt.

Dyami (Native American) soaring eagle.

Dyer (English) fabric dyer.

Dyke (English) dike; ditch.
Dike

Dylan ☆ BG (Welsh) sea. See also Dillon.
Dylane, Dylann, Dylen, Dylian, Dylin, Dyllan, Dyllen, Dyllian, Dyllin, Dyllyn, Dylon, Dylyn

Dylon (Welsh) a form of Dylan.
Dyllion, Dyllon

Dyonis (German) a form of Dionisio.

Dyre (Norwegian) dear heart.

Dyson (English) a short form of Dennison.
Dysen, Dysonn

E [GB](American) an initial used as a first name.

Ea (Irish) a form of Hugh.

Eachan (Irish) horseman.

Eadberto (Teutonic) outstanding for his riches.

Eagan (Irish) very mighty.
Egan, Egon

Eamon (Irish) a form of Edmond, Edmund.
Aimon, Eammon, Eamonn

Ean (English) a form of Ian.
Eaen, Eann, Eayon, Eion, Eon, Eyan, Eyon

Earl (Irish) pledge. (English) nobleman.
Airle, Earld, Earle, Earlie, Earlson, Early, Eorl, Erl, Erle, Errol

Earnest (English) a form of Ernest.
Earn, Earnesto, Earnie, Eranest

Easton (English) eastern town.
Eason, Easten, Eastin, Eastton

Eaton (English) estate on the river.
Eatton, Eton, Eyton

Eb (Hebrew) a short form of Ebenezer.
Ebb, Ebbie, Ebby

Eben (Hebrew) rock.
Eban, Ebin, Ebon

Ebenezer (Hebrew) foundation stone. Literature: Ebenezer Scrooge is a miserly character in Charles Dickens's *A Christmas Carol*.
Eb, Ebbaneza, Eben, Ebeneezer, Ebeneser, Ebenezar, Eveneser

Eberhard (German) courageous as a boar. See also Everett.
Eber, Ebere, Eberardo, Eberhardt, Evard, Everard, Everardo, Everhardt, Everhart

Ebner (English) a form of Abner.

Ebo (Fante) born on Tuesday.

Ebony [GB] (Greek) a hard, dark wood.

Ecio (Latin) possessor of great strength.

Eco (Greek) sound, resonance.

Ed (English) a short form of
Edgar, Edsel, Edward.
Edd

Edan (Scottish) fire.
Edain

Edbert (English) wealthy; bright.
Ediberto

Edberto (Germanic) he whose
blade makes him shine.

Edco (Greek) he who blows with
force.

Eddie (English) a familiar form of
Edgar, Edsel, Edward.
Eddee, Eddy, Edi, Edie

Eddy BG (English) a form of
Eddie.
Eddye, Edy

Edel (German) noble.
Adel, Edell, Edelmar, Edelweiss

Edelberto (Teutonic) descendant
of nobles.

Edelio (Greek) person who
always remains young.

Edelmiro (Germanic) celebrated
for the nobility that he represents.

Eden GB (Hebrew) delightful.
Bible: the garden that was first
home to Adam and Eve.
*Eaden, Eadin, Edan, Edenson,
Edin, Edyn, Eiden*

Eder (Hebrew) flock.
Ederick, Edir

Edgar BG (English) successful
spearman. See also Garek, Gerik,
Medgar.
*Ed, Eddie, Edek, Edgard, Edgardo,
Edgars*

Edgardo (Spanish) a form of
Edgar.

Edilio (Greek) he who is like a
statue.

Edipo (Greek) he who has
swollen feet.

Edison (English) son of Edward.
Eddison, Edisen, Edson

Edmond (English) a form of
Edmund.
*Eamon, Edmon, Edmonde,
Edmondo, Edmondson, Esmond*

Edmund (English) prosperous
protector.
*Eadmund, Eamon, Edmand,
Edmaund, Edmond, Edmun,
Edmundo, Edmunds*

Edmundo (Spanish) a form of
Edmund.
Edmando, Mundo

Edo (Czech) a form of Edward.

Edoardo (Italian) a form of
Edward.

Edorta (Basque) a form of
Edward.

Edouard (French) a form of
Edward.
Édoard, Édouard

Edric (English) prosperous ruler.
*Eddric, Eddrick, Ederick, Edrek,
Edrice, Edrick, Edrico*

Edsel (English) rich man's house.
Ed, Eddie, Edsell

Edson (English) a short form of
Edison.
Eddson, Edsen

Eduardo 🅱🅶 (Spanish) a form of
Edward.
Estuardo, Estvardo

Edur (Basque) snow.

Edward (English) prosperous
guardian. See also Audie, Duarte,
Ekewaka, Ned, Ted, Teddy.
*Ed, Eddie, Edik, Edko, Edo,
Edoardo, Edorta, Édouard, Eduard,
Eduardo, Edus, Edvard, Edvardo,
Edwardo, Edwards, Edwy, Edzio,
Ekewaka, Etzio, Ewart*

Edwin 🅱🅶 (English) prosperous
friend. See also Ned, Ted.
*Eadwinn, Edik, Edlin, Eduino,
Edwan, Edwen, Edwon, Edwyn*

Efrain (Hebrew) fruitful.
*Efran, Efrane, Efrayin, Efren,
Efrian, Eifraine*

Efraín (Hebrew) a form of Efrain.

Efrat (Hebrew) honored.

Efreín, Efrén (Spanish) a form of
Efraín.

Efrem (Hebrew) a short form of
Ephraim.
Efe, Efraim, Efrim, Efrum

Efren (Hebrew) a form of Efrain,
Ephraim.

Egan (Irish) ardent, fiery.
Egann, Egen, Egon

Egbert (English) bright sword.
See also Bert, Bertie.

Egerton (English) Edgar's town.
*Edgarton, Edgartown, Edgerton,
Egeton*

Egidio (Greek) he who, in battle,
carries the goatskin sword.

Egil (Norwegian) awe inspiring.
Eigil

Eginhard (German) power of the
sword.
*Eginhardt, Einhard, Einhardt,
Enno*

Egisto (Greek) raised on goat's
milk.

Egon (German) formidable.

Egor (Russian) a form of George.
See also Igor, Yegor.

Ehren (German) honorable.

Eikki (Finnish) ever powerful.

Eileen 🅶🅱 (Irish) a form of
Helen.

Einar (Scandinavian) individualist.
Ejnar, Inar

Eion (Irish) a form of Ean, Ian.
Eann, Eian, Ein, Eine, Einn

Eitan (Hebrew) a form of Ethan.
Eita, Eithan, Eiton

Ejau (Ateso) we have received.

Ekewaka (Hawaiian) a form of Edward.

Ekon (Nigerian) strong.

Eladio (Greek) he who came from Greece.

Elam (Hebrew) highlands.

Elan (Hebrew) tree. (Native American) friendly.
Elann

Elbert (English) a form of Albert.
Elberto

Elbio (Celtic) he who comes from the mountain.

Elchanan (Hebrew) a form of John.
Elchan, Elchonon, Elhanan, Elhannan

Elden (English) a form of Alden, Aldous.
Eldan, Eldin

Elder (English) dweller near the elder trees.

Eldon (English) holy hill.

Eldred (English) a form of Aldred.
Eldrid

Eldridge (English) a form of Aldrich.
El, Eldred, Eldredge, Eldrege, Eldrid, Eldrige, Elric

Eldwin (English) a form of Aldwin.
Eldwinn, Eldwyn, Eldwynn

Eleanor GB (Greek) light.

Eleazar (Hebrew) God has helped. See also Lazarus.
Elazar, Elazaro, Eleasar, Eléazar, Eliazar, Eliezer

Eleazaro (Hebrew) God will help me.

Elek (Hungarian) a form of Alec, Alex.
Elec, Elic, Elik

Elenio (Greek) he who shines like the sun.

Eleodoro (Greek) he who comes from the sun.

Eleuterio (Greek) he who enjoys liberty for being honest.

Elger (German) a form of Alger.
Elger, Ellgar, Ellger

Elgin (English) noble; white.
Elgan, Elgen

Eli BG (Hebrew) uplifted. A short form of Elijah, Elisha. Bible: the high priest who trained the prophet Samuel. See also Elliot.
Elie, Elier, Ellie, Eloi, Eloy, Ely

Elia GB (Zuni) a short form of Elijah.
Eliah, Elio, Eliya, Elya

Elian (English) a form of Elijah. See also Trevelyan.
Elion

Elias (Greek) a form of Elijah.
Elia, Eliasz, Elice, Eliyas, Ellias, Ellice, Ellis, Elyas, Elyes

Elías (Hebrew) a form of Elias.

Eliazar (Hebrew) a form of Eleazar.
Eliasar, Eliazer, Elizar, Elizardo

Elido (Greek) native of Elida.

Elie (Hebrew) a form of Eli.

Eliecer (Hebrew) God is his constant aid.

Eliezer (Hebrew) a form of Eleazar.
Elieser

Eligio (Latin) he who has been elected by God.

Elihu (Hebrew) a short form of Eliyahu.
Elih, Eliu, Ellihu

Elijah ☀️ 🅱️🅶 (Hebrew) a form of Eliyahu. Bible: a Hebrew prophet. See also Eli, Elisha, Elliot, Ilias, Ilya.
El, Elia, Elian, Elias, Elija, Elijha, Elijiah, Elijio, Elijuah, Elijuo, Elisjsha, Eliya, Eliyah, Ellis

Elika (Hawaiian) a form of Eric.

Elisabeth 🅶🅱️ (Hebrew) a form of Elizabeth.

Elisandro (Greek) liberator of men.

Eliseo (Hebrew) a form of Elisha.
Elisee, Elisée, Elisei, Elisiah, Elisio

Elisha 🅱️🅶 (Hebrew) God is my salvation. Bible: a Hebrew

prophet, successor to Elijah. See also Eli, Elijah.
Elijsha, Eliseo, Elish, Elishah, Elisher, Elishia, Elishua, Elysha, Lisha

Eliyahu (Hebrew) the Lord is my God.
Eliyahou, Elihu

Elizabeth 🅶🅱️ (Hebrew) consecrated to God

Elkan (Hebrew) God is jealous.
Elkana, Elkanah, Elkin, Elkins

Elki (Moquelumnan) hanging over the top.

Ella 🅶🅱️ (English) elfin; beautiful. (Greek) a short form of Eleanor.

Ellard (German) sacred; brave.
Allard, Ellerd

Ellery (English) from a surname derived from the name Hilary.
Ellary, Ellerey

Ellie 🅶🅱️ (Hebrew) a form of Eli.

Elliot, Elliott 🅱️🅶 (English) forms of Eli, Elijah.
Elio, Eliot, Eliott, Eliud, Eliut, Elliotte, Elyot, Elyott

Ellis 🅱️🅶 (English) a form of Elias (see Boys' Names).
Elis

Ellison (English) son of Ellis.
Elison, Ellson, Ellyson, Elson

Ellsworth (English) nobleman's estate.
Ellswerth, Elsworth

Elman (German) like an elm tree.
Elmen

Elmer (English) noble; famous.
Aylmer, Elemér, Ellmer, Elmir, Elmo

Elmo (Greek) lovable, friendly.
(Italian) guardian. (Latin) a
familiar form of Anselm.
(English) a form of Elmer.

Elmore (English) moor where the
elm trees grow.

Elonzo (Spanish) a form of
Alonzo.
Elon, Élon, Elonso

Eloy (Latin) chosen.
Eloi

Elpidio (Greek) he who has
hopes.

Elrad (Hebrew) God rules.
Rad, Radd

Elroy (French) a form of Delroy,
Leroy.
Elroi

Elsdon (English) nobleman's hill.

Elston (English) noble's town.
Ellston

Elsu (Native American) swooping,
soaring falcon.

Elsworth (English) noble's estate.

Elton (English) old town.
*Alton, Eldon, Ellton, Elthon,
Eltonia*

Eluney (Mapuche) gift.

Elvern (Latin) a form of Alvern.
Elver, Elverne

Elvin (English) a form of Alvin.
El, Elvyn, Elwin, Elwyn, Elwynn

Elvio (Spanish) light skinned;
blond.

Elvis (Scandinavian) wise.
El, Elviz, Elvys

Elvy (English) elfin warrior.

Elwell (English) old well.

Elwood (English) old forest. See
also Wood, Woody.

Ely (Hebrew) a form of Eli.
Geography: a region of England
with extensive drained fens.
Elya, Elyie

Eman (Czech) a form of
Emmanuel.
Emaney, Emani

Emanuel Bg (Hebrew) a form of
Emmanuel.
*Emaniel, Emannual, Emannuel,
Emanual, Emanueal, Emanuele,
Emanuell, Emanuelle*

Emerenciano (Latin) to be
deserving, to acquire the rights to
something.

Emerson Bg (German, English)
son of Emery.
Emmerson, Emreson

Emery Bg (German) industrious
leader.
*Aimery, Emari, Emarri, Emeri,
Emerich, Emerio, Emmerich,*

Emmerie, Emmery, Emmo, Emory, Emrick, Emry, Inre, Imrich

Emesto (Spanish) serious.

Emeterio (Greek) he who deserves affection.

Emigdio (Greek) he who has brown skin.

Emil (Latin) flatterer. (German) industrious. See also Milko, Milo.
Aymil, Emiel, Émile, Emilek, Emiliano, Emilio, Emill, Emils, Emilyan, Emlyn

Emile 🅱🅶 (French) a form of Émile.

Émile (French) a form of Emil.
Emiel, Emile, Emille

Emiliano (Italian) a form of Emil.
Emilian, Emilion

Emilien (Latin) friendly; industrious.

Emilio 🅱🅶 (Italian, Spanish) a form of Emil.
Emielio, Emileo, Emilio, Emilios, Emillio, Emilo

Emillen (Latin) hard-working man.

Emily 🅶🅱 (Latin) flatterer. (German) industrious.

Emir (Arabic) chief, commander.

Emlyn (Welsh) waterfall.
Emelen, Emlen, Emlin

Emma 🅶🅱 (German) a short form of Emily.

Emmanuel 🅱🅶 (Hebrew) God is with us. See also Immanuel, Maco, Mango, Manuel.
Eman, Emanuel, Emanuell, Emek, Emmahnuel, Emmanel, Emmaneuol, Emmanle, Emmanual, Emmanueal, Emmanuele, Emmanuell, Emmanuelle, Emmanuil, Enmanuel

Emmanuelle 🅶🅱 (Hebrew) a form of Emmanuel.

Emmett (German) industrious; strong. (English) ant. History: Robert Emmett was an Irish patriot.
Em, Emet, Emett, Emitt, Emmet, Emmette, Emmitt, Emmot, Emmott, Emmy

Emmitt (German, English) a form of Emmett.
Emmit

Emory 🅱🅶 (German) a form of Emery.
Amory, Emmory, Emorye

Emre (Turkish) brother.
Emra, Emrah, Emreson

Emrick (German) a form of Emery.
Emeric, Emerick, Emric, Emrique, Emryk

Enapay (Sioux) brave appearance; he appears.

Endre (Hungarian) a form of Andrew.
Ender

Eneas (Greek) a form of Aeneas.
Eneias, Enné

Engelbert (German) bright as an angel. See also Ingelbert.
Bert, Englebert

Engelberto (Germanic) shining of the Anglos.

Enio (Spanish) second divinity of war.

Enli (Dene) that dog over there.

Ennis (Greek) mine. (Scottish) a form of Angus.
Eni, Enni

Enoch (Hebrew) dedicated, consecrated. Bible: the father of Methuselah.
Enoc, Enock, Enok

Enol (Asturian) referring to lake Enol.

Enon (Hebrew) very strong.

Enos (Hebrew) man.
Enosh

Enric (Romanian) a form of Henry.
Enrica

Enrick (Spanish) a form of Henry.
Enricky

Enrico (Italian) a form of Henry.
Enzio, Enzo, Rico

Enrikos (Greek) a form of Henry.

Enrique (Spanish) a form of Henry. See also Quiqui.
Enrigué, Enriqué, Enriquez, Enrrique

Enver (Turkish) bright; handsome.

Enyeto (Native American) walks like a bear.

Enzi (Swahili) powerful.

Eoin (Welsh) a form of Evan.

Ephraim (Hebrew) fruitful. Bible: the second son of Joseph.
Efraim, Efrayim, Efrem, Efren, Ephraen, Ephrain, Ephram, Ephrem, Ephriam

Epicuro (Greek) he who helps.

Epifanio (Greek) he who gives off brilliance because of his form.

Epimaco (Greek) easy to attack, easy to wipe out.

Epulef (Mapuche) two races, two quick trips.

Eraclio (Spanish) a form of Heraclio.

Erardo (Greek) he who is the guest of honor, to whom homage is paid.

Erasmus (Greek) lovable.
Érasme, Erasmo, Rasmus

Erastus (Greek) beloved.
Éraste, Erastious, Ras, Rastus

Erato (Greek) kind, pleasant.

Erbert (German) a short form of Herbert.
Ebert, Erberto

Ercole (Italian) splendid gift.

Erek (Scandinavian) a form of Eric.
Erec

Erhard (German) strong; resolute.
Erhardt, Erhart

Eri (Teutonic) vigilant.

Eriberto (Italian) a form of Herbert.
Erberto, Heriberto

Eric ☀ B̄Ḡ (Scandinavian) ruler of all. (English) brave ruler. (German) a short form of Frederick. History: Eric the Red was a Norwegian explorer who founded Greenland's first colony.
Aric, Ehrich, Elika, Erek, Éric, Ericc, Erich, Erick, Erico, Erik, Erikur, Erric, Eryc, Rick

Erica ḠB̄ (Scandinavian) a form of Eric.

Erich (Czech, German) a form of Eric.

Erick (English) a form of Eric.
Errick, Eryck

Erickson (English) son of Eric.
Erickzon, Erics, Ericson, Ericsson, Erikson, Erikzzon, Eriqson

Erik B̄Ḡ (Scandinavian) a form of Eric.
Erek, Erike, Eriks, Erikur, Errick, Errik, Eryk

Erika ḠB̄ (Scandanavian) a form of Erica.

Erikur (Icelandic) a form of Eric, Erik.

Erin ḠB̄ (Irish) peaceful. History: an ancient name for Ireland.
Erine, Erinn, Erino, Eron, Errin, Eryn, Erynn

Erland (English) nobleman's land.
Erlend

Erling (English) nobleman's son.

Ermanno (Italian) a form of Herman.
Erman

Ermano (Spanish) a form of Herman.
Ermin, Ermine, Erminio, Ermon

Ermelindo (Teutonic) offers sacrifices to God.

Ermino (Spanish) a form of Erminia (see Girls' names).

Erminoldo (Germanic) government of strength.

Ernest (English) earnest, sincere. See also Arno.
Earnest, Ernestino, Ernesto, Ernestus, Ernie, Erno, Ernst

Ernesto (Spanish) a form of Ernest.
Ernester, Neto

Ernie (English) a familiar form of Ernest.
Earnie, Erney, Erny

Erno (Hungarian) a form of Ernest.
Ernö

Ernst (German) a form of Ernest.
  Erns

Erol (Turkish) strong, courageous.
  Eroll

Eron (Irish) a form of Erin.
  Erran, Erren, Errion, Erron

Eros (Greek) love.

Errando (Basque) bold.

Errol (Latin) wanderer. (English)
  a form of Earl.
  Erol, Erold, Erroll, Erryl

Erroman (Basque) from Rome.

Erskine (Scottish) high cliff.
  (English) from Ireland.
  Ersin, Erskin, Kinny

Ervin, Erwin (English) sea friend.
  Forms of Irving, Irwin.
  *Earvin, Erv, Erven, Ervyn, Erwan,
  Erwinek, Erwinn, Erwyn, Erwynn*

Ervine (English) a form of Irving.
  Erv, Ervin, Ervince, Erving, Ervins

Ervino (Germanic) he who is
  consistent with honors.

Eryn GB (Irish) a form of Erin.

Esau (Hebrew) rough; hairy.
  Bible: Jacob's twin brother.
  Esaw

Esaú (Hebrew) a form of Esau.

Escipión (Latin) man who uses a
  cane.

Escolástico (Latin) man who
  teaches all that he knows.

Esculapio (Greek) doctor.

Esequiel (Hebrew) a form of
  Ezekiel.

Eshkol (Hebrew) grape clusters.

Eskil (Norwegian) god vessel.

Esleban (Hebrew) bearer of
  children.

Esmond (English) rich protector.

Esopo (Greek) he who brings
  good luck.

Espartaco (Greek) he who
  plants.

Espen (Danish) bear of the gods.

Essien (Ochi) sixth-born son.

Estanislao (Slavic) glory of his
  village.

Estanislau (Slavic) glory.

Este (Italian) east.
  Estes

Esteban (Spanish) crowned.

Estéban (Spanish) a form of
  Stephen.
  *Estabon, Esteben, Estefan,
  Estefano, Estefen, Estephan,
  Estephen*

Estebe (Basque) a form of
  Stephen.

Estevan (Spanish) a form of
  Stephen.
  Esteven, Estevon, Estiven

Estevao (Spanish) a form of Stephen.
Estevez

Estraton (Greek) man of the army.

Etelberto (Spanish) a form of Adalberto.

Eterio (Greek) as clean and pure as heaven.

Ethan ☀ BG (Hebrew) strong; firm.
Eathan, Eathen, Eathon, Eeathen, Eitan, Etan, Ethaen, Ethe, Ethen, Ethian

Etienne BG (French) a form of Stephen.

Étienne (French) a form of Stephen.
Etian, Etien, Étienn, Ettien

Ettore (Italian) steadfast.
Etor, Etore

Etu (Native American) sunny.

Eubulo (Greek) good counselor.

Eucario (Greek) gracious, generous.

Eucarpo (Greek) he who bears good fruit.

Euclid (Greek) intelligent. History: the founder of Euclidean geometry.

Eudoro (Greek) beautiful gift.

Eudoxio (Greek) good thought, he who is famous.

Eufemio (Greek) he who has a good reputation.

Eufrasio (Greek) he who uses words well, who is full of happiness.

Eufronio (Greek) having a good mind; he who makes others happy, who gives pleasure.

Eugen (German) a form of Eugene.

Eugene BG (Greek) born to nobility. See also Ewan, Gene, Gino, Iukini, Jenö, Yevgenyi, Zenda.
Eoghan, Eugen, Eugéne, Eugeni, Eugenio, Eugenius, Evgeny, Ezven

Eugenio (Spanish) a form of Eugene.

Eulalio (Greek) good speaker.

Eulises (Latin) a form of Ulysses.

Eulogio (Greek) he who speaks well.

Eumenio (Greek) opportune, favorable; the kind-hearted one.

Euniciano (Spanish) happy victory.

Euno (Greek) intellect, reason, understanding.

Eupilo (Greek) warmly welcomed.

Euprepio (Greek) decent, comfortable.

Eupsiquio (Greek) having a good soul; valiant.

Euquerio (Greek) sure handed.

Eurico (Germanic) prince to whom all pay homage.

Eusebio (Greek) with good feelings.

Eusiquio (Greek) a form of Eupsiquio.

Eustace (Greek) productive. (Latin) stable, calm. See also Stacey.
Eustache, Eustachius, Eustachy, Eustashe, Eustasius, Eustatius, Eustazio, Eustis, Eustiss

Eustacio, Eustasio (Greek) healthy and strong.

Eustaquio (Greek) he who has many heads of wheat.

Eustoquio (Greek) good marksman; a skillful man.

Eustorgio (Greek) well-loved.

Eustrato (Greek) good soldier.

Eutiquio (Greek) fortunate.

Eutrapio (Greek) returning; changing, transforming.

Eva GB (Greek) a short form of Evangelina. (Hebrew) a form of Eve (see Girls' Names).

Evan ☆ BG (Irish) young warrior. (English) a form of John. See also Bevan, Owen.
Eavan, Eoin, Ev, Evaine, Evann, Evans, Even, Evens, Evin, Evon, Evyn, Ewan, Ewen

Evando (Greek) he is considered a good man.

Evangelino (Greek) he who brings glad tidings.

Evangelos (Greek) a form of Andrew.
Evagelos, Evaggelos, Evangelo

Evaristo (Greek) excellent one.

Evelio (Hebrew) he who gives life.

Evelyn GB (English) hazelnut.
Evelin

Evencio (Latin) successful.

Everardo (German) strong as a boar.
Everado

Everett BG (English) a form of Eberhard.
Ev, Evered, Everet, Everette, Everhett, Everit, Everitt, Everrett, Evert, Evrett

Everley (English) boar meadow.
Everlea, Everlee

Everton (English) boar town.

Evgeny (Russian) a form of Eugene. See also Zhek.
Evgeni, Evgenij, Evgenyi

Evin (Irish) a form of Evan.
Evian, Evinn, Evins

Evodio (Greek) he who follows a good road.

Ewald (German) always powerful. (English) powerful lawman.

Ewan (Scottish) a form of Eugene, Evan. See also Keon.
Euan, Euann, Euen, Ewen, Ewhen

Ewert (English) ewe herder, shepherd.
Ewart

Ewing (English) friend of the law.
Ewin, Ewynn

Exavier (Basque) a form of Xavier.
Exaviar, Exavior, Ezavier

Exequiel (Hebrew) God is my strength.

Expedito (Latin) unencumbered, free of hindrances.

Exuperancio (Latin) he who is outstanding, excellent, superior.

Exuperio (Latin) he who exceeds expectations.

Eyota (Native American) great.

Ezekiel (Hebrew) strength of God. Bible: a Hebrew prophet. See also Haskel, Zeke.
Esequiel, Ezakeil, Ezéchiel, Ezeck, Ezeckiel, Ezeeckel, Ezekeial, Ezekeil, Ezekeyial, Ezekial, Ezekielle, Ezell, Ezequiel, Eziakah, Eziechiele

Ezequias (Hebrew) Yahweh is my strength.

Ezequías (Hebrew) one to whom God gave powers; the one has divine power.

Ezequiel (Hebrew) a form of Ezekiel.
Esequiel, Eziequel

Ezer (Hebrew) a form of Ezra.

Ezio (Latin) he who has a nose like an eagle.

Ezra BG (Hebrew) helper; strong. Bible: a Jewish priest who led the Jews back to Jerusalem.
Esdras, Esra, Ezer, Ezera, Ezrah, Ezri, Ezry

Ezven (Czech) a form of Eugene.
Esven, Esvin, Ezavin, Ezavine

Faber (German) a form of Fabian.

Fabian BG (Latin) bean grower.
Fabain, Fabayan, Fabe, Fabein, Fabek, Fabeon, Faber, Fabert, Fabi, Fabiano, Fabien, Fabin, Fabio, Fabion, Fabius, Fabiyan, Fabiyus, Fabyan, Fabyen, Faybian, Faybien

Fabián (Spanish) a form of Fabio.

Fabiano (Italian) a form of Fabian.
Fabianno, Fabio

Fabio (Latin) a form of Fabian. (Italian) a short form of Fabiano.
Fabbio

Fabrizio (Italian) craftsman.
Fabrice, Fabricio, Fabrizius

Fabron (French) little blacksmith; apprentice.
Fabre, Fabroni

Facundo (Latin) he who puts forth arguments that convince people.

Fadey (Ukrainian) a form of Thaddeus.
Faday, Faddei, Faddey, Faddy, Fade, Fadeyka, Fadie, Fady

Fadi (Arabic) redeemer.
Fadhi

Fadil (Arabic) generous.
Fadeel, Fadel

Fadrique (Spanish) a form of Federico.

Fagan (Irish) little fiery one.
Fagin

Fahd (Arabic) lynx.
Fahaad, Fahad

Fai (Chinese) beginning.

Fairfax (English) blond.
Fair, Fax

Faisal (Arabic) decisive.
Faisel, Faisil, Faisl, Faiyaz, Faiz, Faizal, Faize, Faizel, Faizi, Fasel, Fasil, Faysal, Fayzal, Fayzel

Faith **GB** (English) faithful; fidelity.

Fakhir (Arabic) excellent.
Fahkry, Fakher

Fakih (Arabic) thinker; reader of the Koran.

Falco (Latin) falconer.
Falcon, Falk, Falke, Falken

Falito (Italian) a familiar form of Rafael, Raphael.

Falkner (English) trainer of falcons. See also Falco.
Falconer, Falconner, Faulconer, Faulconner, Faulkner

Fallon **GB** (Irish) grandchild of the ruler.

Fane (English) joyful, glad.
Fanes, Faniel

Fantino (Latin) infant-like; innocent.

Fanuel (Hebrew) vision of God.

Faraji (Swahili) consolation.

Faraón (Egyptian) pharaoh; inhabitant of the grand palace.

Farid (Arabic) unique.

Faris (Arabic) horseman.
Faraz, Fares, Farhaz, Farice, Fariez, Farris

Farley (English) bull meadow; sheep meadow. See also Lee.
Fairlay, Fairlee, Fairleigh, Fairley, Fairlie, Far, Farlay, Farlee, Farleigh, Farlie, Farly, Farrleigh, Farrley

Farnell (English) fern-covered hill.
Farnall, Fernald, Fernall, Furnald

Farnham (English) field of ferns.
Farnam, Farnum, Fernham

Farnley (English) fern meadow.
*Farnlea, Farnlee, Farnleigh,
Farnly, Fernlea, Fernlee,
Fernleigh, Fernley*

Faro (Spanish) reference to the
card game faro.

Faroh (Latin) a form of Pharaoh.

Farold (English) mighty traveler.

Farquhar (Scottish) dear.
*Fark, Farq, Farquar, Farquarson,
Farque, Farquharson, Farquy,
Farqy*

Farr (English) traveler.
*Faer, Farran, Farren, Farrin,
Farrington, Farron*

Farrell (Irish) heroic;
courageous.
Farrel, Farrill, Farryll, Ferrell

Farrow (English) piglet.

Farruco (Spanish) a form of
Francis, Francisco.
Frascuelo

Faruq (Arabic) honest.
*Farook, Farooq, Faroque, Farouk,
Faruqh*

Faste (Norwegian) firm.

Fath (Arabic) victor.

Fatin (Arabic) clever.

Fauac (Quechua) he who flies.

Fauacuaipa (Quechua) rooster
in flight.

Faust (Latin) lucky, fortunate.
History: the sixteenth-century
German necromancer who
inspired many legends.
Faustino, Faustis, Fausto, Faustus

Faustiniano (Latin) a form of
Faustinus.

Faustino (Italian) a form of Faust.

Fausto (Italian) a form of Faust.

Favian (Latin) understanding.
Favain, Favio, Favyen

Faxon (German) long-haired.

Febe, Febo (Latin) he who
shines, who stands out.

Federico (Italian, Spanish) a
form of Frederick.
Federic, Federigo, Federoquito

Fedro (Greek) splendid man.

Feivel (Yiddish) God aids.

Feliks (Russian) a form of Felix.

Felipe 🅱🅶 (Spanish) a form of
Philip.
*Feeleep, Felipino, Felo, Filip,
Filippo, Filips, Fillip, Flip*

Felippo (Italian) a form of Philip.
*Felip, Filippo, Lipp, Lippo, Pip,
Pippo*

Felisardo (Latin) valiant and
skillful man.

Felix (Latin) fortunate; happy. See
also Pitin.
Fee, Felic, Félice, Feliciano,

Felicio, Felike, Feliks, Felo, Félix, Felizio, Phelix

Félix (Latin) a form of Felix.

Felton (English) field town.
Felten, Feltin

Fenton (English) marshland farm.
Fen, Fennie, Fenny, Fintan, Finton

Feo (Spanish) ugly.

Feodor (Slavic) a form of Theodore.
Dorek, Fedar, Fedinka, Fedor, Fedya, Fyodor

Feoras (Greek) smooth rock.

Ferdinand (German) daring, adventurous. See also Hernando.
Feranado, Ferd, Ferda, Ferdie, Ferdinánd, Ferdy, Ferdynand, Fernando, Nando

Ferenc (Hungarian) a form of Francis.
Feri, Ferke, Ferko

Fergus (Irish) strong; manly.
Fearghas, Fearghus, Feargus, Ferghus, Fergie, Ferguson, Fergusson

Fermin (French, Spanish) firm, strong.
Ferman, Firmin, Furman

Fermín (Spanish) a form of Fermin.

Fernán (Spanish) a form of Fernando.

Fernando (Spanish) a form of Ferdinand.
Ferando, Ferdinando, Ferdnando, Ferdo, Fernand, Fernandez, Fernendo

Feroz (Persian) fortunate.

Ferran (Arabic) baker.
Feran, Feron, Ferrin, Ferron

Ferrand (French) iron gray hair.
Farand, Farrand, Farrant, Ferrant

Ferrell (Irish) a form of Farrell.
Ferrel, Ferrill, Ferryl

Ferris (Irish) a form of Peter.
Fares, Faris, Fariz, Farris, Farrish, Feris, Ferriss

Feta-plom (Mapuche) high and large plain.

Fiacro (Latin) soldier, combatant.

Fico (Spanish) a familiar form of Frederick.

Fidel (Latin) faithful. History: Fidel Castro was the Cuban revolutionary who overthrew a dictatorship in 1959 and established a communist regime in Cuba.
Fidele, Fidèle, Fidelio, Fidelis, Fidell, Fido

Fidencio (Latin) trusting; fearless, self-assured.

Field (English) a short form of Fielding.
Fields

Fielding (English) field; field worker.
Field

Fife (Scottish) from Fife, Scotland.
Fyfe

Fifi GB (Fante) born on Friday.

Fil (Polish) a form of Phil.
Filipek

Filadelfo, Filademo (Greek) man who loves his brothers.

Filbert (English) brilliant. See also Bert.
Filberte, Filberto, Filiberto, Philbert

Fileas (Greek) he who loves deeply.

Filelio (Latin) he who is trustworthy.

Filemón (Greek) horse-lover; he who is spirited and friendly.

Filiberto (Spanish) a form of Filbert.

Filip (Greek) a form of Philip.
Filip, Filippo

Fillipp (Russian) a form of Philip.
Filip, Filipe, Filipek, Filips, Fill, Fillip, Filya

Filmore (English) famous.
Fillmore, Filmer, Fyllmer, Fylmer, Philmore

Filón (Greek) philosophical friend.

Filya (Russian) a form of Philip.

Fineas (Irish) a form of Phineas.
Finneas

Finian (Irish) light skinned; white.
Finnen, Finnian, Fionan, Fionn, Phinean

Finlay (Irish) blond-haired soldier.
Findlay, Findley, Finlea, Finlee, Finley, Finn, Finnlea, Finnley

Finn (German) from Finland. (Irish) blond haired; light skinned. A short form of Finlay. (Norwegian) from the Lapland.
Fin, Finnie, Finnis, Finny

Finnegan (Irish) light skinned; white.
Finegan

Fiorello (Italian) little flower.
Fiore

Firas (Arabic) persistent.

Firman (French) firm; strong.
Ferman, Firmin

Firmino (Latin) firm, sure.

Firmo (Latin) morally and physically firm.

Firth (English) woodland.

Fischel (Yiddish) a form of Phillip.

Fiske (English) fisherman.
Fisk

Fitch (English) weasel, ermine.
Fitche

Fito (Spanish) a form of Adolfo.

Fitz (English) son.
Filz

Fitzgerald (English) son of Gerald.

Fitzhugh (English) son of Hugh.
Hugh

Fitzpatrick (English) son of Patrick.

Fitzroy (Irish) son of Roy.

Fiz (Latin) happy, fertile.

Flaminio (Spanish) Religion: Marcantonio Flaminio coauthored one of the most important texts of the Italian Reformation.

Flann (Irish) redhead.
Flainn, Flannan, Flannery

Flavian (Latin) blond, yellow haired.
Flavel, Flavelle, Flavien, Flavio, Flawiusz

Flaviano (Latin) belonging to the old Roman family, Flavia; one of the blonde ones.

Flavio (Italian) a form of Flavian.
Flabio, Flavious, Flavius

Fleming (English) from Denmark; from Flanders.
Flemming, Flemmyng, Flemyng

Fletcher (English) arrow featherer, arrow maker.
Flecher, Fletch

Flint (English) stream; flint stone.
Flynt

Flip (Spanish) a short form of Felipe. (American) a short form of Philip.

Floreal (Latin) alludes to the eighth month of the French Revolution.

Florencio (Italian) a form of Florent.

Florent (French) flowering.
Florenci, Florencio, Florentin, Florentino, Florentyn, Florentz, Florinio, Florino

Florente (Latin) to bloom.

Florian (Latin) flowering, blooming.
Florien, Florrian, Flory, Floryan

Florián (Latin) a form of Florian.

Floriano (Spanish) a form of Florian.

Florio (Spanish) a form of Florián.

Floyd BG (English) a form of Lloyd.

Flurry (English) flourishing, blooming.

Flynn (Irish) son of the red-haired man.
Flin, Flinn, Flyn

Focio (Latin) illuminated, shining.

Folke (German) a form of Volker.
Folker

Foluke (Yoruba) given to God.

Foma (Bulgarian, Russian) a form of Thomas.
Fomka

Fonso (German, Italian) a short form of Alphonso.
Fonzo

Fontaine (French) fountain.

Fonzie (German) a familiar form of Alphonse.
Fons, Fonsie, Fonsy, Fonz

Forbes (Irish) prosperous.
Forbe

Ford (English) a short form of names ending in "ford."

Fordel (Gypsy) forgiving.

Forest BG (French) a form of Forrest.
Forestt, Foryst

Forester (English) forest guardian.
Forrester, Forrie, Forry, Forster, Foss, Foster

Formerio (Latin) beauty.

Forrest BG (French) forest; woodsman.
Forest, Forester, Forrestar, Forrester, Forrestt, Forrie

Fortino (Italian) fortunate, lucky.

Fortune (French) fortunate, lucky.
Fortun, Fortunato, Fortuné, Fortunio

Foster (Latin) a short form of Forester.

Fowler (English) trapper of wildfowl.

Fran GB (Latin) a short form of Francis.
Franh

Frances GB (Latin) a form of Francis.

Francesca GB (Italian) a form of Frances.

Francesco (Italian) a form of Francis.

Franchot (French) a form of Francis.

Francis BG (Latin) free; from France. Religion: Saint Francis of Assisi was the founder of the Franciscan order. See also Farruco, Ferenc.
Fran, France, Frances, Francesco, Franchot, Francisco, Franciskus, Franco, François, Frang, Frank, Frannie, Franny, Frans, Franscis, Fransis, Franta, Frantisek, Frants, Franus, Frantisek, Franz, Frencis

Francisco (Portuguese, Spanish) a form of Francis. See also Chilo, Cisco, Farruco, Paco, Pancho.
Franco, Fransisco, Fransysco, Frasco, Frisco

Franco (Latin) a short form of Francis.
Franko

François (French) a form of Francis.
Francoise

Frank (English) a short form of Francis, Franklin. See also Palani, Pancho.
Franc, Franck, Franek, Frang, Franio, Franke, Frankie, Franko

Frankie 🅱🅶 (English) a familiar form of Frank.
Francky, Franke, Frankey, Franki, Franky, Franqui

Franklin 🅱🅶 (English) free landowner.
Fran, Francklen, Francklin, Francklyn, Francylen, Frank, Frankin, Franklen, Franklinn, Franklyn, Franquelin

Franklyn (English) a form of Franklin.
Franklynn

Frans (Swedish) a form of Francis.
Frants

Frantisek (Czech) a form of Francis.
Franta

Franz (German) a form of Francis.
Fransz, Frantz, Franzen, Franzie, Franzin, Franzl, Franzy

Fraser 🅱🅶 (French) strawberry. (English) curly haired.
Fraizer, Frasier, Fraze, Frazer, Frazier

Fraterno (Latin) relating to the brother.

Frayne (French) dweller at the ash tree. (English) stranger.
Fraine, Frayn, Frean, Freen, Freyne

Fred (German) a short form of Alfred, Frederick, Manfred.
Fredd, Fredde, Fredo, Fredson

Freddie 🅱🅶 (German) a familiar form of Frederick.
Freddi, Freddy, Fredi, Fredy

Freddy, Fredy (German) familiar forms of Frederick.

Frederic (German) a form of Frederick.
Frédéric, Frederich, Frederric, Fredric, Fredrich

Frederick (German) peaceful ruler. See also Dick, Eric, Fico, Peleke, Rick.
Federico, Fico, Fred, Fredderick, Freddie, Freddrick, Freddy, Fredek, Frederic, Fréderick, Frédérick, Frederik, Frederique, Frederrick, Fredo, Fredrick, Fredwick, Fredwyck, Fredy, Friedrich, Fritz

Frederico (Spanish) a form of Frederick.
Fredrico, Frederigo

Frederik (German) a form of Frederick.
Frédérik, Frederrik, Fredrik

Frederique 🅶🅱 (French) a form of Frederick.

Fredo (Spanish) a form of Fred.

Fredrick 🅱🅶 (German) a form of Frederick.
Fredric, Fredricka, Fredricks

Freeborn (English) child of freedom.
Free

Freeman (English) free.
Free, Freedman, Freemin, Freemon, Friedman, Friedmann

Fremont (German) free; noble protector.

Fresco (Spanish) fresh.

Frewin (English) free; noble friend.
Frewen

Frey (English) lord. (Scandinavian) Mythology: the Norse god who dispenses peace and prosperity.

Frick (English) bold.

Fridolf (English) peaceful wolf.
Freydolf, Freydulf, Fridulf

Fridolino (Teutonic) he who loves peace.

Friedrich (German) a form of Frederick.
Friedel, Friedrick, Fridrich, Fridrick, Friedrike, Friedryk, Fryderyk

Frisco (Spanish) a short form of Francisco.

Fritz (German) a familiar form of Frederick.
Fritson, Fritts, Fritzchen, Fritzl

Froberto (Spanish) a form of Roberto.

Frode (Norwegian) wise.

Froilan (Teutonic) rich and beloved young master.

Froilán (Germanic) a form of Froilan.

Fronton (Latin) he who thinks.

Fructuoso (Latin) he who bears much fruit.

Frumencio (Latin) he who provides wheat.

Fulberto (Germanic) he who shines amongst all in the village.

Fulbright (German) very bright.
Fulbert

Fulco (Spanish) village.

Fulgencio (Latin) he who shines and stands out because of his goodness.

Fuller (English) cloth thickener.

Fulton (English) field near town.

Fulvio (Latin) he who has reddish hair.

Funsoni (Nguni) requested.

Fyfe (Scottish) a form of Fife.
Fyffe

Fynn (Ghanaian) Geography: another name for the Offin River in Ghana.

Fyodor (Russian) a form of Theodore.

G

G BG (American) an initial used as a first name.

Gabby (American) a familiar form of Gabriel.
Gabbi, Gabbie, Gabi, Gabie, Gaby

Gabe (Hebrew) a short form of Gabriel.

Gabino (American) a form of Gabriel.
Gabin, Gabrino

Gábor (Hungarian) God is my strength.
Gabbo, Gabko, Gabo

Gabrial (Hebrew) a form of Gabriel.
Gaberial, Gabrael, Gabraiel, Gabrail, Gabreal, Gabriael, Gabrieal, Gabryalle

Gabriel ⭐ BG (Hebrew) devoted to God. Bible: the angel of the Annunciation.
Gab, Gabe, Gabby, Gabino, Gabis, Gábor, Gabreil, Gabrel, Gabrell, Gabrial, Gabriël, Gabriele, Gabriell, Gabrielle, Gabrielli,
Gabrile, Gabris, Gabryel, Gabys, Gavril, Gebereal, Ghabriel, Riel

Gabriela, Gabriella GB (Italian) forms of Gabrielle.

Gabrielle GB (Hebrew) a form of Gabriel.

Gabrielli (Italian) a form of Gabriel.
Gabriello

Gabrio (Spanish) God is my strength.

Gabryel BG (Hebrew) a form of Gabriel.

Gadi (Arabic) God is my fortune.
Gad, Gaddy, Gadiel

Gaetan (Italian) from Gaeta, a region in southern Italy.
Gaetano, Gaetono

Gagandeep BG (Sikh) sky's light.

Gage BG (French) pledge.
Gager, Gaige, Gaje

Gaige (French) a form of Gage.

Gair (Irish) small.
Gaer, Gearr, Geir

Gaius (Latin) rejoicer. See also Cai.

Galbraith (Irish) Scotsman in Ireland.
Galbrait, Galbreath

Gale (Greek) a short form of Galen.
Gael, Gail, Gaile, Gayle

Galeaso (Latin) he who is protected by the helmet.

Galen BG (Greek) healer; calm. (Irish) little and lively.
Gaelan, Gaelen, Gaelin, Gaelyn, Gailen, Galan, Gale, Galeno, Galin, Galyn, Gaylen

Galeno (Spanish) illuminated child. (Greek, Irish) a form of Galen.

Galileo (Hebrew) he who comes from Galilee.

Gallagher (Irish) eager helper.

Galloway (Irish) Scotsman in Ireland.
Gallway, Galway

Galo (Latin) native of Galilee.

Galt (Norwegian) high ground.

Galton (English) owner of a rented estate.
Gallton

Galvin (Irish) sparrow.
Gal, Gall, Gallven, Gallvin, Galvan, Galven

Gamal (Arabic) camel. See also Jamal.
Gamall, Gamel, Gamil

Gamaliel (Hebrew) God is your reward.

Gamble (Scandinavian) old.

Gamelberto (Germanic) distinguished because of his advancing age.

Gan (Chinese) daring, adventurous. (Vietnamese) near.

Gandolfo (Germanic) valiant warrior.

Ganimedes (Spanish) he was the most beautiful of the mortals.

Gannon (Irish) light skinned, white.
Gannan, Gannen, Gannie, Ganny

Ganya BG (Zulu) clever.

Gar (English) a short form of Gareth, Garnett, Garrett, Garvin.
Garr

Garcia (Spanish) mighty with a spear.

García (Spanish) a form of Garcia.

Garcilaso (Spanish) a form of García.

Gardner (English) gardener.
Gard, Gardener, Gardie, Gardiner, Gardy

Garek (Polish) a form of Edgar.

Garen (English) a form of Garry.
Garan, Garen, Garin, Garion, Garon, Garyn, Garyon

Gareth (Welsh) gentle.
Gar, Garith, Garreth, Garrith, Garth, Garyth

Garett BG (Irish) a form of Garrett.
Gared, Garet, Garette, Garhett, Garit, Garitt, Garritt

Garfield (English) field of spears; battlefield.

Garibaldo (Germanic) he who is bold with a lance.

Garland **BG** (French) wreath of flowers; prize. (English) land of spears; battleground.
Garlan, Garlen, Garllan, Garlund, Garlyn

Garman (English) spearman.
Garmann, Garrman

Garner (French) army guard, sentry.
Garnier

Garnett (Latin) pomegranate seed; garnet stone. (English) armed with a spear.
Gar, Garnet, Garnie, Garrnett

Garnock (Welsh) dweller by the alder river.

Garrad (English) a form of Garrett.
Gared, Garrard, Garred, Garrod, Gerred, Gerrid, Gerrod, Garrode, Jared

Garren, Garrin (English) forms of Garry.
Garran, Garrion, Garron, Garyn, Gerren, Gerron, Gerryn

Garret (Irish) a form of Garrett.
Garrit, Garyt, Gerret, Garrid, Gerrit, Gerrot

Garrett **BG** (Irish) brave spearman. See also Jarrett.
Gar, Gareth, Garett, Garrad, Garret, Garrette, Gerrett, Gerritt, Gerrott

Garrick (English) oak spear.
Gaerick, Garek, Garick, Garik, Garreck, Garrek, Garric, Garrik, Garryck, Garryk, Gerreck, Gerrick

Garrison **BG** (French) troops stationed at a fort; garrison.
Garison, Garisson, Garris

Garroway (English) spear fighter.
Garraway

Garry (English) a form of Gary.
Garen, Garrey, Garri, Garrie, Garren, Garrin

Garson (English) son of Gar.

Garth (Scandinavian) garden, gardener. (Welsh) a short form of Gareth.

Garvey (Irish) rough peace.
Garbhán, Garrvey, Garrvie, Garv, Garvan, Garvie, Garvy

Garvin (English) comrade in battle.
Gar, Garvan, Garven, Garvyn, Garwen, Garwin, Garwyn, Garwynn

Garwood (English) evergreen forest. See also Wood, Woody.
Garrwood

Gary **BG** (German) mighty spearman. (English) a familiar form of Gerald. See also Kali.
Gare, Garey, Gari, Garry

Gaspar (French) a form of Casper.
Gáspár, Gaspard, Gaspare, Gaspari, Gasparo, Gasper, Gazsi

Gaston (French) from Gascony, France.
Gascon, Gastaun

Gastón (Germanic) a form of Gaston.

Gaudencio (Latin) he who is happy and content.

Gaudioso (Latin) happy, joyful.

Gausberto (Germanic) Gothic brightness.

Gaute (Norwegian) great.

Gautier (French) a form of Walter.
Galtero, Gaulterio, Gaultier, Gaultiero, Gauthier

Gavin ☀ BG (Welsh) white hawk.
Gav, Gavan, Gaven, Gavinn, Gavino, Gavn, Gavohn, Gavon, Gavyn, Gavynn, Gawain

Gavriel (Hebrew) man of God.
Gav, Gavi, Gavrel, Gavril, Gavy

Gavril (Russian) a form of Gavriel.
Ganya, Gavrilo, Gavrilushka

Gawain (Welsh) a form of Gavin.
Gawaine, Gawayn, Gawayne, Gawen, Gwayne

Gaylen (Greek) a form of Galen.
Gaylin, Gaylinn, Gaylon, Gaylyn

Gaylord (French) merry lord; jailer.
Gaillard, Gallard, Gay, Gayelord, Gayler, Gaylor

Gaynor (Irish) son of the fair-skinned man.
Gainer, Gainor, Gay, Gayner, Gaynnor

Geary (English) variable, changeable.
Gearey, Gery

Gedeon (Bulgarian, French) a form of Gideon.

Gedeón (Hebrew) a form of Gideon.

Geffrey (English) a form of Geoffrey. See also Jeffrey.
Gefery, Geff, Geffery, Geffrard

Gelasio (Greek) cheerful and happy, enjoys having fun.

Gellert (Hungarian) a form of Gerald.

Gemelo (Latin) fraternal twin.

Geminiano (Latin) identical twin.

Gena GB (Russian) a short form of Yevgenyi.
Genka, Genya, Gine

Genaro (Latin) consecrated to God.
Genereo, Genero, Gennaro

Gene BG (Greek) a short form of Eugene.
Genek

Genek (Polish) a form of Gene.

Generos, Generoso (Spanish) generous.

Genesis **GB** (Latin) origin; birth.

Genevieve **GB** (German, French) a form of Guinevere (see Girls' Names).

Geno (Italian) a form of John. A short form of Genovese.
Genio, Jeno

Genovese (Italian) from Genoa, Italy.
Geno, Genovis

Gent (English) gentleman.
Gentle, Gentry

Genty (Irish, English) snow.

Geoff (English) a short form of Geoffrey.

Geoffery (English) a form of Geoffrey.
Geofery

Geoffrey (English) a form of Jeffrey. See also Giotto, Godfrey, Gottfried, Jeff.
Geffrey, Geoff, Geoffery, Geoffre, Geoffrie, Geoffroi, Geoffroy, Geoffry, Geofrey, Geofri, Gofery

Geordan (Scottish) a form of Gordon.
Geordann, Geordian, Geordin, Geordon

Geordie (Scottish) a form of George.
Geordi, Geordy

Georg (Scandinavian) a form of George.

George (Greek) farmer. See also Durko, Egor, Iorgos, Jerzy, Jiri, Joji, Jörg, Jorge, Jorgen, Joris, Jorrín, Jur, Jurgis, Keoki, Mahiái, Semer, Yegor, Yorgos, Yoyi, Yrjo, Yuri, Zhora.
Geordie, Georg, Georgas, Georges, Georget, Georgi, Georgii, Georgio, Georgios, Georgiy, Georgy, Gevork, Gheorghe, Giorgio, Giorgos, Goerge, Goran, Gordios, Gorge, Gorje, Gorya, Grzegorz, Gyorgy

Georges (French) a form of George.
Geórges

Georgia **GB** (Greek) a form of George.

Georgio (Italian) a form of George.

Georgios (Greek) a form of George.
Georgious, Georgius

Georgy (Greek) a familiar form of George.
Georgie

Geovanni, Geovanny (Italian) forms of Giovanni.
Geovan, Geovani, Geovanne, Geovannee, Geovannhi, Geovany

Geraint (English) old.

Gerald 🅱🅶 (German) mighty spearman. See also Fitzgerald, Jarell, Jarrell, Jerald, Jerry, Kharald.
Garald, Garold, Garolds, Gary, Gearalt, Gellert, Gérald, Geralde, Geraldo, Gerale, Geraud, Gerek, Gerick, Gerik, Gerold, Gerrald, Gerrell, Gérrick, Gerrild, Gerrin, Gerrit, Gerrold, Gerry, Geryld, Giraldo, Giraud, Girauld

Geraldo (Italian, Spanish) a form of Gerald.

Gerard (English) brave spearman. See also Jerard, Jerry.
Garrard, Garrat, Garratt, Gearard, Gerad, Gerar, Gérard, Gerardo, Geraro, Géraud, Gerd, Gerek, Gerhard, Gerrard, Gerrit, Gerry, Girard

Gerardo 🅱🅶 (Spanish) a form of Gerard.
Gherardo

Gerasimo (Greek) award, recompense.

Géraud (French) a form of Gerard.
Gerrad, Gerraud

Gerbrando (Germanic) sword.

Gerek (Polish) a form of Gerard.

Geremia (Hebrew) exalted by God. (Italian) a form of Jeremiah.

Geremiah (Italian) a form of Jeremiah.
Geremia, Gerimiah, Geromiah

Gerhard (German) a form of Gerard.
Garhard, Gerhardi, Gerhardt, Gerhart, Gerhort

Gerik (Polish) a form of Edgar.
Geric, Gerick

Germain (French) from Germany. (English) sprout, bud. See also Jermaine.
Germaine, German, Germane, Germano, Germayn, Germayne

Germán (Germanic) male warrior.

Germinal (Latin) he who sprouts.

Geroldo (Germanic) commander of the lance.

Gerome (English) a form of Jerome.

Geronimo (Greek, Italian) a form of Jerome. History: a famous Apache chief.
Geronemo

Gerónimo (Greek) a form of Geronimo.

Gerrit (Dutch) a form of Gerald.

Gerry (English) a familiar form of Gerald, Gerard. See also Jerry.
Geri, Gerre, Gerri, Gerrie, Gerryson

Gershom (Hebrew) exiled. (Yiddish) stranger in exile.
Gersham, Gersho, Gershon, Gerson, Geurson, Gursham, Gurshan

Gerson (English) son of Gar.
Gersan, Gershawn

Gert (German, Danish) fighter.

Gervaise BG (French)
honorable. See also Jervis.
*Garvais, Garvaise, Garvey,
Gervais, Gervase, Gervasio,
Gervaso, Gervayse, Gervis,
Gerwazy*

Gerwin (Welsh) fair love.

Gesualdo (Germanic) prisoner of
the king.

Gethin (Welsh) dusky.
Geth

Getulio (Latin) he who came
from Getulia in the northern
region of Africa.

Ghazi (Arabic) conqueror.

Ghilchrist (Irish) servant of
Christ. See also Gil.
*Gilchrist, Gilcrist, Gilie, Gill,
Gilley, Gilly*

Ghislain (French) pledge.

Gi (Korean) brave.

Gia (Vietnamese) family.

Giacinto (Portuguese, Spanish) a
form of Jacinto.
Giacintho

Giacomo (Italian) a form of
Jacob.
*Gaimo, Giacamo, Giaco,
Giacobbe, Giacobo, Giacopo*

Gian (Italian) a form of Giovanni,
John.
*Gianetto, Giann, Gianne, Giannes,
Gianni, Giannis, Giannos, Ghian*

Giancarlo (Italian) a combination of John + Charles.
Giancarlos, Gianncarlo

Gianluca (Italian) a combination
of John + Lucas.

Gianni (Italian) a form of Johnny.
Giani, Gionni

Gianpaolo (Italian) a combination of John + Paul.
Gianpaulo

Gib (English) a short form of
Gilbert.
Gibb, Gibbie, Gibby

Gibor (Hebrew) powerful.

Gibson (English) son of Gilbert.
*Gibbon, Gibbons, Gibbs, Gillson,
Gilson*

Gideon (Hebrew) tree cutter.
Bible: the judge who defeated the
Midianites.
Gedeon, Gideone, Gidon, Hedeon

Gidon (Hebrew) a form of
Gideon.

Gifford (English) bold giver.
Giff, Giffard, Gifferd, Giffie, Giffy

Gig (English) horse-drawn carriage.

Gil (Greek) shield bearer.
(Hebrew) happy. (English) a
short form of Ghilchrist, Gilbert.
Gili, Gill, Gilli, Gillie, Gillis, Gilly

Gilad (Arabic) camel hump; from Giladi, Saudi Arabia.
Giladi, Gilead

Gilamu (Basque) a form of William.
Gillen

Gilbert (English) brilliant pledge; trustworthy. See also Gil, Gillett.
Gib, Gilberto, Gilburt, Giselbert, Giselberto, Giselbertus, Guilbert

Gilberto (Spanish) a form of Gilbert.

Gilby (Scandinavian) hostage's estate. (Irish) blond boy.
Gilbey, Gillbey, Gillbie, Gillby

Gilchrist (Irish) a form of Ghilchrist.

Gildo (Spanish) a form of Hermenegildo.

Gilen (Basque, German) illustrious pledge.

Giles (French) goatskin shield.
Gide, Gilles, Gyles

Gillean (Irish) Bible: Saint John's servant.
Gillan, Gillen, Gillian

Gillermo (Spanish) resolute protector.

Gillespie (Irish) son of the bishop's servant.
Gillis

Gillett (French) young Gilbert.
Gelett, Gelette, Gillette

Gillian GB (Irish) a form of Gillean.

Gilmer (English) famous hostage.
Gilmar

Gilmore (Irish) devoted to the Virgin Mary.
Gillmore, Gillmour, Gilmour

Gilon (Hebrew) circle.

Gilroy (Irish) devoted to the king.
Gilderoy, Gildray, Gildroy, Gillroy, Roy

Gines (Greek) he who produces life.

Gino (Greek) a familiar form of Eugene. (Italian) a short form of names ending in "gene," "gino."
Ghino

Giona (Italian) a form of Jonah.

Giordano (Italian) a form of Jordan.
Giordan, Giordana, Giordin, Guordan

Giorgio (Italian) a form of George.

Giorgos (Greek) a form of George.
Georgos, Giorgios

Giosia (Italian) a form of Joshua.

Giotto (Italian) a form of Geoffrey.

Giovani (Italian) a form of Giovanni.
Giavani, Giovan, Giovane, Giovanie, Giovon

Giovanni BG (Italian) a form of
John. See also Jeovanni, Jiovanni.
*Geovanni, Geovanny, Gian,
Gianni, Giannino, Giovani,
Giovann, Giovannie, Giovanno,
Giovanny, Giovonathon, Giovonni,
Giovonnia, Giovonnie, Givonni*

Giovanny (Italian) a form of
Giovanni.
Giovany

Gipsy (English) wanderer.
Gipson, Gypsy

Girvin (Irish) small; tough.
Girvan, Girven, Girvon

Gisberto (Germanic) he who
shines in battle with his sword.

Giselle GB (German) pledge;
hostage.

Gitano (Spanish) gypsy.

Giuliano (Italian) a form of
Julius.
Giulano, Giulino, Giulliano

Giulio (Italian) a form of Julius.
Guilano

Giuseppe (Italian) a form of
Joseph.
*Giuseppi, Giuseppino, Giusseppe,
Guiseppe, Guiseppi, Guiseppie,
Guisseppe*

Giustino (Italian) a form of
Justin.
Giusto

Givon (Hebrew) hill; heights.
Givan, Givawn, Givyn

Gladwin (English) cheerful. See
also Win.
*Glad, Gladdie, Gladdy, Gladwinn,
Gladwyn, Gladwynne*

Glanville (English) village with
oak trees.

Glen BG (Irish) a form of Glenn.
Glyn

Glendon (Scottish) fortress in the
glen.
*Glenden, Glendin, Glenn,
Glennden, Glennton, Glenton*

Glendower (Welsh) from
Glyndwr, Wales.

Glenn BG (Irish) a short form of
Glendon.
*Gleann, Glen, Glennie, Glennis,
Glennon, Glenny, Glynn*

Glentworth (English) from
Glenton, England.

Glenville (Irish) village in the
glen.

Gloria GB (Latin) glory.

Glyn (Welsh) a form of Glen.
Glin, Glynn

Goddard (German) divinely firm.
*Godard, Godart, Goddart,
Godhardt, Godhart, Gothart,
Gotthard, Gotthardt, Gotthart*

Godfredo (Spanish) friend of
God.

Godfrey (Irish) God's peace.
(German) a form of Jeffrey. See
also Geoffrey, Gottfried.
*Giotto, Godefroi, Godfree, Godfry,
Godofredo, Godoired, Godrey,
Goffredo, Gofraidh, Gofredo, Gorry*

Godwin (English) friend of God.
See also Win.
*Godewyn, Godwinn, Godwyn,
Goodwin, Goodwyn, Goodwynne,
Goodwynne*

Goel (Hebrew) redeemer.

Goldwin (English) golden friend.
See also Win.
*Golden, Goldewin, Goldewinn,
Goldewyn, Goldwyn, Goldwynn*

Goliard (Spanish) rebel.

Goliat (Hebrew) he who lives his
life making pilgrimages.

Goliath (Hebrew) exiled. Bible:
the giant Philistine whom David
slew with a slingshot.
Golliath

Gomda (Kiowa) wind.

Gomer (Hebrew) completed,
finished. (English) famous battle.

Gonza (Rutooro) love.

Gonzalo (Spanish) wolf.
*Goncalve, Gonsalo, Gonsalve,
Gonzales, Gonzelee, Gonzolo*

Gordon (English) triangular-
shaped hill.
*Geordan, Gord, Gordain, Gordan,
Gorden, Gordonn, Gordy*

Gordy (English) a familiar form of
Gordon.
Gordie

Gore (English) triangular-shaped
land; wedge-shaped land.

Gorgonio (Greek) violent one.

Gorman (Irish) small; blue eyed.

Goro (Japanese) fifth.

Gosheven (Native American)
great leaper.

Gosvino (Teutonic) friend of God.

Gotardo (Germanic) he who is
valiant because of the strength
that he receives from God.

Gottfried (German) a form of
Geoffrey, Godfrey.
Gotfrid, Gotfrids, Gottfrid

Gotzon (German) a form of Angel.

Govert (Dutch) heavenly peace.

Gower (Welsh) pure.

Gowon (Tiv) rainmaker.
Gowan

Goyo (Spanish) a form of
Gerardo.

Gozol (Hebrew) soaring bird.
Gozal

Gracián (Latin) possessor of
grace.

Graciano (Latin) one recognized
by God; he has love and divine
blessing.

Graciliano (Latin) name comes from Gados, the useful martyr from Faleria, Italy.

Grady (Irish) noble; illustrious.
Gradea, Gradee, Gradey, Gradleigh, Graidey, Graidy

Graeme (Scottish) a form of Graham.
Graem

Graham BG (English) grand home.
Graeham, Graehame, Graehme, Graeme, Grahamme, Grahm, Grahame, Grahme, Gram, Grame, Gramm, Grayeme, Grayham

Granger (French) farmer.
Grainger, Grange

Grant BG (English) a short form of Grantland.
Grand, Grantham, Granthem, Grantley

Grantland (English) great plains.
Grant

Granville (French) large village.
Gran, Granvel, Granvil, Granvile, Granvill, Grenville, Greville

Grato (Latin) one recognized by God; he has love and divine blessing.

Grau (Spanish) a form of Gerardo.

Gray (English) gray haired.
Graye, Grey, Greye

Grayden (English) gray haired.
Graden, Graydan, Graydyn, Greyden

Graydon (English) gray hill.
Gradon, Grayton, Greydon

Grayson BG (English) bailiff's son. See also Sonny.
Graysen, Greyson

Grazián (Spanish) a form of Graciano.

Greeley (English) gray meadow.
Greelea, Greeleigh, Greely

Greenwood (English) green forest.
Green, Greener

Greg, Gregg (Latin) short forms of Gregory.
Graig, Greig, Gregson

Greggory (Latin) a form of Gregory.
Greggery

Gregor (Scottish) a form of Gregory.
Gregoor, Grégor, Gregore

Gregorio (Italian, Portuguese) a form of Gregory.
Gregorios

Gregory BG (Latin) vigilant watchman. See also Jörn, Krikor.
Gergely, Gergo, Greagoir, Greagory, Greer, Greg, Gregary, Greger, Gregery, Greggory, Grégoire, Gregor, Gregorey, Gregori, Grégorie, Gregorio, Gregorius, Gregors, Gregos, Gregrey, Gregroy, Gregry, Greogry, Gries, Grisha, Grzegorz

Gresham (English) village in the pasture.

Greyson (English) a form of Grayson.
Greysen, Greysten, Greyston

Griffin BG (Latin) hooked nose.
Griff, Griffen, Griffie, Griffon, Griffy, Gryphon

Griffith (Welsh) fierce chief; ruddy.
Grifen, Griff, Griffeth, Griffie, Griffy, Griffyn, Griffynn, Gryphon

Grigori (Bulgarian) a form of Gregory.
Grigoi, Grigor, Grigore, Grigorios, Grigorov, Grigory

Grimoaldo (Spanish) confessor.

Grimshaw (English) dark woods.

Grisha (Russian) a form of Gregory.

Griswold (German, French) gray forest.
Gris, Griz, Grizwald

Grosvener (French) big hunter.

Grover (English) grove.
Grove

Guacraya (Quechua) strong and brave like a bull.

Guadalberto (Germanic) he is all-powerful and shines because of it.

Guadalupe GB (Arabic) river of black stones.
Guadalope

Guaina (Quechua) young; friend.

Gualberto (Spanish) a form of Walter.
Gualterio

Gualtar (Spanish) a form of Gerardo.

Gualtiero (Italian) a form of Walter.
Gualterio

Guaman (Quechua) falcon.

Guamanachachi (Quechua) he who has valorous ancestors such as the falcon.

Guamancapac (Quechua) lord falcon.

Guamancaranca (Quechua) he who fights like a thousand falcons.

Guamanchaua (Quechua) cruel as a falcon.

Guamanchuri (Quechua) son of the falcon.

Guamanpuma (Quechua) strong and powerful as a puma and a falcon.

Guamantiupac (Quechua) glorious falcon.

Guamanyana (Quechua) black falcon.

Guamanyurac (Quechua) white falcon.

Guamay (Quechua) young, fresh, new.

Guanca, Guancar (Quechua) rock; summit; drum.

Guanpú (Aymara) born in a festive time; he who arrives in an opportune moment.

Guari (Quechua) savage, untamable, untiring; wild like the vicuna; protected by the gods.

Guarino (Teutonic) he who defends well.

Guariruna (Quechua) untamed and wild man.

Guarititu, Guartito (Quechua) untamed and difficult to deal with, like the vicuna.

Guascar (Quechua) he of the chain, rope of bindweed.

Guaual (Quechua) myrtle.

Guayasamin (Quechua) happy, white bird in flight.

Guayau (Quechua) royal willow.

Guaynacapac (Quechua) young master.

Guaynarimac (Quechua) young speaker.

Guaynay (Quechua) my youngster; my beloved.

Guaypa, Guaypaya (Quechua) rooster; creator, inventor.

Guayra (Quechua) wind, fast as the wind.

Guayua (Aymara) restless, mischievous; fast as the wind.

Guglielmo (Italian) a form of William.

Guido (Italian) a form of Guy.

Guilford (English) ford with yellow flowers.
Guildford

Guilherme (Portuguese) a form of William.

Güillac (Quechua) he who warns.

Guillaume (French) a form of William.
Guillaums, Guilleaume, Guilem, Guyllaume

Guillermo (Spanish) a form of William.
Guillerrmo

Güiracocha, Güiracucha (Quechua) sea foam; the sea's vital energy.

Güisa (Quechua) prophet; he is a sorcerer for having been a twin.

Güiuyac (Quechua) brilliant, luminous.

Güiyca (Quechua) sacred.

Güiycauaman (Quechua) sacred falcon.

Gumaro (Germanic) army of men; disciplined man.

Gumersindo (Germanic) excellent man.

Gundelberto (Teutonic) he who shines in battle.

Gunnar (Scandinavian) a form of Gunther.
Guner, Gunner

Gunther (Scandinavian) battle army; warrior.
Guenter, Guenther, Gun, Gunnar, Guntar, Gunter, Guntero, Gunthar, Günther

Guotin (Chinese) polite; strong leader.

Gurion (Hebrew) young lion.
Gur, Guri, Guriel

Gurjot BG (Sikh) light of the guru.

Gurpreet BG (Sikh) devoted to the guru; devoted to the Prophet.
Gurjeet, Gurmeet, Guruprit

Gurvir BG (Sikh) guru's warrior.
Gurveer

Gus (Scandinavian) a short form of Angus, Augustine, Gustave.
Guss, Gussie, Gussy, Gusti, Gustry, Gusty

Gustaf (Swedish) a form of Gustave.
Gustaaf, Gustaff

Gustave (Scandinavian) staff of the Goths. History: Gustavus Adolphus was a king of Sweden. See also Kosti, Tabo, Tavo.
Gus, Gustaf, Gustaff, Gustaof, Gustav, Gustáv, Gustava, Gustaves, Gustavo, Gustavs, Gustavus, Gustik, Gustus, Gusztav

Gustavo (Italian, Spanish) a form of Gustave.
Gustabo

Guthrie (German) war hero. (Irish) windy place.
Guthrey, Guthry

Gutierre (Spanish) a form of Walter.

Guy BG (Hebrew) valley. (German) warrior. (French) guide. See also Guido.
Guyon

Guyapi (Native American) candid.

Guzman (Gothic) good man; man of God.

Guzmán (Teutonic) a form of Guzman.

Gwayne (Welsh) a form of Gawain.
Gwaine, Gwayn

Gwidon (Polish) life.

Gwilym (Welsh) a form of William.
Gwillym

Gwyn GB (Welsh) fair; blessed.
Gwynn, Gwynne

Gyasi (Akan) marvelous baby.

Gyorgy (Russian) a form of George.
Gyoergy, György, Gyuri, Gyurka

Gyula (Hungarian) youth.
Gyala, Gyuszi

H **GB** (American) an initial used as a first name.

Habib (Arabic) beloved.

Habid (Arabic) appreciated one.

Hacan (Quechua) brilliant, splendorous.

Hacanpoma, Hacanpuma (Quechua) brilliant puma.

Hackett (German, French) little wood cutter.
Hacket, Hackit, Hackitt

Hackman (German, French) wood cutter.

Hadar (Hebrew) glory.

Haddad (Arabic) blacksmith.

Hadden (English) heather-covered hill.
Haddan, Haddon, Haden

Haden (English) a form of Hadden.
Hadin, Hadon, Hadyn, Haeden

Hadi (Arabic) guiding to the right.
Hadee, Hady

Hadley **GB** (English) heather-covered meadow.
Had, Hadlea, Hadlee, Hadleigh, Hadly, Lee, Leigh

Hadrian (Latin, Swedish) dark.
Adrian, Hadrien

Hadrián (Latin) a form of Hadrian.

Hadulfo (Germanic) combat wolf.

Hadwin (English) friend in a time of war.
Hadwinn, Hadwyn, Hadwynn, Hadwynne

Hagan (German) strong defense.
Haggan

Hagen (Irish) young, youthful.

Hagley (English) enclosed meadow.

Hagos (Ethiopian) happy.

Hahnee (Native American) beggar.

Hai (Vietnamese) sea.

Haidar (Arabic) lion.
Haider

Haiden **BG** (English) a form of Hayden.
Haidyn

Haig (English) enclosed with hedges.

Hailey **GB** (Irish) a form of Haley.
Haile, Haille, Haily, Halee

Haji (Swahili) born during the pilgrimage to Mecca.

Hakan (Native American) fiery.

Hakeem **BG** (Arabic) a form of Hakim.
Hakam, Hakem

Hakim (Arabic) wise. (Ethiopian) doctor.
Hakeem, Hakiem

Hakon (Scandinavian) of Nordic ancestry.
Haaken, Haakin, Haakon, Haeo, Hak, Hakan, Hako

Hal (English) a short form of Halden, Hall, Harold.

Halbert (English) shining hero.
Bert, Halburt

Halden (Scandinavian) half-Danish. See also Dane.
Hal, Haldan, Haldane, Halfdan, Halvdan

Hale (English) a short form of Haley. (Hawaiian) a form of Harry.
Hayle, Heall

Halee GB (Irish) a form of Hailey.

Halen (Swedish) hall.
Hale, Hallen, Haylan, Haylen

Haley GB (Irish) ingenious.
Hailey, Hale, Haleigh, Halley, Hayleigh, Hayley, Hayli

Halford (English) valley ford.

Hali GB (Greek) sea.

Halian (Zuni) young.

Halil (Turkish) dear friend.
Halill

Halim (Arabic) mild, gentle.
Haleem

Hall (English) manor, hall.
Hal, Halstead, Halsted

Hallam (English) valley.

Hallan (English) dweller at the hall; dweller at the manor.
Halin, Hallene, Hallin

Halley GB (English) meadow near the hall; holy.

Hallie GB (English) a form of Halley.

Halliwell (English) holy well.
Hallewell, Hellewell, Helliwell

Hallward (English) hall guard.

Halsey GB (English) Hal's island.

Halstead (English) manor grounds.
Halsted

Halton (English) estate on the hill.

Halvor (Norwegian) rock; protector.
Halvard

Ham (Hebrew) hot. Bible: one of Noah's sons.

Hamal (Arabic) lamb. Astronomy: a bright star in the constellation of Aries.

Hamar (Scandinavian) hammer.

Hamid (Arabic) praised. See also Muhammad.
Haamid, Hamaad, Hamadi, Hamd, Hamdrem, Hamed, Hamedo, Hameed, Hamidi, Hammad, Hammed, Humayd

Hamill (English) scarred.
Hamel, Hamell, Hammill

Hamilton (English) proud estate.
Hamel, Hamelton, Hamil, Hamill, Tony

Hamish (Scottish) a form of Jacob, James.

Hamisi (Swahili) born on Thursday.

Hamlet (German, French) little village; home. Literature: one of Shakespeare's tragic heroes.

Hamlin (German, French) loves his home.
Hamblin, Hamelen, Hamelin, Hamlen, Hamlyn, Lin

Hammet (English, Scandinavian) village.
Hammett, Hamnet, Hamnett

Hammond (English) village.
Hamond

Hampton (English) Geography: a town in England.
Hamp

Hamza (Arabic) powerful.
Hamzah, Hamze, Hamzeh, Hamzia

Hanale (Hawaiian) a form of Henry.
Haneke

Hanan (Hebrew) grace.
Hananel, Hananiah, Johanan

Hanbal (Arabic) pure. History: Ahmad Ibn Hanbal founded an Islamic school of thought.

Handel (German, English) a form of John. Music: George Frideric Handel was a German composer whose works include *Messiah* and *Water Music*.

Hanford (English) high ford.

Hanif (Arabic) true believer.
Haneef, Hanef

Hank (American) a familiar form of Henry.

Hanley (English) high meadow.
Handlea, Handleigh, Handley, Hanlea, Hanlee, Hanleigh, Hanly, Henlea, Henlee, Henleigh, Henley

Hanna, Hannah **GB** (German) forms of Hanno.

Hannes (Finnish) a form of John.

Hannibal (Phoenician) grace of God. History: a famous Carthaginian general who fought the Romans.
Anibal

Hanno (German) a short form of Johan.
Hannon, Hannu, Hanon

Hans (Scandinavian) a form of John.
Hanschen, Hansel, Hants, Hanz

Hansel (Scandinavian) a form of Hans.
Haensel, Hansell, Hansl, Hanzel

Hansen (Scandinavian) son of Hans.
Hanson

Hansh (Hindi) god; godlike.

Hanson (Scandinavian) a form of Hansen.
Hansen, Hanssen, Hansson

Hanus (Czech) a form of John.

Haoa (Hawaiian) a form of Howard.

Hara GB (Hindi) seizer. Religion: another name for the Hindu god Shiva.

Harald (Scandinavian) a form of Harold.
Haraldo, Haralds, Haralpos

Harb (Arabic) warrior.

Harbin (German, French) little bright warrior.
Harben, Harbyn

Harcourt (French) fortified dwelling.
Court, Harcort

Hardeep (Punjabi) a form of Harpreet.

Harden (English) valley of the hares.
Hardian, Hardin

Harding (English) brave; hardy.
Hardin

Hardwin (English) brave friend.

Hardy (German) bold, daring.
Hardie

Harel (Hebrew) mountain of God.
Harell, Hariel, Harrell

Harford (English) ford of the hares.

Hargrove (English) grove of the hares.
Hargreave, Hargreaves

Hari (Hindi) tawny.
Hariel, Harin

Harith (Arabic) cultivator.

Harjot (Sikh) light of God.
Harjeet, Harjit, Harjodh

Harkin (Irish) dark red.
Harkan, Harken

Harlan (English) hare's land; army land.
Harland, Harlen, Harlenn, Harlin, Harlon, Harlyn, Harlynn

Harland (English) a form of Harlan.
Harlend

Harley BG (English) hare's meadow; army meadow.
Arley, Harlea, Harlee, Harleigh, Harly

Harlow (English) hare's hill; army hill. See also Arlo.

Harman, Harmon (English) forms of Herman.
Harm, Harmen, Harmond, Harms

Harold (Scandinavian) army ruler. See also Jindra.
Araldo, Garald, Garold, Hal, Harald, Haraldas, Haraldo,

*Haralds, Harry, Heraldo, Herold,
Heronim, Herrick, Herryck*

Haroldo (Germanic) he who
dominates the region with his
army.

Haroun (Arabic) lofty; exalted.
*Haarun, Harin, Haron, Haroon,
Harron, Harun*

Harper (English) harp player.
Harp, Harpo

Harpreet GB (Punjabi) loves
God, devoted to God.
Hardeep

Harris (English) a short form of
Harrison.
Haris, Hariss

Harrison BG (English) son of
Harry.
*Harison, Harreson, Harris,
Harrisen, Harrisson*

Harrod (Hebrew) hero; conqueror.

Harry (English) a familiar form of
Harold. See also Arrigo, Hale,
Parry.
*Harm, Harray, Harrey, Harri,
Harrie*

Hart (English) a short form of
Hartley.

Hartley (English) deer meadow.
*Hart, Hartlea, Hartlee, Hartleigh,
Hartly*

Hartman (German) hard; strong.

Hartwell (English) deer well.
Harwell, Harwill

Hartwig (German) strong advisor.

Hartwood (English) deer forest.
Harwood

Harvey (German) army warrior.
*Harv, Hervé, Hervey, Hervie,
Hervy*

Harvir BG (Sikh) God's warrior.
Harvier

Hasad (Turkish) reaper,
harvester.

Hasan (Arabic) a form of Hassan.
*Hasaan, Hasain, Hasaun,
Hashaan, Hason*

Hasani (Swahili) handsome.
*Hasan, Hasanni, Hassani,
Heseny, Hassen, Hassian, Husani*

Hashim (Arabic) destroyer of evil.
*Haashim, Hasham, Hasheem,
Hashem*

Hasin (Hindi) laughing.
*Haseen, Hasen, Hassin, Hazen,
Hesen*

Haskel (Hebrew) a form of
Ezekiel.
Haskell

Haslett (English) hazel-tree land.
Haze, Hazel, Hazlett, Hazlitt

Hassan (Arabic) handsome.
Hasan, Hassen, Hasson

Hassel (German, English)
witches' corner.
*Hassal, Hassall, Hassell, Hazael,
Hazell*

Hastin (Hindi) elephant.

Hastings (Latin) spear. (English) house council.
Hastie, Hasty

Hastu (Quechua) bird of the Andes.

Hatim (Arabic) judge.
Hateem, Hatem

Hatuntupac (Quechua) magnificent, great and majestic.

Hauk (Norwegian) hawk.
Haukeye

Havelock (Norwegian) sea battler.

Haven 🇬🇧 (Dutch, English) harbor, port; safe place.
Haeven, Havin, Hevin, Hevon, Hovan

Havika (Hawaiian) a form of David.

Hawk (English) hawk.
Hawke, Hawkin, Hawkins

Hawley (English) hedged meadow.
Hawleigh, Hawly

Hawthorne (English) hawthorn tree.

Hayden ☆ 🇧🇬 (English) hedged valley.
Haiden, Haydan, Haydenn, Haydn, Haydon

Hayes (English) hedged valley.
Hayse

Hayley 🇬🇧 (Irish) a form of Haley.

Hayward (English) guardian of the hedged area.
Haward, Heyvard, Heyward

Haywood (English) hedged forest.
Heywood, Woody

Haziel (Hebrew) vision of God.

Hearn (Scottish, English) a short form of Ahearn.
Hearne, Herin, Hern

Heath 🇧🇬 (English) heath.
Heathe, Heith

Heathcliff (English) cliff near the heath. Literature: the hero of Emily Brontë's novel *Wuthering Heights*.

Heather 🇬🇧 (English) flowering heather.

Heaton (English) high place.

Heaven 🇬🇧 (English) place of beauty and happiness. Bible: where God and angels are said to dwell.

Heber (Hebrew) ally, partner.

Hector (Greek) steadfast. Mythology: the greatest hero of the Trojan War in Homer's epic poem *Iliad*.

Héctor (Greek) a form of Hector.

Hedley (English) heather-filled meadow.
Headley, Headly, Hedly

Hegesipo (Greek) horse rider.

Heinrich (German) a form of Henry.
Heindrick, Heiner, Heinreich, Heinrick, Heinrik, Hinrich

Heinz (German) a familiar form of Henry.

Heladio (Greek) native of Halade, Greece.

Helaku (Native American) sunny day.

Heldrado (Germanic) counselor of warriors.

Helen **GB** (Greek) light.

Helge (Russian) holy.

Heli (Hebrew) he who offers himself to God.

Helio (Spanish) gift of the sun god.

Heliodoro (Greek) gift of god.

Heliogabalo (Syrian) he who adores the sun.

Helki **BG** (Moquelumnan) touching.

Helmer (German) warrior's wrath.

Helmut (German) courageous.
Helmuth

Helvecio (Latin) ancient inhabitants of present-day Switzerland.

Heman (Hebrew) faithful.

Henderson (Scottish, English) son of Henry.
Hendrie, Hendries, Hendron, Henryson

Hendrick (Dutch) a form of Henry.
Hendricks, Hendrickson, Hendrik, Hendriks, Hendrikus, Hendrix, Henning

Heniek (Polish) a form of Henry.
Henier

Henley (English) high meadow.

Henning (German) a form of Hendrick, Henry.

Henoch (Yiddish) initiator.
Enoch, Henock, Henok

Henri (French) a form of Henry.
Henrico, Henrri

Henrick (Dutch) a form of Henry.
Heinrick, Henerik, Henrich, Henrik, Henryk

Henrique (Portuguese) a form of Henry.

Henry (German) ruler of the household. See also Arrigo, Enric, Enrick, Enrico, Enrikos, Enrique, Hanale, Honok, Kiki.
Hagan, Hank, Harro, Harry, Heike, Heinrich, Heinz, Hendrick, Henery, Heniek, Henning, Henraoi, Henri, Henrick, Henrim, Henrique, Henrry, Heromin, Hersz

Heracleos, Heraclio (Greek) belonging to Hercules.

Heraclito, Heráclito (Greek) he who is drawn to the sacred.

Heraldo (Spanish) a form of Harold.
Herald, Hiraldo

Herb (German) a short form of Herbert.
Herbie, Herby

Herbert (German) glorious soldier.
Bert, Erbert, Eriberto, Harbert, Hebert, Hébert, Heberto, Herb, Heriberto, Hurbert

Herculano (Latin) belonging to Hercules.

Hercules (Latin) glorious gift. Mythology: a Greek hero of fabulous strength, renowned for his twelve labors.
Herakles, Herc, Hercule, Herculie

Hércules (Etruscan) a form of Hercules.

Heriberto (Spanish) a form of Herbert.
Heribert

Hermagoras (Greek) disciple of Hermes.

Hermalindo, Hermelindo (German) he who is like a shield of strength.

Herman (Latin) noble. (German) soldier. See also Armand, Ermanno, Ermano, Mandek.
Harmon, Hermaan, Hermann, Hermie, Herminio, Hermino, Hermon, Hermy, Heromin

Hermán (Germanic) a form of Herman.

Hermenegildo (Germanic) he who offers sacrifices to God.

Hermes (Greek) messenger. Mythology: the divine herald of Greek mythology.

Hermógenes (Greek) sent from Hermes.

Hernan (German) peacemaker.

Hernán (Germanic) a form of Herman.

Hernando (Spanish) a form of Ferdinand.
Hernandes, Hernandez

Herodes (Greek) fire dragon.

Herodoto (Greek) sacred talent.

Heródoto (Greek) divine talent; gift.

Herón, Heros (Latin) hero.

Herrick (German) war ruler.
Herrik, Herryck

Herschel (Hebrew) a form of Hershel.
Herchel, Hersch, Herschel, Herschell

Hersh (Hebrew) a short form of Hershel.
Hersch, Hirsch

Hershel (Hebrew) deer.
Herschel, Hersh, Hershal,
Hershall, Hershell, Herzl,
Hirschel, Hirshel

Hertz (Yiddish) my strife.
Herzel

Herve (Breton) active in combat.

Hervé (French) a form of Harvey.

Hesiquio (Greek) tranquil.

Hesperos (Greek) evening star.
Hespero

Hesutu (Moquelumnan) picking
up a yellow jacket's nest.

Hew (Welsh) a form of Hugh.
Hewe, Huw

Hewitt (German, French) little
smart one.
Hewe, Hewet, Hewett, Hewie,
Hewit, Hewlett, Hewlitt, Hugh

Hewson (English) son of Hugh.

Hezekiah (Hebrew) God gives
strength.
Hezekyah, Hazikiah, Hezikyah

Hiamovi (Cheyenne) high chief.

Hibah (Arabic) gift.

Hidalgo (Spanish) noble one.

Hideaki (Japanese) smart, clever.
Hideo

Hieremias (Greek) God will
uplift.

Hieronymos (Greek) a form of
Jerome. Art: Hieronymus Bosch
was a fifteenth-century Dutch
painter.
Hierome, Hieronim, Hieronimo,
Hieronimos, Hieronymo,
Hieronymus

Hieu (Vietnamese) respectful.

Higinio (Greek) he who has good
health.

Hilario (Spanish) a form of Hilary.

Hilary **GB** (Latin) cheerful. See
also Ilari.
Hi, Hilair, Hilaire, Hilarie, Hilario,
Hilarion, Hilarius, Hil, Hill, Hillary,
Hillery, Hilliary, Hillie, Hilly

Hildebrand (German) battle
sword.
Hildebrando, Hildo

Hildemaro (Germanic) famous in
combat.

Hilel (Arabic) new moon.

Hillary **GB** (Latin) a form of
Hilary.

Hillel (Hebrew) greatly praised.
Religion: Rabbi Hillel originated
the Talmud.

Hilliard (German) brave warrior.
Hillard, Hiller, Hillier, Hillierd,
Hillyard, Hillyer, Hillyerd

Hilmar (Swedish) famous noble.

Hilton (English) town on a hill.
Hylton

Hinto (Dakota) blue.

Hinun (Native American) spirit of the storm.

Hipacio (Spanish) confessor.

Hipócrates (Greek) powerful because of his cavalry.

Hipólito (Greek) a form of Hippolyte.

Hippolyte (Greek) horseman.
Hipolito, Hippolit, Hippolitos, Hippolytus, Ippolito

Hiram (Hebrew) noblest; exalted.
Hi, Hirom, Huram, Hyrum

Hiromasa (Japanese) fair, just.

Hiroshi (Japanese) generous.

Hisoka (Japanese) secretive, reserved.

Hiu (Hawaiian) a form of Hugh.

Ho (Chinese) good.

Hoang (Vietnamese) finished.

Hobart (German) Bart's hill.
Hobard, Hobbie, Hobby, Hobie, Hoebart

Hobert (German) Bert's hill.
Hobey

Hobson (English) son of Robert.
Hobbs, Hobs

Hoc (Vietnamese) studious.

Hod (Hebrew) a short form of Hodgson.

Hodgson (English) son of Roger.
Hod

Hogan (Irish) youth.
Hogin

Holbrook (English) brook in the hollow.
Brook, Holbrooke

Holden BG (English) hollow in the valley.
Holdan, Holdin, Holdon, Holdun, Holdyn

Holic (Czech) barber.

Holland (French) Geography: a former province of the Netherlands.

Holleb (Polish) dove.
Hollub, Holub

Hollie GB (English) a form of Hollis.

Hollis BG (English) grove of holly trees.

Holly GB (English) a form of Hollis.

Holmes (English) river islands.

Holt (English) forest.
Holten, Holton

Homer (Greek) hostage; pledge; security. Literature: a renowned Greek epic poet.
Homar, Homere, Homère, Homero, Homeros, Homerus

Hondo (Shona) warrior.

Honesto (Filipino) honest.

Honi (Hebrew) gracious.
Choni

Honok (Polish) a form of Henry.

Honon (Moquelumnan) bear.

Honorato (Spanish) honorable.

Honoré (Latin) honored.
Honor, Honoratus, Honoray,
Honorio, Honorius

Honovi (Native American) strong.

Honza (Czech) a form of John.

Hop (Chinese) agreeable.

Hope **GB** (English) hope.

Horace (Latin) keeper of the
hours. Literature: a famous
Roman lyric poet and satirist.
Horacio, Horaz

Horacio (Latin) a form of Horace.

Horado (Spanish) timekeeper.

Horangel (Greek) messenger
from the heights or from the
mountain.

Horatio (Latin) clan name. See
also Orris.
Horatius, Oratio

Horst (German) dense grove;
thicket.
Hurst

Hortencio (Latin) he who has a
garden and loves it.

Hortensio (Latin) gardener.

Horton (English) garden estate.
Hort, Horten, Orton

Hosa (Arapaho) young crow.

Hosea (Hebrew) salvation. Bible:
a Hebrew prophet.
Hose, Hoseia, Hoshea, Hosheah

Hospicio (Spanish) he who is
accommodating.

Hotah (Lakota) white.

Hototo (Native American)
whistler.

Houghton (English) settlement on
the headland.

Houston **BG** (English) hill town.
Geography: a city in Texas.
Housten, Houstin, Hustin, Huston

Howard (English) watchman. See
also Haoa.
Howie, Ward

Howe (German) high.
Howey, Howie

Howell (Welsh) remarkable.
Howel

Howi (Moquelumnan) turtledove.

Howie (English) a familiar form
of Howard, Howland.
Howey

Howin (Chinese) loyal swallow.

Howland (English) hilly land.
Howie, Howlan, Howlen

Hoyt (Irish) mind; spirit.

Hu (Chinese) tiger.

Huaiquilaf (Mapuche) good, straight lance.

Huapi (Mapuche) island.

Hubbard (German) a form of Hubert.

Hubert (German) bright mind; bright spirit. See also Beredei, Uberto.
Bert, Hobart, Hubbard, Hubbert, Huber, Hubertek, Huberto, Hubertson, Hubie, Huey, Hugh, Hugibert, Huibert, Humberto

Huberto (Spanish) a form of Hubert.
Humberto

Hubie (English) a familiar form of Hubert.
Hube, Hubi

Hucsuncu (Quechua) he who has only one love; faithful.

Hud (Arabic) Religion: a Muslim prophet.

Hudson (English) son of Hud.

Huechacura (Mapuche) sharp rock; peak.

Huenchulaf (Mapuche) healthy man; happy, joyous, festive.

Huenchuleo (Mapuche) brave; handsome river; having grown up near the river.

Huenchuman (Mapuche) proud male condor.

Huenchumilla (Mapuche) ascending light; lucent point.

Huenchuñir (Mapuche) male fox.

Huentemil (Mapuche) light from above, beam of light; possessor of much silver and gold.

Huenuhueque (Mapuche) lamb from heaven.

Huenullan (Mapuche) heavenly altar.

Huenuman (Mapuche) condor from the sky; from heaven.

Huenupan (Mapuche) branch from heaven; lion from heaven.

Huey (English) a familiar form of Hugh.
Hughey, Hughie, Hughy, Hui

Hueypín (Mapuche) broken, odd land.

Hugh (English) a short form of Hubert. See also Ea, Hewitt, Huxley, Maccoy, Ugo.
Fitzhugh, Hew, Hiu, Hue, Huey, Hughes, Hugo, Hugues

Hugo 🅱🅶 (Latin) a form of Hugh.
Ugo

Hugolino (Germanic) he who has spirit and intelligence.

Huichacura (Mapuche) rock with just one ridge, just one side.

Huichahue (Mapuche) battlefield.

Huichalef (Mapuche) he who
runs on just one side; one
straight line.

Huichañir (Mapuche) fox from
another region.

Huidaleo (Mapuche) branch in
the river; the river separates.

Huinculche (Mapuche) people
that live on the hill.

Huircalaf (Mapuche) cry of joy;
healthy shout.

Huircaleo (Mapuche) whisper of
the river, noise from the river.

Hulbert (German) brilliant grace.
*Bert, Hulbard, Hulburd, Hulburt,
Hull*

Hullen (Mapuche) spring.

Humbaldo (Germanic) daring as
a lion cub.

Humbert (German) brilliant
strength. See also Umberto.
Hum, Humberto

Humberto (Portuguese) a form of
Humbert.

Humphrey (German) peaceful
strength. See also Onofrio,
Onufry.
*Hum, Humfredo, Humfrey,
Humfrid, Humfried, Humfry,
Hump, Humph, Humphery,
Humphry, Humphrys, Hunfredo*

Hung (Vietnamese) brave.

Hunt (English) a short form of
names beginning with "Hunt."

Hunter ☀ BG (English) hunter.
Hunt, Huntur

Huntington (English) hunting
estate.
Hunt, Huntingdon

Huntley (English) hunter's
meadow.
*Hunt, Huntlea, Huntlee,
Huntleigh, Huntly*

Hurley (Irish) sea tide.
Hurlee, Hurleigh

Hurst (English) a form of Horst.
Hearst, Hirst

Husai (Hebrew) hurried one.

Husam (Arabic) sword.

Husamettin (Turkish) sharp
sword.

Huslu (Native American) hairy
bear.

Hussain (Arabic) a form of
Hussein.
*Hossain, Husain, Husani, Husayn,
Hussan, Hussayn*

Hussein (Arabic) little;
handsome.
*Hossein, Houssein, Houssin,
Huissien, Huossein, Husein,
Husien, Hussain, Hussien*

Hussien (Arabic) a form of
Hussein.
Husian, Hussin

Hutchinson (English) son of the hutch dweller.
Hutcheson

Hute (Native American) star.

Hutton (English) house on the jutting ledge.
Hut, Hutt, Huttan

Huxley (English) Hugh's meadow.
Hux, Huxlea, Huxlee, Huxleigh, Lee

Huy (Vietnamese) glorious.

Hy (Vietnamese) hopeful.
(English) a short form of Hyman.

Hyacinthe (French) hyacinth.

Hyatt (English) high gate.
Hyat

Hyde (English) cache; measure of land equal to 120 acres; animal hide.

Hyder (English) tanner, preparer of animal hides for tanning.

Hyman (English) a form of Chaim.
Haim, Hayim, Hayvim, Hayyim, Hy, Hyam, Hymie

Hyun-Ki (Korean) wise.

Hyun-Shik (Korean) clever.

Iago (Spanish, Welsh) a form of Jacob, James. Literature: the villain in Shakespeare's *Othello*.
Jago

Iain (Scottish) a form of Ian.

Iakobos (Greek) a form of Jacob.
Iakov, Iakovos, Iakovs

Ian ☀ 🅱🅶 (Scottish) a form of John. See also Ean, Eion.
Iain, Iane, Iann

Ianos (Czech) a form of John.
Iannis

Ib (Phoenician, Danish) oath of Baal.

Iban (Basque) a form of John.

Iber, Ibérico, Iberio, Ibero (Latin) native of Iberia or who comes from the Iberian peninsula.

Ibi (Latin) at another place.

Ibon (Basque) a form of Ivor.

Ibrahim (Hausa) my father is exalted.
Ibrahaim, Ibraham, Ibraheem, Ibrahem, Ibrahiem, Ibrahiim, Ibrahmim

Ichabod (Hebrew) glory is gone. Literature: Ichabod Crane is the main character of Washington

Irving's story "The Legend of Sleepy Hollow."

Idi (Swahili) born during the Idd festival.

Idris (Welsh) eager lord. (Arabic) Religion: a Muslim prophet.
Idrease, Idrees, Idres, Idress, Idreus, Idriece, Idriss, Idrissa, Idriys

Idumeo (Latin) red.

Iestyn (Welsh) a form of Justin.

Igashu (Native American) wanderer; seeker.
Igasho

Iggy (Latin) a familiar form of Ignatius.

Ignacio (Italian) a form of Ignatius.
Ignazio

Ignado (Spanish) fiery or ardent.

Ignatius (Latin) fiery, ardent. Religion: Saint Ignatius of Loyola founded the Jesuit order. See also Inigo, Neci.
Iggie, Iggy, Ignac, Ignác, Ignace, Ignacio, Ignacius, Ignatios, Ignatious, Ignatz, Ignaz, Ignazio

Igor (Russian) a form of Inger, Ingvar. See also Egor, Yegor.
Igoryok

Ihsan (Turkish) compassionate.

Ike (Hebrew) a familiar form of Isaac. History: the nickname of the thirty-fourth U.S. president

Dwight D. Eisenhower.
Ikee, Ikey

Iker (Basque) visitation.

Ilan (Hebrew) tree. (Basque) youth.

Ilari (Basque) a form of Hilary.
Ilario

Ilias (Greek) a form of Elijah.
Illias, Illyas, Ilyas, Ilyes

Ilidio (Latin) troop.

Illan (Basque, Latin) youth.

Illayuc (Quechua) luminous; fortunate, touched by the gods.

Ilom (Ibo) my enemies are many.

Iluminado (Latin) he who receives the inspiration of God.

Ilya (Russian) a form of Elijah.
Ilia, Ilie, Ilija, Iliya, Ilja, Illia, Illya

Imad (Arabic) supportive; mainstay.

Iman **GB** (Hebrew) a short form of Immanuel.

Imani **GB** (Hebrew) a form of Iman.
Imanni

Immanuel (Hebrew) a form of Emmanuel.
Iman, Imanol, Imanuel, Immanual, Immanuele, Immuneal

Imran (Arabic) host.
Imraan

Imre (Hungarian) a form of Emery.
Imri

Imrich (Czech) a form of Emery.
Imrus

Inalef (Mapuche) swift reinforcement; he who follows behind.

Inay (Hindi) god; godlike.

Inca (Quechua) king; prince or male-child of royal heritage.

Incaurco, Incaurcu (Quechua) hill; Incan god.

Ince (Hungarian) innocent.

Indalecio (Arabic) same as the master.

Inder (Hindi) god; godlike.
Inderbir, Inderdeep, Inderjeet, Inderjit, Inderpal, Inderpreet, Inderveer, Indervir, Indra, Indrajit

Indiana (American) land of Indians. Geography: name of a U.S. state.
Indi, Indy

Indíbil (Spanish) he who is very black.

Indro (Spanish) victor.

Inek (Welsh) a form of Irvin.

Ing (Scandinavian) a short form of Ingmar.
Inge

Ingelbert (German) a form of Engelbert.
Inglebert

Inger (Scandinavian) son's army.
Igor, Ingemar, Ingmar

Ingmar (Scandinavian) famous son.
Ing, Ingamar, Ingamur, Ingemar

Ingram (English) angel.
Inglis, Ingra, Ingraham, Ingrim

Ingvar (Scandinavian) Ing's soldier.
Igor, Ingevar

Inigo (Basque) a form of Ignatius.
Iñaki, Iniego, Iñigo

Iniko (Ibo) born during bad times.

Innis (Irish) island.
Innes, Inness, Inniss

Innocenzio (Italian) innocent.
Innocenty, Inocenci, Inocencio, Inocente, Inosente

Inteus (Native American) proud; unashamed.

Intiauqui (Quechua) sun prince.

Intichurin (Quechua) child of the sun.

Intiguaman (Quechua) sun falcon.

Intiyafa (Quechua) ray of sunlight.

Ioakim (Russian) a form of Joachim.
Ioachime, Ioakimo, Iov

Ioan (Greek, Bulgarian, Romanian) a form of John.
Ioane, Ioann, Ioannes, Ioannikios, Ioannis, Ionel

Iokepa (Hawaiian) a form of Joseph.
Keo

Iolo (Welsh) the Lord is worthy.
Iorwerth

Ionakana (Hawaiian) a form of Jonathan.

Iorgos (Greek) a form of George.

Iosif (Greek, Russian) a form of Joseph.

Iosua (Romanian) a form of Joshua.

Ipyana (Nyakyusa) graceful.

Ira (Hebrew) watchful.

Iram (English) bright.

Irene GB (Greek) peaceful.

Ireneo, Irineo (Greek) lover of peace.

Iris GB (Greek) rainbow.

Irumba (Rutooro) born after twins.

Irv (Irish, Welsh, English) a short form of Irvin, Irving.

Irvin (Irish, Welsh, English) a short form of Irving. See also Ervine.
Inek, Irv, Irven, Irvine, Irvinn, Irvon

Irving (Irish) handsome. (Welsh) white river. (English) sea friend. See also Ervin, Ervine.
Irv, Irvin, Irvington, Irwin, Irwing

Irwin (English) a form of Irving. See also Ervin.
Irwinn, Irwyn

Isa (Arabic) a form of Jesus.
Isaah

Isaac ☆ (Hebrew) he will laugh. Bible: the son of Abraham and Sarah. See also Itzak, Izak, Yitzchak.
Aizik, Icek, Ike, Ikey, Ikie, Isaak, Isaakios, Isac, Isacc, Isacco, Isack, Isaic, Ishaq, Isiac, Isiacc, Issac, Issca, Itzak, Izak, Izzy

Isaak (Hebrew) a form of Isaac.
Isack, Isak, Isik, Issak

Isabel GB (Spanish) consecrated to God.

Isabella GB (Italian) a form of Isabel.

Isabelle GB (French) a form of Isabel.

Isacar (Hebrew) he was given for a favor.

Isadoro (Spanish) gift of Isis.

Isaiah ☆ **BG** (Hebrew) God is my salvation. Bible: a Hebrew prophet.
Isa, Isai, Isaia, Isaias, Isaid, Isaih, Isaish, Ishaq, Isia, Isiah, Isiash, Issia, Issiah, Izaiah, Izaiha, Izaya, Izayah, Izayaih, Izayiah, Izeyah, Izeyha

Isaias (Hebrew) a form of Isaiah.
Isaiahs, Isais, Izayus

Isaías (Hebrew) a form of Isaias.

Isam (Arabic) safeguard.

Isamar GB (Hebrew) a form of Itamar.

Isas (Japanese) meritorious.

Iscay (Quechua) second child.

Iscaycuari (Quechua) doubly savage and untamable.

Isekemu (Native American) slow-moving creek.

Isham (English) home of the iron one.

Ishan (Hindi) direction.
Ishaan, Ishaun

Ishaq (Arabic) a form of Isaac.
Ishaac, Ishak

Ishmael (Hebrew) God will hear. Literature: the narrator of Herman Melville's novel *Moby-Dick*.
Isamael, Isamail, Ishma, Ishmail, Ishmale, Ishmeal, Ishmeil, Ishmel, Ishmil, Ismael, Ismail

Isidore (Greek) gift of Isis. See also Dorian, Ysidro.
Isador, Isadore, Isadorios, Isidor, Isidro, Issy, Ixidor, Izadore, Izidor, Izidore, Izydor, Izzy

Isidro (Greek) a form of Isidore.
Isidoro, Isidoros

Iskander (Afghan) a form of Alexander.

Ismael (Arabic) a form of Ishmael.

Ismail (Arabic) a form of Ishmael.
Ismeil, Ismiel

Isocrates (Greek) he who can do as much as the next man.

Isod (Hebrew) God fights and prevails; the angel's antagonist.

Israel (Hebrew) prince of God; wrestled with God. History: the nation of Israel took its name from the name given Jacob after he wrestled with the angel of the Lord. See also Yisrael.
Iser, Isreal, Israhel, Isrell, Isrrael, Isser, Izrael, Izzy, Yisrael

Isreal (Hebrew) a form of Israel.
Isrieal

Issa (Swahili) God is our salvation.

Issac (Hebrew) a form of Isaac.
Issacc, Issaic, Issiac

Issiah (Hebrew) a form of Isaiah.
Issaiah, Issia

Istu (Native American) sugar pine.

István (Hungarian) a form of Stephen.
Isti, Istvan, Pista

Itaete (Guarani) blade.

Italo (Latin) he came from the land that is between the seas.

Ithel (Welsh) generous lord.

Itamar, Ittamar (Hebrew) island of palms.

Itzak (Hebrew) a form of Isaac, Yitzchak.
Itzik

Iukini (Hawaiian) a form of Eugene.
Kini

Iustin (Bulgarian, Russian) a form of Justin.

Ivan (Russian) a form of John.
Iván, Ivanchik, Ivanichek, Ivann, Ivano, Ivas, Iven, Ivin, Ivon, Ivyn, Vanya

Ivar BG (Scandinavian) a form of Ivor. See also Yves, Yvon.
Iv, Iva

Ives (English) young archer.
Ive, Iven, Ivey, Yves

Ivey GB (English) a form of Ives.

Ivo (German) yew wood; bow wood.
Ibon, Ivar, Ives, Ivon, Ivonnie, Ivor, Yvo

Ivor (Scandinavian) a form of Ivo.
Ibon, Ifor, Ivar, Iver, Ivory, Ivry

Ivy GB (English) ivy tree.

Iwan (Polish) a form of John.

Iyafa, Iyapa (Quechua) lightning.

Iyapo (Yoruba) many trials; many obstacles.

Iyapoma, Iyapuma (Quechua) puma of light.

Iyapu (Quechua) lightning.

Iyatecsi, Iyaticsi (Quechua) eternal light; origin of light.

Iye (Native American) smoke.

Izak (Czech) a form of Isaac.
Itzhak, Ixaka, Izaac, Izaak, Izac, Izaic, Izak, Izec, Izeke, Izick, Izik, Izsak, Izsák, Izzak

Izzy (Hebrew) a familiar form of Isaac, Isidore, Israel.
Issy

J BG (American) an initial used as a first name.
J.

Ja (Korean) attractive, magnetic.

Ja'far (Sanskrit) little stream.
Jafar, Jafari, Jaffar, Jaffer, Jafur

Jaali (Swahili) powerful.

Jaan (Estonian) a form of Christian.

Jaap (Dutch) a form of Jim.

Jabari (Swahili) fearless, brave.
Jabaar, Jabahri, Jabar, Jabarae, Jabare, Jabaree, Jabarei, Jabarie, Jabarri, Jabarrie, Jabary, Jabbar, Jabbaree, Jabbari, Jaber, Jabiari, Jabier, Jabori, Jaborie

Jabel (Hebrew) like the arrow that flies.

Jabez (Hebrew) born in pain.
Jabe, Jabes, Jabesh

Jabin (Hebrew) God has created.
Jabain, Jabien, Jabon

Jabir (Arabic) consoler, comforter.
Jabiri, Jabori

Jabril (Arabic) a form of Jibril.
Jabrail, Jabree, Jabreel, Jabrel, Jabrell, Jabrelle, Jabri, Jabrial, Jabrie, Jabriel, Jabrielle, Jabrille

Jabulani (Shona) happy.

Jacan (Hebrew) trouble.
Jachin

Jacari (American) a form of Jacorey.
Jacarey, Jacaris, Jacarius, Jacarre, Jacarri, Jacarrus, Jacarus, Jacary, Jacaure, Jacauri, Jaccar, Jaccari

Jace BG (American) a combination of the initials J. + C.
JC, J.C., Jacee, Jacek, Jacey, Jacie, Jaice, Jaicee

Jacen (Greek) a form of Jason.
Jaceon

Jacey GB (American) a form of Jace.

Jacinto (Portuguese, Spanish) hyacinth. See also Giacinto.
Jacindo, Jacint, Jacinta

Jack ☆ (American) a familiar form of Jacob, John. See also Keaka.
Jackie, Jacko, Jackub, Jak, Jax, Jock, Jocko

Jackie, Jacky BG (American) familiar forms of Jack.
Jackey

Jackson ☆ BG (English) son of Jack.
Jacksen, Jacksin, Jacson, Jakson, Jaxon

Jaclyn GB (American) a short form of Jacqueline (see Girls' Names).

Jaco (Portuguese) a form of Jacob.

Jacob ☆ BG (Hebrew) supplanter, substitute. Bible: son of Isaac, brother of Esau. See also Akiva, Chago, Checha, Coby, Diego, Giacomo, Hamish, Iago, Iakobos, James, Kiva, Koby, Kuba, Tiago, Yakov, Yasha, Yoakim.
Jaap, Jachob, Jack, Jackob, Jackub, Jaco, Jacobb, Jacobe, Jacobi, Jacobo, Jacoby, Jacolbi, Jacolby, Jacque, Jacques, Jacub, Jaecob, Jago, Jaicob, Jaime, Jake, Jakob, Jalu, Jasha, Jaycob, Jecis, Jeks, Jeska, Jim, Jocek,

Jock, Jocob, Jocobb, Jocoby, Jocolby, Jokubas

Jacobi, Jacoby B̄G (Hebrew) forms of Jacob.
Jachobi, Jacobbe, Jacobee, Jacobey, Jacobie, Jacobii, Jacobis

Jacobo (Hebrew) a form of Jacob.

Jacobson (English) son of Jacob.
Jacobs, Jacobsen, Jacobsin, Jacobus

Jacorey (American) a combination of Jacob + Corey.
Jacari, Jacori, Jacoria, Jacorie, Jacoris, Jacorius, Jacorrey, Jacorrien, Jacorry, Jacory, Jacouri, Jacourie, Jakari

Jacque (French) a form of Jacob.
Jacquay, Jacqui, Jocque, Jocqui

Jacques B̄G (French) a form of Jacob, James. See also Coco.
Jackque, Jackques, Jackquise, Jacot, Jacquan, Jacquees, Jacquese, Jacquess, Jacquet, Jacquett, Jacquez, Jacquis, Jacquise, Jaquez, Jarques, Jarquis

Jacquez, Jaquez (French) forms of Jacques.
Jaques, Jaquese, Jaqueus, Jaqueze, Jaquis, Jaquise, Jaquze, Jocquez

Jacy (Tupi-Guarani) moon.
Jaicy, Jaycee

Jada ḠB (American) a short form of Jadrien.

Jade ḠB (Spanish) jade, precious stone.
Jaeid, Jaid, Jaide

Jaden ☆ B̄G (Hebrew) a form of Jadon.
Jadee, Jadeen, Jadenn, Jadeon, Jadin, Jaeden

Jadon (Hebrew) God has heard.
Jaden, Jadyn, Jaedon, Jaiden, Jaydon

Jadrien (American) a combination of Jay + Adrien.
Jad, Jada, Jadd, Jader, Jadrian

Jadyn ḠB (Hebrew) a form of Jadon.
Jadyne, Jaedyn

Jae-Hwa (Korean) rich, prosperous.

Jaegar (German) hunter.
Jaager, Jaeger, Jagur

Jael ḠB (Hebrew) mountain goat.
Yael

Jaelen (American) a form of Jalen.
Jaelan, Jaelaun, Jaelin, Jaelon, Jaelyn

Jagger (English) carter.
Jagar, Jager, Jaggar

Jago (English) a form of James.

Jaguar (Spanish) jaguar.
Jagguar

Jahi (Swahili) dignified.

Jahlil (Hindi) a form of Jalil.
Jahlal, Jahlee, Jahleel, Jahliel

Jahmar (American) a form of Jamar.
Jahmare, Jahmari, Jahmarr, Jahmer

Jahvon (Hebrew) a form of Javan.
Jahvan, Jahvine, Jahwaan, Jahwon

Jai 🅱🅶 (Tai) heart.
Jaie, Jaii

Jaiden 🅱🅶 (Hebrew) a form of Jadon.
Jaidan, Jaidon, Jaidyn

Jailen (American) a form of Jalen.
Jailan, Jailani, Jaileen, Jailen, Jailon, Jailyn, Jailynn

Jaime 🅱🅶 (Spanish) a form of Jacob, James.
Jaimey, Jaimie, Jaimito, Jaimy, Jayme, Jaymie

Jaimee 🅶🅱 (Spanish) a form of Jaime.

Jaimie 🅶🅱 (English) a form of Jamie. (Spanish) a form of Jaime.

Jaír (Spanish) a form of Jairo.

Jairo (Spanish) God enlightens.
Jair, Jairay, Jaire, Jairus, Jarius

Jaison (Greek) a form of Jason.
Jaisan, Jaisen, Jaishon, Jaishun

Jaivon (Hebrew) a form of Javan.
Jaiven, Jaivion, Jaiwon

Jaja (Ibo) honored.

Jajuan (American) a combination of the prefix Ja + Juan.
Ja Juan, Jauan, Jawaun, Jejuan, Jujuan, Juwan

Jakari (American) a form of Jacorey.
Jakaire, Jakar, Jakaray, Jakarie, Jakarious, Jakarius, Jakarre, Jakarri, Jakarus

Jake ☀ (Hebrew) a short form of Jacob.
Jakie, Jayk, Jayke

Jakeem (Arabic) uplifted.

Jakob (Hebrew) a form of Jacob.
Jaekob, Jaikab, Jaikob, Jakab, Jakeb, Jakeob, Jakeub, Jakib, Jakiv, Jakobe, Jakobi, Jakobus, Jakoby, Jakov, Jakovian, Jakub, Jakubek, Jekebs

Jakome (Basque) a form of James.
Xanti

Jal (Gypsy) wanderer.

Jalan (American) a form of Jalen.
Jalaan, Jalaen, Jalain, Jaland, Jalane, Jalani, Jalanie, Jalann, Jalaun, Jalean, Jallan

Jaleel 🅱🅶 (Hindi) a form of Jalil.
Jaleell, Jaleil, Jalel

Jalen BG (American) a combination of the prefix Ja + Len.
Jaelen, Jailen, Jalan, Jaleen, Jalend, Jalene, Jalin, Jallen, Jalon, Jalyn

Jalil (Hindi) revered.
Jahlil, Jalaal, Jalal

Jalin, Jalyn (American) forms of Jalen.
Jalian, Jaline, Jalynn, Jalynne

Jalisat (Arabic) he who receives little, gives more.

Jalon (American) a form of Jalen.
Jalone, Jaloni, Jalun

Jam (American) a short form of Jamal, Jamar.
Jama

Jamaal BG (Arabic) a form of Jamal.

Jamaine (Arabic) a form of Germain.

Jamal BG (Arabic) handsome.
See also Gamal.
Jahmal, Jahmall, Jahmalle, Jahmeal, Jahmeel, Jahmeil, Jahmel, Jahmelle, Jahmil, Jahmile, Jaimal, Jam, Jamaal, Jamael, Jamahl, Jamail, Jamaile, Jamala, Jamale, Jamall, Jamalle, Jamar, Jamaul, Jamel, Jamil, Jammal, Jamor, Jamual, Jarmal, Jaumal, Jemal, Jermal, Jomal, Jomall

Jamar BG (American) a form of Jamal.
Jam, Jamaar, Jamaari, Jamahrae, Jamair, Jamara, Jamaras, Jamaraus, Jamarl, Jamarr, Jamarre, Jamarrea, Jamarree, Jamarri, Jamarvis, Jamaur, Jamir, Jamire, Jamiree, Jammar, Jarmar, Jarmarr, Jaumar, Jemaar, Jemar, Jimar, Jomar

Jamarcus BG (American) a combination of the prefix Ja + Marcus.
Jamarco, Jamarkus, Jemarcus, Jimarcus

Jamari (American) a form of Jamario.
Jamare, Jamarea, Jamaree, Jamareh, Jamaria, Jamarie, Jamaul

Jamario (American) a combination of the prefix Ja + Mario.
Jamareo, Jamari, Jamariel, Jamarious, Jamaris, Jamarius, Jamariya, Jemario, Jemarus

Jamarquis (American) a combination of the prefix Ja + Marquis.
Jamarkees, Jamarkeus, Jamarkis, Jamarqese, Jamarqueis, Jamarques, Jamarquez, Jamarquios, Jamarqus

Jamel (Arabic) a form of Jamal.
Jameel, Jamele, Jamell, Jamelle, Jammel, Jamuel, Jamul, Jarmel, Jaumal, Jaumell, Je-Mell, Jimell

James ☀ B🄶 (Hebrew)
supplanter, substitute. (English) a
form of Jacob. Bible: James the
Great and James the Less were
two of the Twelve Apostles. See
also Diego, Hamish, Iago, Kimo,
Santiago, Seamus, Seumas, Yago,
Yasha.
*Jacques, Jago, Jaime, Jaimes,
Jakome, Jamesie, Jamesy,
Jamez, Jameze, Jamie, Jamies,
Jamse, Jamyes, Jamze, Jas,
Jasha, Jay, Jaymes, Jem, Jemes,
Jim*

Jameson B🄶 (English) son of
James.
*Jamerson, Jamesian, Jamison,
Jaymeson*

Jami G🄱 (English) a form of
Jamie.

Jamie G🄱 (English) a familiar
form of James.
*Jaime, Jaimey, Jaimie, Jame,
Jamee, Jamey, Jameyel, Jami,
Jamia, Jamiah, Jamian, Jamme,
Jammie, Jamiee, Jammy, Jamy,
Jamye, Jayme, Jaymee, Jaymie*

Jamil B🄶 (Arabic) a form of
Jamal.
*Jamiel, Jamiell, Jamielle, Jamile,
Jamill, Jamille, Jamyl, Jarmil*

Jamin (Hebrew) favored.
*Jamen, Jamian, Jamien, Jamion,
Jamionn, Jamon, Jamun, Jamyn,
Jarmin, Jarmon, Jaymin*

Jamison B🄶 (English) son of
James.
*Jamiesen, Jamieson, Jamis,
Jamisen, Jamyson, Jaymison*

Jamon (Hebrew) a form of Jamin.
Jamohn, Jamone, Jamoni

Jamond (American) a
combination of James +
Raymond.
*Jamod, Jamont, Jamonta,
Jamontae, Jamontay, Jamonte,
Jarmond*

Jamor (American) a form of
Jamal.
*Jamoree, Jamori, Jamorie,
Jamorius, Jamorrio, Jamorris,
Jamory, Jamour*

Jamsheed (Persian) from Persia.
Jamshaid, Jamshed

Jan B🄶 (Dutch, Slavic) a form of
John.
*Jaan, Jana, Janae, Jann, Janne,
Jano, Janson, Jenda, Yan*

Jana G🄱 (Dutch, Slavic) a form of
Jan.

Janae G🄱 (Dutch, Slavic) a form
of Jan.

Janco (Czech) a form of John.
Jancsi, Janke, Janko

Jando (Spanish) a form of
Alexander.
Jandino

Jane G🄱 (Hebrew) God is
gracious.

Janeil (American) a combination of the prefix Ja + Neil.
Janal, Janel, Janell, Janelle, Janiel, Janielle, Janile, Janille, Jarnail, Jarneil, Jarnell

Janek (Polish) a form of John.
Janak, Janik, Janika, Janka, Jankiel, Janko

Janell, Janelle **GB** (American) forms of Janeil.

Janessa **GB** (American) a form of Jane.

Janette **GB** (French) a form of Janet (see Girls' Names).

Janine **GB** (French) a form of Jane.

Janis **GB** (Latvian) a form of John.
Ansis, Jancis, Zanis

Janne (Finnish) a form of John.
Jann, Jannes

János (Hungarian) a form of John.
Jancsi, Jani, Jankia, Jano

Janson (Scandinavian) son of Jan.
Janse, Jansen, Jansin, Janssen, Jansun, Jantzen, Janzen, Jensen, Jenson

Jantzen (Scandinavian) a form of Janson.
Janten, Jantsen, Jantson

Janus (Latin) gate, passageway; born in January. Mythology: the Roman god of beginnings and endings.
Jannese, Jannus, Januario, Janusz

Japheth (Hebrew) handsome. (Arabic) abundant. Bible: a son of Noah. See also Yaphet.
Japeth, Japhet

Jaquan **BG** (American) a combination of the prefix Ja + Quan.
Jaequan, Jaiqaun, Jaiquan, Jaqaun, Jaqawan, Jaquaan, Jaquain, Ja'quan, Jaquane, Jaquann, Jaquanne, Jaquavius, Jaquawn, Jaquin, Jaquon, Jaqwan

Jaquarius (American) a combination of Jaquan + Darius.
Jaquari, Jaquarious, Jaquaris

Jaquavius (American) a form of Jaquan.
Jaquavas, Jaquaveis, Jaquaveius, Jaquaveon, Jaquaveous, Jaquavias, Jaquavious, Jaquavis, Jaquavus

Jaquon (American) a form of Jaquan.
Jaequon, Jaqoun, Jaquinn, Jaqune, Jaquoin, Jaquone, Jaqwon

Jarad (Hebrew) a form of Jared.
Jaraad, Jaraed

Jarah (Hebrew) sweet as honey.
Jerah

Jardan (Hebrew) a form of Jordan.
Jarden, Jardin, Jardon

Jareb (Hebrew) contending.
Jarib

Jared BG (Hebrew) a form of Jordan.
Jahred, Jaired, Jarad, Jaredd, Jareid, Jarid, Jarod, Jarred, Jarrett, Jarrod, Jarryd, Jerad, Jered, Jerod, Jerrad, Jerred, Jerrod, Jerryd, Jordan

Jarek (Slavic) born in January.
Janiuszck, Januarius, Januisz, Jarec, Jarrek, Jarric, Jarrick

Jarell (Scandinavian) a form of Gerald.
Jairell, Jarael, Jareil, Jarel, Jarelle, Jariel, Jarrell, Jarryl, Jayryl, Jerel, Jerell, Jerrell, Jharell

Jaren (Hebrew) a form of Jaron.
Jarian, Jarien, Jarin, Jarion

Jareth (American) a combination of Jared + Gareth.
Jarreth, Jereth, Jarreth

Jarett (English) a form of Jarrett.
Jaret, Jarette

Jarl (Scandinavian) earl, nobleman.

Jarlath (Latin) in control.
Jarl, Jarlen

Jarman (German) from Germany.
Jerman

Jarod BG (Hebrew) a form of Jared.
Jarodd, Jaroid

Jaron (Hebrew) he will sing; he will cry out.
Jaaron, Jairon, Jaren, Jarone, Jarren, Jarron, Jaryn, Jayron, Jayronn, Je Ronn, J'ron

Jaroslav (Czech) glory of spring.
Jarda

Jarred BG (Hebrew) a form of Jared.
Ja'red, Jarrad, Jarrayd, Jarrid, Jarrod, Jarryd, Jerrid

Jarrell (English) a form of Gerald.
Jarel, Jarell, Jarrel, Jerall, Jerel, Jerell

Jarren (Hebrew) a form of Jaron.
Jarrain, Jarran, Jarrian, Jarrin

Jarrett BG (English) a form of Garrett, Jared.
Jairett, Jareth, Jarett, Jaretté, Jarhett, Jarratt, Jarret, Jarrette, Jarrot, Jarrott, Jerrett

Jarrod (Hebrew) a form of Jared.
Jarod, Jerod, Jerrod

Jarryd (Hebrew) a form of Jared.
Jarrayd, Jaryd

Jarvis (German) skilled with a spear.
Jaravis, Jarv, Jarvaris, Jarvas, Jarvaska, Jarvey, Jarvez, Jarvie, Jarvios, Jarvious, Jarvius, Jarvorice, Jarvoris, Jarvous, Jarvus, Javaris, Jervey, Jervis

Jaryn (Hebrew) a form of Jaron.
Jarryn, Jarynn, Jaryon

Jas BG (Polish) a form of John.
(English) a familiar form of James.
Jasio

Jasha (Russian) a familiar form
of Jacob, James.
Jascha

Jashawn (American) a combi-
nation of the prefix Ja + Shawn.
*Jasean, Jashan, Jashaun,
Jashion, Jashon*

Jaskaran BG (Sikh) sings praises
to the Lord.
Jaskaren, Jaskarn, Jaskiran

Jaskarn BG (Sikh) a form of
Jaskaran.

Jasleen GB (Latin) a form of
Jocelyn.

Jasmeet BG (Persian) a form of
Jasmine.

Jasmin GB (Persian) jasmine
flower.
*Jasman, Jasmanie, Jasmine,
Jasmon, Jasmond*

Jasmine GB (Persian) a form of
Jasmin.

Jason ☀ (Greek) healer.
Mythology: the hero who led the
Argonauts in search of the
Golden Fleece.
*Jacen, Jaeson, Jahson, Jaison,
Jasan, Jasaun, Jase, Jasen, Jasin,
Jasson, Jasten, Jasun, Jasyn,
Jathan, Jathon, Jay, Jayson*

Jasón (Greek) a form of Jason.

Jaspal (Punjabi) living a virtuous
lifestyle.

Jasper BG (French) brown, red,
or yellow ornamental stone.
(English) a form of Casper. See
also Kasper.
Jaspar, Jazper, Jespar, Jesper

Jaspreet BG (Punjabi) virtuous.

Jasson (Greek) a form of Jason.
Jassen, Jassin

Jatinra (Hindi) great Brahmin sage.

Javan (Hebrew) Bible: son of
Japheth.
*Jaewan, Jahvaughan, Jahvon,
Jaivon, Javante, Javaon,
JaVaughn, Javen, Javian, Javien,
Javin, Javine, Javoanta, Javon,
Javona, Javone, Javonte, Jayvin,
Jayvion, Jayvon, Jevan, Jevon*

Javante (American) a form of
Javan.
*Javantae, Javantai, Javantée,
Javanti*

Javaris (English) a form of Jarvis.
*Javaor, Javar, Javaras, Javare,
Javares, Javari, Javarias,
Javaries, Javario, Javarius,
Javaro, Javaron, Javarous,
Javarre, Javarreis, Javarri,
Javarrious, Javarris, Javarro,
Javarte, Javarus, Javorious,
Javoris, Javorius, Javouris*

Javas (Sanskrit) quick, swift.
Jayvas, Jayvis

Javier (Spanish) owner of a new house. See also Xavier.
Jabier, Javer, Javere, Javiar

Javiero (Spanish) born in January.

Javon 🅱🅶 (Hebrew) a form of Javan.
Jaavon, Jaevin, Jaevon, Jaewon, Javeon, Javion, Javionne, Javohn, Javona, Javone, Javoney, Javoni, Javonn, Javonne, Javonni, Javonnie, Javonnte, Javoun, Jayvon

Javonte 🅱🅶 (American) a form of Javan.
Javona, Javontae, Javontai, Javontay, Javontaye, Javonté, Javontee, Javonteh, Javontey

Jawaun (American) a form of Jajuan.
Jawaan, Jawan, Jawann, Jawn, Jawon, Jawuan

Jawhar (Arabic) jewel; essence.

Jaxon (English) a form of Jackson.
Jaxen, Jaxsen, Jaxson, Jaxsun, Jaxun

Jay 🅱🅶 (French) blue jay. (English) a short form of James, Jason.
Jae, Jai, Jave, Jaye, Jeays, Jeyes

Jayce (American) a combination of the initials J. + C.
JC, J.C., Jayc, Jaycee, Jay Cee, Jaycey, Jecie

Jaycob (Hebrew) a form of Jacob.
Jaycub, Jaykob

Jayde 🅶🅱 (American) a combination of the initials J. + D.
JD, J.D., Jayd, Jaydee, Jayden

Jayden ☀ 🅱🅶 (American) a form of Jayde.
Jaydan, Jaydin, Jaydn, Jaydon

Jayla 🅶🅱 (American) a form of Jaylee.

Jaylee (American) a combination of Jay + Lee.
Jayla, Jayle, Jaylen

Jaylen 🅱🅶 (American) a combination of Jay + Len.
Jaylaan, Jaylan, Jayland, Jayleen, Jaylend, Jaylin, Jayln, Jaylon, Jaylun, Jaylund, Jaylyn

Jaylin 🅱🅶 (American) a form of Jaylen.
Jaylian, Jayline

Jaylon 🅱🅶 (American) a form of Jaylen.
Jayleon

Jaylyn 🅱🅶 (American) a form of Jaylen.
Jaylynd, Jaylynn, Jaylynne

Jayme 🅶🅱 (English) a form of Jamie.
Jaymie

Jaymes (English) a form of James.
Jaymis, Jayms, Jaymz

Jayquan (American) a combination of Jay + Quan.
Jaykwan, Jaykwon, Jayqon, Jayquawn, Jayqunn

Jayson (Greek) a form of Jason.
Jaycent, Jaysean, Jaysen, Jayshaun, Jayshawn, Jayshon, Jayshun, Jaysin, Jaysn, Jayssen, Jaysson, Jaysun

Jayvon (American) a form of Javon.
Jayvion, Jayvohn, Jayvone, Jayvonn, Jayvontay, Jayvonte, Jaywan, Jaywaun, Jaywin

Jazmine **GB** (Persian) a form of Jasmine.

Jazz (American) jazz.
Jaz, Jazze, Jazzlee, Jazzman, Jazzmen, Jazzmin, Jazzmon, Jazztin, Jazzton, Jazzy

Jean **BG** (French) a form of John.
Jéan, Jeane, Jeannah, Jeannie, Jeannot, Jeano, Jeanot, Jeanty, Jene

Jeanette **GB** (French) a form of Jean.

Jeb (Hebrew) a short form of Jebediah.
Jebb, Jebi, Jeby

Jebediah (Hebrew) a form of Jedidiah.
Jeb, Jebadia, Jebadiah, Jebadieh, Jebidiah

Jed (Hebrew) a short form of Jedidiah. (Arabic) hand.
Jedd, Jeddy, Jedi

Jediah (Hebrew) hand of God.
Jedaia, Jedaiah, Jedeiah, Jedi, Yedaya

Jedidiah **BG** (Hebrew) friend of God, beloved of God. See also **Didi.**
Jebediah, Jed, Jedadiah, Jeddediah, Jedediah, Jedediha, Jedidia, Jedidiah, Jedidiyah, Yedidya

Jedrek (Polish) strong; manly.
Jedric, Jedrik, Jedrus

Jeff (English) a short form of Jefferson, Jeffrey. A familiar form of Geoffrey.
Jef, Jefe, Jeffe, Jeffey, Jeffie, Jeffy, Jhef

Jefferson **BG** (English) son of Jeff. History: Thomas Jefferson was the third U.S. president.
Jeferson, Jeff, Jeffers

Jeffery **BG** (English) a form of Jeffrey.
Jefery, Jeffari, Jeffary, Jeffeory, Jefferay, Jeffereoy, Jefferey, Jefferie, Jeffory

Jefford (English) Jeff's ford.

Jeffrey **BG** (English) divinely peaceful. See also **Geffrey, Geoffrey, Godfrey.**
Jeff, Jefferies, Jeffery, Jeffre, Jeffree, Jeffrery, Jeffrie, Jeffries, Jeffry, Jefre, Jefri, Jefry, Jeoffroi, Joffre, Joffrey

Jeffry (English) a form of Jeffrey.

Jehan (French) a form of John.
Jehann

Jehová (Hebrew) I am what I am.

Jehu (Hebrew) God lives. Bible: a military commander and king of Israel.
Yehu

Jelani (Swahili) mighty.
Jel, Jelan, Jelanie, Jelaun

Jem ☐ (English) a short form of James, Jeremiah.
Jemmie, Jemmy

Jemal (Arabic) a form of Jamal.
Jemaal, Jemael, Jemale, Jemel

Jemel (Arabic) a form of Jemal.
Jemeal, Jemehl, Jemehyl, Jemell, Jemelle, Jemello, Jemeyle, Jemile, Jemmy

Jemond (French) worldly.
Jemon, Jémond, Jemonde, Jemone

Jenaro (Latin) born in January.

Jenkin (Flemish) little John.
Jenkins, Jenkyn, Jenkyns, Jennings

Jenna ☐ (Arabic) small bird. (Welsh) a short form of Jennifer.

Jennifer ☐ (Welsh) white wave; white phantom. A form of Guinevere (see Girls' Names).

Jenny ☐ (Welsh) a familiar form of Jennifer.

Jenö (Hungarian) a form of Eugene.
Jenci, Jency, Jenoe, Jensi, Jensy

Jenofonte (Greek) he who comes from another country and is eloquent.

Jens (Danish) a form of John.
Jense, Jensen, Jenson, Jenssen, Jensy, Jentz

Jeovanni (Italian) a form of Giovanni.
Jeovahny, Jeovan, Jeovani, Jeovany

Jequan (American) a combination of the prefix Je + Quan.
Jeqaun, Jequann, Jequon

Jerad, Jerrad (Hebrew) forms of Jared.
Jeread, Jeredd

Jerahmy (Hebrew) a form of Jeremy.
Jerahmeel, Jerahmeil, Jerahmey

Jerald (English) a form of Gerald.
Jeraldo, Jerold, Jerral, Jerrald, Jerrold, Jerry

Jerall (English) a form of Jarrell.
Jerael, Jerai, Jerail, Jeraile, Jeral, Jerale, Jerall, Jerrail, Jerral, Jerrel, Jerrell, Jerrelle

Jeramie, Jeramy (Hebrew) forms of Jeremy.
Jerame, Jeramee, Jeramey, Jerami, Jerammie

Jerard (French) a form of
Gerard.
Jarard, Jarrard, Jerardo, Jeraude,
Jerrard

Jere (Hebrew) a short form of
Jeremiah, Jeremy.
Jeré, Jeree

Jered, Jerred (Hebrew) forms of
Jared.
Jereed, Jerid, Jerryd, Jeryd

Jerel, Jerell, Jerrell (English)
forms of Jarell.
Jerelle, Jeriel, Jeril, Jerrail,
Jerral, Jerrall, Jerrel, Jerrill,
Jerrol, Jerroll, Jerryl, Jerryll,
Jeryl, Jeryle

Jereme, Jeremey (Hebrew)
forms of Jeremy.
Jarame

Jeremiah ✡ BG (Hebrew) God
will uplift. Bible: a Hebrew
prophet. See also Dermot,
Yeremey, Yirmaya.
Geremiah, Jaramia, Jem,
Jemeriah, Jemiah, Jeramiah,
Jeramiha, Jere, Jereias,
Jeremaya, Jeremi, Jeremia,
Jeremial, Jeremias, Jeremija,
Jeremy, Jerimiah, Jerimiha,
Jerimya, Jermiah, Jermija, Jerry

Jeremías (Hebrew) a form of
Jeremiah.

Jeremie, Jérémie (Hebrew)
forms of Jeremy.
Jeremi, Jérémie, Jeremii

Jeremy BG (English) a form of
Jeremiah.
Jaremay, Jaremi, Jaremy, Jem,
Jemmy, Jerahmy, Jeramie,
Jeramy, Jere, Jereamy, Jereme,
Jeremee, Jeremey, Jeremie,
Jérémie, Jeremry, Jérémy,
Jeremye, Jereomy, Jeriemy,
Jerime, Jerimy, Jermey, Jeromy,
Jerremy

Jeriah (Hebrew) Jehovah has
seen.

Jericho (Arabic) city of the
moon. Bible: a city conquered by
Joshua.
Jeric, Jerick, Jerico, Jerik, Jerric,
Jerrick, Jerrico, Jerricoh, Jerryco

Jermaine BG (French) a form of
Germain. (English) sprout, bud.
Jarman, Jeremaine, Jeremane,
Jerimane, Jermain, Jerman,
Jermane, Jermanie, Jermanne,
Jermany, Jermayn, Jermayne,
Jermiane, Jermine, Jer-Mon,
Jermone, Jermoney, Jhirmaine

Jermal (Arabic) a form of Jamal.
Jermael, Jermail, Jermall,
Jermaul, Jermel, Jermell, Jermil,
Jermol, Jermyll

Jermey (English) a form of
Jeremy.
Jerme, Jermee, Jermere,
Jermery, Jermie, Jermy, Jhermie

Jermiah (Hebrew) a form of
Jeremiah.
Jermiha, Jermiya

Jerney (Slavic) a form of Bartholomew.

Jerod, Jerrod (Hebrew) forms of Jarrod.
Jerode, Jeroid

Jerolin (Basque, Latin) holy.

Jerome (Latin) holy. See also Geronimo, Hieronymos.
Gerome, Jere, Jeroen, Jerom, Jérome, Jérôme, Jeromo, Jeromy, Jeron, Jerónimo, Jerrome, Jerromy

Jeromy (Latin) a form of Jerome.
Jeromee, Jeromey, Jeromie

Jeron (English) a form of Jerome.
Jéron, Jerone, Jeronimo, Jerrin, Jerrion, Jerron, Jerrone, J'ron

Jerrett (Hebrew) a form of Jarrett.
Jeret, Jerett, Jeritt, Jerret, Jerrette, Jerriot, Jerritt, Jerrot, Jerrott

Jerrick (American) a combination of Jerry + Derrick.
Jaric, Jarrick, Jerick, Jerrik

Jerry B⃞G⃞ (German) mighty spearman. (English) a familiar form of Gerald, Gerard. See also Gerry, Kele.
Jehri, Jere, Jeree, Jeris, Jerison, Jerri, Jerrie, Jery

Jerusalén (Hebrew) peaceful place.

Jervis (English) a form of Gervaise, Jarvis.

Jerzy (Polish) a form of George.
Jersey, Jerzey, Jurek

Jesabel, Jezabel (Hebrew) oath of God.

Jeshua (Hebrew) a form of Joshua.
Jeshuah

Jess B⃞G⃞ (Hebrew) a short form of Jesse.

Jesse ☀ B⃞G⃞ (Hebrew) wealthy. Bible: the father of David. See also Yishai.
Jese, Jesee, Jesi, Jess, Jessé, Jessee, Jessie, Jessy

Jessenia G⃞B⃞ (Arabic) flower.

Jessi G⃞B⃞ (Hebrew) a form of Jessie.

Jessica G⃞B⃞ (Hebrew) wealthy.

Jessie B⃞G⃞ (Hebrew) a form of Jesse.
Jesie

Jessika G⃞B⃞ (Hebrew) a form of Jessica.

Jessy B⃞G⃞ (Hebrew) a form of Jesse.
Jescey, Jessey, Jessye, Jessyie, Jesy

Jestin (Welsh) a form of Justin.
Jessten, Jesten, Jeston, Jesstin, Jesston

Jesualdo (Germanic) he who takes the lead.

Jesus ✦ BG (Hebrew) a form of Joshua. Bible: son of Mary and Joseph, believed by Christians to be the Son of God. See also Chucho, Isa, Yosu.
Jecho, Jessus, Jesu, Jesús, Josu

Jesús (Hispanic) a form of Jesus.

Jethro (Hebrew) abundant. Bible: the father-in-law of Moses. See also Yitro.
Jeth, Jethroe, Jetro, Jett

Jett (English) hard, black mineral. (Hebrew) a short form of Jethro.
Jet, Jetson, Jetter, Jetty

Jevan (Hebrew) a form of Javan.
Jevaun, Jeven, Jevin

Jevon (Hebrew) a form of Javan.
Jevion, Jevohn, Jevone, Jevonn, Jevonne, Jevonnie

Jevonte (American) a form of Jevon.
Jevonta, Jevontae, Jevontaye, Jevonté

Jibade (Yoruba) born close to royalty.

Jibben (Gypsy) life.
Jibin

Jibril (Arabic) archangel of Allah.
Jabril, Jibreel, Jibriel

Jill GB (English) a short form of Jillian.

Jillian GB (Latin) youthful.

Jilt (Dutch) money.

Jim (Hebrew, English) a short form of James. See also Jaap.
Jimbo, Jimm, Jimmy

Jimbo (American) a familiar form of Jim.
Jimboo

Jimell (Arabic) a form of Jamel.
Jimel, Jimelle, Jimill, Jimmell, Jimmelle, Jimmiel, Jimmil

Jimeno (Spanish) a form of Simeón.

Jimiyu (Abaluhya) born in the dry season.

Jimmie BG (English) a form of Jimmy.
Jimi, Jimie, Jimmee, Jimmi

Jimmy BG (English) a familiar form of Jim.
Jimmey, Jimmie, Jimmye, Jimmyjo, Jimy

Jimoh (Swahili) born on Friday.

Jin BG (Chinese) gold.
Jinn

Jindra (Czech) a form of Harold.

Jing-Quo (Chinese) ruler of the country.

Jiovanni (Italian) a form of Giovanni.
Jio, Jiovani, Jiovanie, Jiovann, Jiovannie, Jiovanny, Jiovany, Jiovoni, Jivan

Jirair (Armenian) strong; hard working.

Jiri (Czech) a form of George.
Jirka

Jiro (Japanese) second son.

Jivin (Hindi) life giver.
Jivanta

Jo GB (Hebrew, Japanese) a form of Joe.

Joab (Hebrew) God is father. See also Yoav.
Joabe, Joaby

Joachim (Hebrew) God will establish. See also Akeem, Ioakim, Yehoyakem.
Joacheim, Joakim, Joaquim, Joaquín, Jokin, Jov

Joanna GB (English) a form of Joan (see Girls' Names).

João (Portuguese) a form of John.

Joaquim (Portuguese) a form of Joachim.

Joaquín (Spanish) a form of Joachim, Yehoyakem.
Jehoichin, Joaquin, Jocquin, Jocquinn, Juaquin

Job (Hebrew) afflicted. Bible: a righteous man whose faith in God survived the test of many afflictions.
Jobe, Jobert, Jobey, Jobie, Joby

Joben (Japanese) enjoys cleanliness.
Joban, Jobin

Jobo (Spanish) a familiar form of Joseph.

Joby BG (Hebrew) a familiar form of Job.
Jobie

Jocelyn GB (Latin) joyous.

Jock (American) a familiar form of Jacob.
Jocko, Joco, Jocoby, Jocolby

Jocquez (French) a form of Jacquez.
Jocques, Jocquis, Jocquise

Jodan (Hebrew) a combination of Jo + Dan.
Jodahn, Joden, Jodhan, Jodian, Jodin, Jodon, Jodonnis

Jodi, Jodie GB (Hebrew) forms of Jody.

Jody BG (Hebrew) a familiar form of Joseph.
Jodey, Jodi, Jodie, Jodiha, Joedy

Joe BG (Hebrew) a short form of Joseph.
Jo, Joely, Joey

Joel BG (Hebrew) God is willing. Bible: an Old Testament Hebrew prophet.
Jôel, Joël, Joell, Joelle, Joely, Jole, Yoel

Joelle BG (Hebrew) a form of Joel.

Joeseph (Hebrew) a form of Joseph.
Joesph

Joey BG (Hebrew) a familiar form of Joe, Joseph.

Johan, Johann (German) forms of John. See also Anno, Hanno, Yoan, Yohan.
Joahan, Joannes, Johahn, Johan, Johanan, Johane, Johannan, Johannes, Johanthan, Johatan, Johathan, Johathon, Johaun, Johon

Johannes (German) a form of Johan, Johann.
Johanes, Johannas, Johannus, Johansen, Johanson, Johonson

John ★ BG (Hebrew) God is gracious. Bible: the name honoring John the Baptist and John the Evangelist. See also Elchanan, Evan, Geno, Gian, Giovanni, Handel, Hannes, Hans, Hanus, Honza, Ian, Ianos, Iban, Ioan, Ivan, Iwan, Keoni, Kwam, Ohannes, Sean, Ugutz, Yan, Yanka, Yanni, Yochanan, Yohance, Zane,
Jack, Jacsi, Jaenda, Jahn, Jan, Janak, Janco, Janek, Janis, Janne, János, Jansen, Jantje, Jantzen, Jas, Jean, Jehan, Jen, Jenkin, Jenkyn, Jens, Jhan, Jhanick, Jhon, Jian, Joáo, João, Jock, Joen, Johan, Johann, Johne, Johnl, Johnlee, Johnnie, Johnny, Johnson, Jon, Jonam, Jonas, Jone, Jones, Jonny, Jonté, Jovan, Juan, Juhana

Johnathan (Hebrew) a form of Jonathan.
Jhonathan, Johathe, Johnatan, Johnathann, Johnathaon, Johnathen, Johnathyne, Johnatten, Johniathin, Johnothan, Johnthan

Johnathon (Hebrew) a form of Jonathon. See also Yanton.
Johnaton

Johnnie BG (Hebrew) a familiar form of John.
Johnie, Johnier, Johnni, Johnsie, Jonni, Jonnie

Johnny BG (Hebrew) a familiar form of John. See also Gianni.
Jantje, Jhonny, Johney, Johnney, Johny, Jonny

Johnson (English) son of John.
Johnston, Jonson

Joi GB (Latin) a form of Joy.

Joji (Japanese) a form of George.

Jojo (Fante) born on Monday.

Jokim (Basque) a form of Joachim.

Jolene GB (Hebrew) God will add, God will increase. (English) a form of Josephine.

Jolon (Native American) valley of the dead oaks.
Jolyon

Jomar (American) a form of Jamar.
Jomari, Jomarie, Jomarri

Jomei (Japanese) spreads light.

Jon BG (Hebrew) a form of John. A short form of Jonathan.
J'on, Joni, Jonn, Jonnie, Jonny, Jony

Jonah BG (Hebrew) dove. Bible: an Old Testament prophet who was swallowed by a large fish.
Giona, Jona, Yonah, Yunus

Jonas (Hebrew) he accomplishes. (Lithuanian) a form of John.
Jonahs, Jonass, Jonaus, Jonelis, Jonukas, Jonus, Jonutis, Joonas

Jonás (Hebrew) a form of Jonas.

Jonatan BG (Hebrew) a form of Jonathan.
Jonatane, Jonate, Jonattan, Jonnattan

Jonathan ☆ BG (Hebrew) gift of God. Bible: the son of King Saul who became a loyal friend of David. See also Ionakana, Yanton, Yonatan.
Janathan, Johnathan, Johnathon, Jon, Jonatan, Jonatha, Jonathen, Jonathin, Jonathon, Jonathun, Jonathyn, Jonethen, Jonnatha, Jonnathan, Jonnathun, Jonothan, Jonthan

Jonathon (Hebrew) a form of Jonathan.
Joanathon, Johnathon, Jonnathon, Jonothon, Jonthon, Jounathon, Yanaton

Jones (Welsh) son of John.
Joenns, Joness, Jonesy

Jonny (Hebrew) a familiar form of John.
Jonhy, Joni, Jonnee, Jony

Jontae (French) a combination of Jon + the suffix Tae.
Johntae, Jontay, Jontea, Jonteau, Jontez

Jontay (American) a form of Jontae.
Johntay, Johnte, Johntez, Jontai, Jonte, Jonté, Jontez

Joop (Dutch) a familiar form of Joseph.
Jopie

Joost (Dutch) just.

Joquin (Spanish) a form of Joaquín.
Joquan, Joquawn, Joqunn, Joquon

Jora GB (Hebrew) teacher.
Yora, Jorah

Joram (Hebrew) Jehovah is exalted.
Joran, Jorim

Jordan ☆ BG (Hebrew) descending. See also Giordano, Yarden.
Jardan, Jared, Jordaan, Jordae, Jordain, Jordaine, Jordane, Jordani, Jordanio, Jordann, Jordanny, Jordano, Jordany, Jordáo, Jordayne, Jorden, Jordian, Jordin, Jordon, Jordun, Jordy, Jordyn, Jorrdan, Jory, Jourdan

Jordán (Hebrew) a form of Jordan.

Jorden BG (Hebrew) a form of Jordan.
Jordenn

Jordon BG (Hebrew) a form of Jordan.
Jeordon, Johordan

Jordy (Hebrew) a familiar form of Jordan.
Jordi, Jordie

Jordyn GB (Hebrew) a form of Jordan.

Jorell (American) he saves. Literature: a name inspired by the fictional character Jor-El, Superman's father.
Jorel, Jor-El, Jorelle, Jorl, Jorrel, Jorrell

Jörg (German) a form of George.
Jeorg, Juergen, Jungen, Jürgen

Jorge BG (Spanish) a form of George.
Jorrín

Jorgen (Danish) a form of George.
Joergen, Jorgan, Jörgen

Joris (Dutch) a form of George.

Jörn (German) a familiar form of Gregory.

Jorrín (Spanish) a form of George.
Jorian, Jorje

Jory (Hebrew) a familiar form of Jordan.
Joar, Joary, Jorey, Jori, Jorie, Jorrie

Josafat (Hebrew) God's judgment.

Jose ☆ BG (Spanish) a form of Joseph.

José (Spanish) a form of Joseph. See also Ché, Pepe.
Josean, Josecito, Josee, Joseito, Joselito, Josey

Josee GB (Spanish) a form of José.

Josef (German, Portuguese, Czech, Scandinavian) a form of Joseph.
Joosef, Joseff, Josif, Jozef, József, Juzef

Joseluis (Spanish) a combination of Jose + Luis.

Joseph ☆ BG (Hebrew) God will add, God will increase. Bible: in the Old Testament, the son of Jacob who came to rule Egypt; in the New Testament, the husband of Mary. See also Beppe, Cheche, Chepe, Giuseppe, Iokepa, Iosif, Osip, Pepa, Peppe, Pino, Sepp, Yeska, Yosef, Yousef, Youssel, Yusif, Yusuf, Zeusef.
Jazeps, Jo, Jobo, Jody, Joe, Joeseph, Joey, Jojo, Joop, Joos, Jooseppi, Jopie, José, Joseba, Josef, Josep, Josephat, Josephe, Josephie, Josephus, Josheph, Josip, Jóska, Joza, Joze, Jozef, Jozeph, Jozhe, Jozio, Jozka, Jozsi, Jozzepi, Jupp, Juziu

Josephine GB (French) a form of Joseph.

Josh (Hebrew) a short form of Joshua.
Joshe

Josha (Hindi) satisfied.

Joshi (Swahili) galloping.

Joshua ☀ BG (Hebrew) God is my salvation. Bible: led the Israelites into the Promised Land. See also Giosia, Iosua, Jesus, Yehoshua.
Jeshua, Johsua, Johusa, Josh, Joshau, Joshaua, Joshauh, Joshawa, Joshawah, Joshia, Joshu, Joshuaa, Joshuah, Joshuea, Joshuia, Joshula, Joshus, Joshusa, Joshuwa, Joshwa, Josue, Jousha, Jozshua, Jozsua, Jozua, Jushua

Josiah BG (Hebrew) fire of the Lord. See also Yoshiyahu.
Joshiah, Josia, Josiahs, Josian, Josias, Josie

Josie GB (Hebrew) a form of Josiah.

Joss (Chinese) luck; fate.
Josse, Jossy

Josue (Hebrew) a form of Joshua.
Joshue, Jossue, Josu, Josua, Josuha, Jozus

Josué (Hebrew) a form of Josue.

Jotham (Hebrew) may God complete. Bible: a king of Judah.

Jourdan (Hebrew) a form of Jordan.
Jourdain, Jourden, Jourdin, Jourdon, Jourdyn

Jovan (Latin) Jove-like, majestic. (Slavic) a form of John. Mythology: Jove, also known as Jupiter, was the supreme Roman deity.
Johvan, Johvon, Jovaan, Jovane, Jovani, Jovanic, Jovann, Jovanni, Jovannis, Jovanny, Jovany, Jovaughn, Jovaun, Joven, Jovenal, Jovenel, Jovi, Jovian, Jovin, Jovito, Jovoan, Jovon, Jovone, Jovonn, Jovonne, Jowan, Jowaun, Yovan, Yovani

Jovani, Jovanni BG (Latin) forms of Jovan.
Jovanie, Jovannie, Jovoni, Jovonie, Jovonni

Jovanny, Jovany (Latin) forms of Jovan.
Jovony

Joy GB (Latin) joyous.

Jr (Latin) a short form of Junior.
Jr.

Juan ☀ BG (Spanish) a form of John. See also Chan.
Juanch, Juanchito, Juane, Juanito, Juann, Juaun

Juancarlos (Spanish) a combination of Juan + Carlos.

Juanelo (Spanish) a form of Juan.

Juanjo (Spanish) a combination of Juan and José.

Juanma (Spanish) a combination of Juan and Manuel.

Juaquin (Spanish) a form of Joaquín.
Juaqin, Juaqine, Juquan, Juaquine

Jubal (Hebrew) ram's horn. Bible: a musician and a descendant of Cain.

Jucundo (Latin) happy, joyous one.

Judah (Hebrew) praised. Bible: the fourth of Jacob's sons. See also Yehudi.
Juda, Judas, Judd, Jude

Judas (Latin) a form of Judah. Bible: Judas Iscariot was the disciple who betrayed Jesus.
Jude

Judd (Hebrew) a short form of Judah.
Jud, Judson

Jude (Latin) a short form of Judah, Judas. Bible: one of the Twelve Apostles, author of "The Epistle of Jude."

Judson (English) son of Judd.

Judy GB (Hebrew) a familiar form of Judith (see Girls' Names).

Juhana (Finnish) a form of John.
Juha, Juho

Juku (Estonian) a form of Richard.
Jukka

Jules (French) a form of Julius.
Joles, Jule

Julia GB (Latin) youthful.

Julian ☆ BG (Greek, Latin) a form of Julius.
Jolyon, Julean, Juliaan, Julianne, Juliano, Julien, Jullian, Julyan

Julián (Spanish) a form of Julio.

Julianna GB (Czech, Spanish, Hungarian) a form of Julia.

Julianne GB (Greek, Latin) a form of Julian.

Julie GB (Greek, Latin) a familiar form of Julius.

Julien BG (Latin) a form of Julian.
Juliene, Julienn, Julienne, Jullien, Jullin

Juliet GB (French) a form of Julia.

Julio BG (Hispanic) a form of Julius.

Julius BG (Greek, Latin) youthful, downy bearded. History: Julius Caesar was a great Roman dictator. See also Giuliano.
Jolyon, Julas, Jule, Jules, Julen, Jules, Julian, Julias, Julie, Julio, Juliusz, Jullius, Juluis

Jumaane (Swahili) born on Tuesday.

Jumah (Arabic, Swahili) born on Friday, a holy day in the Islamic religion.
Jimoh, Juma

Jumoke (Yoruba) loved by everyone.

Jun 🅱🅶 (Chinese) truthful. (Japanese) obedient; pure.
Junnie

Junior (Latin) young.
Jr, Junious, Junius, Junor

Júpiter (Latin) origin or source of light.
Jupiter

Jupp (German) a form of Joseph.

Jur (Czech) a form of George.
Juraz, Jurek, Jurik, Jurko, Juro

Jurgis (Lithuanian) a form of George.
Jurgi, Juri

Juro (Japanese) best wishes; long life.

Jurrien (Dutch) God will uplift.
Jore, Jurian, Jurre

Justen (Latin) a form of Justin.
Jasten

Justice 🅶🅱 (Latin) a form of Justis.
Justic, Justiz, Justyc, Justyce

Justin ✻ 🅱🅶 (Latin) just, righteous. See also Giustino, Iestyn, Iustin, Tutu, Ustin, Yustyn.
Jastin, Jaston, Jestin, Jobst, Joost, Jost, Jusa, Just, Justain,

Justan, Justas, Justek, Justen, Justian, Justinas, Justine, Justinian, Justinius, Justinn, Justino, Justins, Justinus, Justo, Juston, Justton, Justukas, Justun, Justyn

Justina 🅶🅱 (Italian) a form of Justine.

Justine 🅶🅱 (Latin) a form of Justin.

Justiniano (Spanish) a form of Justino.

Justino (Latin) a form of Justin.

Justis (French) just.
Justice, Justs, Justus, Justyse

Justyn 🅱🅶 (Latin) a form of Justin.
Justn, Justyne, Justynn

Juven, Juvencio, Juventino (Latin) he is the one that represents youth.

Juvenal (Latin) young. Literature: a Roman satirist.
Juvon, Juvone

Juwan 🅱🅶 (American) a form of Jajuan.
Juvon, Juvone, Juvaun, Juwaan, Juwain, Juwane, Juwann, Juwaun, Juwon, Juwonn, Juwuan, Juwuane, Juwvan, Jwan, Jwon

K

K GB (American) an initial used as a first name.

Ka'eo (Hawaiian) victorious.

Kabiito (Rutooro) born while foreigners are visiting.

Kabil (Turkish) a form of Cain.
Kabel

Kabir (Hindi) History: an Indian mystic poet.
Kabar, Kabeer, Kabier

Kabonero (Runyankore) sign.

Kabonesa (Rutooro) difficult birth.

Kacey GB (Irish) a form of Casey. (American) a combination of the initials K. + C. See also KC.
Kace, Kacee, Kaci, Kacy, Kaesy, Kase, Kasey, Kasie, Kasy, Kaycee

Kaci GB (Irish) a form of Kacey.

Kadar (Arabic) powerful.
Kader

Kadarius (American) a combination of Kade + Darius.
Kadairious, Kadarious, Kadaris, Kadarrius, Kadarus, Kaddarrius, Kaderious, Kaderius

Kade BG (Scottish) wetlands. (American) a combination of the initials K. + D.
Kadee, Kady, Kaid, Kaide, Kaydee

Kadeem BG (Arabic) servant.
Kadim, Khadeem

Kaden BG (Arabic) a form of Kadin.
Kadeen, Kadein, Kaidan, Kaiden

Kadin (Arabic) friend, companion.
Caden, Kaden, Kadyn, Kaeden, Kayden

Kadir (Arabic) spring greening.
Kadeer

Kado (Japanese) gateway.

Kaeden (Arabic) a form of Kadin.
Kaedin, Kaedon, Kaedyn

Kaelan, Kaelin (Irish) forms of Kellen.
Kael, Kaelen, Kaelon, Kaelyn

Kaeleb (Hebrew) a form of Kaleb.
Kaelib, Kaelob, Kaelyb, Kailab, Kaileb

Kaelyn GB (Irish) a form of Kaelan.

Kaemon (Japanese) joyful; right-handed.
Kaeman, Kaemen, Kaemin

Kaenan (Irish) a form of Keenan.
Kaenen, Kaenin, Kaenyn

Kafele (Nguni) worth dying for.

Kaga (Native American) writer.

Kagan (Irish) a form of Keegan.
Kage, Kagen, Kaghen, Kaigan

Kahale (Hawaiian) home.

Kahil (Turkish) young;
inexperienced; naive.
Cahil, Kaheel, Kale, Kayle

Kahlil BG (Arabic) a form of
Khalíl.
*Kahleal, Kahlee, Kahleel, Kahleil,
Kahli, Kahliel, Kahlill, Kalel, Kalil*

Kaholo (Hawaiian) runner.

Kahraman (Turkish) hero.

Kai BG (Welsh) keeper of the
keys. (German) a form of Kay.
(Hawaiian) sea.
Kae, Kaie, Kaii

Kaikara (Runyoro) Religion: a
Banyoro deity.

Kailen (Irish) a form of Kellen.
*Kail, Kailan, Kailey, Kailin, Kailon,
Kailyn*

Kaili (Hawaiian) Religion: a
Hawaiian god.
Kailli

Kailyn GB (Irish) a form of
Kailen.

Kain (Welsh, Irish) a form of
Kane.
*Kainan, Kaine, Kainen, Kainin,
Kainon*

Kainoa (Hawaiian) name.

Kaipo (Hawaiian) sweetheart.

Kairo (Arabic) a form of Cairo.
Kaire, Kairee, Kairi

Kaiser (German) a form of
Caesar.
Kaesar, Kaisar, Kaizer

Kaitlin GB (Irish) pure.

Kaiven (American) a form of Kevin.
Kaivan, Kaiven, Kaivon, Kaiwan

Kaj (Danish) earth.
Kai, Kaje

Kakar (Hindi) grass.

Kala GB (Hindi) black; phase.
(Hawaiian) sun.

Kalama BG (Hawaiian) torch.
Kalam

Kalan (Irish) a form of Kalen.
Kalane, Kallan

Kalani GB (Hawaiian) sky; chief.
Kalan

Kale (Arabic) a short form of
Kahlil. (Hawaiian) a familiar
form of Carl.
*Kalee, Kalen, Kaleu, Kaley, Kali,
Kalin, Kalle, Kayle*

Kaleb BG (Hebrew) a form of
Caleb.
*Kaeleb, Kal, Kalab, Kalabe, Kalb,
Kale, Kaleob, Kalev, Kalib, Kalieb,
Kallb, Kalleb, Kalob, Kaloeb,
Kalub, Kalyb, Kilab*

Kaleigh GB (American) a form of
Caley.

Kalen, Kalin (Arabic, Hawaiian)
forms of Kale. (Irish) forms of
Kellen.
Kalan

Kalevi (Finnish) hero.

Kaley **GB** (Arabic) a familiar form of Kale.

Kali **GB** (Arabic) a short form of Kalil. (Hawaiian) a form of Gary.

Kalil (Arabic) a form of Khalíl.
Kaleel, Kalell, Kali, Kaliel, Kaliil

Kaliq (Arabic) a form of Khaliq.
Kalic, Kalique

Kalkin (Hindi) tenth. Religion: Kalki is the final incarnation of the Hindu god Vishnu.
Kalki

Kalle **BG** (Scandinavian) a form of Carl. (Arabic, Hawaiian) a form of Kale.

Kallen (Irish) a form of Kellen.
Kallan, Kallin, Kallion, Kallon, Kallun, Kalun

Kalon (Irish) forms of Kellen.
Kalone, Kalonn, Kalyen, Kalyne, Kalynn

Kaloosh (Armenian) blessed event.

Kalvin (Latin) a form of Calvin.
Kal, Kalv, Kalvan, Kalven, Kalvon, Kalvyn, Vinny

Kalyn **GB** (Irish) a form of Kellen.

Kamaka (Hawaiian) face.

Kamakani (Hawaiian) wind.

Kamal (Hindi) lotus. (Arabic) perfect, perfection.
Kamaal, Kamel, Kamil

Kamau (Kikuyu) quiet warrior.

Kamden (Scottish) a form of Camden.
Kamdon

Kameron **BG** (Scottish) a form of Cameron.
Kam, Kamaren, Kamaron, Kameran, Kameren, Kamerin, Kamerion, Kamerron, Kamerun, Kameryn, Kamey, Kammeren, Kammeron, Kammy, Kamoryn, Kamran, Kamron

Kami **GB** (Hindi) loving.

Kamil **BG** (Arabic) a form of Kamal.
Kameel

Kamran, Kamron (Scottish) forms of Kameron.
Kammron, Kamrein, Kamren, Kamrin, Kamrun, Kamryn

Kamuela (Hawaiian) a form of Samuel.

Kamuhanda (Runyankore) born on the way to the hospital.

Kamukama (Runyankore) protected by God.

Kamuzu (Nguni) medicine.

Kamya (Luganda) born after twin brothers.

Kana (Japanese) powerful; capable. (Hawaiian) Mythology: a demigod.

Kanaiela (Hawaiian) a form of Daniel.
Kana, Kaneii

Kandace 🇬🇧 (Greek) glittering white; glowing. (American) a form of Candice.

Kane 🇧🇬 (Welsh) beautiful. (Irish) tribute. (Japanese) golden. (Hawaiian) eastern sky. (English) a form of Keene. See Kahan, Kain, Kaney, Kayne.

Kange (Lakota) raven.
Kang, Kanga

Kaniel (Hebrew) stalk, reed.
Kan, Kani, Kannie, Kanny

Kannan (Hindi) Religion: another name for the Hindu god Krishna.
Kanaan, Kanan, Kanen, Kanin, Kanine, Kannen

Kannon (Polynesian) free. (French) A form of Cannon.
Kanon

Kanoa 🇧🇬 (Hawaiian) free.

Kantu (Hindi) happy.

Kanu (Swahili) wildcat.

Kaori (Japanese) strong.

Kapila (Hindi) ancient prophet.
Kapil

Kapono (Hawaiian) righteous.
Kapena

Kara 🇬🇧 (Greek, Danish) pure.

Kardal (Arabic) mustard seed.
Karandal, Kardell

Kare (Norwegian) enormous.
Karee

Kareem 🇧🇬 (Arabic) noble; distinguished.
Karee, Karem, Kareme, Karim, Karriem

Karel 🇧🇬 (Czech) a form of Carl.
Karell, Karil, Karrell

Karen 🇬🇧 (Greek) pure.

Karey (Greek) a form of Carey.
Karee, Kari, Karry, Kary

Kari 🇬🇧 (Greek) a form of Karey.

Karif (Arabic) born in autumn.
Kareef

Kariisa (Runyankore) herdsman.

Karim (Arabic) a form of Kareem.

Karina 🇬🇧 (Russian) a form of Karen.

Karl (German) a form of Carl.
Kaarle, Kaarlo, Kale, Kalle, Kalman, Kálmán, Karcsi, Karel, Kari, Karlen, Karlitis, Karlo, Karlos, Karlton, Karlus, Karol, Kjell

Karla 🇬🇧 (German) a form of Carla. (Slavic) a short form of Karoline (see Girls' Names).

Karlen (Latvian, Russian) a form of Carl.
Karlan, Karlens, Karlik, Karlin, Karlis, Karlon

Karly 🇬🇧 (Latin) little and strong. (American) a form of Carly.

Karmel **BG** (Hebrew) a form of Carmel.

Karney (Irish) a form of Carney.

Karol (Czech, Polish) a form of Carl.
Karal, Karolek, Karolis, Karalos, Károly, Karrel, Karrol

Karr (Scandinavian) a form of Carr.

Karson (English) a form of Carson.
Karrson, Karsen

Karsten (Greek) anointed.
Carsten, Karstan, Karston

Karu (Hindi) cousin.
Karun

Karutunda (Runyankore) little.

Karwana (Rutooro) born during wartime.

Kaseem (Arabic) divided.
Kasceem, Kaseam, Kaseym, Kasim, Kasseem, Kassem, Kazeem

Kaseko (Rhodesian) mocked, ridiculed.

Kasem (Tai) happiness.

Kasen (Basque) protected with a helmet.
Kasean, Kasene, Kaseon, Kasin, Kason, Kassen

Kasey **GB** (Irish) a form of Casey.
Kaese, Kaesy, Kasay, Kassey

Kashawn (American) a combination of the prefix Ka + Shawn.
Kashain, Kashan, Kashaun, Kashen, Kashon

Kasib (Arabic) fertile.

Kasim (Arabic) a form of Kaseem.
Kassim

Kasimir (Arabic) peace. (Slavic) a form of Casimir.
Kasim, Kazimierz, Kazimir, Kazio, Kazmer, Kazmér, Kázmér

Kasiya (Nguni) separate.

Kasper (Persian) treasurer. (German) a form of Casper.
Jasper, Kaspar, Kaspero

Kass (German) blackbird.
Kaese, Kasch, Kase

Kassandra **GB** (Greek) a form of Cassandra.

Kassidy **GB** (Irish) a form of Cassidy.
Kassady, Kassie, Kassy

Kate **GB** (Greek) pure. (English) a short form of Katherine.

Kateb (Arabic) writer.

Katelyn **GB** (Irish) a form of Caitlin.

Katerina **GB** (Slavic) a form of Katherine.

Katherine **GB** (Greek) pure.

Kathrine **GB** (Greek) a form of Katherine.

Kathryn GB (English) a form of Katherine.

Kathy GB (English) a familiar form of Katherine.

Katia GB (Russian) a form of Katherine.

Katie GB (English) a familiar form of Kate.

Katlin GB (Irish) a form of Katlyn (see Girls' Names).

Kato (Runyankore) second of twins.

Katungi (Runyankore) rich.

Kavan (Irish) handsome.
Cavan, Kavanagh, Kavaugn, Kaven, Kavenaugh, Kavin, Kavon, Kayvan

Kaveh (Persian) ancient hero.

Kavi (Hindi) poet.

Kavin, Kavon (Irish) forms of Kavan.
Kaveon, Kavion, Kavone, Kayvon, Kaywon

Kawika (Hawaiian) a form of David.

Kay GB (Greek) rejoicing. (German) fortified place. Literature: one of King Arthur's knights of the Round Table.
Kai, Kaycee, Kaye, Kayson

Kaycee GB (Greek, German) a form of Kay. (American, Irish) a form of Kacey.

Kayden BG (Arabic) a form of Kadin.
Kayde, Kaydee, Kaydin, Kaydn, Kaydon

Kayin (Nigerian) celebrated. (Yoruba) long-hoped-for child.

Kayla GB (Hebrew, Arabic) a form of Kayle.

Kaylan GB (Irish) a form of Kaylen.

Kayle (Hebrew) faithful dog. (Arabic) a short form of Kahlil.
Kayl, Kayla, Kaylee

Kayleb (Hebrew) a form of Caleb.
Kaylib, Kaylob, Kaylub

Kaylee GB (Hebrew, Arabic) a form of Kayle.

Kaylen (Irish) a form of Kellen.
Kaylan, Kaylin, Kaylon, Kaylyn, Kaylynn

Kaylin GB (Irish) a form of Kaylen.

Kaylon BG (Irish) a form of Kaylen.

Kaylyn, Kaylynn GB (Irish) forms of Kaylen.

Kayne (Hebrew) a form of Cain.
Kaynan, Kaynen, Kaynon

Kayode (Yoruba) he brought joy.

Kayonga (Runyankore) ash.

Kazio (Polish) a form of Casimir, Kasimir. See also Cassidy.

Kazuo (Japanese) man of peace.

KC (American) a combination of the initials K. + C. See also Kacey.
Kc, K.C., Kcee, Kcey

Keagan (Irish) a form of Keegan.
Keagean, Keagen, Keaghan, Keagyn

Keahi (Hawaiian) flames.

Keaka (Hawaiian) a form of Jack.

Kealoha (Hawaiian) fragrant.
Ke'ala

Keanan (Irish) a form of Keenan.
Keanen, Keanna, Keannan, Keanon

Keandre (American) a combination of the prefix Ke + Andre.
Keandra, Keandray, Keandré, Keandree, Keandrell, Keondre

Keane (German) bold; sharp. (Irish) handsome. (English) a form of Keene.
Kean

Keanna GB (Irish) a form of Keanan.

Keanu BG (Irish) a form of Keenan.
Keaneu, Keani, Keanno, Keano, Keanue, Keeno, Keenu, Kianu

Kearn (Irish) a short form of Kearney.
Kearne

Kearney (Irish) a form of Carney.
Kar, Karney, Karny, Kearn, Kearny

Keary (Irish) a form of Kerry.
Kearie

Keaton BG (English) where hawks fly.
Keatan, Keaten, Keatin, Keatton, Keatyn, Keeton, Keetun

Keaven (Irish) a form of Kevin.
Keavan, Keavon

Keawe (Hawaiian) strand.

Keb (Egyptian) earth. Mythology: an ancient earth god, also known as Geb.

Kedar (Hindi) mountain lord. (Arabic) powerful. Religion: another name for the Hindu god Shiva.
Kadar, Kedaar, Keder

Keddy (Scottish) a form of Adam.
Keddie

Kedem (Hebrew) ancient.

Kedrick (English) a form of Cedric.
Keddrick, Kederick, Kedrek, Kedric, Kiedric, Kiedrick

Keefe (Irish) handsome; loved.

Keegan BG (Irish) little; fiery.
Kaegan, Kagan, Keagan, Keagen, Keeghan, Keegon, Keegun, Kegan, Keigan

Keelan (Irish) little; slender.
Keelen, Keelin, Keelyn, Keilan, Kelan

Keeley GB (Irish) handsome.
Kealey, Kealy, Keeli, Keelian, Keelie

Keely GB (Irish) a form of Keeley.

Keenan BG (Irish) little Keene.
Kaenan, Keanan, Keanu, Keenen, Keennan, Keenon, Kenan, Keynan, Kienan, Kienon

Keene (German) bold; sharp.
(English) smart. See also Kane.
Kaene, Keane, Keen, Keenan

Keenen (Irish) a form of Keenan.
Keenin, Kienen

Kees (Dutch) a form of Kornelius.
Keese, Keesee, Keyes

Keevon (Irish) a form of Kevin.
Keevan, Keeven, Keevin, Keewan, Keewin

Kegan (Irish) a form of Keegan.
Kegen, Keghan, Kegon, Kegun

Kehind (Yoruba) second-born twin.
Kehinde

Keiffer (German) a form of Cooper.
Keefer, Keifer, Kiefer

Keigan (Irish) a form of Keegan.
Keighan, Keighen

Keiji (Japanese) cautious ruler.

Keilan (Irish) a form of Keelan.
Keilen, Keilin, Keillene, Keillyn, Keilon, Keilynn

Keir (Irish) a short form of Kieran.

Keitaro (Japanese) blessed.
Keita

Keith (Welsh) forest. (Scottish) battle place. See also Kika.
Keath, Keeth, Keithen

Keithen (Welsh, Scottish) a form of Keith.
Keithan, Keitheon, Keithon

Keivan (Irish) a form of Kevin.
Keiven, Keivn, Keivon, Keivone

Kekapa (Hawaiian) tapa cloth.

Kekipi (Hawaiian) rebel.

Kekoa (Hawaiian) bold, courageous.

Kelby (German) farm by the spring.
Keelby, Kelbee, Kelbey, Kelbi, Kellby

Kele (Hopi) sparrow hawk.
(Hawaiian) a form of Jerry.
Kelle

Kelemen (Hungarian) gentle; kind.
Kellman

Kelevi (Finnish) hero.

Keli (Hawaiian) a form of Terry.

Keli'i (Hawaiian) chief.

Kelile (Ethiopian) protected.

Kell (Scandinavian) spring.

Kellan (Irish) a form of Kellen.
Keillan

Kellen BG (Irish) mighty warrior.
*Kaelan, Kailen, Kalan, Kalen,
Kalin, Kallen, Kalon, Kalyn,
Kaylen, Keelan, Kelden, Kelin,
Kellan, Kelle, Kellin, Kellyn,
Kelyn, Kelynn*

Keller (Irish) little companion.

Kelley GB (Irish) a form of Kelly.

Kelli, Kellie GB (Irish) forms of
Kelly.

Kelly GB (Irish) warrior.
*Kelle, Kellen, Kelley, Kelli, Kellie,
Kely*

Kelmen (Basque) merciful.
Kelmin

Kelsea GB (Scandinavian) a form
of Kelsey.

Kelsey GB (Scandinavian) island
of ships.
*Kelcy, Kelse, Kelsea, Kelsi,
Kelsie, Kelso, Kelsy, Kesley, Kesly*

Kelsi, Kelsy GB (Scandinavian)
forms of Kelsey.

Kelton BG (English) keel town;
port.
*Kelden, Keldon, Kelson, Kelston,
Kelten, Keltin, Keltonn, Keltyn*

Kelvin BG (Irish, English) narrow
river. Geography: a river in
Scotland.
*Kelvan, Kelven, Kelvon, Kelvyn,
Kelwin, Kelwyn*

Kemal (Turkish) highest honor.

Kemen (Basque) strong.

Kemp (English) fighter; champion.

Kempton (English) military town.

Ken (Japanese) one's own kind.
(Scottish) a short form of
Kendall, Kendrick, Kenneth.
Kena, Kenn, Keno

Kenan (Irish) a form of Keenan.

Kenaz (Hebrew) bright.

Kendal GB (English) a form of
Kendall.
*Kendale, Kendali, Kendel, Kendul,
Kendyl*

Kendall GB (English) valley of the
river Kent.
*Ken, Kendal, Kendell, Kendrall,
Kendryll, Kendyll, Kyndall*

Kendarius (American) a combi-
nation of Ken + Darius.
*Kendarious, Kendarrious,
Kendarrius, Kenderious,
Kenderius, Kenderyious*

Kendell (English) a form of
Kendall.
Kendelle, Kendrel, Kendrell

Kendra GB (English) a form of
Kenda (see Girls' Names).

Kendrew (Scottish) a form of
Andrew.

Kendrick 🅱🅶 (Irish) son of
Henry. (Scottish) royal chieftain.
*Ken, Kenderrick, Kendric,
Kendrich, Kenedrick, Kendricks,
Kendrik, Kendrix, Kendryck,
Kenndrick, Keondric, Keondrick*

Kenia 🅶🅱 (Hebrew) a form of
Kenya.

Kenley (English) royal meadow.
*Kenlea, Kenlee, Kenleigh, Kenlie,
Kenly*

Kenn (Scottish) a form of Ken.

Kenna 🅶🅱 (Scottich) a form of
Kennan.

Kennan (Scottish) little Ken.
*Kenna, Kenan, Kenen, Kennen,
Kennon*

Kennard (Irish) brave chieftain.
Kenner

Kennedy 🅶🅱 (Irish) helmeted
chief. History: John F. Kennedy
was the thirty-fifth U.S. president.
*Kenedy, Kenidy, Kennady,
Kennedey*

Kenneth 🅱🅶 (Irish) handsome.
(English) royal oath.
*Ken, Keneth, Kenneith, Kennet,
Kennethen, Kennett, Kennieth,
Kennith, Kennth, Kenny, Kennyth,
Kenya*

Kenny 🅱🅶 (Scottish) a familiar
form of Kenneth.
*Keni, Kenney, Kenni, Kennie,
Kinnie*

Kenrick (English) bold ruler;
royal ruler.
Kenric, Kenricks, Kenrik

Kent 🅱🅶 (Welsh) white; bright.
(English) a short form of Kenton.
Geography: a region in England.

Kentaro (Japanese) big boy.

Kenton (English) from Kent,
England.
Kent, Kenten, Kentin, Kentonn

Kentrell 🅱🅶 (English) king's
estate.
Kenreal, Kentrel, Kentrelle

Kenward (English) brave; royal
guardian.

Kenya 🅶🅱 (Hebrew) animal horn.
(Russian) a form of Kenneth.
Geography: a country in east-
central Africa.
Kenyatta

Kenyatta (American) a form of
Kenya.
*Kenyata, Kenyatae, Kenyatee,
Kenyatter, Kenyatti, Kenyotta*

Kenyon (Irish) white haired,
blond.
Kenyan, Kenynn, Keonyon

Kenzie 🅶🅱 (Scottish) wise leader.
See also Mackenzie.
Kensie

Keoki (Hawaiian) a form of
George.

Keola (Hawaiian) life.

Keon BG (Irish) a form of Ewan.
*Keeon, Keion, Keionne, Keondre,
Keone, Keonne, Keonte, Keony,
Keyon, Kian, Kion*

Keoni (Hawaiian) a form of John.

Keonte (American) a form of
Keon.
*Keonntay, Keonta, Keontae,
Keontay, Keontaye, Keontez,
Keontia, Keontis, Keontrae,
Keontre, Keontrey, Keontrye*

Kerbasi (Basque) warrior.

Kerel (Afrikaans) young.
Kerell

Kerem (Turkish) noble; kind.
Kereem

Kerey (Gypsy) homeward bound.
Ker

Keri GB (Irish) a form of Kerry.

Kerman (Basque) from Germany.

Kermit (Irish) a form of Dermot.
Kermey, Kermie, Kermitt, Kermy

Kern (Irish) a short form of
Kieran.
Kearn, Kerne

Kerr (Scandinavian) a form of
Carr.
Karr

Kerri (Irish) a form of Kerry.

Kerrick (English) king's rule.

Kerry (Irish) dark; dark haired.
Keary, Keri, Kerrey, Kerri, Kerrie

Kers (Todas) Botany: an Indian
plant.

Kersen (Indonesian) cherry.

Kerstan (Dutch) a form of
Christian.

Kerwin (Irish) little; dark.
(English) friend of the
marshlands.
*Kervin, Kervyn, Kerwinn, Kerwyn,
Kerwynn, Kirwin, Kirwyn*

Kesar (Russian) a form of Caesar.
Kesare

Keshawn (American) a
combination of the prefix Ke +
Shawn.
*Keeshaun, Keeshawn, Keeshon,
Kesean, Keshan, Keshane,
Keshaun, Keshayne, Keshion,
Keshon, Keshone, Keshun,
Kishan*

Kesin (Hindi) long-haired beggar.

Kesse GB (Ashanti, Fante)
chubby baby.
Kessie

Kester (English) a form of
Christopher.

Kestrel (English) falcon.
Kes

Keung (Chinese) universe.

Kevan (Irish) a form of Kevin.
*Kavan, Kewan, Kewane, Kewaun,
Keyvan, Kiwan, Kiwane*

Keven BG (Irish) a form of Kevin.
Keve, Keveen, Kiven

Kevin ☆ **BG** (Irish) handsome.
See also Cavan.
*Kaiven, Keaven, Keevon, Keivan,
Kev, Kevan, Keven, Keverne,
Kevian, Kevien, Kévin, Kevinn,
Kevins, Kevis, Kevn, Kevon,
Kevvy, Kevyn, Kyven*

Kevon **BG** (Irish) a form of Kevin.
*Keveon, Kevion, Kevone,
Kevonne, Kevontae, Kevonte,
Kevoyn, Kevron, Kewon, Kewone,
Keyvon, Kivon*

Kevyn **BG** (Irish) a form of Kevin.
Kevyon

Key (English) key; protected.

Keyana **GB** (American) a form of
Kiana.

Keyon (Irish) a form of Keon.
Keyan, Keyen, Keyin, Keyion

Keyonna **GB** (American) a form
of Kiana.

Keyshawn (American) a
combination of Key + Shawn.
*Keyshan, Keyshaun, Keyshon,
Keyshun*

Khachig (Armenian) small cross.
Khachik

Khadijah **GB** (Arabic)
trustworthy.

Khaim (Russian) a form of Chaim.

Khaldun (Arabic) forever.
Khaldoon, Khaldoun

Khalfani (Swahili) born to lead.
Khalfan

Khälid (Arabic) eternal.
Khaled, Khallid, Khalyd

Khalíl (Arabic) friend.
*Kahlil, Kaleel, Kalil, Khahlil,
Khailil, Khailyl, Khalee, Khaleel,
Khaleil, Khali, Khalial, Khaliel,
Khalihl, Khalill, Khaliyl*

Khaliq (Arabic) creative.
Kaliq, Khalique

Khamisi (Swahili) born on
Thursday.
Kham

Khan (Turkish) prince.
Khanh

Kharald (Russian) a form of
Gerald.

Khayru (Arabic) benevolent.
Khiri, Khiry, Kiry

Khoury (Arabic) priest.
Khory

Khristian (Greek) a form of
Christian, Kristian.
*Khris, Khristan, Khristin, Khriston,
Khrystian*

Khristopher (Greek) a form of
Kristopher.
*Khristofer, Khristophar,
Khrystopher*

Khristos (Greek) a form of
Christos.
Khris, Khristophe, Kristo, Kristos

Kia **GB** (African) season's
beginning. (American) a short
form of Kiana.

Kiana **GB** (American) a combination of the prefix Ki + Anna.

Kiara **GB** (Irish) little and dark.

Kibo (Uset) worldly; wise.

Kibuuka (Luganda) brave warrior. History: a Ganda warrior deity.

Kidd (English) child; young goat.

Kiefer (German) a form of Keifer.
Kief, Kieffer, Kiefor, Kiffer, Kiiefer

Kiel (Irish) a form of Kyle.
Kiell

Kiele **GB** (Hawaiian) gardenia.

Kieran **BG** (Irish) little and dark; little Keir.
Keiran, Keiren, Keiron, Kiaron, Kiarron, Kier, Kieren, Kierian, Kierien, Kierin, Kiernan, Kieron, Kierr, Kierre, Kierron, Kyran

Kiernan (Irish) a form of Kieran.
Kern, Kernan, Kiernen

Kiersten **GB** (Scandanavian) a form of Kirsten.

Kiet (Tai) honor.

Kifeda (Luo) only boy among girls.

Kiho (Rutooro) born on a foggy day.

Kijika (Native American) quiet walker.

Kika (Hawaiian) a form of Keith.

Kiki **GB** (Spanish) a form of Henry.

Kile (Irish) a form of Kyle.
Kilee, Kilen, Kiley, Kiyl, Kiyle

Kiley **GB** (Irish) a form of Kile, Kyle.

Killian (Irish) little Kelly.
Kilean, Kilian, Kilien, Killie, Killien, Killiean, Killion, Killy

Kim **GB** (English) a short form of Kimball.
Kimie, Kimmy

Kimball (Greek) hollow vessel. (English) warrior chief.
Kim, Kimbal, Kimbel, Kimbell, Kimble

Kimberly **GB** (English) chief, ruler.

Kimo (Hawaiian) a form of James.

Kimokeo (Hawaiian) a form of Timothy.

Kin (Japanese) golden.

Kincaid (Scottish) battle chief.
Kincade, Kinkaid

Kindin (Basque) fifth.

King (English) king. A short form of names beginning with "King."

Kingsley (English) king's meadow.
King, Kings, Kingslea, Kingslie, Kingsly, Kingzlee, Kinslea, Kinslee, Kinsley, Kinslie, Kinsly

Kingston (English) king's estate.
King, Kinston

Kingswell (English) king's well.
King

Kini GB (Hawaiian) a short form
of Iukini.

Kinnard (Irish) tall slope.

Kinsey GB (English) victorious
royalty.
Kinze, Kinzie

Kinton (Hindi) crowned.

Kion (Irish) a form of Keon.
Kione, Kionie, Kionne

Kioshi (Japanese) quiet.

Kipp (English) pointed hill.
Kip, Kippar, Kipper, Kippie, Kippy

Kir (Bulgarian) a familiar form of
Cyrus.

Kira GB (Persian) sun. (Latin)
light.

Kiral (Turkish) king; supreme
leader.

Kiran GB (Sanskrit) beam of light.
Kyran

Kirby BG (Scandinavian) church
village. (English) cottage by the
water.
*Kerbey, Kerbie, Kerby, Kirbey,
Kirbie, Kirkby*

Kiri (Cambodian) mountain.

Kiril (Slavic) a form of Cyril.
Kirill, Kiryl, Kyrillos

Kirios (Greek) supreme being, the
Lord.

Kiritan (Hindi) wearing a crown.

Kirk (Scandinavian) church.
Kerk

Kirkland (English) church land.
Kirklin, Kirklind, Kirklynd

Kirkley (English) church
meadow.

Kirklin (English) a form of
Kirkland.
*Kirklan, Kirklen, Kirkline, Kirkloun,
Kirklun, Kirklyn, Kirklynn*

Kirkwell (English) church well;
church spring.

Kirkwood (English) church
forest.

Kirsten GB (Greek) Christian;
anointed. (Scandinavian) a form
of Christine.

Kirton (English) church town.

Kishan (American) a form of
Keshawn.
*Kishaun, Kishawn, Kishen,
Kishon, Kyshon, Kyshun*

Kistna (Hindi) sacred, holy.
Geography: a sacred river in
India.

Kistur (Gypsy) skillful rider.

Kit (Greek) a familiar form of
Christian, Christopher, Kristopher.
Kitt, Kitts

Kito (Swahili) jewel; precious child.

Kitwana (Swahili) pledged to live.

Kiva (Hebrew) a short form of Akiva, Jacob.
Kiba, Kivi, Kiwa

Kiyoshi (Japanese) quiet; peaceful.

Kizza (Luganda) born after twins.
Kizzy

Kjell (Swedish) a form of Karl.
Kjel

Klaus (German) a short form of Nicholas. A form of Claus.
Klaas, Klaes, Klas, Klause

Klay (English) a form of Clay.

Klayton (English) a form of Clayton.

Kleef (Dutch) cliff.

Klement (Czech) a form of Clement.
Klema, Klemenis, Klemens, Klemet, Klemo, Klim, Klimek, Kliment, Klimka

Kleng (Norwegian) claw.

Knight (English) armored knight.
Knightly

Knoton (Native American) a form of Nodin.

Knowles (English) grassy slope.
Knolls, Nowles

Knox (English) hill.

Knute (Scandinavian) a form of Canute.
Knud, Knut

Koby (Polish) a familiar form of Jacob.
Kobby, Kobe, Kobey, Kobi, Kobia, Kobie

Kodi **BG** (English) a form of Kody.
Kode, Kodee, Kodie

Kody **BG** (English) a form of Cody.
Kodey, Kodi, Kodye, Koty

Kofi (Twi) born on Friday.

Kohana (Lakota) swift.

Koi (Choctaw) panther. (Hawaiian) a form of Troy.

Kojo (Akan) born on Monday.

Koka (Hawaiian) Scotsman.

Kokayi (Shona) gathered together.

Kolby **BG** (English) a form of Colby.
Kelby, Koalby, Koelby, Kohlbe, Kohlby, Kolbe, Kolbey, Kolbi, Kolbie, Kolebe, Koleby, Kollby

Kole (English) a form of Cole.
Kohl, Kohle

Koleman (English) a form of Coleman.
Kolemann, Kolemen

Kolin (English) a form of Colin.
Kolen, Kollen, Kollin, Kollyn, Kolyn

Kolton (English) a form of Colton.
Kolt, Koltan, Kolte, Kolten, Koltin, Koltn, Koltyn

Kolya (Russian) a familiar form of Nikolai, Nikolos.
Kola, Kolenka, Kolia, Kolja

Kona 🅱🅶 (Hawaiian) a form of Don.
Konala

Konane (Hawaiian) bright moonlight.

Kondo (Swahili) war.

Kong (Chinese) glorious; sky.

Konner (Irish) a form of Conner, Connor.
Konar, Koner

Konnor (Irish) a form of Connor.
Kohner, Kohnor, Konor

Kono (Moquelumnan) squirrel eating a pine nut.

Konrad (German) a form of Conrad.
Khonrad, Koen, Koenraad, Kon, Konn, Konney, Konni, Konnie, Konny, Konrád, Konrade, Konrado, Kord, Kort, Kunz

Konstantin (German, Russian) a form of Constantine. See also Dinos.
Konstancji, Konstadine, Konstadino, Konstandinos, Konstantinas, Konstantine, Konstantinos, Konstantio, Konstanty, Konstantyn, Konstanz, Konstatino, Kostadino, Kostadinos, Kostandino, Kostandinos, Kostantin, Kostantino, Kostas, Kostenka, Kostya, Kotsos

Kontar (Akan) only child.

Korb (German) basket.

Korbin (English) a form of Corbin.
Korban, Korben, Korbyn

Kordell (English) a form of Cordell.
Kordel

Korey 🅱🅶 (Irish) a form of Corey, Kory.
Kore, Koree, Korei, Korio, Korre, Korria, Korrye

Kori 🅶🅱 (Irish) a form of Kory.

Kornel (Latin) a form of Cornelius, Kornelius.
Kees, Korneil, Kornél, Korneli, Kornelisz, Kornell, Krelis, Soma

Kornelius (Latin) a form of Cornelius. See also Kees, Kornel.
Karnelius, Korneilius, Korneliaus, Kornelious, Kornellius

Korrigan (Irish) a form of Corrigan.
Korigan, Korigan, Korrigon, Korrigun

Kort (German, Dutch) a form of Cort, Kurt.
Kourt

Kortney 🅶🅱 (English) a form of Courtney.
Kortni, Kourtney

Korudon (Greek) helmeted one.

Kory BG (Irish) a form of Corey.
Korey, Kori, Korie, Korrey, Korri, Korrie, Korry

Kosey (African) lion.
Kosse

Kosmo (Greek) a form of Cosmo.
Kosmy, Kozmo

Kostas (Greek) a short form of Konstantin.

Kosti (Finnish) a form of Gustave.

Kosumi (Moquelumnan) spear fisher.

Koukalaka (Hawaiian) a form of Douglas.

Kourtland (English) a form of Courtland.
Kortlan, Kortland, Kortlend, Kortlon, Kourtlin

Kourtney GB (American) a form of Courtney.

Kovit (Tai) expert.

Kraig (Irish, Scottish) a form of Craig.
Kraggie, Kraggy, Krayg, Kreg, Kreig, Kreigh

Krikor (Armenian) a form of Gregory.

Kris BG (Greek) a form of Chris. A short form of Kristian, Kristofer, Kristopher.
Kriss, Krys

Krischan (German) a form of Christian.
Krishan, Krishaun, Krishawn, Krishon, Krishun

Krishna (Hindi) delightful, pleasurable. Religion: the eighth and principal avatar of the Hindu god Vishnu.
Kistna, Kistnah, Krisha, Krishnah

Krispin (Latin) a form of Crispin.
Krispian, Krispino, Krispo

Krista GB (Czech) a form of Christina.

Kristen GB (Greek) a form of Kristian, Kristyn. (French, English) a form of Christine.

Krister (Swedish) a form of Christian.
Krist, Kristar

Kristian BG (Greek) a form of Christian, Khristian.
Kerstan, Khristos, Kit, Kris, Krischan, Krist, Kristan, Kristar, Kristek, Kristen, Krister, Kristien, Kristin, Kristine, Kristinn, Kristion, Kristjan, Kristo, Kristos, Krists, Krystek, Krystian, Khrystiyan

Kristin GB (Greek) a form of Kristian.

Kristina GB (Greek) Christian; anointed. (Scandinavian) a form of Christina.

Kristine GB (Greek) a form of Kristian.

Kristo (Greek) a short form of Khristos.

Kristofer (Swedish) a form of Kristopher.
Kris, Kristafer, Kristef, Kristifer, Kristoff, Kristoffer, Kristofo, Kristofor, Kristofyr, Kristufer, Kristus, Krystofer

Kristoff (Greek) a short form of Kristofer, Kristopher.
Kristof, Kristóf

Kristophe (French) a form of Kristopher.

Kristopher ☒☒ (Greek) a form of Christopher. See also Topher.
Khristopher, Kit, Kris, Krisstopher, Kristapher, Kristepher, Kristfer, Kristfor, Kristo, Kristofer, Kristoff, Kristoforo, Kristoph, Kristophe, Kristophor, Kristos, Krists, Krisus, Krystopher, Krystupas, Krzysztof

Kristy ☒☒ (American) a familiar form of Kristine, Krystal.

Kristyn ☒☒ (Greek) a form of Kristen.

Kruz (Spanish) a form of Cruz.
Kruise, Kruize, Kruse, Kruze

Krystal ☒☒ (American) clear, brilliant glass.

Krystian ☒☒ (Polish) a form of Christian.
Krys, Krystek, Krystien, Krystin

Kuba (Czech) a form of Jacob.
Kubo, Kubus

Kueng (Chinese) universe.

Kugonza (Rutooro) love.

Kuiril (Basque) lord.

Kumar (Sanskrit) prince.

Kunle (Yoruba) home filled with honors.

Kuper (Yiddish) copper.

Kurt (Latin, German, French) a short form of Kurtis. A form of Curt.
Kirt, Kort, Kuno, Kurtt

Kurtis (Latin, French) a form of Curtis.
Kirtis, Kirtus, Kurt, Kurtes, Kurtez, Kurtice, Kurties, Kurtiss, Kurtus, Kurtys

Kuruk (Pawnee) bear.

Kuzih (Carrier) good speaker.

Kwabena (Akan) born on Tuesday.

Kwacha (Nguni) morning.

Kwako (Akan) born on Wednesday.
Kwaka, Kwaku

Kwam (Zuni) a form of John.

Kwame (Akan) born on Saturday.
Kwamen, Kwami, Kwamin

Kwan (Korean) strong.
Kwane

Kwasi (Akan) born on Sunday. (Swahili) wealthy.
Kwasie, Kwazzi, Kwesi

Kwayera (Nguni) dawn.

Kwende (Nguni) let's go.

Kyele (Irish) a form of Kyle.

Kyla GB (Irish) attractive.
(Yiddish) crown; laurel.

Kylan (Irish) a form of Kyle.
*Kyelen, Kyleen, Kylen, Kylin,
Kyline, Kylon, Kylun*

Kyle ☼ BG (Irish) narrow piece
of land; place where cattle graze.
(Yiddish) crowned with laurels.
*Cyle, Kiel, Kilan, Kile, Kilen, Kiley,
Ky, Kye, Kyel, Kyele, Kylan, Kylee,
Kyler, Kyley, Kylie, Kyll, Kylle,
Kyrell*

Kylee (GB Irish) a form of Kyle.

Kyler BG (English) a form of Kyle.
Kylar, Kylor

Kylie GB (West Australian
Aboriginal) curled stick;
boomerang. (Irish) a familiar
form of Kyle.

Kym GB (English, Vietnamese) a
form of Kim.

Kynan (Welsh) chief.

Kyndall GB (English) a form of
Kendall.
Kyndal, Kyndel, Kyndell, Kyndle

Kyne (English) royal.

Kyran (Sanskrit) a form of Kiran.
Kyren, Kyron, Kyrone

Kyros (Greek) master.

Kyven (American) a form of Kevin.
*Kyvan, Kyvaun, Kyvon, Kywon,
Kywynn*

L BG (American) an initial used as
a first name.

Laban (Hawaiian) white.
Labon, Lebaan, Leban, Liban

Labaron (American) a combi-
nation of the prefix La + Baron.
*Labaren, Labarren, Labarron,
Labearon, Labron*

Labib (Arabic) sensible; intelligent.

Labrentsis (Russian) a form of
Lawrence.
Labhras, Labhruinn, Labrencis

Lacey GB (Latin) cheerful.
(Greek) a familiar form of Larissa.

Lachlan (Scottish) land of lakes.
*Lache, Lachlann, Lachunn,
Lakelan, Lakeland*

Lacy GB (Latin) a form of Lacey.

Ladarian (American) a combi-
nation of the prefix La + Darian.
*Ladarien, Ladarin, Ladarion,
Ladarren, Ladarrian, Ladarrien,
Ladarrin, Ladarrion, Laderion,
Laderrian, Laderrion*

Ladarius (American) a combination of the prefix La + Darius.
Ladarious, Ladaris, Ladarrius, Ladauris, Laderius, Ladirus

Ladarrius (American) a form of Ladarius.
Ladarrias, Ladarries, Ladarrious, Laderrious, Laderris

Ladd (English) attendant.
Lad, Laddey, Laddie, Laddy

Laderrick (American) a combination of the prefix La + Derrick.
Ladarrick, Ladereck, Laderic, Laderricks

Ladio (Slavic) he who governs with glory.

Ladislao (Slavic) he who governs with glory.

Ladislav (Czech) a form of Walter.
Laco, Lada, Ladislaus

Lado (Fante) second-born son.

Ladolfo, Landolfo (Germanic) skillful as a wolf in the city.

Laertes (Greek) rock-picker.

Lafayette (French) History: Marquis de Lafayette was a French soldier and politician who aided the American Revolution.
Lafaiete, Lafayett, Lafette, Laffyette

Lahual (Araucanian) larch tree.

Laine 🅱🅶 (English) a form of Lane.
Lain

Laird (Scottish) wealthy landowner.

Lais (Arabic) lion.

Lajos (Hungarian) famous; holy.
Lajcsi, Laji, Lali

Lake (English) lake.
Lakan, Lakane, Lakee, Laken, Lakin

Laken 🅶🅱 (English) a form of Lake.

Lakota 🅱🅶 (Dakota) a tribal name.
Lakoda

Lal (Hindi) beloved.

Lamar 🅱🅶 (German) famous throughout the land. (French) sea, ocean.
Lamair, Lamario, Lamaris, Lamarr, Lamarre, Larmar, Lemar

Lambert (German) bright land.
Bert, Lambard, Lamberto, Lambirt, Lampard, Landbert

Lamond (French) world.
Lammond, Lamon, Lamonde, Lamondo, Lamondre, Lamund, Lemond

Lamont 🅱🅶 (Scandinavian) lawyer.
Lamaunt, Lamonta, Lamonte, Lamontie, Lamonto, Lamount, Lemont

Lance BG (German) a short form
of Lancelot.
Lancy, Lantz, Lanz, Launce

Lancelot (French) attendant.
Literature: the knight who loved
King Arthur's wife, Queen
Guinevere.
*Lance, Lancelott, Launcelet,
Launcelot*

Landelino (Teutonic) he who is a
friend of the earth.

Landen (English) a form of Landon.
Landenn

Lander (Basque) lion man.
(English) landowner.
Landers, Landor

Landerico (Teutonic) powerful in
the region; he who exercises
power in the region.

Landin BG (English) a form of
Landon.

Lando (Portuguese, Spanish) a
short form of Orlando, Rolando.

Landon ☆ BG (English) open,
grassy meadow.
Landan, Landen, Landin, Landyn

Landrada (Teutonic) counselor in
his village.

Landry (French, English) ruler.
Landre, Landré, Landrue

Lane BG (English) narrow road.
Laine, Laney, Lanie, Layne

Lang (Scandinavian) tall man.
Lange

Langdon (English) long hill.
Landon, Langsdon, Langston

Langford (English) long ford.
Lanford, Lankford

Langley (English) long meadow.
*Langlea, Langlee, Langleigh,
Langly*

Langston (English) long, narrow
town.
Langsden, Langsdon

Langundo (Native American)
peaceful.

Lani GB (Hawaiian) heaven.

Lanny (American) a familiar form
of Lawrence, Laurence.
Lanney, Lannie, Lennie

Lanu (Moquelumnan) running
around the pole.

Lanz (Italian) a form of Lance.
Lanzo, Lonzo

Lao (Spanish) a short form of
Stanislaus.

Lap (Vietnamese) independent.

Lapidos (Hebrew) torches.
Lapidoth

Laquan (American) a combi-
nation of the prefix La + Quan.
*Laquain, Laquann, Laquanta,
Laquantae, Laquante, Laquawn,
Laquawne, Laquin, Laquinn,
Laqun, Laquon, Laquone, Laqwan,
Laqwon*

Laquintin (American) a combination of the prefix La + Quintin.
Laquentin, Laquenton, Laquintas, Laquinten, Laquintiss, Laquinton

Lara 🇬🇧 (Greek) cheerful. (Latin) shining; famous. Mythology: a Roman nymph. A short form of Laraine, Laura.

Laramie (French) tears of love. Geography: a town in Wyoming on the Overland Trail.
Larami, Laramy, Laremy

Larenzo (Italian, Spanish) a form of Lorenzo.
Larenz, Larenza, Larinzo, Laurenzo

Larissa (Greek) cheerful.

Larkin (Irish) rough; fierce.
Larklin

Larnell (American) a combination of Larry + Darnell.

Laron (French) thief.
Laran, La'ron, La Ron, Larone, Laronn, Larron, La Ruan

Larrimore (French) armorer.
Larimore, Larmer, Larmor

Larry 🇧🇬 (Latin) a familiar form of Lawrence.
Larrie, Lary

Lars (Scandinavian) a form of Lawrence.
Laris, Larris, Larse, Larsen, Larson, Larsson, Larz, Lasse, Laurans, Laurits, Lavrans, Lorens

LaSalle (French) hall.
Lasal, Lasalle, Lascell, Lascelles

Lash (Gypsy) a form of Louis.
Lashi, Lasho

Lashawn (American) a combination of the prefix La + Shawn.
Lasaun, Lasean, Lashajaun, Lashan, Lashane, Lashaun, Lashon, Lashun

Lashon (American) a form of Lashawn.
Lashone, Lashonne

Lasse (Finnish) a form of Nicholas.

László (Hungarian) famous ruler.
Laci, Lacko, Laslo, Lazlo

Lateef (Arabic) gentle; pleasant.
Latif, Letif

Latham (Scandinavian) barn. (English) district.
Laith, Lathe, Lay

Lathan (American) a combination of the prefix La + Nathan.
Lathaniel, Lathen, Lathyn, Leathan

Lathrop (English) barn, farmstead.
Lathe, Lathrope, Lay

Latimer (English) interpreter.
Lat, Latimor, Lattie, Latty, Latymer

Latravis (American) a combination of the prefix La + Travis.
Latavious, Latavius, Latraveus,

Latraviaus, Latravious, Latravius, Latrayvious, Latrayvous, Latrivis

Latrell (American) a combination of the prefix La + Kentrell.
Latreal, Latreil, Latrel, Latrelle, Letreal, Letrel, Letrell, Letrelle

Laudalino (Portuguese) praised.
Lino

Laughlin (Irish) servant of Saint Secundinus.
Lanty, Lauchlin, Leachlainn

Laura GB (Latin) crowned with laurel.

Laurelino, Laurentino (Latin) winner; worthy of honors.

Lauren GB (Latin) a form of Laurence.

Laurence GB (Latin) crowned with laurel. A form of Lawrence. See also Rance, Raulas, Raulo, Renzo.
Lanny, Lauran, Laurance, Laureano, Laurencho, Laurencio, Laurens, Laurent, Laurentij, Laurentios, Laurentiu, Laurentius, Laurentz, Laurentzi, Laurie, Laurin, Lauris, Laurits, Lauritz, Laurnet, Lauro, Laurus, Lavrenti, Lurance

Laurencio (Spanish) a form of Laurence.

Laurens (Dutch) a form of Laurence.
Laurenz

Laurent (French) a form of Laurence.
Laurente

Laurie GB (English) a familiar form of Laurence.
Lauri, Laury, Lorry

Lauris (Swedish) a form of Laurence.

Lauro (Filipino) a form of Laurence.

Laury GB (English) a form of Laurie.

Lautaro (Araucanian) daring and enterprising.

LaValle (French) valley.
Lavail, Laval, Lavalei, Lavalle, Lavell

Lavan (Hebrew) white.
Lavane, Lavaughan, Laven, Lavon, Levan

Lavaughan (American) a form of Lavan.
Lavaughn, Levaughan, Levaughn

Lave (Italian) lava. (English) lord.

Lavell (French) a form of LaValle.
Lavel, Lavele, Lavelle, Levele, Levell, Levelle

Lavi (Hebrew) lion.

Lavon (American) a form of Lavan.
Lavion, Lavone, Lavonn, Lavonne, Lavont, Lavonte

Lavrenti (Russian) a form of Lawrence.
Larenti, Lavrentij, Lavrusha, Lavrik, Lavro

Lawerence (Latin) a form of Lawrence.
Lawerance

Lawford (English) ford on the hill.
Ford, Law

Lawler (Irish) soft-spoken.
Lawlor, Lollar, Loller

Lawrence 🅱🅶 (Latin) crowned with laurel. See also Brencis, Chencho.
Labrentsis, Laiurenty, Lanny, Lanty, Larance, Laren, Larian, Larien, Laris, Larka, Larrance, Larrence, Larry, Lars, Larya, Laurence, Lavrenti, Law, Lawerence, Lawrance, Lawren, Lawrey, Lawrie, Lawron, Lawry, Lencho, Lon, Lóránt, Loreca, Loren, Loretto, Lorenzo, Lorne, Lourenco, Lowrance

Lawson (English) son of Lawrence.
Lawsen, Layson

Lawton (English) town on the hill.
Laughton, Law

Layne 🅱🅶 (English) a form of Lane.
Layn, Laynee

Layton 🅱🅶 (English) a form of Leighton.
Laydon, Layten, Layth, Laythan, Laython

Lazaro, Lázaro (Italian) forms of Lazarus.
Lazarillo, Lazarito, Lazzaro

Lazarus (Greek) a form of Eleazar. Bible: Lazarus was raised from the dead by Jesus.
Lazar, Lázár, Lazare, Lazarius, Lazaro, Lazaros, Lazorus

Leah 🅶🅱 (Hebrew) weary.

Leal (Spanish) loyal and faithful worker.

Leander (Greek) lion-man; brave as a lion.
Ander, Leandro

Leandre (Greek) calm, serene man.

Leandro (Spanish) a form of Leander.
Leandra, Léandre, Leandrew, Leandros

Leanne 🅶🅱 (English) a form of Leeann, Lian (see Girls' Names).

Learco (Greek) judge of his village.

Leben (Yiddish) life.
Laben, Lebon

Lebna (Ethiopian) spirit; heart.

Ledarius (American) a combination of the prefix Le + Darius.
Ledarrious, Ledarrius, Lederious, Lederris

Lee 🅱🅶 (English) a short form of Farley, Leonard, and names

containing "lee."
Leigh

Leggett (French) one who is sent; delegate.
Legate, Legette, Leggitt, Liggett

Lei BG (Chinese) thunder. (Hawaiian) a form of Ray.

Leib (Yiddish) roaring lion.
Leibel

Leif (Scandinavian) beloved.
Laif, Leife, Lief

Leigh GB (English) a form of Lee.

Leighton (English) meadow farm.
Lay, Layton, Leigh, Leyton

Leith (Scottish) broad river.

Lek (Tai) small.

Lekeke (Hawaiian) powerful ruler.

Leks (Estonian) a familiar form of Alexander.
Leksik, Lekso

Lel (Gypsy) taker.

Leland BG (English) meadowland; protected land.
Lealand, Lee, Leeland, Leigh, Leighland, Lelan, Lelann, Lelend, Lelund, Leyland

Lelio (Latin) he who is talkative.

Lemar (French) a form of Lamar.
Lemario, Lemarr

Lemuel (Hebrew) devoted to God.
Lem, Lemmie, Lemmy

Len (Hopi) flute. (German) a short form of Leonard.

Lenard (German) a form of Leonard.
Lennard

Lencho (Spanish) a form of Lawrence.
Lenci, Lenzy

Lennart (Swedish) a form of Leonard.
Lennerd

Lenno (Native American) man.

Lennon (Irish) small cloak; cape.
Lenon

Lennor (Gypsy) spring; summer.

Lennox (Scottish) with many elms.
Lennix, Lenox

Lenny (German) a familiar form of Leonard.
Leni, Lennie, Leny

Leo (Latin) lion. (German) a short form of Leon, Leopold.
Lavi, Leão, Lee, Leib, Leibel, Léo, Léocadie, Leos, Leosko, Leosoko, Lev, Lio, Lion, Liutas, Lyon, Nardek

Leobardo (Italian) a form of Leonard.

Leocadio (Greek) he who shines because of his whiteness.

Leodoualdo (Teutonic) he who governs his village.

Leofrido (Teutonic) he who brings peace to his village.

Leon (Greek, German) a short form of Leonard, Napoleon.
Leo, Léon, Leonas, Léonce, Leoncio, Leondris, Leone, Leonek, Leonetti, Leoni, Leonid, Leonidas, Leonirez, Leonizio, Leonon, Leons, Leontes, Leontios, Leontrae, Liutas

León (Latin) a form of Leon.

Leonard (German) brave as a lion.
Leanard, Lee, Len, Lena, Lenard, Lennart, Lenny, Leno, Leobardo, Leon, Léonard, Leonardis, Leonardo, Leonart, Leonerd, Leonhard, Leonidas, Leonnard, Leontes, Lernard, Lienard, Linek, Lnard, Lon, Londard, Lonnard, Lonya, Lynnard

Leonardo (Italian) a form of Leonard.
Leonaldo, Lionardo

Leonel (English) little lion. See also Lionel.
Leonell

Leonelo (Spanish) a form of Leonel.

Leonhard (German) a form of Leonard.
Leonhards

Leonid (Russian) a form of Leonard.
Leonide, Lyonechka, Lyonya

Leonidas (Greek) a form of Leonard.
Leonida, Leonides

Leónidas (Spanish) a form of León.

Leontino (German) strong as a lion.

Leopold (German) brave people.
Leo, Leopoldo, Leorad, Lipót, Lopolda, Luepold, Luitpold, Poldi

Leopoldo (Italian) a form of Leopold.

Leor (Hebrew) my light.
Leory, Lior

Lequinton (American) a combination of the prefix Le + Quinton.
Lequentin, Lequenton, Lequinn

Leron (French) round, circle. (American) a combination of the prefix Le + Ron.
Leeron, Le Ron, Lerone, Liron, Lyron

Leroy (French) king. See also Delroy, Elroy.
Lee, Leeroy, LeeRoy, Leigh, Lerai, Leroi, LeRoi, LeRoy, Roy

Les (Scottish, English) a short form of Leslie, Lester.
Lessie

Lesharo (Pawnee) chief.

Leshawn (American) a combination of the prefix Le + Shawn.
Lashan, Lesean, Leshaun, Leshon, Leshun

Lesley **GB** (Scottish) a form of Leslie.

Leslie **GB** (Scottish) gray fortress.
Lee, Leigh, Les, Leslea, Leslee, Lesley, Lesli, Lesly, Lezlie, Lezly

Lesly **GB** (Scottish) a form of Leslie.

Lesmes (Teutonic) he whose nobility protects him.

Lester **BG** (Latin) chosen camp. (English) from Leicester, England.
Leicester, Les

Leto (Latin) he who is always happy.

Leuco (Greek) luminous one.

Lev (Hebrew) heart. (Russian) a form of Leo. A short form of Leverett, Levi.
Leb, Leva, Levka, Levko, Levushka

Leverett (French) young hare.
Lev, Leveret, Leverit, Leveritt

Levi **BG** (Hebrew) joined in harmony. Bible: the third son of Jacob; Levites are the priestly tribe of the Israelites.
Leavi, Leevi, Leevie, Lev, Levey, Levie, Levin, Levitis, Levy, Lewi, Leyvi

Levin (Hebrew) a form of Levi.
Levine, Levion

Levon (American) a form of Lavon.
Leevon, Levone, Levonn, Levonne, Levonte, Lyvonne

Lew (English) a short form of Lewis.

Lewin (English) beloved friend.

Lewis **BG** (Welsh) a form of Llewellyn. (English) a form of Louis.
Lew, Lewes, Lewie, Lewy

Lex (English) a short form of Alexander.
Lexi, Lexin

Lexie **GB** (English) a form of Lex.

Lexus **GB** (Greek) a short form of Alexander.
Lexis, Lexius, Lexxus

Leyati (Moquelumnan) shape of an abalone shell.

Lí (Chinese) strong.

Lia **GB** (Greek) bringer of good news. (Hebrew, Dutch, Italian) dependent.

Liam **BG** (Irish) a form of William.
Liem, Lliam, Lyam

Liana **GB** (Latin) youth. (French) bound, wrapped up; tree covered with vines. (English) meadow. (Hebrew) short form of Eliana (see Girls' Names).

Liang (Chinese) good, excellent.

Liban 🅱🅶 (Hawaiian) a form of Laban.
Libaan, Lieban

Líbano (Latin) white.

Liber (Latin) he who spreads abundance.

Liberal (Latin) lover of liberty.

Liberato (Latin) liberated one.

Liberio (Portuguese) liberation.
Liberaratore, Liborio

Liberto (Latin) a form of Liberal.

Libiac, Llipiac (Quechua) ray of light; brilliant, glowing.

Libio, Livio (Latin) born in a dry place; comes from the desert.

Licas (Greek) wolf.

Licurgo (Greek) he who frightens off wolves.

Lidio (Greek, Portuguese) ancient.

Ligongo (Yao) who is this?

Likeke (Hawaiian) a form of Richard.

Liko (Chinese) protected by Buddha. (Hawaiian) bud.
Like

Lin 🅶🅱 (Burmese) bright. (English) a short form of Lyndon.
Linh, Linn, Linny, Lyn, Lynn

Linc (English) a short form of Lincoln.
Link

Lincoln 🅱🅶 (English) settlement by the pool. History: Abraham Lincoln was the sixteenth U.S. president.
Linc, Lincon, Lyncoln

Linda 🅶🅱 (Spanish) pretty.

Lindberg (German) mountain where linden grow.
Lindbergh, Lindburg, Lindy

Lindell (English) valley of the linden.
Lendall, Lendel, Lendell, Lindall, Lindel, Lyndale, Lyndall, Lyndel, Lyndell

Linden (English) a form of Lyndon.

Lindley (English) linden field.
Lindlea, Lindlee, Lindleigh, Lindly

Lindon (English) a form of Lyndon.
Lin, Lindan

Lindor (Latin) he who seduces, likes to seduce.

Lindsay 🅶🅱 (English) a form of Lindsey.
Linsay

Lindsey 🅶🅱 (English) linden-tree island.
Lind, Lindsay, Lindsee, Lindsie, Lindsy, Lindzy, Linsey, Linzie, Linzy, Lyndsay, Lyndsey, Lyndsie, Lynzie

Linford (English) linden ford.
Lynford

Linfred (German) peaceful, calm.

Linley (English) flax meadow.
Linlea, Linlee, Linleigh, Linly

Linton (English) flax town.
Lintonn, Lynton, Lyntonn

Linu (Hindi) lily.

Linus (Greek) flaxen haired.
Linas, Linux

Linwood (English) flax wood.

Lio (Hawaiian) a form of Leo.

Lionel (French) lion cub. See also
Leonel.
*Lional, Lionell, Lionello, Lynel,
Lynell, Lyonel*

Liron BG (Hebrew) my song.
Lyron

Lisa GB (Hebrew) consecrated to
God. (English) a short form of
Elizabeth.

Lisandro, Lisias (Spanish)
liberator.

Lisardo (Hebrew) defender of the
faith, fights for God.

Lise GB (Moquelumnan) salmon's
head coming out of the water.

Lisette GB (French) a form of
Lisa. (English) a familiar form of
Elise, Elizabeth.

Lisimba (Yao) lion.
Simba

Lisístrato (Greek) he who fights
for the liberating army.

Lister (English) dyer.

Litton (English) town on the hill.
Liton

Liu (African) voice.

Liuz (Polish) light.
Lius

Livingston (English) Leif's town.
Livingstone

Liwanu (Moquelumnan) growling
bear.

Lizbeth GB (English) a short form
of Elizabeth.

Llacsa (Quechua) he who is the
color of bronze.

Llallaua (Aymara) magnificent.

Llancamil (Mapuche) shining
stone, gold and silver pearl.

Llancañir (Mapuche) fox that is
pearl-colored.

Llanqui (Quechua) potter's clay.

Llarico, Llaricu (Aymara)
indomitable; he who does not
allow himself to be humiliated
nor does he to bow to anyone.

Llashapoma, Llashapuma
(Quechua) heavy puma; slow.

Llewellyn (Welsh) lionlike.
*Lewis, Llewelin, Llewellen,
Llewelleyn, Llewellin, Llewlyn,
Llywellyn, Llywellynn, Llywelyn*

Lloque, Lluqui (Quechua) left-handed, from the left side.

Lloqueyupanqui,
Lluquiyupanqui (Quechua) left-handed, memorable.

Lloyd 🅱🅶 (Welsh) gray haired; holy. See also Floyd.
Loy, Loyd, Loyde, Loydie

Lobo (Spanish) wolf.

Lochlain (Irish, Scottish) land of lakes.
Laughlin, Lochlan, Lochlann, Lochlin, Locklynn

Locke (English) forest.
Lock, Lockwood

Loe (Hawaiian) a form of Roy.

Logan ☀ 🅱🅶 (Irish) meadow.
Llogan, Loagan, Loagen, Loagon, Logann, Logen, Loggan, Loghan, Logon, Logn, Logun, Logunn, Logyn

Lok (Chinese) happy.

Lokela (Hawaiian) a form of Roger.

Lokni (Moquelumnan) raining through the roof.

Lomán (Irish) bare. (Slavic) sensitive.

Lombard (Latin) long bearded.
Bard, Barr

Lon (Irish) fierce. (Spanish) a short form of Alonso, Alonzo, Leonard, Lonnie.
Lonn

Lonan (Zuni) cloud.

Lonato (Native American) flint stone.

Loncopan (Mapuche) puma's head; leader of the pumas; principal branch or capitol.

London 🅱🅶 (English) fortress of the moon. Geography: the capital of the United Kingdom.
Londen, Londyn, Lunden, Lundon

Long (Chinese) dragon. (Vietnamese) hair.

Lonnie (German, Spanish) a familiar form of Alonso, Alonzo.
Lon, Loni, Lonie, Lonnell, Lonney, Lonni, Lonniel, Lonny

Lono (Hawaiian) Mythology: the god of learning and intellect.

Lonzo (German, Spanish) a short form of Alonso, Alonzo.
Lonso

Lootah (Lakota) red.

Lopaka (Hawaiian) a form of Robert.

Loránd (Hungarian) a form of Roland.

Lóránt (Hungarian) a form of Lawrence.
Lorant

Lorcan (Irish) little; fierce.

Lord (English) noble title.

Loren **GB** (Latin) a short form of Lawrence.
Lorin, Lorren, Lorrin, Loryn

Lorena **GB** (English) a form of Lauren.

Lorenzo (Italian, Spanish) a form of Lawrence.
Larenzo, Lerenzo, Lewrenzo, Lorenc, Lorence, Lorenco, Lorencz, Lorens, Lorenso, Lorentz, Lorenz, Lorenza, Loretto, Lorinc, Lörinc, Lorinzo, Loritz, Lorrenzo, Lorrie, Lorry, Lourenza, Lourenzo, Lowrenzo, Renzo, Zo

Loretto (Italian) a form of Lawrence.
Loreto

Lori **GB** (English) a form of Lorry.

Lorién (Aragonese) a form of Lorenzo.

Lorimer (Latin) harness maker.
Lorrie, Lorrimer, Lorry

Loring (German) son of the famous warrior.
Lorrie, Lorring, Lorry

Loris **BG** (Dutch) clown.

Loritz (Latin, Danish) laurel.
Lauritz

Lorne (Latin) a short form of Lawrence.
Lorn, Lornie

Lorry (English) a form of Laurie.
Lori, Lorri, Lory

Lot (Hebrew) hidden, covered. Bible: Lot fled from Sodom, but his wife glanced back upon its destruction and was transformed into a pillar of salt.
Lott

Lotario (Germanic) distinguished warrior.

Lothar (German) a form of Luther.
Lotaire, Lotarrio, Lothair, Lothaire, Lothario, Lotharrio

Lou **BG** (German) a short form of Louis.

Loudon (German) low valley.
Loudan, Louden, Loudin, Lowden

Louie (German) a familiar form of Louis.

Louis (German) famous warrior. See also Aloisio, Aloysius, Clovis, Luigi.
Lash, Lashi, Lasho, Lewis, Lou, Loudovicus, Louie, Louies, Louise, Lucho, Lude, Ludek, Ludirk, Ludis, Ludko, Ludwig, Lughaidh, Lui, Luigi, Luis, Luiz, Luki, Lutek

Louise **GB** (German) famous warrior.

Lourdes **GB** (French) from Lourdes, France. Religion: a place where the Virgin Mary was said to have appeared.

Louvain (English) Lou's vanity. Geography: a city in Belgium.
Louvin

Lovell (English) a form of Lowell.
Louvell, Lovel, Lovelle, Lovey

Lowell (French) young wolf.
(English) beloved.
Lovell, Lowe, Lowel

Loyal (English) faithful, loyal.
Loy, Loyall, Loye, Lyall, Lyell

Loyola (Latin) has a wolf in his shield.

Luano (Latin) fountain.

Lubomir (Polish) lover of peace.

Luboslaw (Polish) lover of glory.
Lubs, Lubz

Luc (French) a form of Luke.
Luce

Luca BG (Italian) a form of Lucius.
Lucca, Luka

Lucas ☆ BG (German, Irish, Danish, Dutch) a form of Lucius.
Lucais, Lucassie, Lucaus, Luccas, Luccus, Luckas, Lucus

Lucero (Spanish) bringer of light.

Lucian (Latin) a form of Lucius.
Liuz, Lucan, Lucanus, Luciano, Lucianus, Lucias, Lucjan, Lukianos, Lukyan

Luciano (Italian) a form of Lucian.
Luca, Lucca, Lucino, Lucio

Lucien (French) a form of Lucius.

Lucila (Latin) bringer of light.

Lucio (Italian) a form of Lucius.

Lucius (Latin) light; bringer of light.
Loukas, Luc, Luca, Lucais, Lucanus, Lucas, Luce, Lucian, Lucien, Lucio, Lucious, Lucis, Luke, Lusio

Lucky (American) fortunate.
Luckee, Luckie, Luckson, Lucson

Lucrecio (Latin) twilight of dawn.

Ludlow (English) prince's hill.

Ludovic (German) a form of Ludwig.
Ludovick, Ludovico

Ludwig (German) a form of Louis. Music: Ludwig van Beethoven was a famous nineteenth-century German composer.
Ludovic, Ludvig, Ludvik, Ludwik, Lutz

Lui (Hawaiian) a form of Louis.

Luigi (Italian) a form of Louis.
Lui, Luiggi, Luigino, Luigy

Luis ☆ BG (Spanish) a form of Louis.
Luise

Luís (Spanish) a form of Luis.

Luisa GB (Spanish) a form of Louisa (see Girls' Names).

Luiz (Spanish) a form of Louis.

Lukas, Lukus (Greek, Czech, Swedish) forms of Luke.
Loukas, Lukais, Lukash, Lukasha, Lukass, Lukasz, Lukaus, Lukkas

Luke ⭐ BG (Latin) a form of Lucius. Bible: companion of Saint Paul and author of the third Gospel of the New Testament.
Luc, Luchok, Luck, Lucky, Luk, Luka, Lúkács, Lukas, Luken, Lukes, Lukus, Lukyan, Lusio

Lukela (Hawaiian) a form of Russel.

Luken (Basque) bringer of light.
Lucan, Lucane, Lucano, Luk

Luki (Basque) famous warrior.

Lukman (Arabic) prophet.
Luqman

Lulani BG (Hawaiian) highest point in heaven.

Lumo (Ewe) born facedown.

Lundy (Scottish) grove by the island.

Lunn (Irish) warlike.
Lon, Lonn

Lunt (Swedish) grove.

Lupercio (Latin) name given to people from Lupercus.

Luperco (Latin) he who frightens off wolves.

Lusila (Hindi) leader.

Lusio (Zuni) a form of Lucius.

Lusorio (Latin) he enjoys games.

Lutalo (Luganda) warrior.

Lutardo (Teutonic) he who is valiant in his village.

Lutfi (Arabic) kind, friendly.

Luther (German) famous warrior. History: Martin Luther was one of the central figures of the Reformation.
Lothar, Lutero, Luthor

Lutherum (Gypsy) slumber.

Luyu BG (Moquelumnan) head shaker.

Luz GB (Spanish) light.

Lyall, Lyell (Scottish) loyal.

Lydia GB (Greek) from Lydia, an ancient land in Asia. (Arabic) strife.

Lyle (French) island.
Lisle, Ly, Lysle

Lyman (English) meadow.
Leaman, Leeman, Lymon

Lynch (Irish) mariner.
Linch

Lyndal (English) valley of lime trees.
Lyndale, Lyndall, Lyndel, Lyndell

Lyndon (English) linden hill. History: Lyndon B. Johnson was the thirty-sixth U.S. president.
Lin, Linden, Lindon, Lyden, Lydon, Lyn, Lyndan, Lynden, Lynn

Lyndsay GB (English) a form of Lindsey.

Lynn GB (English) waterfall; brook.
Lyn, Lynell, Lynette, Lynnard, Lynoll

Lyron (Hebrew) a form of Leron, Liron.

Lysander (Greek) liberator.
Lyzander, Sander

M GB (American) an initial used as a first name.

Maalik (Punjabi) a form of Malik.
Maalek, Maaliek

Mac (Scottish) son.
Macs

Macabeo (Hebrew) progressing.

Macadam (Scottish) son of Adam.
MacAdam, McAdam

Macallister (Irish) son of Alistair.
Macalaster, Macalister, MacAlister, McAlister, McAllister

Macario (Spanish) a form of Makarios.

Macarthur (Irish) son of Arthur.
MacArthur, McArthur

Macaulay (Scottish) son of righteousness.
Macaulee, Macauley, Macaully, Macauly, Maccauley, Mackauly, Macualay, McCauley

Macbride (Scottish) son of a follower of Saint Brigid.
Macbryde, Mcbride, McBride

Maccoy (Irish) son of Hugh, Coy.
MacCoy, Mccoy, McCoy

Maccrea (Irish) son of grace.
MacCrae, MacCray, MacCrea, Macrae, Macray, Makray, Mccrea, McCrea

Macdonald (Scottish) son of Donald.
MacDonald, Mcdonald, McDonald, Mcdonna, Mcdonnell, McDonnell

Macdougal (Scottish) son of Dougal.
MacDougal, Mcdougal, McDougal, McDougall, Dougal

Mace (French) club. (English) a short form of Macy, Mason.
Macean, Maceo, Macer, Macey, Macie, Macy

Macedonio (Greek) he who triumphs and grows in stature.

Macerio (Spanish) blessed.

Macgregor (Scottish) son of Gregor.
Macgreggor

Machas (Polish) a form of Michael.

Macías (Hebrew) a form of Matías.

Macie **GB** (French, English) a form of Mace.

Maciel (Latin) very slender, skeleton-like.

Mack (Scottish) a short form of names beginning with "Mac" and "Mc."
Macke, Mackey, Mackie, Macklin, Macks, Macky

Mackenzie **GB** (Irish) son of Kenzie.
Mackensy, Mackenxo, Mackenze, Mackenzey, Mackenzi, MacKenzie, Mackenzly, Mackenzy, Mackienzie, Mackinsey, Mackinzie, Makenzie, McKenzie, Mickenzie

Mackinnley (Irish) son of the learned ruler.
Mackinley, MacKinnley, Mackinnly, Mckinley

Macklain (Irish) a form of Maclean.
Macklaine, Macklane

Maclean (Irish) son of Leander.
Machlin, Macklain, MacLain, MacLean, Maclin, Maclyn, Makleen, McLaine, McLean

Macmahon (Irish) son of Mahon.
MacMahon, McMahon

Macmurray (Irish) son of Murray.
McMurray

Macnair (Scottish) son of the heir.
Macknair

Maco (Hungarian) a form of Emmanuel.

Macon (German, English) maker.

Macrobio (Greek) he who enjoys a long life.

Macy **GB** (French) Matthew's estate.
Mace, Macey

Maddison **GB** (English) a form of Madison.

Maddock (Welsh) generous.
Madoc, Madock, Madog

Maddox (Welsh, English) benefactor's son.
Maddux, Madox

Madeline **GB** (Greek) high tower.

Madhar (Hindi) full of intoxication; relating to spring.

Madisen **GB** (English) a form of Madison.

Madison **GB** (English) son of Maude; good son.
Maddie, Maddison, Maddy, Madisen, Madisson, Madisyn, Madsen, Son, Sonny

Madongo (Luganda) uncircumcised.

Madu (Ibo) people.

Mael (Celtic) prince.

Magar (Armenian) groom's attendant.
Magarious

Magee (Irish) son of Hugh.
MacGee, MacGhee, McGee

Magen (Hebrew) protector.

Magín (Latin) he who is imaginative.

Magnar (Norwegian) strong; warrior.
Magne

Magno (Latin) great, of great fame; magnificent.

Magnus (Latin) great.
Maghnus, Magnes, Manius, Mayer

Magomu (Luganda) younger of twins.

Maguire (Irish) son of the beige one.
MacGuire, McGuire, McGwire

Mahammed (Arabic) a form of Muhammad.
Mahamad, Mahamed

Mahdi (Arabic) guided to the right path.
Mahde, Mahdee, Mahdy

Mahesa (Hindi) great lord. Religion: another name for the Hindu god Shiva.

Mahi'ai (Hawaiian) a form of George.

Mahir (Arabic, Hebrew) excellent; industrious.
Maher

Mahkah (Lakota) earth.

Mahmoud (Arabic) a form of Muhammad.
Mahamoud, Mahmmoud, Mahmuod

Mahmúd (Arabic) a form of Muhammad.
Mahmed, Mahmood, Mahmut

Mahoma (Arabic) worthy of being praised.

Mahomet (Arabic) a form of Muhammad.
Mehemet, Mehmet

Mahon (Irish) bear.

Mahpee (Lakota) sky.

Maicu (Quechua) eagle.

Maimun (Arabic) lucky.
Maimon

Maiqui (Quechua) tree.

Maira GB (Irish) a form of Mary.

Mairtin (Irish) a form of Martin.
Martain, Martainn

Maitias (Irish) a form of Mathias.
Maithias

Maitiú (Irish) a form of Matthew.

Maitland (English) meadowland.

Majencio (Latin) he who becomes more and more famous.

Majid (Arabic) great, glorious.
Majd, Majde, Majdi, Majdy, Majed, Majeed

Major (Latin) greater; military rank.
Majar, Maje, Majer, Mayer, Mayor

Makaio (Hawaiian) a form of Matthew.

Makalani (Mwera) writer.

Makani BG (Hawaiian) wind.

Makarios (Greek) happy; blessed.
Macario, Macarios, Maccario, Maccarios

Makell GB (Hebrew) a form of Michael.

Makenna GB (American) a form of Mackenna (see Girls' Names).

Makenzie GB (Irish) a form of Mackenzie.
Makensie, Makenzy

Makin (Arabic) strong.
Makeen

Makis (Greek) a form of Michael.

Makoto (Japanese) sincere.

Maks (Hungarian) a form of Max.
Makszi

Maksim (Russian) a form of Maximilian.
Maksimka, Maksym, Maxim

Maksym (Polish) a form of Maximilian.
Makimus, Maksim, Maksymilian

Makyah (Hopi) eagle hunter.

Mal (Irish) a short form of names beginning with "Mal."

Malachi (Hebrew) angel of God. Bible: the last canonical Hebrew prophet.
Maeleachlainn, Mal, Malachai, Malachia, Malachie, Malachy, Malakai, Malake, Malaki, Malchija, Malechy, Málik

Malachy (Irish) a form of Malachi.

Malajitm (Sanskrit) garland of victory.

Malaquias, Malaquías (Hebrew) my messenger.

Malco, Malcon (Hebrew) he who is like a king.

Malcolm (Scottish) follower of Saint Columba who Christianized North Scotland. (Arabic) dove.
Mal, Malcalm, Malcohm, Malcolum, Malcom, Malkolm

Malcom (Scottish) a form of Malcolm.
Malcome, Malcum, Malkom, Malkum

Malden (English) meeting place in a pasture.
Mal, Maldon

Malek (Arabic) a form of Málik.
Maleak, Maleek, Maleik, Maleka, Maleke, Mallek

Maleko (Hawaiian) a form of Mark.

Malik 🆖 (Punjabi, Arabic) a form of Málik.

Málik (Punjabi) lord, master. (Arabic) a form of Malachi.
Maalik, Mailik, Malak, Malic, Malick, Malicke, Maliek, Maliik, Malik, Malike, Malikh, Maliq, Malique, Mallik, Malyk, Malyq

Malin (English) strong, little warrior.
Mal, Mallin, Mallon

Mallory 🆖 (German) army counselor. (French) wild duck.
Lory, Mal, Mallery, Mallori, Mallorie, Malory

Maloney (Irish) church going.
Malone, Malony

Malvern (Welsh) bare hill.
Malverne

Malvin (Irish, English) a form of Melvin.
Mal, Malvinn, Malvyn, Malvynn

Mamani (Aymara) falcon.

Mamertino (Latin) name given to inhabitants of Mesina in Sicily.

Mamerto (Latin) native of Mamertium, an ancient city in the south of Italy.

Mamo 🆖 (Hawaiian) yellow flower; yellow bird.

Man-Shik (Korean) deeply rooted.

Man-Young (Korean) ten thousand years of prosperity.

Manases (Hebrew) he who forgets everything.

Manchu (Chinese) pure.

Mancio (Latin) he who foretells the future.

Manco (Peruvian) supreme leader. History: a sixteenth-century Incan king.

Mandala (Yao) flowers.
Manda, Mandela

Mandeep 🆖 (Punjabi) mind full of light.
Mandieep

Mandek (Polish) a form of Armand, Herman.
Mandie

Mandel (German) almond.
Mandell

Mander (Gypsy) from me.

Mandy 🆖 (Latin) lovable. A familiar form of Amanda.

Manford (English) small ford.

Manfred (English) man of peace.
See also Fred.
Manfret, Manfrid, Manfried, Maniferd, Mannfred, Mannfryd

Manfredo (Germanic) he who has power to safeguard the peace.

Manger (French) stable.

Mango (Spanish) a familiar form of Emmanuel, Manuel.

Manheim (German) servant's home.

Manipi (Native American) living marvel.

Manius (Scottish) a form of Magnus.
Manus, Manyus

Manjot BG (Indian) light of the mind.

Manley (English) hero's meadow.
Manlea, Manleigh, Manly

Manlio (Latin) he who was born in the morning.

Mann (German) man.
Manin

Manning (English) son of the hero.

Mannix (Irish) monk.
Mainchin

Manny (German, Spanish) a familiar form of Manuel.
Mani, Manni, Mannie, Many

Mano (Hawaiian) shark.
(Spanish) a short form of Manuel.
Manno, Manolo

Manoj (Sanskrit) cupid.

Manolito (Spanish) God is with us.

Manpreet GB (Punjabi) mind full of love.

Manque (Mapuche) condor.

Manquecura (Mapuche) refuge from the condor; two-colored rock.

Manquepan (Mapuche) condor's branch; spotted puma.

Mansa (Swahili) king. History: a fourteenth-century king of Mali.

Mansel (English) manse; house occupied by a clergyman.
Mansell

Mansfield (English) field by the river; hero's field.

Manso (Latin) delivered, trusted one.

Mansueto (Latin) he who is peaceful, docile.

Mansür (Arabic) divinely aided.
Mansoor, Mansour

Manton (English) man's town; hero's town.
Mannton, Manten

Manu (Hindi) lawmaker. History: the reputed writer of the Hindi compendium of sacred laws and customs. (Hawaiian) bird. (Ghanaian) second-born son.

Manuel (Hebrew) a short form of Emmanuel.
Maco, Mango, Mannuel, Manny, Mano, Manolón, Manual, Manuale, Manue, Manuelli, Manuelo, Manuil, Manyuil, Minel

Manville (French) worker's village. (English) hero's village.
Mandeville, Manvel, Manvil

Manzo (Japanese) third son.

Manzur (Arabic) winner, he who defeats all.

Maona (Winnebago) creator, earth maker.

Mapira (Yao) millet.

Marc (French) a form of Mark.

Marcel ☀G (French) a form of Marcellus.
Marcell, Marsale, Marsel

Marceliano (Spanish) a form of Marcelo.

Marcelino (Italian) a form of Marcellus.
Marceleno, Marcelin, Marcellin, Marcellino

Marcellus (Latin) a familiar form of Marcus.
Marceau, Marcel, Marceles,

Marcelias, Marcelino, Marcelis, Marcelius, Marcellas, Marcelleous, Marcellis, Marcellous, Marcelluas, Marcelo, Marcelus, Marcely, Marciano, Marcilka, Marcsseau, Marquel, Marsalis

Marcelo, Marcello (Italian) forms of Marcellus.
Marchello, Marsello, Marselo

March (English) dweller by a boundary.

Marcial (Spanish) a form of Marcio.

Marciano (Italian) a form of Martin.
Marci, Marcio

Marcilka (Hungarian) a form of Marcellus.
Marci, Marcilki

Marcin (Polish) a form of Martin.

Marcio (Italian) a form of Marciano.

Marco ☀G (Italian) a form of Marcus. History: Marco Polo was a thirteenth-century Venetian traveler who explored Asia.
Marcko, Marko

Marcos (Spanish) a form of Marcus.
Marckos, Marcous, Markos, Markose

Marcus ☀G (Latin) martial, warlike.
Marc, Marcas, Marcellus,

Marcio, Marckus, Marco,
Marcos, Marcous, Marcuss,
Marcuus, Marcux, Marek, Mark,
Markov, Markus

Mardonio (Persian) male
warrior.

Mardoqueo (Hebrew) he who
adores the god of war.

Marek (Slavic) a form of Marcus.

Maren **GB** (Basque) sea.

Mareo (Japanese) uncommon.

Margaret **GB** (Greek) pearl.

Maria **GB** (Hebrew) bitter; sea of
bitterness. (Italian, Spanish) a
form of Mary.

Mariah **GB** (Hebrew) a form of
Mary.

Mariam **GB** (Hebrew) a form of
Miriam.

Marian **GB** (Polish) a form of
Mark.

Marianne **GB** (English) a form of
Marian.

Mariano (Italian) a form of
Mark.

Marid (Arabic) rebellious.

Marie **GB** (French) a form of
Mary.

Marin (French) sailor.
Marine, Mariner, Marino, Marius,
Marriner

Marina **GB** (Latin) sea.

Marino (Italian) a form of Marin.
Marinos, Marinus, Mario,
Mariono

Mario **BG** (Italian) a form of
Marino.
Marios, Marrio

Marion **GB** (French) bitter; sea of
bitterness.
Mareon, Mariano

Marisela **GB** (Latin) a form of
Marisa (see Girls' Names).

Marissa **GB** (Latin) a form of
Marisa (see Girls' Names).

Marius (Latin) a form of Marin.
Marious

Marjolaine **GB** (French)
marjoram.

Mark **BG** (Latin) a form of
Marcus. Bible: author of the
second Gospel in the New
Testament. See also Maleko.
Marc, Marek, Marian, Mariano,
Marke, Markee, Markel, Markell,
Markey, Marko, Markos, Márkus,
Markusha, Marque, Martial,
Marx

Markanthony (Italian) a
combination of Mark + Anthony.

Marke (Polish) a form of Mark.

Markel, Markell **BG** (Latin)
forms of Mark.
Markelle, Markelo

Markes (Portuguese) a form of Marques.
Markess, Markest

Markese (French) a form of Marquis.
Markease, Markeece, Markees, Markeese, Markei, Markeice, Markeis, Markeise, Markes, Markez, Markeze, Markice

Markham (English) homestead on the boundary.

Markis (French) a form of Marquis.
Markies, Markiese, Markise, Markiss, Markist

Marko (Latin) a form of Marco, Mark.
Markco

Markus (Latin) a form of Marcus.
Markas, Markcus, Markcuss, Markys, Marqus

Marland (English) lake land.

Marlen 🅶🅱 (English) a form of Marlin.

Marley 🅶🅱 (English) lake meadow.
Marlea, Marleigh, Marly, Marrley

Marlin (English) deep-sea fish.
Marlion, Marlyn

Marlon 🅱🅶 (French) a form of Merlin.

Marlow (English) hill by the lake.
Mar, Marlo, Marlowe

Marlyn 🅶🅱 (English) a form of Marlin.

Marmion (French) small.
Marmyon

Marnin (Hebrew) singer; bringer of joy.

Maro (Japanese) myself.

Marón (Arabic) male saint.

Marquan (American) a combination of Mark + Quan.
Marquane, Marquante

Marquel (American) a form of Marcellus.
Marqueal, Marquelis, Marquell, Marquelle, Marquellis, Marquiel, Marquil, Marquiles, Marquill, Marquille, Marquillus, Marqwel, Marqwell

Marques (Portuguese) nobleman.
Markes, Markqes, Markques, Markquese, Marqese, Marqesse, Marqez, Marqeze, Marquees, Marquese, Marquess, Marquesse, Marquest, Markqueus, Marquez, Marqus

Marquez 🅱🅶 (Portuguese) a form of Marques.
Marqueze, Marquiez

Marquice (American) a form of Marquis.
Marquaice, Marquece

Marquis, Marquise 🅱🅶 (French) nobleman.
Marcquis, Marcuis, Markis,

Markquis, Markquise, Markuis,
Marqise, Marquee, Marqui,
Marquice, Marquie, Marquies,
Marquiss, Marquist, Marquiz,
Marquize

Marquon (American) a combination of Mark + Quon.
Marquin, Marquinn, Marqwan,
Marqwon, Marqwyn

Marr (Spanish) divine. (Arabic) forbidden.

Mars (Latin) bold warrior. Mythology: the Roman god of war.

Marsalis (Italian) a form of Marcellus.
Marsalius, Marsallis, Marsellis,
Marsellius, Marsellus

Marsden (English) marsh valley.
Marsdon

Marsh (English) swamp land. (French) a short form of Marshall.

Marshal (French) a form of Marshall.
Marschal, Marshel

Marshall BG (French) caretaker of the horses; military title.
Marsh, Marshal, Marshell

Marshawn (American) a combination of Mark + Shawn.
Marshaine, Marshaun,
Marshauwn, Marshean,
Marshon, Marshun

Marston (English) town by the marsh.

Martell (English) hammerer.
Martel, Martele, Martellis

Marten (Dutch) a form of Martin.
Maarten, Martein

Martez (Spanish) a form of Martin.
Martaz, Martaze, Martes,
Martese, Marteze, Martice,
Martiece, Marties, Martiese,
Martiez, Martis, Martise, Martize

Marti GB (Spanish) a form of Martin.
Martee, Martie

Martial (Latin) martial, warlike. (French) a form of Mark.

Martin BG (Latin, French) a form of Martinus. History: Martin Luther King, Jr. led the Civil Rights movement and won the Nobel Peace Prize. See also Tynek.
Maartin, Mairtin, Marciano,
Marcin, Marinos, Marius, Mart,
Martan, Marten, Martez, Marti,
Martijn, Martinas, Martine,
Martinez, Martinho, Martiniano,
Martinien, Martinka, Martino,
Martins, Marto, Marton, Márton,
Marts, Marty, Martyn, Mattin,
Mertin, Morten, Moss

Martín (Latin) a form of Martin.

Martina GB (Latin) a form of Martin.

Martine GB (Latin, French) a form of Martin.

Martinez (Spanish) a form of Martin.
Martines

Martinho (Portuguese) a form of Martin.

Martino (Italian) a form of Martin.
Martinos

Martiño (Latin) a form of Martin.

Martins (Latvian) a form of Martin.

Martinus (Latin) martial, warlike.
Martin

Martir (Greek) he who gives a testament of faith.

Marty (Latin) a familiar form of Martin.
Martey, Marti, Martie

Marut (Hindi) Religion: the Hindu god of the wind.

Marv (English) a short form of Marvin.
Marve, Marvi, Marvis

Marvin (English) lover of the sea.
Marv, Marvein, Marven, Marvion, Marvn, Marvon, Marvyn, Marwin, Marwynn, Mervin

Marwan (Arabic) history personage.

Marwood (English) forest pond.

Mary GB (Hebrew) bitter; sea of bitterness.

Masaccio (Italian) twin.
Masaki

Masahiro (Japanese) broad-minded.

Masamba (Yao) leaves.

Masao (Japanese) righteous.

Masato (Japanese) just.

Mashama (Shona) surprising.

Maska (Native American) powerful. (Russian) mask.

Maslin (French) little Thomas.
Maslen, Masling

Mason ☆ BG (French) stone worker.
Mace, Maison, Masson, Masun, Masyn, Sonny

Masou (Native American) fire god.

Massey (English) twin.
Massi

Massimo BG (Italian) greatest.
Massimiliano

Masud (Arabic, Swahili) fortunate.
Masood, Masoud, Mhasood

Matai (Basque, Bulgarian) a form of Matthew.
Máté, Matei

Matalino (Filipino) bright.

Mateo (Spanish) a form of Matthew.
Matías, Matteo

Mateos, Mathías (Hebrew) offered up to God.

Mateusz (Polish) a form of Matthew.
Matejs, Mateus

Mathe (German) a short form of Matthew.

Mather (English) powerful army.

Matheu (German) a form of Matthew.
Matheau, Matheus, Mathu

Mathew **BG** (Hebrew) a form of Matthew.

Mathias, Matthias (German, Swedish) forms of Matthew.
Maitias, Mathi, Mathia, Mathis, Matías, Matthia, Matthieus, Mattia, Mattias, Matus

Mathieu, Matthieu **BG** (French) forms of Matthew.
Mathie, Mathieux, Mathiew, Matthiew, Mattieu, Mattieux

Matías (Spanish) a form of Mathias.
Mattias

Mato (Native American) brave.

Matope (Rhodesian) our last child.

Matoskah (Lakota) white bear.

Mats (Swedish) a familiar form of Matthew.
Matts, Matz

Matson (Hebrew) son of Matt.
Matison, Matsen, Mattison, Mattson

Matt (Hebrew) a short form of Matthew.
Mat

Matteen (Afghan) disciplined; polite.

Matteus (Scandinavian) a form of Matthew.

Matthew ✺ **BG** (Hebrew) gift of God. Bible: author of the first Gospel of the New Testament.
Mads, Makaio, Maitiú, Mata, Matai, Matek, Mateo, Mateusz, Matfei, Mathe, Matheson, Matheu, Mathew, Mathian, Mathias, Mathieson, Mathieu, Matro, Mats, Matt, Matteus, Matthaeus, Matthaios, Matthaus, Matthäus, Mattheus, Matthews, Mattmias, Matty, Matvey, Matyas, Mayhew

Matty (Hebrew) a familiar form of Matthew.
Mattie

Matus (Czech) a form of Mathias.

Matusalén (Hebrew) symbol of longevity.

Matvey (Russian) a form of Matthew.
Matviy, Matviyko, Matyash, Motka, Motya

Matyas (Polish) a form of Matthew.
Mátyás

Mauli (Hawaiian) a form of Maurice.

Maurice (Latin) dark skinned; moor; marshland. See also Seymour.
Mauli, Maur, Maurance, Maureo, Mauricio, Maurids, Mauriece, Maurikas, Maurin, Maurino, Maurise, Mauritz, Maurius, Maurizio, Mauro, Maurrel, Maurtel, Maury, Maurycy, Meurig, Moore, Morice, Moritz, Morrel, Morrice, Morrie, Morrill, Morris

Mauricio 🅱🅶 (Spanish) a form of Maurice.
Mauriccio, Mauriceo, Maurico, Maurisio

Mauritz (German) a form of Maurice.

Maurizio (Italian) a form of Maurice.

Mauro (Latin) a short form of Maurice.
Maur, Maurio

Maury (Latin) a familiar form of Maurice.
Maurey, Maurie, Morrie

Maverick 🅱🅶 (American) independent.
Maverik, Maveryke, Mavric, Mavrick

Mawuli (Ewe) there is a God.

Max 🅱🅶 (Latin) a short form of Maximilian, Maxwell.
Mac, Mack, Maks, Maxe, Maxx, Maxy, Miksa

Maxfield (English) Mack's field.

Maxi (Czech, Hungarian, Spanish) a familiar form of Maximilian, Máximo.
Makszi, Maxey, Maxie, Maxis, Maxy

Maxim (Russian) a form of Maxime.

Maxime 🅱🅶 (French) most excellent.
Maxim, Maxyme

Maximilian (Latin) greatest.
Mac, Mack, Maixim, Maksim, Maksym, Max, Maxamillion, Maxemilian, Maxemilion, Maxi, Maximalian, Maximili, Maximilia, Maximiliano, Maximilianus, Maximilien, Maximillian, Máximo, Maximos, Maxmilian, Maxmillion, Maxon, Maxymilian, Maxymillian, Mayhew, Miksa

Maximiliano (Italian) a form of Maximilian.
Massimiliano, Maximiano, Maximino

Maximillian (Latin) a form of Maximilian.
Maximillan, Maximillano, Maximillien, Maximillion, Maxmillian, Maxximillian, Maxximillion

Máximo (Spanish) a form of Maximilian.
Massimo, Maxi, Maximiano, Maximiliano, Maximino, Máximo

Maximos (Greek) a form of
  Maximilian.

Maxine GB (Latin) greatest.

Maxwell BG (English) great
  spring.
  Max, Maxwel, Maxwill,
  Maxxwell, Maxy

Maxy (English) a familiar form of
  Max, Maxwell.
  Maxi

Mayer (Hebrew) a form of Meir.
  (Latin) a form of Magnus, Major.
  Mahyar, Mayeer, Mayor, Mayur

Mayes (English) field.
  Mayo, Mays

Mayhew (English) a form of
  Matthew.

Maynard (English) powerful;
  brave. See also Meinhard.
  May, Mayne, Maynhard, Maynor,
  Ménard

Mayo (Irish) yew-tree plain.
  (English) a form of Mayes.
  Geography: a county in Ireland.

Mayon (Indian) person of black
  complexion. Religion: another
  name for the Indian god Mal.

Mayonga (Luganda) lake sailor.

Mayta (Quechua) where are you?

Maytacuapac (Quechua) oh,
  Lord, where are you?

Mayua (Quechua) violet, purple.

Mazi (Ibo) sir.
  Mazzi

Mazin (Arabic) proper.
  Mazen, Mazinn, Mazzin

Mbita (Swahili) born on a cold
  night.

Mbwana (Swahili) master.

Mc Kenna GB (American) a
  form of Mackenna (see Girls'
  Names).

Mc Kenzie GB (Irish) a form of
  Mackenzie.

McGeorge (Scottish) son of
  George.
  MacGeorge

Mckade (Scottish) son of Kade.
  Mccade

Mckay BG (Scottish) son of Kay.
  Mackay, MacKay, Mckae, Mckai,
  McKay

Mckayla GB (American) a form
  of Makayla (see Girls' Names).

Mckell (American) a form of
  Makell.

Mckenna GB (American) a form
  of Mackenna (see Girls' Names).

McKenzie, Mckenzie GB
  (Irish) forms of Mackenzie.
  Mccenzie, Mckennzie, Mckensey,
  Mckensie, Mckenson,
  Mckensson, Mckenzi, Mckenzy,
  Mckinzie

Mckinley 🅱🅶 (Irish) a form of Mackinnley.
Mckinely, Mckinnely, Mckinnlee, Mckinnley, McKinnley

Mead 🅱🅶 (English) meadow.
Meade, Meed

Meaghan 🅶🅱 (Welsh) a form of Megan.

Medardo (Germanic) boldly powerful; he who is worthy of honors.

Medarno (Saxon) he who deserves to be honored, distinguished, awarded.

Medgar (German) a form of Edgar.

Medwin (German) faithful friend.

Megan 🅶🅱 (Greek) pearl; great. (Irish) a form of Margaret.

Meghan 🅶🅱 (Welsh) a form of Megan.

Meginardo (Teutonic) he who is a strong leader.

Mehetabel (Hebrew) who God benefits.

Mehrdad (Persian) gift of the sun.

Mehtar (Sanskrit) prince.
Mehta

Meinhard (German) strong, firm. See also Maynard.
Meinhardt, Meinke, Meino, Mendar

Meinrad (German) strong counsel.

Meir (Hebrew) one who brightens, shines; enlightener. History: Golda Meir was the prime minister of Israel.
Mayer, Meyer, Muki, Myer

Meka 🅶🅱 (Hawaiian) eyes.

Mel 🅱🅶 (English, Irish) a familiar form of Melvin.

Melanie 🅶🅱 (Greek) dark skinned.

Melanio (Greek) having black skin.

Melbourne (English) mill stream.
Melborn, Melburn, Melby, Milborn, Milbourn, Milbourne, Milburn, Millburn, Millburne

Melchior (Hebrew) king.
Meilseoir, Melchor, Melker, Melkior

Meldon (English) mill hill.
Melden

Melecio (Greek) careful and attentive.

Melibeo (Greek) he who takes care of the mentally handicapped.

Melissa 🅶🅱 (Greek) honey bee.

Meliton, Melitón (Greek) from the island of Malta.

Melivilu (Mapuche) four snakes.

Melquíades (Hebrew) king of God.

Melrone (Irish) servant of Saint Ruadhan.

Melvern (Native American) great chief.

Melville (French) mill town. Literature: Herman Melville was a well-known nineteenth-century American writer.
Milville

Melvin (Irish) armored chief. (English) mill friend; council friend. See also Vinny.
Malvin, Mel, Melvino, Melvon, Melvyn, Melwin, Melwyn, Melwynn

Menachem (Hebrew) comforter.
Menahem, Nachman

Menandro (Greek) he who remains a man.

Menas (Greek) related to the months.

Menassah (Hebrew) cause to forget.
Menashe, Menashi, Menashia, Menashiah, Menashya, Manasseh

Mendel (English) repairman.
Mendeley, Mendell, Mendie, Mendy

Mendo (Spanish) a form of Hermenegildo.

Menelao (Greek) he who goes to the village to fight.

Mengesha (Ethiopian) kingdom.

Menico (Spanish) a short form of Domenico.

Mensah (Ewe) third son.

Mentor (Greek) teacher.

Menz (German) a short form of Clement.

Mercer (English) storekeeper.
Merce

Mercurio (Latin) he who pays attention to business.

Mered (Hebrew) revolter.

Meredith GB (Welsh) guardian from the sea.
Meredyth, Merideth, Meridith, Merry

Merion (Welsh) from Merion, Wales.
Merrion

Merle BG (French) a short form of Merlin, Merrill.
Meryl

Merlin (English) falcon. Literature: the magician who served as counselor in King Arthur's court.
Marlon, Merle, Merlen, Merlinn, Merlyn, Merlynn

Merlín (Spanish) a form of Merlin.

Merlino (Spanish) a form of Merlín.

Merrick (English) ruler of the sea.
Merek, Meric, Merick, Merik, Merric, Merrik, Meryk, Meyrick, Myrucj

Merrill (Irish) bright sea. (French) famous.
Meril, Merill, Merle, Merrel, Merrell, Merril, Meryl

Merritt (Latin, Irish) valuable; deserving.
Merit, Meritt, Merrett

Merton (English) sea town.
Murton

Merulo (Latin) he who is fine as a blackbird.

Merv (Irish) a short form of Mervin.

Merville (French) sea village.

Mervin (Irish) a form of Marvin.
Merv, Mervyn, Mervynn, Merwin, Merwinn, Merwyn, Murvin, Murvyn, Myrvyn, Myrvynn, Myrwyn

Meshach (Hebrew) artist. Bible: one of Daniel's three friends who emerged unharmed from the fiery furnace of Babylon.

Mesut (Turkish) happy.

Metikla (Moquelumnan) reaching a hand underwater to catch a fish.

Metrenco (Mapuche) still water, without a current; stagnant.

Metrofanes (Greek) he who resembles his mother.

Mette (Greek, Danish) pearl.
Almeta, Mete

Meulén (Mapuche) whirlwind.

Meurig (Welsh) a form of Maurice.

Meyer (German) farmer.
Mayer, Meier, Myer

Mhina (Swahili) delightful.

Micah ⒷⒼ (Hebrew) a form of Michael. Bible: a Hebrew prophet.
Mic, Micaiah, Michiah, Mika, Mikah, Myca, Mycah

Micha (Hebrew) a short form of Michael.
Mica, Micha, Michah

Michael ☆ ⒷⒼ (Hebrew) who is like God? See also Micah, Miguel, Mika, Miles.
Machael, Machas, Mahail, Maichail, Maikal, Makael, Makal, Makel, Makell, Makis, Meikel, Mekal, Mekhail, Mhichael, Micael, Micah, Micahel, Mical, Micha, Michaele, Michaell, Michail, Michak, Michal, Michale, Michalek, Michalel, Michau, Micheal, Micheil, Michel, Michele, Michelet, Michiel, Micho, Michoel, Mick, Mickael, Mickey, Mihail, Mihalje, Mihkel, Mika, Mikael, Mikáele, Mikal, Mike, Mikeal, Mikel, Mikelis, Mikell, Mikhail, Mikkel,

Mikko, Miksa, Milko, Miquel, Misael, Misi, Miska, Mitchell, Mychael, Mychajlo, Mychal, Mykal, Mykhas

Michaela GB (Hebrew) who is like God?

Michail (Russian) a form of Michael.
Mihas, Mikail, Mikale, Misha

Michal BG (Polish) a form of Michael.
Michak, Michalek, Michall

Micheal BG (Irish) a form of Michael.

Michel BG (French) a form of Michael.
Michaud, Miche, Michee, Michell, Michelle, Michon

Michelangelo (Italian) a combination of Michael + Angelo. Art: Michelangelo Buonarroti was one of the greatest Renaissance painters.
Michelange, Miguelangelo

Michele GB (Italian) a form of Michael.

Michelle GB (French) a form of Michele.

Michio (Japanese) man with the strength of three thousand.

Mick (English) a short form of Michael, Mickey.
Mickerson

Mickael BG (English) a form of Michael.
Mickaele, Mickal, Mickale, Mickeal, Mickel, Mickell, Mickelle, Mickle

Mickenzie (Irish) a form of Mackenzie.
Mickenze, Mickenzy, Mikenzie

Mickey (Irish) a familiar form of Michael.
Mick, Micki, Mickie, Micky, Miki, Mique

Micu (Hungarian) a form of Nick.

Midas (Greek) fleeting and admirable business.

Miguel ⭐ BG (Portuguese, Spanish) a form of Michael.
Migeel, Migel, Miguelly, Migui

Miguelangel (Spanish) a combination of Miguel + Angel.

Mihail (Greek, Bulgarian, Romanian) a form of Michael.
Mihailo, Mihal, Mihalis, Mikail

Mijaíl (Russian) a form of Miguel.

Mika GB (Ponca) raccoon. (Hebrew) a form of Micah. (Russian) a familiar form of Michael.
Miika, Mikah

Mikael BG (Swedish) a form of Michael.
Mikaeel, Mikaele

Mikáele (Hawaiian) a form of Michael.
Mikele

Mikal (Hebrew) a form of Michael.
Mekal, Mikahl, Mikale

Mikasi (Omaha) coyote.

Mike (Hebrew) a short form of Michael.
Mikey, Myk

Mikeal (Irish) a form of Michael.

Mikel BG (Basque) a form of Michael.
Mekel, Mikele, Mekell, Mikell, Mikelle

Mikelis (Latvian) a form of Michael.
Mikus, Milkins

Mikhail (Greek, Russian) a form of Michael.
Mekhail, Mihály, Mikhael, Mikhale, Mikhalis, Mikhalka, Mikhall, Mikhel, Mikhial, Mikhos

Miki GB (Japanese) tree.
Mikio

Mikkel (Norwegian) a form of Michael.
Mikkael, Mikle

Mikko (Finnish) a form of Michael.
Mikk, Mikka, Mikkohl, Mikkol, Miko, Mikol

Mikolaj (Polish) a form of Nicholas.
Mikolai

Mikolas (Greek) a form of Nicholas.
Miklós, Milek

Miksa (Hungarian) a form of Max.
Miks

Milagro (Spanish) miracle.

Milan (Italian) northerner. Geography: a city in northern Italy.
Milaan, Milano, Milen, Millan, Millen, Mylan, Mylen, Mylon, Mylynn

Milap (Native American) giving.

Milborough (English) middle borough.
Milbrough

Milcíades (Greek) he of reddish complexion.

Milek (Polish) a familiar form of Nicholas.

Miles (Greek) millstone. (Latin) soldier. (German) merciful. (English) a short form of Michael.
Milas, Milles, Milo, Milson, Myles

Milford (English) mill by the ford.

Mililani BG (Hawaiian) heavenly caress.

Milko (Czech) a form of Michael. (German) a familiar form of Emil.
Milkins

Millán (Latin) belonging to the Emilia family.

Millañir (Mapuche) silver fox.

Millard (Latin) caretaker of the mill.
Mill, Millar, Miller, Millward, Milward, Myller

Miller (English) miller; grain grinder.
Mellar, Millard, Millen

Mills (English) mills.

Milo (German) a form of Miles. A familiar form of Emil.
Millo, Mylo

Milos (Greek, Slavic) pleasant.

Miloslav (Czech) lover of glory.
Milda

Milt (English) a short form of Milton.

Milton (English) mill town.
Milt, Miltie, Milty, Mylton

Mimis (Greek) a familiar form of Demetrius.

Min (Burmese) king.

Mina GB (Burmese) a form of Min.

Mincho (Spanish) a form of Benjamin.

Minel (Spanish) a form of Manuel.

Miner (English) miner.

Mingan (Native American) gray wolf.

Mingo (Spanish) a short form of Domingo.

Minh (Vietnamese) bright.
Minhao, Minhduc, Minhkhan, Minhtong, Minhy

Minkah (Akan) just, fair.

Minor (Latin) junior; younger.
Mynor

Minoru (Japanese) fruitful.

Mio (Spanish) mine.

Mique (Spanish) a form of Mickey.
Mequel, Mequelin, Miquel

Miracle GB (Latin) wonder, marvel.

Miranda GB (Latin) strange; wonderful; admirable.

Mirco (Spanish) he who assures the peace.

Miriam GB (Hebrew) bitter; sea of bitterness.

Miron (Polish) peace.

Miroslav (Czech) peace; glory.
Mirek, Miroslaw, Miroslawy

Mirwais (Afghan) noble ruler.

Misael BG (Hebrew) a form of Michael.
Mischael, Mishael, Missael

Misha GB (Russian) a short form of Michail.
Misa, Mischa, Mishael, Mishal, Mishe, Mishenka, Mishka

Miska (Hungarian) a form of Michael.
Misi, Misik, Misko, Miso

Mister (English) mister.
Mistur

Misty GB (English) shrouded by mist.

Misu (Moquelumnan) rippling water.

Mitch (English) a short form of Mitchell.

Mitchel (English) a form of Mitchell.
Mitchael, Mitchal, Mitcheal, Mitchele, Mitchil, Mytchel

Mitchell BG (English) a form of Michael.
Mitch, Mitchall, Mitchel, Mitchelle, Mitchem, Mytch, Mytchell

Mitsos (Greek) a familiar form of Demetrius.

Modesto (Latin) modest.

Moe (English) a short form of Moses.
Mo

Mogens (Dutch) powerful.

Mohamad (Arabic) a form of Muhammad.
Mohamid

Mohamed BG (Arabic) a form of Muhammad.
Mohamd, Mohameed

Mohamet (Arabic) a form of Muhammad.
Mahomet, Mehemet, Mehmet

Mohammad (Arabic) a form of Muhammad.
Mahammad, Mohammadi, Mohammd, Mohammid, Mohanad, Mohmad

Mohammed (Arabic) a form of Muhammad.
Mahammed, Mahomet, Mohammad, Mohaned, Mouhamed, Muhammad

Mohamud (Arabic) a form of Muhammad.
Mohammud, Mohamoud

Mohan (Hindi) delightful.

Moises (Portuguese, Spanish) a form of Moses.
Moices, Moise, Moisés, Moisey, Moisis

Moishe (Yiddish) a form of Moses.
Moshe

Mojag (Native American) crying baby.

Molimo (Moquelumnan) bear going under shady trees.

Molly GB (Irish) a familiar form of Mary.

Momuso (Moquelumnan) yellow jackets crowded in their nests for the winter.

Mona GB (Moquelumnan) gathering jimsonweed seed.

Monahan (Irish) monk.
Monaghan, Monoghan

Mongo (Yoruba) famous.

Monica GB (Greek) solitary.
(Latin) advisor.

Monitor (Latin) he who counsels.

Monroe (Irish) Geography: the mouth of the Roe River.
Monro, Munro, Munroe

Montague (French) pointed mountain.
Montagne, Montagu, Monte

Montana GB (Spanish) mountain. Geography: a U.S. state.
Montaine, Montanna

Montaro (Japanese) big boy.
Montario, Monterio, Montero

Monte (Spanish) a short form of Montgomery.
Montae, Montaé, Montay, Montea, Montee, Monti, Montoya, Monty

Montego (Spanish) mountainous.

Montel (American) a form of Montreal.
Montele, Montell, Montelle

Montenegro (Spanish) black mountain.

Montes (Spanish) mountains.

Montez (Spanish) dweller in the mountains.
Monteiz, Monteze, Montezz, Montisze

Montgomery (English) rich man's mountain.
Monte, Montgomerie, Monty

Montre (French) show.
Montra, Montrae, Montray, Montraz, Montres, Montrey, Montrez, Montreze

Montreal (French) royal mountain. Geography: a city in Quebec.
Montel, Monterial, Monterrell, Montrail, Montrale, Montrall, Montreall, Montrell, Montrial

Montrell BG (French) a form of Montreal.
Montral, Montrel, Montrele, Montrelle

Montsho (Tswana) black.

Monty (English) a familiar form of Montgomery.

Moore (French) dark; moor; marshland.
Moor, Mooro, More

Mordecai (Hebrew) martial, warlike. Mythology: Marduk was the Babylonian god of war. Bible: wise counselor to Queen Esther.
Mord, Mordachai, Mordechai, Mordie, Mordy, Mort

Mordred (Latin) painful.
Literature: the bastard son of King Arthur.
Modred

Morel (French) an edible mushroom.
Morrel

Moreland (English) moor; marshland.
Moorland, Morland

Morell (French) dark; from Morocco.
Moor, Moore, Morelle, Morelli, Morill, Morrell, Morrill, Murrel, Murrell

Morey (Greek) a familiar form of Moris. (Latin) a form of Morrie.
Morrey, Morry

Morfeo (Greek) he who makes you see beautiful figures.

Morgan 🎗 (Scottish) sea warrior.
Morgen, Morghan, Morgin, Morgon, Morgun, Morgunn, Morgwn, Morgyn, Morrgan

Moriah 🎗 (Hebrew) God is my teacher. (French) dark skinned.

Morio (Japanese) forest.

Moris (Greek) son of the dark one. (English) a form of Morris.
Morey, Morisz, Moriz

Moritz (German) a form of Maurice, Morris.
Morisz

Morley (English) meadow by the moor.
Moorley, Moorly, Morlee, Morleigh, Morlon, Morly, Morlyn, Morrley

Morrie (Latin) a familiar form of Maurice, Morse.
Maury, Morey, Mori, Morie, Morry, Mory, Morye

Morris (Latin) dark skinned; moor; marshland. (English) a form of Maurice.
Moris, Moriss, Moritz, Morrese, Morrise, Morriss, Morry, Moss

Morse (English) son of Maurice.
Morresse, Morrie, Morrison, Morrisson

Mort (French, English) a short form of Morten, Mortimer, Morton.
Morte, Mortey, Mortie, Mortty, Morty

Morten (Norwegian) a form of Martin.
Mort

Mortimer (French) still water.
Mort, Mortymer

Morton (English) town near the moor.
Mort

Morven (Scottish) mariner.
Morvien, Morvin

Mose (Hebrew) a short form of Moses.

Moses BG (Hebrew) drawn out of the water. (Egyptian) son, child. Bible: the Hebrew lawgiver who brought the Ten Commandments down from Mount Sinai.
Moe, Moise, Moïse, Moisei, Moises, Moishe, Mose, Mosese, Moshe, Mosiah, Mosie, Moss, Mosses, Mosya, Mosze, Moszek, Mousa, Moyses, Moze

Moshe (Hebrew, Polish) a form of Moses.
Mosheh

Mosi BG (Swahili) first-born.

Moss (Irish) a short form of Maurice, Morris. (English) a short form of Moses.

Moswen BG (African) light in color.

Motega (Native American) new arrow.

Mouhamed (Arabic) a form of Muhammad.
Mouhamad, Mouhamadou, Mouhammed, Mouhamoin

Mousa (Arabic) a form of Moses.
Moussa

Moze (Lithuanian) a form of Moses.
Mozes, Mózes

Mpasa (Nguni) mat.

Mposi (Nyakyusa) blacksmith.

Mpoza (Luganda) tax collector.

Msrah (Akan) sixth-born.

Mtima (Nguni) heart.

Muata (Moquelumnan) yellow jackets in their nest.

Mucio (Latin) he who endures silence.

Mugamba (Runyoro) talks too much.

Mugisa (Rutooro) lucky.
Mugisha, Mukisa

Muhammad (Arabic) praised. History: the founder of the Islamic religion. See also Ahmad, Hamid, Yasin.
Mahmoud, Mahmúd, Mohamed, Mohamet, Mohamud, Mohammed, Mouhamed, Muhamad, Muhamed, Muhamet, Muhammadali, Muhammed

Muhannad (Arabic) sword.
Muhanad

Muhsin (Arabic) beneficent; charitable.

Muhtadi (Arabic) rightly guided.

Muir (Scottish) moor; marshland.

Mujahid (Arabic) fighter in the way of Allah.

Mukasa (Luganda) God's chief administrator.

Mukhtar (Arabic) chosen.
Mukhtaar

Mukul (Sanskrit) bud, blossom; soul.

Mullu (Quechua) coral, jewel.

Mulogo (Musoga) wizard.

Mun-Hee (Korean) literate; shiny.

Mundan (Rhodesian) garden.

Mundo (Spanish) a short form of Edmundo.

Mundy (Irish) from Reamonn.

Mungo (Scottish) amiable.

Munir (Arabic) brilliant; shining.

Munny (Cambodian) wise.

Muraco (Native American) white moon.

Murali (Hindi) flute. Religion: the instrument the Hindu god Krishna is usually depicted as playing.

Murat (Turkish) wish come true.

Murdock (Scottish) wealthy sailor.
Murdo, Murdoch, Murtagh

Murphy (Irish) sea warrior.
Murfey, Murfy

Murray (Scottish) sailor.
Macmurray, Moray, Murrey, Murry

Murtagh (Irish) a form of Murdock.
Murtaugh

Musa (Swahili) child.

Musád (Arabic) untied camel.

Musoke (Rukonjo) born while a rainbow was in the sky.

Mustafa (Arabic) chosen; royal.
Mostafa, Mostaffa, Moustafa, Mustafaa, Mustafah, Mustafe, Mustaffa, Mustafo, Mustapha, Mustoffa, Mustofo

Mustafá (Turkish) a form of Mustafa.

Mustapha (Arabic) a form of Mustafa.
Mostapha, Moustapha

Muti (Arabic) obedient.

Mwaka (Luganda) born on New Year's Eve.

Mwamba (Nyakyusa) strong.

Mwanje (Luganda) leopard.

Mwinyi (Swahili) king.

Mwita (Swahili) summoner.

Mya GB (Burmese) emerald. (Italian) a form of Mia (see Girls' Names).

Mychajlo (Latvian) a form of Michael.
Mykhaltso, Mykhas

Mychal (American) a form of Michael.
Mychall, Mychalo, Mycheal

Myer (English) a form of Meir.
Myers, Myur

Mykal, Mykel (American) forms of Michael.
Mykael, Mikele, Mykell

Myles BG (Latin) soldier.
(German) a form of Miles.
Myels, Mylez, Mylles, Mylz

Mynor (Latin) a form of Minor.

Myo (Burmese) city.

Myriam GB (American) a form of
Miriam.

Myron (Greek) fragrant ointment.
*Mehran, Mehrayan, My, Myran,
Myrone, Ron*

Myung-Dae (Korean) right;
great.

Mzuzi (Swahili) inventive.

N

N BG (American) an initial used
as a first name.

N'namdi (Ibo) his father's name
lives on.

Naaman (Hebrew) pleasant.

Nabiha (Arabic) intelligent.

Nabil (Arabic) noble.
Nabeel, Nabiel

Nabor (Hebrew) prophet's light.

Nabucodonosor (Chaldean) God
protects my reign.

Nachman (Hebrew) a short form
of Menachem.
Nachum, Nahum

Nada (Arabic) generous.

Nadav (Hebrew) generous; noble.
Nadiv

Nadidah (Arabic) equal to
anyone else.

Nadim (Arabic) friend.
Nadeem

Nadine GB (French, Slavic) a
form of Nadia (see Girls' Names).

Nadir (Afghan, Arabic) dear, rare.
Nader

Nadisu (Hindi) beautiful river.

Naeem (Arabic) benevolent.
Naem, Naim, Naiym, Nieem

Naftali (Hebrew) wreath.
Naftalie

Nagid (Hebrew) ruler; prince.

Nahele (Hawaiian) forest.

Nahma (Native American)
sturgeon.

Nahuel (Araucanian) tiger.

Naiara (Spanish) reference to the
Virgin Mary.

Nailah (Arabic) successful.

Nairn (Scottish) river with alder
trees.
Nairne

Najee (Arabic) a form of Naji.
Najae, Najée, Najei, Najiee

Naji (Arabic) safe.
Najee, Najih

Najíb (Arabic) born to nobility.
Najib, Nejeeb

Najji (Muganda) second child.

Nakia GB (Arabic) pure.
*Nakai, Nakee, Nakeia, Naki,
Nakiah, Nakii*

Nakos (Arapaho) sage, wise.

Naldo (Spanish) a familiar form
of Reginald.

Nalren (Dene) thawed out.

Nam (Vietnamese) scrape off.

Namaka (Hawaiian) eyes.

Namid (Ojibwa) star dancer.

Namir (Hebrew) leopard.
Namer

Namuncura (Mapuche) foot of
stone, strong foot.

Ñancuvilu (Mapuche) snake that
is the color of lead, off-white.

Nancy GB (English) gracious. A
familiar form of Nan (see Girls'
Names).

Nandin (Hindi) Religion: a
servant of the Hindu god Shiva.
Nandan

Nando (German) a familiar form
of Ferdinand.
Nandor

Nangila (Abaluhya) born while
parents traveled.

Nangwaya (Mwera) don't mess
with me.

Nansen (Swedish) son of Nancy.

Nantai (Navajo) chief.

Nantan (Apache) spokesman.

Naoko (Japanese) straight, honest.

Naolin (Spanish) sun god of the
Mexican people.

Napayshni (Lakota) he does not
flee; courageous.

Napier (Spanish) new city.
Neper

Napoleon (Greek) lion of the
woodland. (Italian) from Naples,
Italy. History: Napoleon Bonaparte
was a famous nineteenth-century
French emperor.
*Leon, Nap, Napolean, Napoléon,
Napoleone, Nappie, Nappy*

Napoleón (Greek) a form of
Napoleon.

Naquan (American) a combi-
nation of the prefix Na + Quan.
*Naqawn, Naquain, Naquen,
Naquon*

Narain (Hindi) protector.
Religion: another name for the
Hindu god Vishnu.
Narayan

Narciso (French) a form of
Narcisse.

Narcisse (French) a form of
Narcissus.
*Narcis, Narciso, Narkis,
Narkissos*

Narcissus (Greek) daffodil.
Mythology: the youth who fell in
love with his own reflection.
Narcisse

Nard (Persian) chess player.

Nardo (German) strong, hardy.
(Spanish) a short form of
Bernardo.

Narno (Latin) he who was born in
the Italian city of Narnia.

Narses (Persian) what the two
martyrs brought from Persia.

Narve (Dutch) healthy, strong.

Nashashuk (Fox, Sauk) loud
thunder.

Nashoba (Choctaw) wolf.

Nasim (Persian) breeze; fresh air.
Naseem, Nassim

Nasser (Arabic) victorious.
*Naseer, Naser, Nasier, Nasir,
Nasr, Nassir, Nassor*

Nat (English) a short form of
Nathan, Nathaniel.
Natt, Natty

Natal (Spanish) a form of Noël.
*Natale, Natalie, Natalino,
Natalio, Nataly*

Natalie **GB** (Spanish) a form of
Natal.

Natan (Hebrew, Hungarian,
Polish, Russian, Spanish) God
has given.
Naten

Natanael (Hebrew) a form of
Nathaniel.
Natanel, Nataniel

Natasha **GB** (Russian) a form of
Natalie.

Nate (Hebrew) a short form of
Nathan, Nathaniel.

Natesh (Hindi) destroyer.
Religion: another name for the
Hindu god Shiva.

Nathan ⭐ **BG** (Hebrew) a short
form of Nathaniel. Bible: a
prophet during the reigns of
David and Solomon.
*Naethan, Nat, Nate, Nathann,
Nathean, Nathen, Nathian,
Nathin, Nathon, Nathyn, Natthan,
Naythan, Nethan*

Nathanael (Hebrew) gift of God.
Bible: one of the Twelve Apostles.
Also known as Bartholomew.
*Nathanae, Nathanal, Nathaneal,
Nathaneil, Nathanel, Nathaneol*

Nathanial (Hebrew) a form of
Nathaniel.
Nathanyal, Nathanual

Nathanie (Hebrew) a familiar
form of Nathaniel.
Nathania, Nathanni

Nathaniel ☀ 🅱🅶 (Hebrew) gift of God.
Nat, Natanael, Nate, Nathan, Nathanael, Nathanial, Nathanie, Nathanielle, Nathanil, Nathanile, Nathanuel, Nathanyel, Nathanyl, Natheal, Nathel, Nathinel, Nethaniel, Thaniel

Nathen (Hebrew) a form of Nathan.

Natividad (Spanish) nativity.

Natori 🅶🅱 (Arabic) a form of Natara (see Girls' Names).

Ñaupac (Quechua) first, principal, first-born; before everyone.

Ñaupari (Quechua) ahead, first.

Ñauque, Ñauqui (Quechua) before everyone.

Nav (Gypsy) name.

Naval (Latin) god of the sailing vessels.

Navarro (Spanish) plains.
Navarre

Navdeep 🅱🅶 (Sikh) new light.
Navdip

Navin (Hindi) new, novel.
Naveen, Naven

Nawat (Native American) left-handed.

Nawkaw (Winnebago) wood.

Nayati (Native American) wrestler.

Nayland (English) island dweller.

Nazareno (Hebrew) he who has separated himself from the rest of the people because he feels constricted, because he has decided to be solitary.

Nazareth (Hebrew) born in Nazareth, Israel.
Nazaire, Nazaret, Nazarie, Nazario, Nazerene, Nazerine

Nazih (Arabic) pure, chaste.
Nazeeh, Nazeem, Nazeer, Nazieh, Nazim, Nazir, Nazz

Ndale (Nguni) trick.

Neal (Irish) a form of Neil.
Neale, Neall, Nealle, Nealon, Nealy

Neandro (Greek) young and manly.

Nebrido (Greek) graceful like the fawn.

Neci 🅱🅶 (Latin) a familiar form of Ignatius.

Nectario (Greek) he who sweetens life with nectar.

Nectarios (Greek) saint. Religion: a saint in the Greek Orthodox Church.

Neculman (Mapuche) swift condor; swift and rapid flight.

Neculqueo (Mapuche) rapid speaker, good with words.

Ned (English) a familiar form of Edward, Edwin.
Neddie, Neddym, Nedrick

Nehemiah (Hebrew) compassion of Jehovah. Bible: a Jewish leader.
Nahemiah, Nechemya, Nehemias, Nehemie, Nehemyah, Nehimiah, Nehmia, Nehmiah, Nemo, Neyamia

Nehru (Hindi) canal.

Neil (Irish) champion.
Neal, Neel, Neihl, Neile, Neill, Neille, Nels, Niall, Niele, Niels, Nigel, Nil, Niles, Nilo, Nils, Nyle

Neka (Native American) wild goose.

Nelek (Polish) a form of Cornelius.

Nelius (Latin) a short form of Cornelius.

Nellie GB (English) a familiar form of Cornelius, Cornell, Nelson.
Nell, Nelly

Nelo (Spanish) a form of Daniel.
Nello, Nilo

Nels (Scandinavian) a form of Neil, Nelson.
Nelse, Nelson, Nils

Nelson BG (English) son of Neil.
Nealson, Neilsen, Neilson, Nellie, Nels, Nelsen, Nilson, Nilsson

Nemesio (Spanish) just.
Nemi

Nemo (Greek) glen, glade. (Hebrew) a short form of Nehemiah.

Nen (Egyptian) ancient waters.

Neofito (Greek) he who began recently.

Neon (Greek) he who is strong.

Neopolo (Spanish) a form of Napoleón.

Nepomuceno (Slavic) he who gives his help.

Neptune (Latin) sea ruler. Mythology: the Roman god of the sea.

Neptuno (Greek) god of the sea.

Nereo (Greek) he who is the captain at sea.

Nerio (Greek) sea traveler.

Nero (Latin, Spanish) stern. History: a cruel Roman emperor.
Neron, Nerone, Nerron

Nerón (Latin) very strong and intrepid.

Nesbit (English) nose-shaped bend in a river.
Naisbit, Naisbitt, Nesbitt, Nisbet, Nisbett

Nesto (Spanish) serious.

Nestor BG (Greek) traveler; wise.
Nester

Néstor (Greek) a form of Nestor.

Nestorio (Greek) a form of Nestor.

Nethaniel (Hebrew) a form of Nathaniel.
Netanel, Netania, Netaniah, Netaniel, Netanya, Nethanel, Nethanial, Nethaniel, Nethanyal, Nethanyel

Neto (Spanish) a short form of Ernesto.

Nevada GB (Spanish) covered in snow. Geography: a U.S. state.
Navada, Nevade

Nevan (Irish) holy.
Nevean

Neville (French) new town.
Nev, Nevil, Nevile, Nevill, Nevyle

Nevin (Irish) worshiper of the saint. (English) middle; herb.
Nefen, Nev, Nevan, Neven, Nevins, Nevyn, Niven

Newbold (English) new tree.

Newell (English) new hall.
Newall, Newel, Newyle

Newland (English) new land.
Newlan

Newlin (Welsh) new lake.
Newlyn

Newman (English) newcomer.
Neiman, Neimann, Neimon, Neuman, Numan, Numen

Newton (English) new town.
Newt

Ngai (Vietnamese) herb.

Nghia (Vietnamese) forever.

Ngoc GB (Vietnamese) jade.

Ngozi (Ibo) blessing.

Ngu (Vietnamese) sleep.

Nguyen (Vietnamese) a form of Ngu.

Nhean (Cambodian) self-knowledge.

Nia GB (Irish) a familiar form of Neila (see Girls' Names).

Niall (Irish) a form of Neil. History: Niall of the Nine Hostages was a famous Irish king.
Nial, Nialle

Nibal (Arabic) arrows.
Nibel

Nibaw (Native American) standing tall.

Nicabar (Gypsy) stealthy.

Nicandro (Greek) he who is victorious amongst men.

Nicasio, Niceto, Nicón (Greek) victorious one.

Níceas (Greek) he of the great victory.

Nicéforo (Greek) he who brings victory.

Nicho (Spanish) a form of Dennis.

Nicholas ⭐ (Greek) victorious
people. Religion: Nicholas of Myra
is a patron saint of children. See
also Caelan, Claus, Cola, Colar,
Cole, Colin, Colson, Klaus, Lasse,
Mikolaj, Mikolas, Milek.
*Niccolas, Nichalas, Nichelas,
Nichele, Nichlas, Nichlos,
Nichola, Nicholaas, Nicholaes,
Nicholase, Nicholaus, Nichole,
Nicholias, Nicholl, Nichollas,
Nicholos, Nichols, Nicholus, Nick,
Nickalus, Nicklaus, Nickolas,
Nicky, Niclas, Niclasse, Nico,
Nicola, Nicolai, Nicolas, Nicoles,
Nicolis, Nicoll, Nicolo, Nikhil,
Niki, Nikili, Nikita, Nikko, Niklas,
Niko, Nikolai, Nikolas, Nikolaus,
Nikolos, Nils, Nioclás, Niocol,
Nycholas*

Nicholaus (Greek) a form of
Nicholas.
*Nichalaus, Nichalous, Nichaolas,
Nichlaus, Nichloas, Nichlous,
Nicholaos, Nicholous*

Nichols, Nicholson (English)
son of Nicholas.
*Nicholes, Nicholis, Nicolls,
Nickelson, Nickoles*

Nick (English) a short form of
Dominic, Nicholas. See also
Micu.
Nic, Nik

Nickalus (Greek) a form of
Nicholas.
*Nickalas, Nickalis, Nickalos,
Nickelas, Nickelus*

Nicklaus, Nicklas (Greek)
forms of Nicholas.
*Nickalaus, Nickalous, Nickelous,
Nicklauss, Nicklos, Nicklous,
Nicklus, Nickolau, Nickolaus,
Nicolaus, Niklaus, Nikolaus*

Nickolas 🅱🅶 (Greek) a form of
Nicholas.
*Nickolaos, Nickolis, Nickolos,
Nickolus, Nickolys, Nickoulas*

Nicky (Greek) a familiar form of
Nicholas.
Nickey, Nicki, Nickie, Niki, Nikki

Nico 🅱🅶 (Greek) a short form of
Nicholas.
Nicco

Nicodemus (Greek) conqueror
of the people.
*Nicodem, Nicodemius, Nikodem,
Nikodema, Nikodemious,
Nikodim*

Nicola 🅶🅱 (Italian) a form of
Nicholas. See also Cola.
Nicolá, Nikolah

Nicolai (Norwegian, Russian) a
form of Nicholas.
*Nicholai, Nickolai, Nicolaj,
Nicolau, Nicolay, Nicoly, Nikalai*

Nicolas 🅱🅶 (Italian) a form of
Nicholas.
*Nico, Nicolaas, Nicolás, Nicolaus,
Nicoles, Nicolis, Nicolus*

Nicole 🅶🅱 (French) a form of
Nicholas.

Nicolette GB (French) a form of Nicole.

Nicolo (Italian) a form of Nicholas.
Niccolo, Niccolò, Nicol, Nicolao, Nicollo

Nicomedes (Greek) he who prepares the victories.

Nicostrato (Greek) general who leads to victory.

Ñielol (Mapuche) eye of the subterranean cavity, eye of the cave.

Niels (Danish) a form of Neil.
Niel, Nielsen, Nielson, Niles, Nils

Nien (Vietnamese) year.

Nigan (Native American) ahead.
Nigen

Nigel BG (Latin) dark night.
Niegel, Nigal, Nigale, Nigele, Nigell, Nigiel, Nigil, Nigle, Nijel, Nye, Nygel, Nyigel, Nyjil

Nika (Yoruba) ferocious.

Nike BG (Greek) victorious.
Nikka

Niki GB (Hungarian) a familiar form of Nicholas.
Nikia, Nikiah, Nikki, Nikkie, Nykei, Nykey

Nikita GB (Russian) a form of Nicholas.
Nakita, Nakitas, Nikula

Nikiti (Native American) round and smooth like an abalone shell.

Nikki GB (Greek) a form of Nicky. (Hungarian) a form of Niki.

Nikko, Niko BG (Hungarian) forms of Nicholas.
Nikoe, Nyko

Niklas (Latvian, Swedish) a form of Nicholas.
Niklaas, Niklaus

Nikola BG (Greek) a short form of Nicholas.
Nikolao, Nikolay, Nykola

Nikolai (Estonian, Russian) a form of Nicholas.
Kolya, Nikolais, Nikolaj, Nikolajs, Nikolay, Nikoli, Nikolia, Nikula, Nikulas

Nikolas (Greek) a form of Nicholas.
Nicanor, Nikalas, Nikalis, Nikalus, Nikholas, Nikolaas, Nikolaos, Nikolis, Nikolos, Nikos, Nilos, Nykolas, Nykolus

Nikolaus (Greek) a form of Nicholas.
Nikalous, Nikolaos

Nikolos (Greek) a form of Nicholas. See also Kolya.
Niklos, Nikolaos, Nikolò, Nikolous, Nikolus, Nikos, Nilos

Nil (Russian) a form of Neil.
Nilya

Nila GB (Hindi) blue.

Niles (English) son of Neil.
Nilesh, Nyles

Nilo (Finnish) a form of Neil.

Nils (Swedish) a short form of Nicholas.

Nimrod (Hebrew) rebel. Bible: a great-grandson of Noah.

Nina GB (Hebrew) a familiar form of Hanna. (Native American) mighty.

Ninacolla (Quechua) flame of fire.

Ninacuyuchi (Quechua) he who moves or stokes the fire; restless and lively like fire.

Ninan (Quechua) fire; restless and lively like fire.

Ninauari (Quechua) llama-like animal of fire; he who is uncontrollable like the vicuna.

Ninauíca (Quechua) sacred fire.

Nino (Chaldean) possessor of palaces.

Niño (Spanish) young child.

Niran (Tai) eternal.

Nishan (Armenian) cross, sign, mark.
Nishon

Nissan (Hebrew) sign, omen; miracle.
Nisan, Nissim, Nissin, Nisson

Nitis (Native American) friend.
Netis

Nixon (English) son of Nick.
Nixan, Nixson

Nizam (Arabic) leader.

Nkunda (Runyankore) loves those who hate him.

Noach (Hebrew) a form of Noah.

Noah ☆ BG (Hebrew) peaceful, restful. Bible: the patriarch who built the ark to survive the Flood.
Noach, Noak, Noe, Noé, Noi

Noam (Hebrew) sweet; friend.

Noble (Latin) born to nobility.
Nobe, Nobie, Noby

Nodin (Native American) wind.
Knoton, Noton

Noe BG (Czech, French) a form of Noah.

Noé (Hebrew, Spanish) quiet, peaceful. See also Noah.

Noel BG (French) a form of Noël.

Noël (French) day of Christ's birth. See also Natal.
Noel, Noél, Noell, Nole, Noli, Nowel, Nowell

Noelino (Spanish) a form of Natal.

Nohea (Hawaiian) handsome.
Noha, Nohe

Nokonyu (Native American) katydid's nose.
Noko, Nokoni

Nolan 🅱🅶 (Irish) famous; noble.
Noland, Nolande, Nolane, Nolen, Nolin, Nollan, Nolyn

Nolasco (Hebrew) he who departs and forgets about promises.

Nolberto (Teutonic) a form of Norberto.

Nollie 🅱🅶 (Latin, Scandinavian) a familiar form of Oliver.
Noll, Nolly

Nora 🅶🅱 (Greek) light.

Norbert (Scandinavian) brilliant hero.
Bert, Norberto, Norbie, Norby

Norberto (Spanish) a form of Norbert.

Norman 🅱🅶 (French) Norseman. History: a name for the Scandinavians who settled in northern France in the tenth century, and who later conquered England in 1066.
Norm, Normand, Normen, Normie, Normy

Normando (Spanish) man from the north.

Norris (French) northerner. (English) Norman's horse.
Norice, Norie, Noris, Norreys, Norrie, Norry, Norrys

Northcliff (English) northern cliff.
Northcliffe, Northclyff, Northclyffe

Northrop (English) north farm.
North, Northup

Norton (English) northern town.

Norville (French, English) northern town.
Norval, Norvel, Norvell, Norvil, Norvill, Norvylle

Norvin (English) northern friend.
Norvyn, Norwin, Norwinn, Norwyn, Norwynn

Norward (English) protector of the north.
Norwerd

Norwood (English) northern woods.

Nostriano (Latin) he who is from our homeland.

Notaku (Moquelumnan) growing bear.

Notelmo (Teutonic) he who protects himself in combat with the helmet.

Nowles (English) a short form of Knowles.

Nsoah (Akan) seventh-born.

Numa (Arabic) pleasant.

Numair (Arabic) panther.

Nuncio (Italian) messenger.
Nunzi, Nunzio

Nuri (Hebrew, Arabic) my fire.
Nery, Noori, Nur, Nuris, Nurism, Nury

Nuriel (Hebrew, Arabic) fire of the Lord.
Nuria, Nuriah, Nuriya

Nuru BG (Swahili) born in daylight.

Nusair (Arabic) bird of prey.

Nwa (Nigerian) son.

Nwake (Nigerian) born on market day.

Nye (English) a familiar form of Aneurin, Nigel.

Nyle (English) island. (Irish) a form of Neil.
Nyal, Nyll

O'neil (Irish) son of Neil.
Oneal, O'neal, Oneil, O'neill, Onel, Oniel, Onil

O'Shea (Irish) son of Shea.
Oshae, Oshai, Oshane, O'Shane, Oshaun, Oshay, Oshaye, Oshe, Oshea, Osheon

Oakes (English) oak trees.
Oak, Oakie, Oaks, Ochs

Oakley (English) oak-tree field.
Oak, Oakes, Oakie, Oaklee, Oakleigh, Oakly, Oaks

Oalo (Spanish) a form of Paul.

Oba BG (Yoruba) king.

Obadele (Yoruba) king arrives at the house.

Obadiah (Hebrew) servant of God.
Obadias, Obed, Obediah, Obie, Ovadiach, Ovadiah, Ovadya

Obdulio (Latin) he who calms in sorrowful moments.

Obed (English) a short form of Obadiah.

Oberon (German) noble; bearlike. Literature: the king of the fairies in the Shakespearean play *A Midsummer Night's Dream*. See also Auberon, Aubrey.
Oberen, Oberron, Oeberon

Obert (German) wealthy; bright.

Oberto (Germanic) a form of Adalberto.

Obie (English) a familiar form of Obadiah.
Obbie, Obe, Obey, Obi, Oby

Ocan (Luo) hard times.

Octavia GB (Latin) a form of Octavio.

Octavio BG (Latin) eighth. See also Tavey, Tavian.
Octave, Octavia, Octavian, Octaviano, Octavien, Octavious, Octavius, Octavo, Octavous, Octavus, Ottavio

Octavious, Octavius (Latin) forms of Octavio.
Octavaius, Octaveous, Octaveus, Octavias, Octaviaus, Octavis, Octavous, Octavus

Odakota (Lakota) friendly.
Oda

Odd (Norwegian) point.
Oddvar

Ode (Benin) born along the road. (Irish, English) a short form of Odell.
Odey, Odie, Ody

Odeberto (Teutonic) he who shines because of his possessions.

Oded (Hebrew) encouraging.

Odell (Greek) ode, melody. (Irish) otter. (English) forested hill.
Dell, Odall, Ode

Odilón (Teutonic) owner of a bountiful inheritance.

Odin (Scandinavian) ruler. Mythology: the Norse god of wisdom and war.
Oden, Odín

Odion (Benin) first of twins.

Odo (Norwegian) a form of Otto.
Audo

Odoacro (German) he who watches over his inheritance.

Odolf (German) prosperous wolf.
Odolff

Odom (Ghanaian) oak tree.

Odon (Hungarian) wealthy protector.
Odi

Odón (Latin) a form of Odon.

Odran (Irish) pale green.
Odhrán, Oran, Oren, Orin, Orran, Orren, Orrin

Odysseus (Greek) wrathful. Literature: the hero of Homer's epic poem *Odyssey*.

Ofer (Hebrew) young deer.

Ofir (Hebrew) ferocious.

Og (Aramaic) king. Bible: the king of Basham.

Ogaleesha (Lakota) red shirt.

Ogbay (Ethiopian) don't take him from me.

Ogbonna (Ibo) image of his father.
Ogbonnia

Ogden (English) oak valley. Literature: Ogden Nash was a twentieth-century American writer of light verse.
Ogdan, Ogdon

Ogima (Chippewa) chief.

Ogun (Nigerian) Mythology: the god of war.
Ogunkeye, Ogunsanwo, Ogunsheye

Ohanko (Native American) restless.

Ohannes (Turkish) a form of John.

Ohanzee (Lakota) comforting shadow.

Ohin (African) chief.
Ohan

Ohitekah (Lakota) brave.

Oistin (Irish) a form of Austin.
Osten, Ostyn, Ostynn

OJ (American) a combination of the initials O. + J.
O.J., Ojay

Ojo (Yoruba) difficult delivery.

Okapi (Swahili) an African animal related to the giraffe but having a short neck.

Oke (Hawaiian) a form of Oscar.

Okechuku (Ibo) God's gift.

Okeke (Ibo) born on market day.
Okorie

Okie (American) from Oklahoma.
Okee, Okey

Oko (Ghanaian) older twin. (Yoruba) god of war.

Okorie (Ibo) a form of Okeke.

Okpara (Ibo) first son.

Okuth (Luo) born in a rain shower.

Ola GB (Yoruba) wealthy, rich.

Olaf (Scandinavian) ancestor. History: a patron saint and king of Norway.
Olaff, Olafur, Olav, Ole, Olef, Olof, Oluf

Olajuwon (Yoruba) wealth and honor are God's gifts.
Olajawon, Olajawun, Olajowuan, Olajuan, Olajuanne, Olajuawon, Olajuwa, Olajuwan, Olaujawon, Oljuwoun

Olamina (Yoruba) this is my wealth.

Olatunji (Yoruba) honor reawakens.

Olav (Scandinavian) a form of Olaf.
Ola, Olave, Olavus, Ole, Olen, Olin, Olle, Olov, Olyn

Ole (Scandinavian) a familiar form of Olaf, Olav.
Olay, Oleh, Olle

Oleg (Latvian, Russian) holy.
Olezka

Olegario (Germanic) he who dominates with his strength and his lance.

Oleksandr (Russian) a form of Alexander.
Olek, Olesandr, Olesko

Olés (Polish) a familiar form of Alexander.

Olimpo (Greek) party; sky; regarding Mount Olympus or the Olympus sanctuary.

Olin (English) holly.
Olen, Olney, Olyn

Olindo (Italian) from Olinthos, Greece.

Oliver ☆ (Latin) olive tree. (Scandinavian) kind; affectionate.
Nollie, Oilibhéar, Oliverio, Oliverios, Olivero, Olivier, Oliviero, Oliwa, Ollie, Olliver, Ollivor, Olvan

Olivia ☆ (Latin) a form of Olive (see Girls' Names).

Olivier ☆ (French) a form of Oliver.

Oliwa (Hawaiian) a form of Oliver.

Ollanta (Aymara) warrior who sees everything from his watchtower.

Ollantay (Quechua) lord Ollanta.

Ollie ☆ (English) a familiar form of Oliver.
Olie, Olle, Olley, Olly

Olo (Spanish) a short form of Orlando, Rolando.

Olubayo (Yoruba) highest joy.

Olufemi (Yoruba) wealth and honor favors me.

Olujimi (Yoruba) God gave me this.

Olushola (Yoruba) God has blessed me.

Omar ☆ (Arabic) highest; follower of the Prophet. (Hebrew) reverent.
Omair, Omari, Omarr, Omer, Umar

Omari (Swahili) a form of Omar.
Omare, Omaree, Omarey

Omaro (Spanish) a form of Omar.

Omer (Arabic) a form of Omar.
Omeer, Omero

Omolara (Benin) child born at the right time.

On (Burmese) coconut. (Chinese) peace.

Onan (Turkish) prosperous.

Onaona (Hawaiian) pleasant fragrance.

Ondro (Czech) a form of Andrew.
Ondra, Ondre, Ondrea, Ondrey

Onesíforo (Greek) he who bears much fruit.

Onésimo (Greek) he who is useful and worthwhile.

Onkar (Hindi) God in his entirety.

Onofrio (German) a form of Humphrey.
Oinfre, Onfre, Onfrio, Onofre, Onofredo

Onslow (English) enthusiast's hill.
Ounslow

Onufry (Polish) a form of Humphrey.

Onur (Turkish) honor.

Ophir (Hebrew) faithful. Bible: an Old Testament people and country.

Opio (Ateso) first of twin boys.

Optato (Latin) desired.

Oral (Latin) verbal; speaker.

Oran (Irish) green.
Odhran, Odran, Ora, Orane, Orran

Orangel (Greek) messenger from the heights or from the mountain.

Oratio (Latin) a form of Horatio.
Orazio

Orbán (Hungarian) born in the city.

Ordell (Latin) beginning.
Orde

Oren (Hebrew) pine tree. (Irish) light skinned, white.
Oran, Orin, Oris, Orono, Orren, Orrin

Orencio (Greek) examining judge.

Orestes (Greek) mountain man. Mythology: the son of the Greek leader Agamemnon.
Aresty, Oreste

Orfeo (Greek) he who has a good voice.

Ori (Hebrew) my light.
Oree, Orie, Orri, Ory

Orien (Latin) visitor from the east.
Orian, Orie, Orin, Oris, Oron, Orono, Orrin, Oryan

Orígenes (Greek) he who comes from Horus, the god of light; born into caring arms.

Oriol (Latin) golden oriole.

Orion BG (Greek) son of fire. Mythology: a giant hunter who was killed by Artemis. See also Zorion.

Orión (Greek) a form of Orion.

Orji (Ibo) mighty tree.

Orlando (German) famous throughout the land. (Spanish) a form of Roland.
Lando, Olando, Olo, Orlan, Orland, Orlanda, Orlandas, Orlandes, Orlandis, Orlandos, Orlandus, Orlo, Orlondo, Orlondon

Orleans (Latin) golden.
Orlean, Orlin

Orman (German) mariner, seaman. (Scandinavian) serpent, worm.
Ormand

Ormond (English) bear mountain; spear protector.
Ormande, Ormon, Ormonde

Oro (Spanish) golden.

Oroncio (Persian) runner.

Orono (Latin) a form of Oren.
Oron

Orosco (Greek) he who lives in the mountains.

Orrick (English) old oak tree.
Orric

Orrin (English) river.
Orin, Oryn, Orynn

Orris (Latin) a form of Horatio.
Oris, Orriss

Orry (Latin) from the Orient.
Oarrie, Orrey, Orrie

Orsino (Italian) a form of Orson.

Orson (Latin) bearlike.
*Orscino, Orsen, Orsin, Orsini,
Orsino, Son, Sonny, Urson*

Orton (English) shore town.

Ortzi (Basque) sky.

Orunjan (Yoruba) born under the
midday sun.

Orval (English) a form of Orville.
Orvel

Orville (French) golden village.
History: Orville Wright and his
brother Wilbur were the first men
to fly an airplane.
Orv, Orval, Orvell, Orvie, Orvil

Orvin (English) spear friend.
Orwin, Owynn

Osahar (Benin) God hears.

Osayaba (Benin) God forgives.

Osaze (Benin) whom God likes.

Osbert (English) divine; bright.

Osborn (Scandinavian) divine
bear. (English) warrior of God.
*Osbern, Osbon, Osborne,
Osbourn, Osbourne, Osburn,
Osburne, Oz, Ozzie*

Oscar 🅱🅶 (Scandinavian) divine
spearman.
Oke, Oskar, Osker, Oszkar

Óscar (Germanic) a form of Oscar.

Oseas, Osías, Ozias (Hebrew)
Lord sustains me; divine
salvation; God is my soul.

Osei (Fante) noble.
Osee

Osgood (English) divinely good.

Osip (Russian, Ukrainian) a form
of Joseph, Yosef. See also Osya.

Osiris (Egyptian) he who
possesses a powerful vision.

Oskar (Scandinavian) a form of
Oscar.
Osker, Ozker

Osman (Turkish) ruler. (English)
servant of God.
*Osmanek, Osmen, Osmin,
Otthmor, Ottmar*

Osmán (Arabic) he who is as
docile as a pigeon chick.

Osmar (English) divine;
wonderful.

Osmaro (Germanic) he who
shines like the glory of God.

Osmond (English) divine
protector.
*Osmand, Osmonde, Osmont,
Osmund, Osmunde, Osmundo*

Osorio (Slavic) killer of wolves.

Osric (English) divine ruler.
Osrick

Ostiano (Spanish) confessor.

Ostin (Latin) a form of Austin.
Ostan, Osten, Ostyn

Osvaldo (Spanish) a form of
Oswald.
*Osbaldo, Osbalto, Osvald,
Osvalda*

Oswald (English) God's power;
God's crest. See also Waldo.
*Osvaldo, Oswaldo, Oswall,
Oswell, Oswold, Oz, Ozzie*

Oswaldo (Spanish) a form of
Oswald.

Oswin (English) divine friend.
Osvin, Oswinn, Oswyn, Oswynn

Osya (Russian) a familiar form of
Osip.

Ota (Czech) prosperous.
Otik

Otadan (Native American) plentiful.

Otaktay (Lakota) kills many;
strikes many.

Otek (Polish) a form of Otto.

Otello (Italian) a form of Othello.

Otelo (Spanish) a form of Otón.

Otem (Luo) born away from home.

Othello (Spanish) a form of Otto.
Literature: the title character in
the Shakespearean tragedy
Othello.
Otello

Othman (German) wealthy.
Ottoman

Otilde (Teutonic) owner of a
bountiful inheritance.

Otis (Greek) keen of hearing.
(German) son of Otto.
*Oates, Odis, Otes, Otess, Otez,
Otise, Ottis, Otys*

Otniel, Otoniel (Hebrew) God is
my strength.

Otoronco (Quechua) jaguar;
tiger; the bravest.

Ottah (Nigerian) thin baby.

Ottar (Norwegian) point warrior;
fright warrior.

Ottmar (Turkish) a form of
Osman.
Otomars, Ottomar

Otto (German) rich.
*Odo, Otek, Otello, Otfried,
Othello, Otho, Othon, Otik, Otilio,
Otman, Oto, Otón, Otton, Ottone*

Ottokar (German) happy warrior.
Otokars, Ottocar

Otu (Native American) collecting
seashells in a basket.

Ouray (Ute) arrow. Astrology:
born under the sign of
Sagittarius.

Oved (Hebrew) worshiper,
follower.

Ovid (Latin) having the shape of
an egg.

Ovidio (Latin) he who takes care of sheep.

Owen ☆ BG (Irish) born to nobility; young warrior. (Welsh) a form of Evan.
Owain, Owens, Owin, Uaine

Owney (Irish) elderly.
Oney

Oxford (English) place where oxen cross the river.
Ford

Oya BG (Moquelumnan) speaking of the jacksnipe.

Oystein (Norwegian) rock of happiness.
Ostein, Osten, Ostin, Øystein

Oz BG (Hebrew) a short form of Osborn, Oswald.

Oziel (Hebrew) he who has divine strength.

Ozturk (Turkish) pure; genuine Turk.

Ozzie (English) a familiar form of Osborn, Oswald.
Ossie, Ossy, Ozee, Ozi, Ozzi, Ozzy

P

P BG (American) an initial used as a first name.

Paavo (Finnish) a form of Paul.
Paaveli

Pabel (Russian) a form of Paul.

Pablo (Spanish) a form of Paul.
Pable, Paublo

Pace (English) a form of Pascal.
Payce

Pachacutec, Pachacutic (Quechua) he who changes the world, who helps bring about a new era.

Pacho (Spanish) free.

Paciano (Latin) he who belongs to the peace.

Paciente (Latin) he who knows how to be patient.

Pacifico (Filipino) peaceful.

Pacífico (Latin) he who searches for peace.

Paco (Italian) pack. (Spanish) a familiar form of Francisco. (Native American) bald eagle. See also Quico.
Pacorro, Panchito, Pancho, Paquito

Pacomio (Greek) he who is robust.

Paddy (Irish) a familiar form of Padraic, Patrick.
Paddey, Paddi, Paddie

Paden (English) a form of Patton.

Padget BG (English) a form of Page.
Padgett, Paget, Pagett

Padraic (Irish) a form of Patrick.
Paddrick, Paddy, Padhraig, Padrai,
Pádraig, Padraigh, Padreic,
Padriac, Padric, Padron, Padruig

Pafnucio (Greek) rich in merits.

Page GB (French) youthful
assistant.
Padget, Paggio, Paige, Payge

Paige GB (English) a form of
Page.

Paillalef (Mapuche) return
quickly, go back.

Painecura (Mapuche) iridescent
stone.

Painevilu (Mapuche) iridescent
snake.

Pakelika (Hawaiian) a form of
Patrick.

Paki (African) witness.

Pal (Swedish) a form of Paul.

Pál (Hungarian) a form of Paul.
Pali, Palika

Palaina (Hawaiian) a form of
Brian.

Palani (Hawaiian) a form of
Frank.

Palash (Hindi) flowery tree.

Palatino (Latin) he who comes
from Mount Palatine.

Palben (Basque) blond.

Palladin (Native American)
fighter.
Pallaton, Palleten

Palmacio (Latin) adorned with
bordered palm leaves.

Palmer (English) palm-bearing
pilgrim.
Pallmer, Palmar

Paloma GB (Spanish) dove.

Palti (Hebrew) God liberates.
Palti-el

Pampín (Latin) he who has the
vigor of a sprouting plant.

Panas (Russian) immortal.

Panayiotis (Greek) a form of
Peter.
Panagiotis, Panajotis, Panayioti,
Panayoti, Panayotis

Pancho (Spanish) a familiar form
of Francisco, Frank.
Panchito

Pancracio (Greek) all-powerful
one.

Panfilo (Greek) friend of all.

Pánfilo (Greek) a form of Panfilo.

Panos (Greek) a form of Peter.
Petros

Pantaleón (Greek) he who is all-
merciful and has everything
under control.

Panteno (Greek) he who is
worthy of all praise.

Panti (Quechua) species of brush.

Paola 🄶🄱 (Italian) a form of Paula (see Girls' Names).

Paolo (Italian) a form of Paul.

Papias (Greek) venerable father.

Paquito (Spanish) a familiar form of Paco.

Paramesh (Hindi) greatest. Religion: another name for the Hindu god Shiva.

Pardeep 🄱🄶 (Sikh) mystic light. *Pardip*

Pardulfo (Germanic) brave warrior, armed with an ax.

Paris 🄶🄱 (Greek) lover. Geography: the capital of France. Mythology: the prince of Troy who started the Trojan War by abducting Helen. *Paras, Paree, Pares, Parese, Parie, Parris, Parys*

París (Greek) a form of Paris.

Parisio (Spanish) a form of Paris.

Pariuana (Quechua) Andean flamingo.

Park (Chinese) cypress tree. (English) a short form of Parker. *Parke, Parkes, Parkey, Parks*

Parker 🄱🄶 (English) park keeper. *Park*

Parkin (English) little Peter. *Perkin*

Parlan (Scottish) a form of Bartholomew. See also Parthalán.

Parménides (Greek) he who is a constant presence.

Parmenio (Greek) he who is loyal and offers his constant presence.

Parnell (French) little Peter. History: Charles Stewart Parnell was a famous Irish politician. *Nell, Parle, Parnel, Parrnell, Pernell*

Parodio (Greek) he who imitates the singing.

Parr (English) cattle enclosure, barn.

Parrish (English) church district. *Parish, Parrie, Parrisch, Parrysh*

Parry (Welsh) son of Harry. *Parrey, Parrie, Pary*

Partemio (Greek) having a pure and virginal appearance.

Parth (Irish) a short form of Parthalán. *Partha, Parthey*

Parthalán (Irish) plowman. See also Bartholomew. *Parlan, Parth*

Parthenios (Greek) virgin. Religion: a Greek Orthodox saint.

Pascal 🄱🄶 (French) born on Easter or Passover. *Pace, Pascale, Pascalle, Paschal,*

Paschalis, Pascoe, Pascow, Pascual, Pasquale

Pascale GB (French) a form of Pascal.

Pascasio (Spanish) a form of Pascual.

Pascua (Hebrew) in reference to Easter, to the sacrifice of the village.

Pascual (Spanish) a form of Pascal.
Pascul

Pasha BG (Russian) a form of Paul.
Pashenka, Pashka

Pasicrates (Greek) he who dominates everyone.

Pasquale (Italian) a form of Pascal.
Pascuale, Pasqual, Pasquali, Pasquel

Pastor (Latin) spiritual leader.

Pat BG (Native American) fish. (English) a short form of Patrick.
Pattie, Patty

Patakusu (Moquelumnan) ant biting a person.

Patamon (Native American) raging.

Patek (Polish) a form of Patrick.
Patick

Paterio (Greek) he who was born in Pateria.

Paterno (Latin) belonging to the father.

Patric (Latin) a form of Patrick.

Patrice GB (French) a form of Patrick.

Patricia GB (Latin) noble.

Patricio (Spanish) a form of Patrick.
Patricius, Patrizio

Patrick ☆ BG (Latin) nobleman. Religion: the patron saint of Ireland. See also Fitzpatrick, Ticho.
Paddy, Padraic, Pakelika, Pat, Patek, Patric, Patrice, Patricio, Patrickk, Patrik, Patrique, Patrizius, Patryk, Pats, Patsy, Pattrick

Patrido (Latin) noble.

Patrin (Gypsy) leaf trail.

Patrocinio (Latin) patronage, protection.

Patryk (Latin) a form of Patrick.
Patryck

Patterson (Irish) son of Pat.
Patteson

Pattin (Gypsy) leaf.

Patton (English) warrior's town.
Paden, Paten, Patin, Paton, Patten, Pattin, Patty, Payton, Peyton

Patwin (Native American) man.

Patxi (Basque, Teutonic) free.

Paucar (Quechua) very refined, excellent.

Paucartupac (Quechua) majestic and excellent.

Paul BG (Latin) small. Bible: Saul, later renamed Paul, was the first to bring the teachings of Christ to the Gentiles.
Oalo, Paavo, Pablo, Pal, Pál, Pall, Paolo, Pasha, Pasko, Pauli, Paulia, Paulin, Paulino, Paulis, Paulo, Pauls, Paulus, Pavel, Pavlos, Pawel, Pol, Poul

Pauli (Latin) a familiar form of Paul.
Pauley, Paulie, Pauly

Paulin (German, Polish) a form of Paul.

Paulino, Pauliño (Spanish) forms of Paul.

Paulo (Portuguese, Swedish, Hawaiian) a form of Paul.

Pausidio (Greek) deliberate, calm man.

Pauyu (Aymara) he who finishes, who brings to a happy ending all work that he undertakes.

Pavel (Russian) a form of Paul.
Paavel, Pasha, Pavils, Pavlik, Pavlo, Pavlusha, Pavlushenka, Pawl

Pavit (Hindi) pious, pure.

Pawel (Polish) a form of Paul.
Pawelek, Pawl

Pax (Latin) peaceful.

Paxton BG (Latin) peaceful town.
Packston, Pax, Paxon, Paxten, Paxtun

Payat (Native American) he is on his way.
Pay, Payatt

Payden (English) a form of Payton.
Paydon

Payne (Latin) from the country.
Paine, Paynn

Paytah (Lakota) fire.
Pay, Payta

Payton GB (English) a form of Patton.
Paiton, Pate, Payden, Peaton, Peighton, Peyton

Paz GB (Spanish) a form of Pax.

Pearce (English) a form of Pierce.
Pears, Pearse

Pearson (English) son of Peter. See also Pierson.
Pearsson, Pehrson, Peirson, Peterson

Peder (Scandinavian) a form of Peter.
Peadar, Pedey

Pedro (Spanish) a form of Peter.
Pedrin, Pedrín, Petronio

Peers (English) a form of Peter.
Peerus, Piers

Peeter (Estonian) a form of Peter.
Peet

Pegaso (Greek) born next to the fountain.

Peirce (English) a form of Peter.
Peirs

Pekelo (Hawaiian) a form of Peter.
Pekka

Pelagio, Pelayo (Greek) excellent sailor.

Peleke (Hawaiian) a form of Frederick.

Pelham (English) tannery town.

Pelí (Latin, Basque) happy.

Pell (English) parchment.
Pall

Pello (Greek, Basque) stone.
Peru, Piarres

Pelope (Greek) having a brown complexion.

Pelton (English) town by a pool.

Pembroke (Welsh) headland. (French) wine dealer. (English) broken fence.
Pembrook

Peniamina (Hawaiian) a form of Benjamin.
Peni

Penley (English) enclosed meadow.

Penn (Latin) pen, quill. (English) enclosure. (German) a short form of Penrod.
Pen, Penna, Penney, Pennie, Penny

Penrod (German) famous commander.
Penn, Pennrod, Rod

Pepa (Czech) a familiar form of Joseph.
Pepek, Pepik

Pepe (Spanish) a familiar form of José.
Pepillo, Pepito, Pequin, Pipo

Pepin (German) determined; petitioner. History: Pepin the Short was an eighth-century king of the Franks.
Pepi, Peppie, Peppy

Peppe (Italian) a familiar form of Joseph.
Peppi, Peppo, Pino

Per (Swedish) a form of Peter.

Perben (Greek, Danish) stone.

Percival (French) pierce the valley. Literature: a knight of the Round Table who first appears in Chrétien de Troyes's poem about the quest for the Holy Grail.
Parsafal, Parsefal, Parsifal, Parzival, Perc, Perce, Perceval, Percevall, Percivall, Percy, Peredur, Purcell

Percy (French) a familiar form of Percival.
Pearcey, Pearcy, Percey, Percie, Piercey, Piercy

Peregrine (Latin) traveler; pilgrim; falcon.
Peregrin, Peregryne, Perine, Perry

Peregrino (Latin) he who travels.

Perfecto (Latin) upright; errorless, without any defects.

Periandro (Greek) worries about men.

Pericles (Greek) just leader. History: an Athenian statesman.

Perico (Spanish) a form of Peter.
Pequin, Perequin

Perine (Latin) a short form of Peregrine.
Perino, Perion, Perrin, Perryn

Perkin (English) little Peter.
Perka, Perkins, Perkyn, Perrin

Pernell (French) a form of Parnell.
Perren, Perrnall

Perpetuo (Latin) having an unchanging goal, who remains faithful to his faith.

Perry BG (English) a familiar form of Peregrine, Peter.
Parry, Perrie, Perrye

Perseo (Greek) destroyer, the destructive one.

Perth (Scottish) thorn-bush thicket. Geography: a burgh in Scotland; a city in Australia.

Pervis (Latin) passage.
Pervez

Pesach (Hebrew) spared. Religion: another name for Passover.
Pessach

Petar (Greek) a form of Peter.

Pete (English) a short form of Peter.
Peat, Peet, Petey, Peti, Petie, Piet, Pit

Peter BG (Greek, Latin) small rock. Bible: Simon, renamed Peter, was the leader of the Twelve Apostles. See also Boutros, Ferris, Takis.
Panayiotos, Panos, Peadair, Peder, Pedro, Peers, Peeter, Peirce, Pekelo, Per, Perico, Perion, Perkin, Perry, Petar, Pete, Péter, Peterke, Peterus, Petr, Petras, Petros, Petru, Petruno, Petter, Peyo, Piaras, Pierce, Piero, Pierre, Pieter, Pietrek, Pietro, Piotr, Piter, Piti, Pjeter, Pyotr

Peterson (English) son of Peter.
Peteris, Petersen

Petiri (Shona) where we are.
Petri

Petr (Bulgarian) a form of Peter.

Petras (Lithuanian) a form of Peter.
Petra, Petrelis

Petros (Greek) a form of Peter.
Petro

Petru (Romanian) a form of Peter.
Petrukas, Petrus, Petruso

Petter (Norwegian) a form of Peter.

Peverell (French) piper.
Peverall, Peverel, Peveril

Peyo (Spanish) a form of Peter.

Peyton BG (English) a form of Patton, Payton.
Peyt, Peyten, Peython, Peytonn

Pharaoh (Latin) ruler. History: a title for the ancient kings of Egypt.
Faroh, Pharo, Pharoah, Pharoh

Phelan (Irish) wolf.

Phelipe (Spanish) a form of Philip.

Phelix (Latin) a form of Felix.

Phelps (English) son of Phillip.

Phil (Greek) a short form of Philip, Phillip.
Fil, Phill

Philander (Greek) lover of mankind.

Philbert (English) a form of Filbert.
Philibert, Phillbert

Philemon (Greek) kiss.
Phila, Philamina, Phileman, Philémon, Philmon

Philip BG (Greek) lover of horses. Bible: one of the Twelve Apostles. See also Felipe, Felippo, Filip, Fillipp, Filya, Fischel, Flip.
Phelps, Phelipe, Phil, Philipp, Philippe, Philippo, Phillip, Phillipos, Phillp, Philly, Philp, Phylip, Piers, Pilib, Pilipo, Pippo

Philipp (German) a form of Philip.
Phillipp

Philippe (French) a form of Philip.
Philipe, Phillepe, Phillipe, Phillippe, Phillippee, Phyllipe

Phillip (Greek) a form of Philip.
Phil, Phillipos, Phillipp, Phillips, Philly, Phyllip

Phillipos (Greek) a form of Phillip.

Philly (American) a familiar form of Philip, Phillip.
Phillie

Philo (Greek) love.

Phinean (Irish) a form of Finian.
Phinian

Phineas (English) a form of Pinchas.
Fineas, Phinehas, Phinny

Phirun (Cambodian) rain.

Phoenix (Latin) phoenix, a legendary bird.
Phenix, Pheonix, Phynix

Phuok (Vietnamese) good.
Phuoc

Pias (Gypsy) fun.

Pichi (Araucanian) small.

Pichiu (Quechua) baby bird.

Pichulman (Mapuche) condor's feather.

Pichunlaf (Mapuche) lucky feather; virtue that brings health and happiness.

Pickford (English) ford at the peak.

Pickworth (English) wood cutter's estate.

Pierce BG (English) a form of Peter.
Pearce, Peerce, Peers, Peirce, Piercy, Piers

Piero (Italian) a form of Peter.
Pero, Pierro

Pierre BG (French) a form of Peter.
Peirre, Piere, Pierrot

Pierre-Luc (French) a combination of Pierre + Luc.
Piere Luc

Piers (English) a form of Philip.

Pierson (English) son of Peter. See also Pearson.
Pierrson, Piersen, Piersson, Piersun

Pieter (Dutch) a form of Peter.
Pietr

Pietro (Italian) a form of Peter.

Pigmalion (Spanish) sculptor.

Pilar (Spanish) pillar.

Pilato (Latin) soldier armed with a lance.

Pilatos (Latin) he who is armed with a pick.

Pili (Swahili) second born.

Pilipo (Hawaiian) a form of Philip.

Pillan (Native American) supreme essence.
Pilan

Pin (Vietnamese) faithful boy.

Pinchas (Hebrew) oracle. (Egyptian) dark skinned.
Phineas, Pincas, Pinchos, Pincus, Pinkas, Pinkus, Pinky

Pinky (American) a familiar form of Pinchas.
Pink

Pino (Italian) a form of Joseph.

Piñon (Tupi-Guarani) Mythology: the hunter who became the constellation Orion.

Pio, Pío (Latin) pious.

Piotr (Bulgarian) a form of Peter.
Piotrek

Pipino (Latin) he who has a small stature.

Pippin (German) father.

Piquichaqui (Quechua) feet of a bug, light-footed.

Piran (Irish) prayer. Religion: the patron saint of miners.
Peran, Pieran

Pirro (Greek, Spanish) flaming hair.

Pista (Hungarian) a familiar form of István.
Pisti

Pitágoras (Greek) he who is like a divine oracle.

Piti (Spanish) a form of Peter.

Pitin (Spanish) a form of Felix.
Pito

Pitney (English) island of the strong-willed man.
Pittney

Pitt (English) pit, ditch.

Piyco, Piycu (Quechua) red bird.

Piycomayu, Piycumayu (Quechua) a river as red as a bright, red bird.

Placido (Spanish) serene.
Placide, Placidus, Placyd, Placydo

Plácido (Latin) a form of Placido.

Plato (Greek) broad shouldered. History: a famous Greek philosopher.
Platon

Platón (Greek) wide-shouldered.

Platt (French) flatland.
Platte

Plauto, Plotino (Greek) he who has flat feet.

Plinio (Latin) he who has many skills, gifts.

Plubio (Greek) man of the sea.

Plutarco (Greek) rich prince.

Plutón (Greek) owner of many riches.

Po Sin (Chinese) grandfather elephant.

Pol (Swedish) a form of Paul.
Pól, Pola, Poul

Poldi (German) a familiar form of Leopold.
Poldo

Poliano (Greek) he who suffers, the sorrowful one.

Policarpo (Greek) he who produces abundant fruit.

Policeto (Greek) he who caused much sorrow.

Polidoro (Greek) having virtues.

Poliecto (Greek) he who is very desired.

Polifemo (Greek) he who is spoken about a lot.

Polión (Greek) powerful Lord who protects.

Pollard (German) close-cropped head.
Poll, Pollerd, Pollyrd

Pollock (English) a form of Pollux. Art: American artist Jackson Pollock was a leader of abstract expressionism.
Pollack, Polloch

Pollux (Greek) crown.
Astronomy: one of the stars in the
constellation Gemini.
Pollock

Polo (Tibetan) brave wanderer.
(Greek) a short form of Apollo.
Culture: a game played on
horseback. History: Marco Polo
was a thirteenth-century Venetian
explorer who traveled throughout
Asia.

Poma, Pomacana (Quechua)
strong and powerful puma.

Pomacaua (Quechua) he who
guards with the quietness of a
puma.

Pomagüiyca (Quechua) sacred
like the puma.

Pomalloque (Quechua) left-
handed puma.

Pomauari (Quechua) indomitable
as a vicuna and strong as a puma.

Pomayauri (Quechua) copper-
colored puma.

Pomeroy (French) apple orchard.
Pommeray, Pommeroy

Pompeyo (Greek) he who heads
the procession.

Pomponio (Latin) lover of
grandeur and the open plains.

Ponce (Spanish) fifth. History:
Juan Ponce de León of Spain
searched for the Fountain of
Youth in Florida.

Poncio (Greek) having come
from the sea.

Ponpey (English) a form of
Pompeyo.

Pony (Scottish) small horse.
Poni

Porcio (Latin) he who earns his
living raising pigs.

Porfirio (Greek, Spanish) purple
stone.
Porphirios, Prophyrios

Porfiro (Greek) purple stone.

Porter (Latin) gatekeeper.
Port, Portie, Porty

Poseidón (Greek) owner of the
waters.

Poshita (Sanskrit) cherished.

Posidio (Greek) he who is
devoted to Poseidon.

Potenciano (Latin) he who
dominates with his empire.

Poul (Danish) a form of Paul.
Poulos, Poulus

Pov (Gypsy) earth.

Powa (Native American) wealthy.

Powell (English) alert.
Powel

Prabhjot 🅱🅶 (Sikh) the light of
God.

Prácido (Latin) tranquil, calm.

Pragnacio (Greek) he who is skillful and practical in business.

Pramad (Hindi) rejoicing.

Pravat (Tai) history.

Prem (Hindi) love.

Prentice (English) apprentice.
Prent, Prentis, Prentiss, Printes, Printiss

Prescott (English) priest's cottage. See also Scott.
Prescot, Prestcot, Prestcott

Presidio (Latin) he who gives pleasant shelter.

Presley GB (English) priest's meadow. Music: Elvis Presley was an influential American rock 'n' roll singer.
Presleigh, Presly, Presslee, Pressley, Prestley, Priestley, Priestly

Preston BG (English) priest's estate.
Prestan, Presten, Prestin, Prestyn

Pretextato (Latin) covered by a toga.

Prewitt (French) brave little one.
Preuet, Prewet, Prewett, Prewit, Pruit, Pruitt

Priamo (Greek) rescued one.

Príamo (Greek) a form of Priamo.

Price (Welsh) son of the ardent one.
Brice, Bryce, Pryce

Pricha (Tai) clever.

Prilidiano (Greek) he who remembers things from the past.

Primeiro (Italian) born first.

Primitivo (Latin) original.

Primo (Italian) first; premier quality.
Preemo, Premo

Prince (Latin) chief; prince.
Prence, Prinz, Prinze

Princeton (English) princely town.
Prenston, Princeston, Princton

Probo (Latin) having moral conduct.

Proceso (Latin) he who moves forward.

Procopio (Greek) he who progresses.

Procoro (Greek) he who prospers.

Proctor (Latin) official, administrator.
Prockter, Procter

Proculo (Latin) he who was born far from home.

Prokopios (Greek) declared leader.

Promaco (Greek) he who prepares for battle.

Prometeo (Greek) he who resembles God.

Prosper (Latin) fortunate.
Prospero, Próspero

Protasio (Greek) he who is in front; the preferred one.

Proteo (Greek) lord of the sea's waves.

Proterio (Greek) he who precedes all the rest.

Proto (Greek) first.

Protólico (Greek) preferred one; he who deserves first place.

Prudenciano (Spanish) humble and honest.

Prudencio (Latin) he who works with sensitivity and modesty.

Pryor (Latin) head of the monastery; prior.
Prior, Pry

Publio (Latin) he who is popular.

Puchac (Quechua) leader; he who leads others down a good path.

Pueblo (Spanish) from the city.

Pulqueria (Latin) beautiful one.

Pulqui (Araucanian) arrow.

Puma, Pumacana (Quechua) strong and powerful puma.

Pumacaua (Quechua) he who guards with the quietness of a puma.

Pumagüiyca (Quechua) sacred like the puma.

Pumalluqui (Quechua) left-handed puma.

Pumasonjo, Pumasuncu (Quechua) courageous heart; heart of a puma.

Pumauari (Quechua) indomitable as a vicuna and strong as a puma.

Pumayauri (Quechua) copper-colored puma.

Pumeet (Sanskrit) pure.

Pupulo (Latin) little boy.

Purdy (Hindi) recluse.

Puric (Quechua) walker, fond of walking.

Purvis (French, English) providing food.
Pervis, Purves, Purviss

Putnam (English) dweller by the pond.
Putnem

Pyotr (Russian) a form of Peter.
Petenka, Petinka, Petrusha, Petya, Pyatr

Qabil (Arabic) able.

Qadim (Arabic) ancient.

Qadir (Arabic) powerful.
*Qaadir, Qadeer, Quaadir, Quadeer,
Quadir*

Qamar (Arabic) moon.
Quamar, Quamir

Qasim (Arabic) divider.
Quasim

Qimat (Hindi) valuable.

Quaashie BG (Ewe) born on
Sunday.

Quadarius (American) a
combination of Quan + Darius.
*Quadara, Quadarious, Quadaris,
Quandarious, Quandarius,
Quandarrius, Qudarius, Qudaruis*

Quade (Latin) fourth.
*Quadell, Quaden, Quadon, Quadre,
Quadrie, Quadrine, Quadrion,
Quaid, Quayd, Quayde, Qwade*

Quamaine (American) a
combination of Quan + Jermaine.
*Quamain, Quaman, Quamane,
Quamayne, Quarmaine*

Quan (Comanche) a short form of
Quanah.

Quanah (Comanche) fragrant.
Quan

Quandre (American) a combination of Quan + Andre.
Quandrae, Quandré

Quant (Greek) how much?
*Quanta, Quantae, Quantai,
Quantas, Quantay, Quante,
Quantea, Quantey, Quantez,
Quantu*

Quantavius (American) a combi-
nation of Quan + Octavius.
*Quantavian, Quantavin,
Quantavion, Quantavious,
Quantavis, Quantavous,
Quatavious, Quatavius*

Quashawn (American) a combi-
nation of Quan + Shawn.
*Quasean, Quashaan, Quashan,
Quashaun, Quashaunn, Quashon,
Quashone, Quashun, Queshan,
Queshon, Qweshawn, Qyshawn*

Qudamah (Arabic) courage.

Quenby BG (Scandinavian) a
form of Quimby.

Quennell (French) small oak.
Quenell, Quennel

Quenten (Latin) a form of Quentin.
Quienten

Quenti, Quinti (Quechua)
hummingbird; shy, small.

Quentin BG (Latin) fifth.
(English) queen's town.
*Qeuntin, Quantin, Quent,
Quentan, Quenten, Quentine,
Quenton, Quentyn, Quentynn,
Quientin, Quinten, Quintin,
Quinton, Qwentin*

Quenton (Latin) a form of Quentin.
Quienton

Querubín (Hebrew) swift, young bull.

Quespi, Quispe, Quispi (Quechua) free, liberated; jewel, shiny like a diamond.

Queupulicán (Mapuche) white stone with a black stripe.

Queupumil (Mapuche) shining stone; brilliant, precious.

Quichuasamin (Quechua) he who brings fortune and happiness to the village.

Quico (Spanish) a familiar form of many names.
Paco

Quidequeo (Mapuche) brilliant; fiery tongue.

Quigley (Irish) maternal side.
Quigly

Quillan (Irish) cub.
Quill, Quillen, Quillin, Quillon

Quillinchu, Quilliyicu (Quechua) sparrow hawk.

Quimby (Scandinavian) woman's estate.
Quenby, Quinby

Quincy 🅱🅶 (French) fifth son's estate.
Quenci, Quency, Quince, Quincee, Quincey, Quinci, Quinn, Quinncy, Quinnsy, Quinsey, Quinzy

Quindarius (American) a combination of Quinn + Darius.
Quindarious, Quindarrius, Quinderious, Quinderus, Quindrius

Quiñelef (Mapuche) a rapid trip, quick race.

Quinlan (Irish) strong; well shaped.
Quindlen, Quinlen, Quinlin, Quinn, Quinnlan, Quinnlin

Quinn 🅱🅶 (Irish) a short form of Quincy, Quinlan, Quinton.
Quin

Quintavius (American) a combination of Quinn + Octavius.
Quintavious, Quintavis, Quintavus, Quintayvious

Quinten (Latin) a form of Quentin.
Quinnten

Quintilian (French) a form of Quintiliano.

Quintiliano (Spanish) a form of Quintilio.

Quintilio (Latin) he who was born in the fifth month.

Quintin (Latin) a form of Quentin.
Quinntin, Quintine, Quintyn

Quintín (Spanish) a form of Quinto.

Quinto (Latin) a form of Quinton.

Quinton BG (Latin) a form of Quentin.
Quinn, Quinneton, Quinnton, Quint, Quintan, Quintann, Quintin, Quintion, Quintus, Quitin, Quito, Quiton, Qunton, Qwinton

Quintrilpe (Mapuche) place of organization.

Quintuillan (Mapuche) searching for the altar.

Quiqui (Spanish) a familiar form of Enrique.
Quinto, Quiquin

Quirino (Latin) he who carries a lance.

Quispiyupanqui (Quechua) he who honors his liberty.

Quisu (Aymara) he who appreciates the value of things.

Quitin (Latin) a short form of Quinton.
Quiten, Quito, Quiton

Quito (Spanish) a short form of Quinton.

Quon (Chinese) bright.

R

R BG (American) an initial used as a first name.

Raanan (Hebrew) fresh; luxuriant.

Rabi BG (Arabic) breeze.
Rabbi, Rabee, Rabeeh, Rabiah, Rabie, Rabih

Race (English) race.
Racel, Rayce

Racham (Hebrew) compassionate.
Rachaman, Rachamim, Rachim, Rachman, Rachmiel, Rachum, Raham, Rahamim

Rachel GB (Hebrew) sheep.

Rad (English) advisor. (Slavic) happy.
Raad, Radd, Raddie, Raddy, Rade, Radee, Radell, Radey, Radi

Radbert (English) brilliant advisor.

Radburn (English) red brook; brook with reeds.
Radborn, Radborne, Radbourn, Radbourne, Radburne

Radcliff (English) red cliff; cliff with reeds.
Radcliffe, Radclyffe

Radford (English) red ford; ford with reeds.

Radley (English) red meadow; meadow of reeds.
Radlea, Radlee, Radleigh, Radly

Radman (Slavic) joyful.
Radmen, Radusha

Radnor (English) red shore; shore with reeds.

Radomil (Slavic) happy peace.

Radoslaw (Polish) happy glory.
Radik, Rado, Radzmir, Slawek

Raegan GB (Irish) a form of
Reagan.

Raekwon (American) a form of
Raquan.
*Raekwan, Raikwan, Rakwane,
Rakwon*

Raequan (American) a form of
Raquan.
*Raequon, Raeqwon, Raiquan,
Raiquen, Raiqoun*

Raeshawn (American) a form of
Rashawn.
*Raesean, Raeshaun, Raeshon,
Raeshun*

Rafael BG (Spanish) a form of
Raphael. See also Falito.
*Rafaelle, Rafaello, Rafaelo, Rafal,
Rafeal, Rafeé, Rafel, Rafello,
Raffael, Raffaelo, Raffeal, Raffel,
Raffiel, Rafiel*

Rafaele (Italian) a form of
Raphael.
Raffaele

Rafal (Polish) a form of Raphael.

Rafe (English) a short form of
Rafferty, Ralph.
Raff

Rafer (Irish) a short form of
Rafferty.
Raffer

Rafferty (Irish) rich, prosperous.
*Rafe, Rafer, Raferty, Raffarty,
Raffer*

Rafi (Arabic) exalted. (Hebrew) a
familiar form of Raphael.
Raffe, Raffee, Raffi, Raffy, Rafi

Rafiq (Arabic) friend.
Raafiq, Rafeeq, Rafic, Rafique

Raghib (Arabic) desirous.
Raquib

Raghnall (Irish) wise power.

Ragnar (Norwegian) powerful
army.
*Ragnor, Rainer, Rainier, Ranieri,
Rayner, Raynor, Reinhold*

Rago (Hausa) ram.

Raguel (Hebrew) everybody's
friend.

Raheem BG (Punjabi)
compassionate God.
Rakeem

Rahim (Arabic) merciful.
*Raaheim, Rahaeim, Raheam,
Raheim, Rahiem, Rahiim, Rahime,
Rahium, Rakim*

Rahman (Arabic) compassionate.
Rahmatt, Rahmet

Rahul (Arabic) traveler.

Rai (Spanish) mighty protector.

Raíd (Arabic) leader.

Raiden (Japanese) Mythology: the
thunder god.
Raidan, Rayden

Railef (Mapuche) a flower that is
bedraggled because of a strong
wind.

Raimi (Quechua) party, celebration.

Raimondo (Italian) a form of Raymond.
Raymondo, Reimundo

Raimund (German) a form of Raymond.
Rajmund

Raimundo (Portuguese, Spanish) a form of Raymond.
Mundo, Raimon, Raimond, Raimonds, Raymundo

Raine GB (English) lord; wise.
Rain, Raines, Rayne

Rainer (German) counselor.
Rainar, Rainey, Rainier, Rainor, Raynier, Reinier

Rainero (Germanic) intelligence that guides.

Rainey (German) a familiar form of Rainer.
Raine, Rainee, Rainie, Rainney, Rainy, Reiny

Raini (Tupi-Guarani) Religion: the god who created the world.

Raishawn (American) a form of Rashawn.
Raishon, Raishun

Rajabu (Swahili) born in the seventh month of the Islamic calendar.

Rajah (Hindi) prince; chief.
Raj, Raja, Rajaah, Rajae, Rajahe, Rajan, Raje, Rajeh, Raji

Rajak (Hindi) cleansing.

Rajan (Hindi) a form of Rajah.
Rajaahn, Rajain, Rajen, Rajin

Rakeem (Punjabi) a form of Raheem.
Rakeeme, Rakeim, Rakem

Rakim (Arabic) a form of Rahim.
Rakiim

Rakin (Arabic) respectable.
Rakeen

Raktim (Hindi) bright red.

Raleigh BG (English) a form of Rawleigh.
Ralegh

Ralph BG (English) wolf counselor.
Radolphus, Rafe, Ralf, Ralpheal, Ralphel, Ralphie, Ralston, Raoul, Raul, Rolf

Ralphie (English) a familiar form of Ralph.
Ralphy

Ralston (English) Ralph's settlement.

Ram (Hindi) god; godlike. Religion: another name for the Hindu god Rama. (English) male sheep. A short form of Ramsey.
Rami, Ramie, Ramy

Ramadan (Arabic) ninth month of the Arabic year in the Islamic calendar.
Rama

Raman GB (Hindi) a short form of Ramanan.

Ramanan (Hindi) god; godlike.
Raman, Ramandeep, Ramanjit, Ramanjot

Rami (Hindi, English) a form of Ram. (Spanish) a short form of Ramiro.
Rame, Ramee, Ramey, Ramih

Ramiro (Portuguese, Spanish) supreme judge.
Ramario, Rameer, Rameir, Ramere, Rameriz, Ramero, Rami, Ramires, Ramirez, Ramos

Ramón (Spanish) a form of Raymond.
Ramon, Remon, Remone, Romone

Ramone (Dutch) a form of Raymond.
Raemon, Raemonn, Ramond, Ramonte, Remone

Ramsden (English) valley of rams.

Ramsey BG (English) ram's island.
Ram, Ramsay, Ramsee, Ramsie, Ramsy, Ramzee, Ramzey, Ramzi, Ramzy

Rance (English) a short form of Laurence. (American) a familiar form of Laurence.
Rancel, Rancell, Rances, Rancey, Rancie, Rancy, Ransel, Ransell

Rancul (Araucanian) plant from the grasslands whose leaves are used to make roofs for huts.

Rand (English) shield; warrior.
Randy

Randal (English) a form of Randall.
Randahl, Randale, Randel, Randl, Randle

Randall BG (English) a form of Randolph.
Randal, Randell, Randy, Randyll

Randi GB (English) a form of Randy.

Randolph (English) shield wolf.
Randall, Randol, Randolf, Randolfo, Randolpho, Randy, Ranolph

Randy BG (English) a familiar form of Rand, Randall, Randolph.
Randdy, Randee, Randey, Randi, Randie, Ranndy

Ranger (French) forest keeper.
Rainger, Range

Rangle (American) cowboy.
Rangler, Wrangle

Rangsey (Cambodian) seven kinds of colors.

Rani GB (Hebrew) my song; my joy.
Ranen, Ranie, Ranon, Roni

Ranieri (Italian) a form of Ragnar.
Raneir, Ranier, Rannier

Ranjan (Hindi) delighted; gladdened.

Rankin (English) small shield.
Randkin

Ransford (English) raven's ford.

Ransley (English) raven's field.

Ransom (Latin) redeemer. (English) son of the shield.
Rance, Ransome, Ranson

Raoul (French) a form of Ralph, Rudolph.
Raol, Raul, Raúl, Reuel

Raphael **BG** (Hebrew) God has healed. Bible: one of the archangels. Art: a prominent painter of the Renaissance. See also Falito, Rafi.
Rafael, Rafaele, Rafal, Rafel, Raphaél, Raphale, Raphaello, Rapheal, Raphel, Raphello, Raphiel, Ray, Rephael

Rapheal (Hebrew) a form of Raphael.
Rafel, Raphiel

Rapier (French) blade-sharp.

Rapiman (Mapuche) condor's vomit; indigestion.

Raquan (American) a combination of the prefix Ra + Quan.
Raaquan, Rackwon, Racquan, Raekwon, Raequan, Rahquan, Raquané, Raquon, Raquwan, Raquwn, Raquwon, Raqwan, Raqwann

Raquel **GB** (French) a form of Rachel.

Rashaad (Arabic) a form of Rashad.

Rashaan (American) a form of Rashawn.
Rasaan, Rashan, Rashann

Rashad (Arabic) wise counselor.
Raashad, Rachad, Rachard, Raeshad, Raishard, Rashaad, Rashadd, Rashade, Rashaud, Rasheed, Rashid, Rashod, Reshad, Rhashad, Rishad, Roshad

Rashard (American) a form of Richard.
Rasharrd

Rashaud (Arabic) a form of Rashad.
Rachaud, Rashaude

Rashaun (American) a form of Rashawn.

Rashawn **BG** (American) a combination of the prefix Ra + Shawn.
Raashawn, Raashen, Raeshawn, Rahshawn, Raishawn, Rasaun, Rasawn, Rashaan, Rashaun, Rashaw, Rashon, Rashun, Raushan, Raushawn, Rhashan, Rhashaun, Rhashawn

Rashean (American) a combination of the prefix Ra + Sean.
Rahsaan, Rahsean, Rahseen, Rasean, Rashane, Rasheen, Rashien, Rashiena

Rasheed 🅱🅶 (Arabic) a form of Rashad.
Rashead, Rashed, Rasheid, Rhasheed

Rashid (Arabic) a form of Rashad.
Rasheyd, Rashida, Rashidah, Rashied, Rashieda, Raushaid

Rashida 🅶🅱 (Swahili) righteous.

Rashidi (Swahili) wise counselor.

Rashod (Arabic) a form of Rashad.
Rashoda, Rashodd, Rashoud, Rayshod, Rhashod

Rashon (American) a form of Rashawn.
Rashion, Rashone, Rashonn, Rashuan, Rashun, Rashunn

Rasmus (Greek, Danish) a short form of Erasmus.

Rauel (Hebrew) friend of God.

Raul (French) a form of Ralph.

Raulas (Lithuanian) a form of Laurence.

Raulo (Lithuanian) a form of Laurence.
Raulas

Raurac (Quechua) burning; ardent.

Raven 🅶🅱 (English) a short form of Ravenel.
Ravan, Ravean, Raveen, Ravin, Ravine, Ravon, Ravyn, Reven, Rhaven

Ravenel (English) raven.
Raven, Ravenell, Revenel

Ravi (Hindi) sun.
Ravee, Ravijot

Ravid (Hebrew) a form of Arvid.

Raviv (Hebrew) rain, dew.

Ravon (English) a form of Raven.
Raveon, Ravion, Ravone, Ravonn, Ravonne, Rayvon, Revon

Rawdon (English) rough hill.

Rawleigh (English) deer meadow.
Raleigh, Rawle, Rawley, Rawling, Rawly, Rawylyn

Rawlins (French) a form of Roland.
Rawlings, Rawlinson, Rawson

Ray 🅱🅶 (French) kingly, royal. (English) a short form of Rayburn, Raymond. See also Lei.
Rae, Raye

Rayan (Irish) a form of Ryan.
Rayaun

Rayburn (English) deer brook.
Burney, Raeborn, Raeborne, Raebourn, Ray, Raybourn, Raybourne, Rayburne

Rayce (English) a form of Race.

Rayden (Japanese) a form of Raiden.
Raidin, Raydun, Rayedon

Rayhan (Arabic) favored by God.
Rayhaan

Rayi (Hebrew) my friend, my companion.

Raymon (English) a form of Raymond.
Rayman, Raymann, Raymen, Raymone, Raymun, Reamonn

Raymond (English) mighty; wise protector. See also Aymon.
Radmond, Raemond, Raimondo, Raimund, Raimundo, Ramón, Ramond, Ramonde, Ramone, Ray, Raymand, Rayment, Raymon, Raymont, Raymund, Raymunde, Raymundo, Redmond, Reymond, Reymundo

Raymundo (Spanish) a form of Raymond.
Raemondo, Raimondo, Raimundo, Raymondo

Raynaldo (Spanish) a form of Reynold.
Raynal, Raynald, Raynold

Raynard (French) a form of Renard, Reynard.
Raynarde

Rayne (English) a form of Raine.
Raynee, Rayno

Raynor (Scandinavian) a form of Ragnar.
Rainer, Rainor, Ranier, Ranieri, Raynar, Rayner

Rayshawn (American) a combination of Ray + Shawn.
Raysean, Rayshaan, Rayshan, Rayshaun, Raysheen, Rayshon, Rayshone, Rayshonn, Rayshun, Rayshunn

Rayshod (American) a form of Rashad.
Raychard, Rayshad, Rayshard, Rayshaud

Rayvon (American) a form of Ravon.
Rayvan, Rayvaun, Rayven, Rayvone, Reyven, Reyvon

Razi BG (Aramaic) my secret.
Raz, Raziel, Raziq

Read (English) a form of Reed, Reid.
Raed, Raede, Raeed, Reaad, Reade

Reading (English) son of the red wanderer.
Redding, Reeding, Reiding

Reagan GB (Irish) little king. History: Ronald Wilson Reagan was the fortieth U.S. president.
Raegan, Reagen, Reaghan, Reegan, Reegen, Regan, Reigan, Reighan, Reign, Rheagan

Rebecca GB (Hebrew) tied, bound.

Rebekah GB (Hebrew) a form of Rebecca.

Rebel (American) rebel.
Reb

Recaredo (Teutonic) counsels his superiors.

Red (American) red, redhead.
Redd

Reda (Arabic) satisfied.
Ridha

Redford (English) red river crossing.
Ford, Radford, Reaford, Red, Redd

Redley (English) red meadow; meadow with reeds.
Radley, Redlea, Redleigh, Redly

Redmond (German) protecting counselor. (English) a form of Raymond.
Radmond, Radmund, Reddin, Redmund

Redpath (English) red path.

Reece ⓑⓖ (Welsh) a form of Rhys.
Reace, Rece, Reice, Reyes, Rhys, Rice, Ryese

Reed ⓑⓖ (English) a form of Reid.
Raeed, Read, Reyde, Rheed

Reese ⓑⓖ (Welsh) a form of Reece.
Rease, Rees, Reis, Reise, Reiss, Riese, Riess

Reeve (English) steward.
Reave, Reaves, Reeves

Reg (English) a short form of Reginald.

Regan ⓖⓑ (Irish) a form of Reagan.
Regen

Reggie ⓑⓖ (English) a familiar form of Reginald.
Regi, Regie

Reginal (English) a form of Reginald.
Reginale, Reginel

Reginald ⓑⓖ (English) king's advisor. A form of Reynold. See also Naldo.
Reg, Reggie, Regginald, Reggis, Reginal, Reginaldo, Reginalt, Reginauld, Reginault, Reginold, Reginuld, Regnauld, Ronald

Regis (Latin) regal.

Regulo, Régulo (Latin) forms of Rex. ⬝

Rehema (Swahili) second-born.

Rei ⓖⓑ (Japanese) rule, law.

Reid ⓑⓖ (English) redhead.
Read, Reed, Reide, Reyd, Ried

Reidar (Norwegian) nest warrior.

Reilly ⓑⓖ (Irish) a form of Riley.
Reiley, Reilley, Reily, Rielly

Reinaldo (Spanish) a form of Reynold.

Reinardo (Teutonic) valiant counselor.

Reinhart (German) a form of Reynard.
Rainart, Rainhard, Rainhardt,

*Rainhart, Reinart, Reinhard,
Reinhardt, Renke*

Reinhold (Swedish) a form of
Ragnar.
Reinold

Reku (Finnish) a form of Richard.

Remi, Rémi **BG** (French) forms
of Remy.
Remie, Remmie

Remigio (Latin) he who mans the
oars.

Remington **BG** (English) raven
estate.
Rem, Reminton, Tony

Remo (Greek) strong one.

Remus (Latin) speedy, quick.
Mythology: Remus and his twin
brother, Romulus, founded
Rome.

Remy (French) from Rheims,
France.
*Ramey, Remee, Remi, Rémi,
Remmy*

Renaldo (Spanish) a form of
Reynold.
Raynaldo, Reynaldo, Rinaldo

Renán (Irish) seal.

Renard (French) a form of
Reynard.
*Ranard, Raynard, Reinard,
Rennard*

Renardo (Italian) a form of
Reynard.

Renato (Italian) reborn.

Renaud (French) a form of
Reynard, Reynold.
*Renauld, Renauldo, Renault,
Renould*

Rendor (Hungarian) policeman.

Rene **BG** (Greek) a short form of
Irene, Renée.

René (French) reborn.
*Renat, Renato, Renatus, Renault,
Renay, Renee, Renny*

Renee **GB** (French) a form of
René.

Renfred (English) lasting peace.

Renfrew (Welsh) raven woods.

Renjiro (Japanese) virtuous.

Renny (Irish) small but strong.
(French) a familiar form of René.
Ren, Renn, Renne, Rennie

Reno (American) gambler.
Geography: a city in Nevada
known for gambling.
Renos, Rino

Renshaw (English) raven woods.
Renishaw

Renton (English) settlement of the
roe deer.

Renzo (Latin) a familiar form of
Laurence. (Italian) a short form
of Lorenzo.
Renz, Renzy, Renzzo

Repucura (Mapuche) jagged
rock; rocky road.

Reshad (American) a form of Rashad.
Reshade, Reshard, Resharrd, Reshaud, Reshawd, Reshead, Reshod

Reshawn (American) a combination of the prefix Re + Shawn.
Reshaun, Reshaw, Reshon, Reshun

Reshean (American) a combination of the prefix Re + Sean.
Resean, Reshae, Reshane, Reshay, Reshayne, Reshea, Resheen, Reshey

Restituto (Latin) he who returns to God.

Reuben (Hebrew) behold a son.
Reuban, Reubin, Reuven, Rheuben, Rhuben, Rube, Ruben, Rubey, Rubin, Ruby, Rueben

Reuven (Hebrew) a form of Reuben.
Reuvin, Rouvin, Ruvim

Rex (Latin) king.
Rexx

Rexford (English) king's ford.

Rexton (English) king's town.

Rey (Spanish) a short form of Reynaldo, Reynard, Reynold.

Reyes (English) a form of Reece.
Reyce

Reyhan 🅱🅖 (Arabic) favored by God.
Reyham

Reymond (English) a form of Raymond.
Reymon, Reymound, Reymund

Reymundo (Spanish) a form of Raymond.
Reimond, Reimonde, Reimundo, Reymon

Reynaldo (Spanish) a form of Reynold.
Renaldo, Rey, Reynauldo

Reynard (French) wise; bold, courageous.
Raynard, Reinhard, Reinhardt, Reinhart, Renard, Renardo, Renaud, Rennard, Rey, Reynardo, Reynaud

Reynold (English) king's advisor. See also Reginald.
Rainault, Rainhold, Ranald, Raynald, Raynaldo, Reinald, Reinaldo, Reinaldos, Reinhart, Reinhold, Reinold, Reinwald, Renald, Renaldi, Renaldo, Renaud, Renauld, Rennold, Renold, Rey, Reynald, Reynaldo, Reynaldos, Reynol, Reynolds, Rinaldo, Ronald

Réz 🅱🅖 (Hungarian) copper; redhead.
Rezsö

Rhett 🅱🅖 (Welsh) a form of Rhys. Literature: Rhett Butler was the hero of Margaret Mitchell's novel *Gone with the Wind*.
Rhet

Rhodes (Greek) where roses grow. Geography: an island of southeast Greece.
Rhoads, Rhodas, Rodas

Rhyan (Irish) a form of Rian.
Rhian

Rhys 🄱🄶 (Welsh) enthusiastic; stream.
Rhett, Rhyce, Rhyse, Rice

Rian (Irish) little king.
Rhyan

Ric (Italian, Spanish) a short form of Rico.
Ricca, Ricci, Ricco

Ricardo 🄱🄶 (Portuguese, Spanish) a form of Richard.
Racardo, Recard, Ricaldo, Ricard, Ricardoe, Ricardos, Riccardo, Riccarrdo, Ricciardo, Richardo

Rice (English) rich, noble. (Welsh) a form of Reece.
Ryce

Rich (English) a short form of Richard.
Ritch

Richard ⭐ 🄱🄶 (English) a form of Richart. See also Aric, Dick, Juku, Likeke.
Rashard, Reku, Ricardo, Rich, Richar, Richards, Richardson, Richart, Richaud, Richer, Richerd, Richie, Richird, Richshard, Rick, Rickard, Rickert, Rickey, Ricky, Rico, Rihardos, Rihards, Rikard, Riocard, Riócard, Risa, Risardas,
Rishard, Ristéard, Ritchard, Rostik, Rye, Rysio, Ryszard

Richart (German) rich and powerful ruler.

Richie (English) a familiar form of Richard.
Richey, Richi, Richy, Rishi, Ritchie

Richman (English) powerful.

Richmond (German) powerful protector.
Richmon, Richmound

Rick (German, English) a short form of Cedric, Frederick, Richard.
Ric, Ricke, Rickey, Ricks, Ricky, Rik, Riki, Rykk

Rickard (Swedish) a form of Richard.

Ricker (English) powerful army.

Rickey 🄱🄶 (English) a familiar form of Richard, Rick, Riqui.

Ricki 🄶🄱 (English) a form of Rickie.

Rickie (English) a form of Ricky.
Rickee, Ricki

Rickward (English) mighty guardian.
Rickwerd, Rickwood

Ricky 🄱🄶 (English) a familiar form of Richard, Rick.
Ricci, Rickie, Riczi, Riki, Rikki, Rikky, Riqui

Rico 🅱🅶 (Spanish) a familiar form
of Richard. (Italian) a short form
of Enrico.
Ric, Ricco

Rida 🅱🅶 (Arabic) favor.

Riddock (Irish) smooth field.
Riddick

Rider (English) horseman.
Ridder, Ryder

Ridge (English) ridge of a cliff.
Ridgy, Rig, Rigg

Ridgeley (English) meadow near
the ridge.
*Ridgeleigh, Ridglea, Ridglee,
Ridgleigh, Ridgley*

Ridgeway (English) path along
the ridge.

Ridley (English) meadow of
reeds.
*Rhidley, Riddley, Ridlea, Ridleigh,
Ridly*

Riel (Spanish) a short form of
Gabriel.

Rigby (English) ruler's valley.

Rigel (Arabic) foot. Astronomy:
one of the stars in the
constellation Orion.

Rigg (English) ridge.
Rigo

Rigoberto (German) splendid;
wealthy.
Rigobert

Rikard (Scandinavian) a form of
Richard.
Rikárd

Riki (Estonian) a form of Rick.
Rikkey, Rikki, Riks, Riky

Rikki 🅶🅱 (English) a form of
Ricky. (Estonian) a form of Riki.

Riley 🅱🅶 (Irish) valiant.
*Reilly, Rhiley, Rhylee, Rhyley,
Rieley, Rielly, Riely, Rilee, Rilley,
Rily, Rilye, Rylee, Ryley*

Rimac (Quechua) speaker,
eloquent.

Rimachi (Quechua) he who
makes us speak.

Rinaldo (Italian) a form of
Reynold.
Rinald, Rinaldi

Ring (English) ring.
Ringo

Ringo (Japanese) apple. (English)
a familiar form of Ring.

Rio (Spanish) river. Geography:
Rio de Janeiro is a city in Brazil.

Riordan (Irish) bard, royal poet.
Rearden, Reardin, Reardon

Rip (Dutch) ripe; full grown.
(English) a short form of Ripley.
Ripp

Ripley (English) meadow near the
river.
Rip, Ripleigh, Ripply

Riqui (Spanish) a form of Rickey.

Rishad (American) a form of Rashad.
Rishaad

Rishawn (American) a combination of the prefix Ri + Shawn.
Rishan, Rishaun, Rishon, Rishone

Rishi (Hindi) sage.

Risley (English) meadow with shrubs.
Rislea, Rislee, Risleigh, Risly, Wrisley

Risto (Finnish) a short form of Christopher.

Riston (English) settlement near the shrubs.
Wriston

Ritchard (English) a form of Richard.
Ritcherd, Ritchyrd, Ritshard, Ritsherd

Ritchie (English) a form of Richie.
Ritchy

Rithisak (Cambodian) powerful.

Ritter (German) knight; chivalrous.
Rittner

River BG (English) river; riverbank.
Rivers, Riviera, Rivor

Riyad (Arabic) gardens.
Riad, Riyaad, Riyadh, Riyaz, Riyod

Roald (Norwegian) famous ruler.

Roan (English) a short form of Rowan.
Rhoan

Roano (Spanish) reddish brown skin.

Roar (Norwegian) praised warrior.
Roary

Roarke (Irish) famous ruler.
Roark, Rorke, Rourke, Ruark

Rob (English) a short form of Robert.
Robb, Robe

Robbie BG (English) a familiar form of Robert.
Robie, Robbi

Robby (English) a familiar form of Robert.
Rhobbie, Robbey, Robhy, Roby

Robert ☆ BG (English) famous brilliance. See also Bobek, Dob, Lopaka.
Bob, Bobby, Rab, Rabbie, Raby, Riobard, Riobart, Rob, Robars, Robart, Robbie, Robby, Rober, Roberd, Robers, Roberte, Roberto, Roberts, Robin, Robinson, Roibeárd, Rosertas, Rubert, Ruberto, Rudbert, Rupert

Robertino (Spanish) a form of Roberto.

Roberto BG (Italian, Portuguese, Spanish) a form of Robert.

Roberts, Robertson (English)
son of Robert.
Roberson, Robertson, Robeson,
Robinson, Robson

Robin 🆖 (English) a short form
of Robert.
Robben, Robbin, Robbins,
Robbyn, Roben, Robinet, Robinn,
Robins, Robyn, Roibín

Robinson (English) a form of
Roberts.
Robbinson, Robens, Robenson,
Robson, Robynson

Robustiano (Latin) strong as the
wood of an oak tree.

Robyn 🆖 (English) a form of
Robin.

Roca, Ruca (Aymara) principal,
chief, prince; strong.

Rocco (Italian) rock.
Rocca, Rocio, Rocko, Rocky, Roko,
Roque

Rochelle 🆖 (French) large
stone. (Hebrew) a form of
Rachel.

Rochester (English) rocky
fortress.
Chester, Chet

Rock (English) a short form of
Rockwell.
Roch, Rocky

Rockford (English) rocky ford.

Rockland (English) rocky land.

Rockledge (English) rocky ledge.

Rockley (English) rocky field.
Rockle

Rockwell (English) rocky spring.
Art: Norman Rockwell was a well-
known twentieth-century
American illustrator.
Rock

Rocky (American) a familiar form
of Rocco, Rock.
Rockey, Rockie

Rod (English) a short form of
Penrod, Roderick, Rodney.
Rodd

Rodas (Greek, Spanish) a form of
Rhodes.

Roddy (English) a familiar form
of Roderick.
Roddie, Rody

Rode (Greek) pink.

Roden (English) red valley. Art:
Auguste Rodin was an innovative
French sculptor.
Rodin

Roderich (German) a form of
Roderick.

Roderick (German) famous ruler.
See also Broderick.
Rhoderick, Rod, Rodderick, Roddy,
Roderic, Roderich, Roderigo,
Roderik, Roderrick, Roderyck,
Rodgrick, Rodrick, Rodricki,
Rodrigo, Rodrigue, Rodrugue,
Roodney, Rory, Rurik, Ruy

Rodger (German) a form of
Roger.
Rodge, Rodgy

Rodman (German) famous man,
hero.
Rodmond

Rodney **BG** (English) island
clearing.
*Rhodney, Rod, Rodnee, Rodnei,
Rodni, Rodnie, Rodnne, Rodny*

Rodolfo (Spanish) a form of
Rudolph.
Rodolpho, Rodulfo

Rodrick (German) a form of
Roderick.
*Roddrick, Rodric, Rodrich, Rodrik,
Rodrique, Rodryck, Rodryk*

Rodrigo (Italian, Spanish) a form
of Roderick.

Rodriguez (Spanish) son of
Rodrigo.
Roddrigues, Rodrigues, Rodriquez

Rodrik (German) famous ruler.

Rodriquez (Spanish) a form of
Rodriguez.
*Rodrigquez, Rodriques,
Rodriquiez*

Roe (English) roe deer.
Row, Rowe

Rogan (Irish) redhead.
Rogein, Rogen

Rogelio **BG** (Spanish) famous
warrior.
Rojelio

Roger (German) famous
spearman. See also Lokela.
*Rodger, Rog, Rogelio, Rogerick,
Rogerio, Rogers, Rogiero, Rojelio,
Rüdiger, Ruggerio, Rutger*

Rogerio (Portuguese, Spanish) a
form of Roger.
Rogerios

Rohan (Hindi) sandalwood.

Rohin (Hindi) upward path.

Rohit (Hindi) big and beautiful
fish.

Roi (French) a form of Roy.

Roja (Spanish) red.
Rojay

Rolán (Spanish) a form of
Rolando.

Roland (German) famous
throughout the land.
*Loránd, Orlando, Rawlins, Rolan,
Rolanda, Rolando, Rolek, Rolland,
Rolle, Rollie, Rollin, Rollo, Rowe,
Rowland, Ruland*

Rolando **BG** (Portuguese,
Spanish) a form of Roland.
*Lando, Olo, Roldan, Roldán,
Rolondo*

Rolf (German) a form of Ralph. A
short form of Rudolph.
Rolfe, Rolle, Rolph, Rolphe

Rolle (Swedish) a familiar form of
Roland, Rolf.

Rollie (English) a familiar form of Roland.
Roley, Rolle, Rolli, Rolly

Rollin (English) a form of Roland.
Rolin, Rollins

Rollo (English) a familiar form of Roland.
Rolla, Rolo

Rolon (Spanish) famous wolf.

Romain (French) a form of Roman.
Romaine, Romane, Romanne

Roman, Román (Latin) from Rome, Italy.
Roma, Romain, Romann, Romanos, Romman, Romochka, Romy

Romanos (Greek) a form of Roman.
Romano

Romario (Italian) a form of Romeo.
Romar, Romarius, Romaro, Romarrio

Romel (Latin) a short form of Romulus.
Romele, Romell, Romello, Rommel

Romelio (Hebrew) God's very beloved one.

Romello (Italian) of Romel.
Romelo, Rommello

Romeo (Italian) pilgrim to Rome; Roman. Literature: the title character of the Shakespearean play *Romeo and Juliet*.
Romario, Roméo, Romero

Romero (Latin) a form of Romeo.
Romario, Romeiro, Romer, Romere, Romerio, Romeris, Romeryo

Romildo (Germanic) glorious hero.

Romney (Welsh) winding river.
Romoney

Romualdo (Germanic) glorious king.

Rómulo (Greek) he who is full of strength.

Romulus (Latin) citizen of Rome. Mythology: Romulus and his twin brother, Remus, founded Rome.
Romel, Romolo, Romono, Romulo

Romy GB (Italian) a familiar form of Roman.
Rommie, Rommy

Ron (Hebrew) a short form of Aaron, Ronald.
Ronn

Ronald BG (Scottish) a form of Reginald.
Ranald, Ron, Ronal, Ronaldo, Ronnald, Ronney, Ronnie, Ronnold, Ronoldo

Ronaldo (Portuguese) a form of Ronald.

Rónán (Irish) seal.
Renan, Ronan, Ronat

Rondel (French) short poem.
Rondal, Rondale, Rondall, Rondeal, Rondell, Rondey, Rondie, Rondrell, Rondy, Ronel

Ronel (American) a form of Rondel.
Ronell, Ronelle, Ronnel, Ronnell, Ronyell

Roni (Hebrew) my song; my joy.
Rani, Roneet, Roney, Ronit, Ronli, Rony

Ronnie **BG** (Scottish) a familiar form of Ronald.
Roni, Ronie, Ronnie, Ronny

Ronny **BG** (Scottish) a form of Ronnie.
Ronney

Ronson (Scottish) son of Ronald.
Ronaldson

Ronté (American) a combination of Ron + the suffix Te.
Rontae, Rontay, Ronte, Rontez

Rooney (Irish) redhead.

Roosevelt (Dutch) rose field. History: Theodore and Franklin D. Roosevelt were the twenty-sixth and thirty-second U.S. presidents, respectively.
Roosvelt, Rosevelt

Roper (English) rope maker.

Rory **BG** (German) a familiar form of Roderick. (Irish) red king.
Rorey, Rori, Rorrie, Rorry

Rosa **GB** (Italian, Spanish) a form of Rose (see Girls' Names).

Rosalio (Spanish) rose.
Rosalino

Rosario **GB** (Portuguese) rosary.

Roscoe (Scandinavian) deer forest.
Rosco

Rosendo (Germanic) excellent master.

Roshad (American) a form of Rashad.
Roshard

Roshean (American) a combination of the prefix Ro + Sean.
Roshain, Roshan, Roshane, Roshaun, Roshawn, Roshay, Rosheen, Roshene

Rosito (Filipino) rose.

Ross **BG** (Latin) rose. (Scottish) peninsula. (French) red.
Rosse, Rossell, Rossi, Rossie, Rossy

Rosswell (English) springtime of roses.
Rosvel

Rostislav (Czech) growing glory.
Rosta, Rostya

Roswald (English) field of roses.
Ross, Roswell

Roth (German) redhead.

Rothwell (Scandinavian) red spring.

Rover (English) traveler.

Rowan **GB** (English) tree with red berries.
Roan, Rowe, Rowen, Rowney, Rowyn

Rowell (English) roe-deer well.

Rowland (English) rough land. (German) a form of Roland.
Rowlando, Rowlands, Rowlandson

Rowley (English) rough meadow.
Rowlea, Rowlee, Rowleigh, Rowly

Rowson (English) son of the redhead.

Roxbury (English) rook's town or fortress.
Roxburghe

Roy (French) king. A short form of Royal, Royce. See also Conroy, Delroy, Fitzroy, Leroy, Loe.
Rey, Roi, Roye, Ruy

Royal (French) kingly, royal.
Roy, Royale, Royall, Royell

Royce 🅱🅶 (English) son of Roy.
Roice, Roy, Royz

Royden (English) rye hill.
Royd, Roydan

Ruben 🅱🅶 (Hebrew) a form of Reuben.
Ruban, Rube, Rubean, Rubens, Rubin, Ruby

Rubén (Hebrew) a form of Ruben.

Rubert (Czech) a form of Robert.

Ruby 🅶🅱 (Hebrew) a familiar form of Reuben, Ruben.

Rucahue (Mapuche) place of construction, field that is used for construction.

Rucalaf (Mapuche) sanitarium, resting home; house of joy.

Ruda (Czech) a form of Rudolph.
Rude, Rudek

Rudd (English) a short form of Rudyard.

Rudecindo (Spanish) a form of Rosendo.

Rudesindo (Teutonic) excellent gentleman.

Rudi (Spanish) a familiar form of Rudolph.
Ruedi

Rudo (Shona) love.

Rudolf (German) a form of Rudolph.
Rodolf, Rodolfo, Rudolfo

Rudolph (German) famous wolf. See also Dolf.
Raoul, Rezsó, Rodolfo, Rodolph, Rodolphe, Rolf, Ruda, Rudek, Rudi, Rudolf, Rudolpho, Rudolphus, Rudy

Rudolpho (Italian) a form of Rudolph.

Rudy 🅱🅶 (English) a familiar form of Rudolph.
Roody, Ruddy, Ruddie, Rudey, Rudi, Rudie

Rudyard (English) red enclosure.
Rudd

Rueben (Hebrew) a form of
Reuben.
Rueban, Ruebin

Rufay (Quechua) warm.

Ruff (French) redhead.

Rufin (Polish) redhead.
Rufino

Rufio (Latin) red-haired.

Ruford (English) red ford; ford
with reeds.
Rufford

Rufus (Latin) redhead.
*Rayfus, Rufe, Ruffis, Ruffus,
Rufino, Rufo, Rufous*

Rugby (English) rook fortress.
History: a famous British school
after which the sport of Rugby
was named.

Ruggerio (Italian) a form of
Roger.
Rogero, Ruggero, Ruggiero

Ruhakana (Rukiga)
argumentative.

Ruland (German) a form of
Roland.
Rulan, Rulon, Rulondo

Rumford (English) wide river
crossing.

Rumi (Quechua) strong and as
eternal as a rock.

Rumimaqui, Rumiñaui
(Quechua) he who has strong
hands, hands of stone.

Rumisonjo, Rumisuncu
(Quechua) hard-hearted, heart of
stone.

Runacatu, Runacoto (Quechua)
short man, small man.

Runako (Shona) handsome.

Rune (German, Swedish) secret.

Runrot (Tai) prosperous.

Runto, Runtu (Quechua)
hailstone.

Rupert (German) a form of
Robert.
Ruperth, Ruperto, Ruprecht

Ruperto (Italian) a form of
Rupert.

Rupinder GB (Sanskrit)
handsome.

Ruprecht (German) a form of
Rupert.

Rush (French) redhead. (English)
a short form of Russell.
Rushi

Rushford (English) ford with
rushes.

Rusk (Spanish) twisted bread.

Ruskin (French) redhead.
Rush, Russ

Russ (French) a short form of
Russell.

Russel (French) a form of
Russell.

Russell (French) redhead; fox colored. See also Lukela.
Roussell, Rush, Russ, Russel, Russelle, Rusty

Rusty (French) a familiar form of Russell.
Ruste, Rusten, Rustie, Rustin, Ruston, Rustyn

Rutger (Scandinavian) a form of Roger.
Ruttger

Rutherford (English) cattle ford.
Rutherfurd

Rutland (Scandinavian) red land.

Rutledge (English) red ledge.

Rutley (English) red meadow.

Ruy (Spanish) a short form of Roderick.
Rui

Ruyan (Spanish) little king.

Ryan ☼ 🅱🅶 (Irish) little king.
Rayan, Rhyan, Rhyne, Ryane, Ryann, Ryen, Ryian, Ryiann, Ryin, Ryne, Ryon, Ryuan, Ryun, Ryyan

Ryann 🅶🅱 (Irish) a form of Ryan.

Rycroft (English) rye field.
Ryecroft

Ryder (English) a form of Rider.
Rydder, Rye

Rye (English) a short form of Ryder. A grain used in cereal and whiskey. (Gypsy) gentleman.
Ry

Ryen (Irish) a form of Ryan.
Ryein, Ryien

Ryerson (English) son of Rider, Ryder.

Ryese (English) a form of Reece.
Reyse, Ryez, Ryse

Ryker (American) a surname used as a first name.
Riker, Ryk

Rylan 🅱🅶 (English) land where rye is grown.
Ryland, Rylean, Rylen, Rylin, Rylon, Rylyn, Rylynn

Ryland (English) a form of Rylan.
Ryeland, Rylund

Ryle (English) rye hill.
Ryal, Ryel

Rylee 🅶🅱 (Irish) a form of Riley.
Ryeleigh, Ryleigh, Rylie, Rillie

Ryley 🅱🅶 (Irish) a form of Riley.
Ryely

Ryman (English) rye seller.

Ryne (Irish) a form of Ryan.
Rynn

Ryon (Irish) a form of Ryan.

S

S 🅶🅱 (American) an initial used as a first name.

Sa'id (Arabic) happy.
*Sa'ad, Saaid, Saed, Sa'eed,
Saeed, Sahid, Saide, Sa'ied,
Saied, Saiyed, Saiyeed, Sajid,
Sajjid, Sayed, Sayeed, Sayid,
Seyed, Shahid*

Sabastian (Greek) a form of
Sebastian.
*Sabastain, Sabastiano,
Sabastien, Sabastin, Sabastion,
Sabaston, Sabbastiun, Sabestian*

Sabelio (Spanish) a form of
Sabino.

Saber (French) sword.
Sabir, Sabre

Sabin (Basque) ancient tribe of
central Italy.
*Saban, Saben, Sabian, Sabien,
Sabino*

Sabino (Basque) a form of Sabin.

Sabiti (Rutooro) born on Sunday.

Sabola (Nguni) pepper.

Sabrina GB (Latin) boundary
line. (English) child of royalty.
(Hebrew) a familiar form of
Sabra (see Girls' Names).

Saburo (Japanese) third-born
son.

Sacha BG (Russian) a form of
Sasha.
Sascha

Sachar (Russian) a form of
Zachary.

Saddam (Arabic) powerful ruler.

Sade GB (Hebrew) a form of
Sarah.

Sadiki (Swahili) faithful.
*Saadiq, Sadeek, Sadek, Sadik,
Sadiq, Sadique*

Sadler (English) saddle maker.
Saddler

Sadoc (Hebrew) just one.

Safari (Swahili) born while
traveling.
Safa, Safarian

Safford (English) willow river
crossing.

Sage BG (English) wise. Botany:
an herb.
Sagen, Sager, Saige, Saje

Sahale (Native American) falcon.
Sael, Sahal, Sahel, Sahil

Sahen (Hindi) above.
Sahan

Sahil (Native American) a form of
Sahale.
Saheel, Sahel

Sahir (Hindi) friend.

Sajag (Hindi) watchful.

Saka (Swahili) hunter.

Sakeri (Danish) a form of
Zachary.
Sakarai, Sakari

Sakima (Native American) king.

Sakuruta (Pawnee) coming sun.

Sal (Italian) a short form of
Salvatore.

Salam (Arabic) lamb.
Salaam

Salamon (Spanish) a form of
Solomon.
Saloman, Salomón

Salaun (French) a form of
Solomon.

Sálih (Arabic) right, good.
Saleeh, Saleh, Salehe

Salim (Swahili) peaceful.

Salím (Arabic) peaceful, safe.
Saleem, Salem, Saliym, Salman

Sally GB (Italian) a familiar form
of Salvatore.

Salmalin (Hindi) taloned.

Salman (Czech) a form of Salím,
Solomon.
Salmaan, Salmaine, Salmon

Salomon (French) a form of
Solomon.
Salomone

Salton (English) manor town;
willow town.

Salustio (Latin) he who offers
salvation.

Salvador (Spanish) savior.
Salvadore

Salvatore (Italian) savior. See
also Xavier.
Sal, Salbatore, Sallie, Sally,

*Salvator, Salvattore, Salvidor,
Sauveur*

Salviano (Spanish) a form of
Salvo.

Salvio (Latin) cured, healthy;
upright.

Salvo (Latin) healthy one.

Sam BG (Hebrew) a short form of
Samuel.
*Samm, Sammy, Sem, Shem,
Shmuel*

Samantha GB (Aramaic) listener.
(Hebrew) told by God.

Sambo (American) a familiar
form of Samuel.
Sambou

Sameer (Arabic) a form of Samír.

Sami, Samy BG (Hebrew) forms
of Sammy.
*Sameeh, Sameh, Samie, Samih,
Sammi*

Samín (Quechua) fortunate,
lucky; adventurous; successful;
happy.

Samír (Arabic) entertaining
companion.
Sameer

Samman (Arabic) grocer.
Saman, Sammon

Sammy BG (Hebrew) a familiar
form of Samuel.
*Saamy, Samey, Sami, Sammee,
Sammey, Sammie, Samy*

Samo (Czech) a form of Samuel.
Samho, Samko

Samson (Hebrew) like the sun. Bible: a judge and powerful warrior betrayed by Delilah.
Sampson, Sansao, Sansom, Sansón, Shem, Shimshon

Samual (Hebrew) a form of Samuel.
Samuael, Samuail

Samuel ✰ BG (Hebrew) heard God; asked of God. Bible: a famous Old Testament prophet and judge. See also Kamuela, Zamiel, Zanvil.
Sam, Samael, Samaru, Samauel, Samaul, Sambo, Sameul, Samiel, Sammail, Sammel, Sammuel, Sammy, Samo, Samouel, Samu, Samual, Samuele, Samuelis, Samuell, Samuello, Samuil, Samuka, Samule, Samuru, Samvel, Sanko, Saumel, Schmuel, Shem, Shmuel, Simão, Simuel, Somhairle, Zamuel

Samuele (Italian) a form of Samuel.
Samulle

Samuelle GB (Hebrew) a form of Samuela (see Girls' Names).

Samuru (Japanese) a form of Samuel.

Sanat (Hindi) ancient.

Sanborn (English) sandy brook.
Sanborne, Sanbourn, Sanbourne, Sanburn, Sanburne, Sandborn, Sandbourne

Sanchez (Latin) a form of Sancho.
Sanchaz, Sancheze

Sancho (Latin) sanctified; sincere. Literature: Sancho Panza was Don Quixote's squire.
Sanchez, Sauncho

Sandeep BG (Punjabi) enlightened.
Sandip

Sander (English) a short form of Alexander, Lysander.
Sandor, Sándor, Saunder

Sanders (English) son of Sander.
Sanderson, Saunders, Saunderson

Sándor (Hungarian) a short form of Alexander.
Sanyi

Sandro (Greek, Italian) a short form of Alexander.
Sandero, Sandor, Sandre, Saundro, Shandro

Sandy GB (English) a familiar form of Alexander.
Sande, Sandey, Sandi, Sandie

Sanford (English) sandy river crossing.
Sandford

Sani (Hindi) the planet Saturn. (Navajo) old.

Sanjay (Sanskrit) triumphant. (American) a combination of Sanford + Jay.
Sanjaya, Sanje, Sanjey, Sanjo

Sanjiv (Hindi) long lived.
Sanjeev

Sankar (Hindi) a form of Shankara, another name for the Hindu god Shiva.

Sansón (Spanish) a form of Samson.
Sanson, Sansone, Sansun

Santana ⚥ (Spanish) Saint Anne. History: Antonio López de Santa Anna was a Mexican general and political leader.
Santanna

Santiago (Spanish) Saint James.

Santino (Spanish) a form of Santonio.
Santion

Santo (Italian, Spanish) holy.
Santos

Santon (English) sandy town.

Santonio (Spanish) a short form of San Antonio or Saint Anthony.
Santino, Santon, Santoni

Santos (Spanish) saint.
Santo

Santosh (Hindi) satisfied.

Sanyu ⚥ (Luganda) happy.

Sapay (Quechua) unique; main.

Saqr (Arabic) falcon.

Saquan (American) a combination of the prefix Sa + Quan.
Saquané, Saquin, Saquon, Saqwan, Saqwone

Sara ⚥ (Hebrew) a form of Sarah.

Sarad (Hindi) born in the autumn.

Sarah ⚥ (Hebrew) child of royalty.

Sargent (French) army officer.
Sargant, Sarge, Sarjant, Sergeant, Sergent, Serjeant

Sarito (Spanish) a form of Caesar.
Sarit

Saritupac (Quechua) glorious prince.

Sariyah (Arabic) clouds at night.

Sarngin (Hindi) archer; protector.

Sarojin (Hindi) like a lotus.
Sarojun

Sasha ⚥ (Russian) a short form of Alexander.
Sacha, Sash, Sashenka, Sashka, Sashok, Sausha

Sasson (Hebrew) joyful.
Sason

Satchel (French) small bag.
Satch

Satordi (French) Saturn.
Satori

Saturio (Latin) protector of the sown fields.

Saturnín (Spanish) gift of Saturn.

Saturnino (Spanish) a form of Saturno.

Saturno (Latin) he who is living an abundant life.

Saul BG (Hebrew) asked for, borrowed. Bible: in the Old Testament, a king of Israel and the father of Jonathan; in the New Testament, Saint Paul's original name was Saul.
Saül, Shaul, Sol, Solly

Saúl (Hebrew) a form of Saul.

Saulo (Greek) he who is tender and delicate.

Savannah GB (Spanish) treeless plain.

Saverio (Italian) a form of Xavier.

Saville (French) willow town.
Savelle, Savil, Savile, Savill, Savylle, Seville, Siville

Savon BG (Spanish) a treeless plain.
Savan, Savaughn, Saveion, Saveon, Savhon, Saviahn, Savian, Savino, Savion, Savo, Savone, Sayvon, Sayvone

Saw (Burmese) early.

Sawyer BG (English) wood worker.
Sawyere

Sax (English) a short form of Saxon.
Saxe

Saxon (English) swordsman. History: the Roman name for the Teutonic raiders who ravaged the Roman British coasts.
Sax, Saxen, Saxsin, Saxxon

Sayani (Quechua) I stay on foot.

Sayarumi (Quechua) erect and strong as stone.

Sayer (Welsh) carpenter.
Say, Saye, Sayers, Sayr, Sayre, Sayres

Sayri (Quechua) prince; he who is always helping those who ask for it.

Sayyid (Arabic) master.
Sayed, Sayid, Sayyad, Sayyed

Scanlon (Irish) little trapper.
Scanlan, Scanlen

Schafer (German) shepherd.
Schaefer, Schaffer, Schiffer, Shaffar, Shäffer

Schmidt (German) blacksmith.
Schmid, Schmit, Schmitt, Schmydt

Schneider (German) tailor.
Schnieder, Snider, Snyder

Schön (German) handsome.
Schoen, Schönn, Shon

Schuyler (Dutch) sheltering.
Schuylar, Schyler, Scoy, Scy, Skuyler, Sky, Skylar, Skyler, Skylor

Schyler GB (Dutch) a form of Schuyler.
Schylar, Schylre, Schylur

Scorpio (Latin) dangerous, deadly. Astronomy: a southern constellation near Libra and Sagittarius. Astrology: the eighth sign of the zodiac.
Scorpeo

Scott BG (English) from Scotland. A familiar form of Prescott.
Scot, Scottie, Scotto, Scotty

Scottie (English) a familiar form of Scott.
Scotie, Scotti

Scotty (English) a familiar form of Scott.
Scottey

Scoville (French) Scott's town.

Scully (Irish) town crier.

Seabert (English) shining sea.
Seabright, Sebert, Seibert

Seabrook (English) brook near the sea.

Seamus (Irish) a form of James.
Seamas, Seumas, Shamus

Sean ☆ BG (Irish) a form of John.
Seaghan, Séan, Seán, Seanán, Seane, Seann, Shaan, Shaine, Shane, Shaun, Shawn, Shayne, Shon, Siôn

Searlas (Irish, French) a form of Charles.
Séarlas, Searles, Searlus

Searle (English) armor.

Seasar (Latin) a form of Caesar.
Seasare, Seazar, Sesar, Sesear, Sezar

Seaton (English) town near the sea.
Seeton, Seton

Sebastian ☆ BG (Greek) venerable. (Latin) revered.
Bastian, Sabastian, Sabastien, Sebashtian, Sebastain, Sebastiane, Sebastiano, Sebastien, Sébastien, Sebastin, Sebastine, Sebaston, Sebbie, Sebestyén, Sebo, Sepasetiano

Sebastián (Greek) a form of Sebastian.

Sebastien, Sébastien BG (French) forms of Sebastian.
Sebasten, Sebastyen

Sebastion (Greek) a form of Sebastian.

Sedgely (English) sword meadow.
Sedgeley, Sedgly

Sedric (Irish) a form of Cedric.
Seddrick, Sederick, Sedrick, Sedrik, Sedriq

Seeley (English) blessed.
Sealey, Seely, Selig

Sef (Egyptian) yesterday. Mythology: one of the two lions that make up the Akeru, guardian of the gates of morning and night.

Sefton (English) village of rushes.

Sefu (Swahili) sword.

Seger (English) sea spear; sea warrior.
Seager, Seeger, Segar

Segismundo (Germanic) victorious protector.

Segun (Yoruba) conqueror.

Segundino (Latin) family's second son.

Segundo (Spanish) second.

Seibert (English) bright sea.
Seabert, Sebert

Seif (Arabic) religion's sword.

Seifert (German) a form of Siegfried.

Sein (Basque) innocent.

Sekaye (Shona) laughter.

Selby (English) village by the mansion.
Selbey, Shelby

Seldon (English) willow tree valley.
Selden, Sellden

Selemías (Hebrew) God rewards.

Selena GB (Greek) moon.

Selig (German) a form of Seeley.
Seligman, Seligmann, Zelig

Selwyn (English) friend from the palace.
Selvin, Selwin, Selwinn, Selwynn, Selwynne, Wyn

Semanda (Luganda) cow clan.

Semarias (Hebrew) God guarded him.

Semer (Ethiopian) a form of George.
Semere, Semier

Semon (Greek) a form of Simon.
Semion

Sempala (Luganda) born in prosperous times.

Sempronio (Latin) name of a Roman family based on male descent.

Sen BG (Japanese) wood fairy.
Senh

Séneca (Latin) venerable elderly man.

Sener (Turkish) bringer of joy.

Senín (Grego) god Jupiter.

Senior (French) lord.

Sennett (French) elderly.
Sennet

Senon (Spanish) living.

Senwe (African) dry as a grain stalk.

Sepp (German) a form of Joseph.
Seppi

Septimio (Latin) seventh child.

Séptimo (Latin) family's seventh son.

Septimus (Latin) seventh.

Serafín (Hebrew) a form of Seraphim.

Serafino (Portuguese) a form of Seraphim.

Seraphim (Hebrew) fiery, burning. Bible: the highest order of angels, known for their zeal and love.
Saraf, Saraph, Serafim, Serafin, Serafino, Seraphimus, Seraphin

Serapio (Latin) consecrated to Serapes, an Egyptian divinity.

Sereno (Latin) calm, tranquil.

Serge (Latin) attendant.
Seargeoh, Serg, Sergei, Sergio, Sergios, Sergius, Sergiusz, Serguel, Sirgio, Sirgios

Sergei (Russian) a form of Serge.
Sergey, Sergeyuk, Serghey, Sergi, Sergie, Sergo, Sergunya, Serhiy, Serhiyko, Serjiro, Serzh

Sergio (Italian) a form of Serge.
Serginio, Serigo, Serjio

Servando (Spanish) to serve.
Servan, Servio

Seth ☆ BG (Hebrew) appointed. Bible: the third son of Adam.
Set, Sethan, Sethe, Shet

Setimba (Luganda) river dweller. Geography: a river in Uganda.

Seumas (Scottish) a form of James.
Seaumus

Severiano (Italian) a form of Séverin.

Séverin (French) severe.
Seve, Sevé, Severan, Severian, Severiano, Severo, Sevien, Sevrin, Sevryn

Severino (Spanish) a form of Severo.

Severn (English) boundary.
Sevearn, Sevren, Sevrnn

Severo (French) a form of Séverin.

Sevilen (Turkish) beloved.

Seward (English) sea guardian.
Sewerd, Siward

Sewati (Moquelumnan) curved bear claws.

Sexton (English) church official; sexton.

Sextus (Latin) sixth.
Sixtus

Seymour (French) prayer. Religion: name honoring Saint Maur. See also Maurice.
Seamor, Seamore, Seamour, See

Shabouh (Armenian) king, noble. History: a fourth-century Persian king.

Shad (Punjabi) happy-go-lucky.
Shadd

Shadi (Arabic) singer.
*Shadde, Shaddi, Shaddy, Shade,
Shadee, Shadeed, Shadey,
Shadie, Shady, Shydee, Shydi*

Shadrach (Babylonian) god;
godlike. Bible: one of three
companions who emerged
unharmed from the fiery furnace
of Babylon.
*Shad, Shadrack, Shadrick,
Sheddrach, Shedrach, Shedrick*

Shadwell (English) shed by a
well.

Shae **GB** (Irish) a form of Shay.

Shah (Persian) king. History: a
title for rulers of Iran.

Shaheem (American) a
combination of Shah + Raheem.
Shaheim, Shahiem, Shahm

Shahid (Arabic) a form of Sa'id.
Shahed, Shaheed

Shai (Hebrew) a short form of
Yeshaya.
Shaie

Shaiming (Chinese) life;
sunshine.

Shaina **GB** (Yiddish) beautiful.

Shaine (Irish) a form of Sean.
Shain

Shaka **BG** (Zulu) founder, first.
History: Shaka Zulu was the
founder of the Zulu empire.

Shakeel (Arabic) a form of
Shaquille.
*Shakeil, Shakel, Shakell, Shakiel,
Shakil, Shakille, Shakyle*

Shakir (Arabic) thankful.
Shaakir, Shakeer, Shakeir, Shakur

Shakur (Arabic) a form of Shakir.
Shakuur

Shalom (Hebrew) peace.
*Shalum, Shlomo, Sholem,
Sholom*

Shalya (Hindi) throne.

Shaman (Sanskrit) holy man,
mystic, medicine man.
*Shamaine, Shamaun, Shamin,
Shamine, Shammon, Shamon,
Shamone*

Shamar (Hebrew) a form of
Shamir.
Shamaar, Shamare, Shamari

Shamir (Hebrew) precious stone.
*Shahmeer, Shahmir, Shamar,
Shameer, Shamyr*

Shamus (American) slang for
detective.
*Shamas, Shames, Shamos,
Shemus*

Shan (Irish) a form of Shane.
Shann, Shanne

Shanahan (Irish) wise, clever.

Shandy (English) rambunctious.
Shandey, Shandie

Shane **BG** (Irish) a form of Sean.
Shan, Shayn, Shayne

Shangobunni (Yoruba) gift from Shango.

Shanley 🄶🄱 (Irish) small; ancient.
Shaneley, Shannley

Shannon 🄶🄱 (Irish) small and wise.
Shanan, Shannan, Shannen, Shannin, Shannone, Shanon

Shantae 🄶🄱 (French) a form of Chante.
Shant, Shanta, Shantai, Shante, Shantell, Shantelle, Shanti, Shantia, Shantie, Shanton, Shanty

Shante 🄶🄱 (French) a form of Shantae.

Shantell 🄶🄱 (American) song.

Shap (English) a form of Shep.

Shaquan (American) a combination of the prefix Sha + Quan.
Shaqaun, Shaquand, Shaquane, Shaquann, Shaquaunn, Shaquawn, Shaquen, Shaquian, Shaquin, Shaqwan

Shaquell (American) a form of Shaquille.
Shaqueal, Shaqueil, Shaquel, Shaquelle, Shaquiel, Shaquiell, Shaquielle

Shaquille 🄱🄶 (Arabic) handsome.
Shakeel, Shaquell, Shaquil, Shaquile, Shaquill, Shaqul

Shaquon (American) a combination of the prefix Sha + Quon.
Shaikwon, Shaqon, Shaquoin, Shaquoné

Sharad (Pakistani) autumn.
Sharod

Sharíf (Arabic) honest; noble.
Shareef, Sharef, Shareff, Shareif, Sharief, Sharife, Shariff, Shariyf, Sharrif, Sharyif

Sharod (Pakistani) a form of Sharad.
Sharrod

Sharon 🄶🄱 (Hebrew) a form of Sharron.

Sharron (Hebrew) flat area, plain.
Sharon, Sharone, Sharonn, Sharonne

Shattuck (English) little shad fish.

Shaun 🄱🄶 (Irish) a form of Sean.
Shaughan, Shaughn, Shaugn, Shauna, Shaunahan, Shaune, Shaunn, Shaunne

Shavar (Hebrew) comet.
Shavit

Shavon 🄶🄱 (American) a combination of the prefix Sha + Yvon.
Shauvan, Shauvon, Shavan, Shavaughn, Shaven, Shavin, Shavone, Shawan, Shawon, Shawun

Shaw (English) grove.

Shawn B G (Irish) a form of Sean.
*Shawen, Shawne, Shawnee,
Shawnn, Shawon*

Shawnta G B (American) a
combination of Shawn + the
suffix Ta.
Shawntae, Shawntel, Shawnti

Shay B G (Irish) a form of Shea.
Shae, Shai, Shaya, Shaye, Shey

Shayan (Cheyenne) a form of
Cheyenne.
Shayaan, Shayann, Shayon

Shayne B G (Hebrew) a form of
Sean.
Shayn, Shaynne, Shean

Shea G B (Irish) courteous.
Shay

Shedrick (Babylonian) a form of
Shadrach.
*Shadriq, Shederick, Shedric,
Shedrique*

Sheehan (Irish) little; peaceful.
Shean

Sheffield (English) crooked field.
Field, Shef, Sheff, Sheffie, Sheffy

Shel (English) a short form of
Shelby, Sheldon, Shelton.

Shelby G B (English) ledge estate.
*Shel, Shelbe, Shelbey, Shelbie,
Shell, Shellby, Shelley, Shelly*

Sheldon B G (English) farm on
the ledge.
Shel, Sheldan, Shelden, Sheldin,

*Sheldyn, Shell, Shelley, Shelly,
Shelton*

Shelley G B (English) a familiar
form of Shelby, Sheldon, Shelton.
Literature: Percy Bysshe Shelley
was a nineteenth-century British
poet.
Shell, Shelly

Shelly G B (English) a form of
Shelby, Sheldon, Shelley.

Shelton B G (English) town on a
ledge.
Shel, Shelley, Shelten

Shem (Hebrew) name; reputation.
(English) a short form of Samuel.
Bible: Noah's oldest son.

Shen (Egyptian) sacred amulet.
(Chinese) meditation.

Shep (English) a short form of
Shepherd.
Shap, Ship, Shipp

Shepherd (English) shepherd.
*Shep, Shepard, Shephard, Shepp,
Sheppard, Shepperd*

Shepley (English) sheep meadow.
*Sheplea, Sheplee, Shepply,
Shipley*

Sherborn (English) clear brook.
*Sherborne, Sherbourn, Sherburn,
Sherburne*

Sheridan G B (Irish) wild.
*Dan, Sheredan, Sheriden,
Sheridon, Sherridan*

Sherill (English) shire on a hill.
Sheril, Sherril, Sherrill

Sherlock (English) light haired.
Literature: Sherlock Holmes is a
famous British detective
character, created by Sir Arthur
Conan Doyle.
Sherlocke, Shurlock, Shurlocke

Sherman (English) sheep
shearer; resident of a shire.
*Scherman, Schermann, Sherm,
Shermain, Shermaine, Shermann,
Shermie, Shermon, Shermy*

Sherrod (English) clearer of the
land.
*Sherod, Sherrad, Sherrard,
Sherrodd*

Sherry 🇬🇧 (French) beloved,
dearest. A familiar form of Sheryl
(see Girls' Names).

Sherwin (English) swift runner,
one who cuts the wind.
*Sherveen, Shervin, Sherwan,
Sherwind, Sherwinn, Sherwyn,
Sherwynd, Sherwynne, Win*

Sherwood (English) bright
forest.
Sherwoode, Shurwood, Woody

Shihab (Arabic) blaze.

Shìlín (Chinese) intellectual.
Shilan

Shiloh (Hebrew) God's gift.
*Shi, Shile, Shiley, Shilo, Shiloe,
Shy, Shyle, Shylo, Shyloh*

Shimon (Hebrew) a form of
Simon.
Shymon

Shimshon (Hebrew) a form of
Samson.
Shimson

Shing (Chinese) victory.
Shingae, Shingo

Shipton (English) sheep village;
ship village.

Shiquan (American) a
combination of the prefix Shi +
Quan.
*Shiquane, Shiquann, Shiquawn,
Shiquoin, Shiqwan*

Shiro (Japanese) fourth-born son.

Shiva (Hindi) life and death.
Religion: the most common name
for the Hindu god of destruction
and reproduction.
Shiv, Shivan, Siva

Shlomo (Hebrew) a form of
Solomon.
*Shelmu, Shelomo, Shelomoh,
Shlomi, Shlomot*

Shmuel (Hebrew) a form of
Samuel.
*Shem, Shemuel, Shmelke,
Shmiel, Shmulka*

Shneur (Yiddish) senior.
Shneiur

Shon (German) a form of Schön.
(American) a form of Sean.
*Shoan, Shoen, Shondae,
Shondale, Shondel, Shone,*

*Shonn, Shonntay, Shontae,
Shontarious, Shouan, Shoun*

Shunnar (Arabic) pheasant.

Shyla **GB** (English) a form of
Sheila (see Girls' Names).

Si (Hebrew) a short form of Silas,
Simon.
Sy

Siañu (Quechua) brown like the
color of coffee.

Sid (French) a short form of
Sidney.
Cyd, Siddie, Siddy, Sidey, Syd

Siddel (English) wide valley.
Siddell

Siddhartha (Hindi) History:
Siddhartha Gautama was the
original name of Buddha, the
founder of Buddhism.
*Sida, Siddartha, Siddhaarth,
Siddhart, Siddharth, Sidh,
Sidharth, Sidhartha, Sidhdharth*

Sidney **GB** (French) from Saint-
Denis, France.
*Cydney, Sid, Sidnee, Sidny, Sidon,
Sidonio, Sydney, Sydny*

Sidonio (Spanish) a form of
Sidney.

Sidwell (English) wide stream.

Siegfried (German) victorious
peace. See also Zigfrid, Ziggy.
*Seifert, Seifried, Siegfred, Siffre,
Sig, Sigfrid, Sigfried, Sigfroi,*

*Sigfryd, Siggy, Sigifredo, Sigvard,
Singefrid, Sygfried, Szygfrid*

Sierra **GB** (Irish) black.
(Spanish) saw-toothed.
Siera

Sig (German) a short form of
Siegfried, Sigmund.

Siggy (German) a familiar form
of Siegfried, Sigmund.

Sigifredo (German) a form of
Siegfried.
Sigefriedo, Sigfrido, Siguefredo

Sigmund (German) victorious
protector. See also Ziggy,
Zsigmond, Zygmunt.
*Siegmund, Sig, Siggy, Sigismond,
Sigismondo, Sigismund,
Sigismundo, Sigismundus,
Sigmond, Sigsmond, Szygmond*

Sigurd (German, Scandinavian)
victorious guardian.
Sigord, Sjure, Syver

Sigwald (German) victorious
leader.

Silas **BG** (Latin) a short form of
Silvan.
Si, Sias, Sylas

Silvan (Latin) forest dweller.
*Silas, Silvain, Silvano, Silvaon,
Silvie, Silvio, Sylvain, Sylvan,
Sylvanus, Sylvio*

Silvano (Italian) a form of Silvan.
Silvanos, Silvanus, Silvino

Silverio (Spanish, Greek) god of trees.

Silvester (Latin) a form of Sylvester.
Silvestr, Silvestre, Silvestro, Silvy

Silvestro (Italian) a form of Sylvester.

Silvio (Italian) a form of Silvan.

Simão (Portuguese) a form of Samuel.

Simba (Swahili) lion. (Yao) a short form of Lisimba.
Sim

Simcha 🅱🅶 (Hebrew) joyful.
Simmy

Simeon (French) a form of Simon.
Simione, Simone

Simeón (Spanish) a form of Simón.

Simms (Hebrew) son of Simon.
Simm, Sims

Simmy (Hebrew) a familiar form of Simcha, Simon.
Simmey, Simmi, Simmie, Symmy

Simon 🅱🅶 (Hebrew) he heard. Bible: one of the Twelve Disciples. See also Symington, Ximenes.
Saimon, Samien, Semon, Shimon, Si, Sim, Simao, Simen, Simeon, Simion, Simm, Simmon, Simmonds, Simmons, Simms, Simmy, Simonas, Simone, Simson, Simyon, Síomón, Symon, Szymon

Simón (Hebrew) a form of Simon.

Simone 🅶🅱 (French) a form of Simeon.

Simplicio (Latin) simple.

Simpson (Hebrew) son of Simon.
Simonson, Simson

Simran 🅶🅱 (Sikh) absorbed in God.

Sinche, Sinchi (Quechua) boss, leader; strong, valorous, hard working.

Sinchipuma (Quechua) strong leader and as valuable as a puma.

Sinchiroca (Quechua) strongest prince amongst the strong ones.

Sinclair (French) prayer. Religion: name honoring Saint Clair.
Sinclare, Synclair

Sinesio (Greek) intelligent one, the shrewd one.

Sinforiano (Spanish) a form of Sinforoso.

Sinforoso (Greek) he who is full of misfortune.

Singh (Hindi) lion.
Sing

Sinjon (English) saint, holy man. Religion: name honoring Saint John.
Sinjin, Sinjun, Sjohn, Syngen, Synjen, Synjon

Siobhan 🅶🅱 (Irish) a form of Joan (see Girls' Names).

Sipatu (Moquelumnan) pulled out.

Sipho (Zulu) present.

Siraj (Arabic) lamp, light.

Sirio (Latin) native of Syria; brilliant like the Syrian sun.

Siro (Latin) native of Syria.

Siseal (Irish) a form of Cecil.

Sisebuto (Teutonic) he who fulfills his leadership role whole-heartedly.

Sisi (Fante) born on Sunday.

Siuca (Quechua) youngest son.

Siva (Hindi) a form of Shiva.
Siv

Sivan (Hebrew) ninth month of the Jewish year.

Siwatu (Swahili) born during a time of conflict.
Siwazuri

Siwili (Native American) long fox's tail.

Sixto (Greek) courteous one; he who has been treated well.

Skah (Lakota) white.
Skai

Skee (Scandinavian) projectile.
Ski, Skie

Skeeter (English) swift.
Skeat, Skeet, Skeets

Skelly (Irish) storyteller.
Shell, Skelley, Skellie

Skelton (Dutch) shell town.

Skerry (Scandinavian) stony island.

Skip (Scandinavian) a short form of Skipper.

Skipper (Scandinavian) shipmaster.
Skip, Skipp, Skippie, Skipton

Skiriki (Pawnee) coyote.

Skule (Norwegian) hidden.

Skye 🅶🅱 (Dutch) a short form of Skylar, Skyler, Skylor.
Sky

Skylar 🅱🅶 (Dutch) a form of Schuyler.
Skilar, Skkylar, Skye, Skyelar, Skylaar, Skylare, Skylarr, Skylayr

Skyler 🅱🅶 (Dutch) a form of Schuyler.
Skieler, Skiler, Skye, Skyeler, Skylee, Skyller

Skylor (Dutch) a form of Schuyler.
Skye, Skyelor, Skyloer, Skylore, Skylour, Skylur, Skylyr

Slade (English) child of the valley.
Slaide, Slayde

Slane (Czech) salty.
Slan

Slater (English) roof slater.
Slader, Slate, Slayter

Slava (Russian) a short form of Stanislav, Vladislav, Vyacheslav.
Slavik, Slavoshka

Slawek (Polish) a short form of Radoslav.

Slevin (Irish) mountaineer.
Slaven, Slavin, Slawin

Sloan (Irish) warrior.
Sloane, Slone

Smedley (English) flat meadow.
Smedleigh, Smedly

Smith (English) blacksmith.
Schmidt, Smid, Smidt, Smitt, Smitty, Smyth, Smythe

Snowden (English) snowy hill.
Snowdon

Socorro (Spanish) helper.

Socrates (Greek) wise, learned. History: a famous ancient Greek philosopher.
Socratis, Sokrates, Sokratis

Sócrates (Greek) a form of Socrates.

Socso (Quechua) blackbird.

Sofanor (Greek) wise man.

Sofia 🇬🇧 (Greek) a form of Sophia.

Sofian (Arabic) devoted.

Sofoclés, Sófocles (Greek) famous for his wisdom.

Sohrab (Persian) ancient hero.

Soja (Yoruba) soldier.

Sol (Hebrew) a short form of Saul, Solomon.
Soll, Sollie, Solly

Solano (Latin) like the eastern wind.

Solly (Hebrew) a familiar form of Saul, Solomon.
Sollie, Zollie, Zolly

Solomon 🇧🇬 (Hebrew) peaceful. Bible: a king of Israel famous for his wisdom. See also Zalman.
Salamen, Salamon, Salamun, Salaun, Salman, Salomo, Salomon, Selim, Shelomah, Shlomo, Sol, Solamh, Solaman, Solly, Solmon, Soloman, Solomonas, Sulaiman

Solon (Greek) wise. History: a noted ancient Athenian lawmaker.

Solón (Greek) a form of Solon.

Somac (Quechua) beautiful.

Somerset (English) place of the summer settlers. Literature: William Somerset Maugham was a well-known British writer.
Sommerset, Sumerset, Summerset

Somerville (English) summer village.
Somerton, Summerton, Summerville

Son (Vietnamese) mountain. (Native American) star. (English) son, boy. A short form of Madison, Orson.
Sonny

Sonco, Sonjoc, Suncu
(Quechua) heart; he who has a good and noble heart.

Soncoyoc, Sonjoyoc
(Quechua) he who has a good heart.

Songan (Native American) strong.
Song

Sonny B**G** (English) a familiar form of Grayson, Madison, Orson, Son.
Soni, Sonnie, Sony

Sono (Akan) elephant.

Sonya G**B** (Greek) wise. (Russian, Slavic) a form of Sophia.

Sophia G**B** (Greek) wise.

Sophie G**B** (Greek) a familiar form of Sophia.

Sören (Danish) thunder; war.
Sorren

Soroush (Persian) happy.

Sorrel G**B** (French) reddish brown.
Sorel, Sorell, Sorrell

Soterios (Greek) savior.
Soteris, Sotero

Southwell (English) south well.

Sovann (Cambodian) gold.

Sowande (Yoruba) wise healer sought me out.

Spalding (English) divided field.
Spaulding

Spangler (German) tinsmith.
Spengler

Spark (English) happy.
Sparke, Sparkie, Sparky

Spear (English) spear carrier.
Speare, Spears, Speer, Speers, Spiers

Speedy (English) quick; successful.
Speed

Spence (English) a short form of Spencer.
Spense

Spencer B**G** (English) dispenser of provisions.
Spence, Spencre, Spenser

Spenser (English) a form of Spencer. Literature: Edmund Spenser was the British poet who wrote *The Faerie Queene*.
Spanser, Spense

Spike (English) ear of grain; long nail.
Spyke

Spiro (Greek) round basket; breath.
Spiridion, Spiridon, Spiros, Spyridon, Spyros

Spoor (English) spur maker.
Spoors

Sproule (English) energetic.
Sprowle

Spurgeon (English) shrub.

Spyros (Greek) a form of Spiro.

Squire (English) knight's assistant; large landholder.

Stacey, Stacy 🇬🇧 (English) familiar forms of Eustace.
Stace, Stacee

Stafford (English) riverbank landing.
Staffard, Stafforde, Staford

Stamford (English) a form of Stanford.

Stamos (Greek) a form of Stephen.
Stamatis, Stamatos

Stan (Latin, English) a short form of Stanley.

Stanbury (English) stone fortification.
Stanberry, Stanbery, Stanburghe, Stansbury

Stancio (Spanish) a form of Constantine.
Stancy

Stancliff (English) stony cliff.
Stanclife, Stancliffe

Standish (English) stony parkland. History: Miles Standish was a leader in colonial America.

Stane (Slavic) a short form of Stanislaus.

Stanfield (English) stony field.
Stansfield

Stanford (English) rocky ford.
Sandy, Stamford, Stan, Standford, Stanfield

Stanislaus (Latin) stand of glory. See also Lao, Tano.
Slavik, Stana, Standa, Stane, Stanislao, Stanislas, Stanislau, Stanislav, Stanislus, Stannes, Stano, Stasik, Stasio

Stanislav (Slavic) a form of Stanislaus. See also Slava.
Stanislaw

Stanley 🇧🇬 (English) stony meadow.
Stan, Stanely, Stanlea, Stanlee, Stanleigh, Stanly

Stanmore (English) stony lake.

Stannard (English) hard as stone.

Stanton (English) stony farm.
Stan, Stanten, Staunton

Stanway (English) stony road.

Stanwick (English) stony village.
Stanwicke, Stanwyck

Stanwood (English) stony woods.

Starbuck (English) challenger of fate. Literature: a character in Herman Melville's novel *Moby-Dick*.

Stark (German) strong, vigorous.
Starke, Stärke, Starkie

Starling 🇧🇬 (English) bird.
Sterling

Starr GB (English) star.
Star, Staret, Starlight, Starlon, Starwin

Stasik (Russian) a familiar form of Stanislaus.
Stas, Stash, Stashka, Stashko, Stasiek

Stasio (Polish) a form of Stanislaus.
Stas, Stasiek, Stasiu, Staska, Stasko

Stavros (Greek) a form of Stephen.

Steadman (English) owner of a farmstead.
Steadmann, Stedman, Stedmen, Steed

Steel (English) like steel.
Steele

Steen (German, Danish) stone.
Steenn, Stein

Steeve (Greek) a short form of Steeven.

Steeven (Greek) a form of Steven.
Steaven, Steavin, Steavon, Steevan, Steeve, Steevn

Stefan (German, Polish, Swedish) a form of Stephen.
Steafan, Steafeán, Stefaan, Stefane, Stefanson, Stefaun, Stefawn, Steffan

Stefano (Italian) a form of Stephen.
Stefanos, Steffano

Stefanos (Greek) a form of Stephen.
Stefans, Stefos, Stephano, Stephanos

Stefen (Norwegian) a form of Stephen.
Steffen, Steffin, Stefin

Steffan (Swedish) a form of Stefan.
Staffan

Stefon (Polish) a form of Stephon.
Staffon, Steffon, Steffone, Stefone, Stefonne

Stein (German) a form of Steen.
Steine, Steiner

Steinar (Norwegian) rock warrior.

Stella GB (Latin) star. (French) a familiar form of Estelle (see Girls' Names).

Stepan (Russian) a form of Stephen.
Stepa, Stepane, Stepanya, Stepka, Stipan

Steph (English) a short form of Stephen.

Stephan (Greek) a form of Stephen.
Stepfan, Stephanas, Stephano, Stephanos, Stephanus, Stephaun

Stephane BG (Greek) a form of Stephanie.

Stéphane (French) a form of Stephen.
Stefane, Stepháne, Stephanne

Stephanie GB (Greek) crowned.

Stephany GB (Greek) a form of Stephanie.

Stephen BG (Greek) crowned.
See also Estéban, Estebe, Estevan, Estevao, Étienne, István, Szczepan, Tapani, Teb, Teppo, Tiennot.
Stamos, Stavros, Stefan, Stefano, Stefanos, Stefen, Stenya, Stepan, Stepanos, Steph, Stephan, Stephanas, Stéphane, Stephens, Stephenson, Stephfan, Stephin, Stephon, Stepven, Steve, Steven, Stevie

Stephon (Greek) a form of Stephen.
Stefon, Stepfon, Stepfone, Stephfon, Stephion, Stephone, Stephonne

Sterling BG (English) valuable; silver penny. A form of Starling.
Sterlen, Sterlin, Stirling

Stern (German) star.

Sterne (English) austere.
Stearn, Stearne, Stearns

Stetson BG (Danish) stepson.
Steston, Steton, Stetsen, Stetzon

Stevan (Greek) a form of Steven.
Stevano, Stevanoe, Stevaughn, Stevean

Steve (Greek) a short form of Stephen, Steven.
Steave, Stevie, Stevy

Steven ☀ BG (Greek) a form of Stephen.
Steeven, Steiven, Stevan, Steve, Stevens, Stevie, Stevin, Stevon, Stiven

Stevens (English) son of Steven.
Stevenson, Stevinson

Stevie GB (English) a familiar form of Stephen, Steven.
Stevey, Stevy

Stevin, Stevon (Greek) forms of Steven.
Stevieon, Stevion, Stevyn

Stewart BG (English) a form of Stuart.
Steward, Stu

Stian (Norwegian) quick on his feet.

Stig (Swedish) mount.

Stiggur (Gypsy) gate.

Stillman (English) quiet.
Stillmann, Stillmon

Sting (English) spike of grain.

Stockman (English) tree-stump remover.

Stockton (English) tree-stump town.

Stockwell (English) tree-stump well.

Stoddard (English) horse keeper.

Stoffel (German) a short form of Christopher.

Stoker (English) furnace tender.
Stoke, Stokes, Stroker

Stone (English) stone.
*Stoen, Stoner, Stoney, Stonie,
Stonie, Stoniy, Stony*

Storm BG (English) tempest,
storm.
*Storme, Stormey, Stormi,
Stormmie, Stormy*

Stormy GB (English) a form of
Storm.

Storr (Norwegian) great.
Story

Stover (English) stove tender.

Stowe (English) hidden; packed
away.

Strahan (Irish) minstrel.
Strachan

Stratford (English) bridge over
the river. Literature: Stratford-
upon-Avon was Shakespeare's
birthplace.
Stradford

Stratton (Scottish) river valley
town.
Straten, Straton

Strephon (Greek) one who turns.

Strom (Greek) bed, mattress.
(German) stream.

Strong (English) powerful.

Stroud (English) thicket.

Struthers (Irish) brook.

Stu (English) a short form of
Stewart, Stuart.
Stew

Stuart BG (English) caretaker,
steward. History: a Scottish and
English royal family.
Stewart, Stu, Stuarrt

Studs (English) rounded nail
heads; shirt ornaments; male
horses used for breeding.
History: Louis "Studs" Terkel is a
famous American journalist.
Stud, Studd

Styles (English) stairs put over a
wall to help cross it.
Stiles, Style, Stylz

Subhi (Arabic) early morning.

Suck Chin (Korean) unshakable
rock.

Sucsu (Quechua) blackbird.

Sudi (Swahili) lucky.
Su'ud

Sued (Arabic) master, chief.
Suede

Suelita (Spanish) little lily.

Suffield (English) southern field.

Sugden (English) valley of sows.

Suhail (Arabic) gentle.
*Sohail, Sohayl, Souhail, Suhael,
Sujal*

Suhay (Quechua) he who is like
yellow corn, fine and abundant;
rock.

Suhuba (Swahili) friend.

Sukhdeep GB (Sikh) light of peace and bliss.

Sukru (Turkish) grateful.

Sulaiman (Arabic) a form of Solomon.
Sulaman, Sulay, Sulaymaan, Sulayman, Suleiman, Suleman, Suleyman, Sulieman, Sulman, Sulomon, Sulyman

Sullivan (Irish) black eyed.
Sullavan, Sullevan, Sully

Sully (Irish) a familiar form of Sullivan. (French) stain, tarnish. (English) south.
Sulleigh, Sulley

Sultan (Swahili) ruler.
Sultaan

Sum (Tai) appropriate.

Sumainca (Quechua) beautiful Inca.

Summer GB (English) a form of Sumner.

Summit (English) peak, top.
Sumeet, Sumit, Summet, Summitt

Sumner (English) church officer; summoner.
Summer

Suncuyuc (Quechua) he who has a good heart.

Sundeep (Punjabi) light; enlightened.
Sundip

Sunny BG (English) sunny, sunshine.
Sun, Sunni

Sunreep (Hindi) pure.
Sunrip

Suri (Quechua) fast like an ostrich.

Susan GB (Hebrew) lily.

Susana GB (Hebrew) a form of Susan.

Sutcliff (English) southern cliff.
Sutcliffe

Sutherland (Scandinavian) southern land.
Southerland, Sutherlan

Sutton (English) southern town.

Suyai, Suyay (Quechua) hope.

Suycauaman (Quechua) youngest son of the falcons.

Suzanne GB (English) a form of Susan.

Sven (Scandinavian) youth.
Svein, Svend, Svenn, Swen, Swenson

Swaggart (English) one who sways and staggers.
Swaggert

Swain (English) herdsman; knight's attendant.
Swaine, Swane, Swanson, Swayne

Swaley (English) winding stream.
Swail, Swailey, Swale, Swales

Sweeney (Irish) small hero.
Sweeny

Swinbourne (English) stream
used by swine.
*Swinborn, Swinborne, Swinburn,
Swinburne, Swinbyrn, Swynborn*

Swindel (English) valley of the
swine.
Swindell

Swinfen (English) swine's mud.

Swinford (English) swine's
crossing.
Swynford

Swinton (English) swine town.

Sy (Latin) a short form of Sylas,
Symon.
Si

Sydnee GB (French) a form of
Sydney.

Sydney GB (French) a form of
Sidney.
Syd, Sydne, Sydnee, Syndey

Syed BG (Arabic) happy.
Syeed, Syid

Sying BG (Chinese) star.

Sylas (Latin) a form of Silas.
Sy, Syles, Sylus

Sylvain (French) a form of Silvan,
Sylvester.
Sylvan, Sylvian

Sylvester (Latin) forest dweller.
*Silvester, Silvestro, Sly, Syl,
Sylvain, Sylverster, Sylvestre*

Symington (English) Simon's
town, Simon's estate.

Symon (Greek) a form of Simon.
*Sy, Syman, Symeon, Symion,
Symms, Symon, Symone*

Szczepan (Polish) a form of
Stephen.

Szygfrid (Hungarian) a form of
Siegfried.
Szigfrid

Szymon (Polish) a form of Simon.

T

T BG (American) an initial used as
a first name.

Taaveti (Finnish) a form of David.
Taavi, Taavo

Tab (German) shining, brilliant.
(English) drummer.
Tabb, Tabbie, Tabby

Tabaré (Tupi) man of the village.

Tabari (Arabic) he remembers.
*Tabahri, Tabares, Tabarious,
Tabarius, Tabarus, Tabur*

Tabatha GB (Greek, Aramaic) a
form of Tabitha (see Girls'
Names).

Tabib (Turkish) physician.
Tabeeb

Tabo (Spanish) a short form of Gustave.

Tabor (Persian) drummer. (Hungarian) encampment.
Tabber, Taber, Taboras, Taibor, Tayber, Taybor, Taver

Taciano, Tácito (Spanish) forms of Tacio.

Tacio (Latin) he who is quiet.

Tad (Welsh) father. (Greek, Latin) a short form of Thaddeus.
Tadd, Taddy, Tade, Tadek, Tadey

Tadan (Native American) plentiful.
Taden

Tadarius (American) a combination of the prefix Ta + Darius.
Tadar, Tadarious, Tadaris, Tadarrius

Taddeo (Italian) a form of Thaddeus.
Tadeo

Taddeus (Greek, Latin) a form of Thaddeus.
Taddeous, Taddeusz, Taddius, Tadeas, Tades, Tadeusz, Tadio, Tadious

Tadi (Omaha) wind.

Tadzi (Carrier) loon.

Tadzio (Polish, Spanish) a form of Thaddeus.
Taddeusz

Taffy GB (Welsh) a form of David. (English) a familiar form of Taft.

Taft (English) river.
Taffy, Tafton

Tage (Danish) day.
Tag

Taggart (Irish) son of the priest.
Tagart, Taggert

Tahír (Arabic) innocent, pure.
Taheer

Tai (Vietnamese) weather; prosperous; talented.

Taima GB (Native American) born during a storm.

Taishawn (American) a combination of Tai + Shawn.
Taisen, Taishaun, Taishon

Tait (Scandinavian) a form of Tate.
Taite, Taitt

Taiwan (Chinese) island; island dweller. Geography: a country off the coast of China.
Taewon, Tahwan, Taivon, Taiwain, Tawain, Tawan, Tawann, Tawaun, Tawon, Taywan, Tywan

Taiwo (Yoruba) first-born of twins.

Taj (Urdu) crown.
Taje, Tajee, Tajeh, Tajh, Taji

Tajo (Spanish) day.
Taio

Tajuan (American) a combination of the prefix Ta + Juan.
Taijuan, Taijun, Taijuon, Tájuan, Tajwan, Taquan, Tyjuan

Takeo (Japanese) strong as bamboo.
Takeyo

Takis (Greek) a familiar form of Peter.
Takias, Takius

Takoda (Lakota) friend to everyone.

Tal (Hebrew) dew; rain.
Tali, Talia, Talley, Talor, Talya

Talbert (German) bright valley.

Talbot (French) boot maker.
Talbott, Tallbot, Tallbott, Tallie, Tally

Talcott (English) cottage near the lake.

Tale (Tswana) green.

Talen (English) a form of Talon.
Talin, Tallen

Talib (Arabic) seeker.

Taliesin (Welsh) radiant brow.
Tallas, Tallis

Taliki (Hausa) fellow.

Talli (Delaware) legendary hero.

Talmadge (English) lake between two towns.
Talmage

Talmai (Aramaic) mound; furrow.
Telem

Talman (Aramaic) injured; oppressed.
Talmon

Talon BG (French, English) claw, nail.
Taelon, Taelyn, Talen, Tallin, Tallon, Talyn

Talor (English) a form of Tal, Taylor.
Taelor, Taelur

Tam BG (Vietnamese) number eight. (Hebrew) honest. (English) a short form of Thomas.
Tama, Tamas, Tamás, Tameas, Tamlane, Tammany, Tammas, Tammen, Tammy

Taman (Slavic) dark, black.
Tama, Tamann, Tamin, Tamon, Tamone

Tamar GB (Hebrew) date; palm tree.
Tamarie, Tamario, Tamarr, Timur

Tambo (Swahili) vigorous.

Tamer (Arabic) he who makes way.

Tamir (Arabic) tall as a palm tree.
Tameer

Tammy GB (English) a familiar form of Thomas.
Tammie

Tamson (Scandinavian) son of Thomas.
Tamsen

Tan (Burmese) million. (Vietnamese) new.
Than

Tancredo (Germanic) he who shrewdly gives advice.

Tanek (Greek) immortal. See also Atek.

Taneli (Finnish) God is my judge.
Taneil, Tanell, Tanella

Taner (English) a form of Tanner.
Tanar

Tanesha 🅖🅑 (American) a combination of the prefix Ta + Nesha (see Girls' Names).

Tanguy (French) warrior.

Tani 🅖🅑 (Japanese) valley.

Tanis 🅖🅑 (Slavic) a form of Tania (see Girls' Names).

Tanmay (Sanskrit) engrossed.

Tanner 🅑🅖 (English) leather worker; tanner.
Tan, Taner, Tanery, Tann, Tannar, Tannir, Tannor, Tanny

Tannin (English) tan colored; dark.
Tanin, Tannen, Tannon, Tanyen, Tanyon

Tanny (English) a familiar form of Tanner.
Tana, Tannee, Tanney, Tannie, Tany

Tano (Spanish) camp glory. (Ghanaian) Geography: a river in Ghana. (Russian) a short form of Stanislaus.
Tanno

Tanton (English) town by the still river.

Tapan (Sanskrit) sun; summer.

Tapani (Finnish) a form of Stephen.
Tapamn, Teppo

Täpko (Kiowa) antelope.

Taquan (American) a combination of the prefix Ta + Quan.
Taquann, Taquawn, Taquon, Taqwan

Taquiri (Quechua) he who creates much music and dance.

Tara 🅖🅑 (Aramaic) throw; carry. (Irish) rocky hill. (Arabic) a measurement.

Tarak (Sanskrit) star; protector.

Taran (Sanskrit) heaven.
Tarran

Tarek (Arabic) a form of Táriq.
Tareek, Tareke

Tarell (German) a form of Terrell.
Tarelle, Tarrel, Tarrell, Taryl

Taren (American) a form of Taron.
Tarren, Tarrin

Tarif (Arabic) uncommon.
Tareef

Tarik (Arabic) a form of Táriq.
Taric, Tarick, Tariek, Tarikh, Tarrick, Tarrik, Taryk

Táriq (Arabic) conqueror. History: Tariq bin Ziyad was the Muslim general who conquered Spain.
Tareck, Tarek, Tarik, Tarique, Tarreq, Tereik

Tarleton (English) Thor's settlement.
Tarlton

Taro (Japanese) first-born male.

Taron (American) a combination of Tad + Ron.
Taeron, Tahron, Taren, Tarone, Tarrion, Tarron, Taryn

Tarquino (Latin) he who was born in Tarquinia, an ancient Italian city.

Tarrant (Welsh) thunder.
Terrant

Tarsicio (Greek) valiant.

Tarun (Sanskrit) young, youth.
Taran

Tarver (English) tower; hill; leader.
Terver

Taryn GB (American) a form of Taron.
Tarryn, Taryon

Tas (Gypsy) bird's nest.

Tasha GB (Greek) born on Christmas day. (Russian) a short form of Natasha.

Tashawn (American) a combination of the prefix Ta + Shawn.
Tashaan, Tashan, Tashaun, Tashon, Tashun

Tass (Hungarian) ancient mythology name.

Tasunke (Dakota) horse.

Tate BG (Scandinavian, English) cheerful. (Native American) long-winded talker.
Tait, Tayte

Tatiano (Latin) he who is quiet.

Tatius (Latin) king, ruler. History: a Sabine king.
Tatianus, Tazio, Titus

Tatum GB (English) cheerful.

Tau (Tswana) lion.

Taua (Quechua) fourth child.

Tauacapac (Quechua) fourth lord; lord of the four regions.

Tauno (Finnish) a form of Donald.

Taurean (Latin) strong; forceful. Astrology: born under the sign of Taurus.
Tauraun, Taurein, Taurin, Taurion, Taurone, Taurus

Taurino (Spanish) bull-like.

Tauro (Spanish) a form of Toro.

Taurus (Latin) Astrology: the second sign of the zodiac.
Taurice, Tauris

Tavares (Aramaic) a form of Tavor.
Tarvarres, Tavarres, Taveress

Tavaris (Aramaic) a form of Tavor.
Tarvaris, Tavar, Tavaras, Tavari, Tavarian, Tavarious, Tavarius, Tavarous, Tavarri, Tavarris, Tavars, Tavarse, Tavarus, Tevaris, Tevarius, Tevarus

Tavey (Latin) a familiar form of Octavio.

Tavi (Aramaic) good.

Tavian (Latin) a form of Octavio.
Taveon, Taviann, Tavien, Tavieon, Tavin, Tavio, Tavion, Tavionne, Tavon, Tayvon

Tavish (Scottish) a form of Thomas.
Tav, Tavi, Tavis

Tavo (Slavic) a short form of Gustave.

Tavon (American) a form of Tavian.
Tavonn, Tavonne, Tavonni

Tavor (Aramaic) misfortune.
Tarvoris, Tavares, Tavaris, Tavores, Tavorious, Tavoris, Tavorise, Tavorres, Tavorris, Tavuris

Tawno (Gypsy) little one.
Tawn

Tayib (Hindi) good; delicate.

Tayler ⚑ (English) a form of Taylor.
Tailer, Taylar, Tayller, Teyler

Taylor ⚑ (English) tailor.
Tailor, Talor, Tayler, Tayllor, Taylour, Taylr, Teylor

Tayshawn (American) a combination of Taylor + Shawn.
Taysean, Tayshan, Tayshun, Tayson

Tayvon (American) a form of Tavian.
Tayvan, Tayvaughn, Tayven, Tayveon, Tayvin, Tayvohn, Taywon

Taz (Arabic) shallow ornamental cup.
Tazz

Tazio (Italian) a form of Tatius.

Teagan ⚑ (Irish) a form of Teague.
Teagen, Teagun, Teegan

Teague (Irish) bard, poet.
Teag, Teagan, Teage, Teak, Tegan, Teige

Tearence (Latin) a form of Terrence.
Tearance, Tearnce, Tearrance

Tearlach (Scottish) a form of Charles.

Tearle (English) stern, severe.

Teasdale (English) river dweller. Geography: a river in England.

Teb (Spanish) a short form of Stephen.

Ted (English) a short form of Edward, Edwin, Theodore.
Tedd, Tedek, Tedik, Tedson

Teddy (English) a familiar form of Edward, Theodore.
Teddey, Teddie, Tedy

Tedmund (English) protector of the land.
Tedman, Tedmond

Tedorik (Polish) a form of Theodore.
Teodoor, Teodor, Teodorek

Tedrick (American) a combination of Ted + Rick.
Teddrick, Tederick, Tedric

Teetonka (Lakota) big lodge.

Tefere (Ethiopian) seed.

Tegan GB (Irish) a form of Teague.
Teghan, Teigan, Tiegan

Tej (Sanskrit) light; lustrous.

Tejas (Sanskrit) sharp.

Tekle (Ethiopian) plant.

Telek (Polish) a form of Telford.

Telem (Hebrew) mound; furrow.
Talmai, Tel

Telémaco (Greek) he who prepares for battle.

Telford (French) iron cutter.
Telek, Telfer, Telfor, Telfour

Teller (English) storyteller.
Tell, Telly

Telly (Greek) a familiar form of Teller, Theodore.

Telmo (English) tiller, cultivator.

Telutci (Moquelumnan) bear making dust as it runs.

Telvin (American) a combination of the prefix Te + Melvin.
Tellvin, Telvan

Tem (Gypsy) country.

Teman (Hebrew) on the right side; southward.

Tembo (Swahili) elephant.

Tempest GB (French) storm.

Temple (Latin) sanctuary.

Templeton (English) town near the temple.
Temp, Templeten

Tennant (English) tenant, renter.
Tenant, Tennent

Tennessee (Cherokee) mighty warrior. Geography: a southern U.S. state.
Tennesee, Tennesy, Tennysee

Tennyson (English) a form of Dennison. Literature: Alfred, Lord Tennyson was a nineteenth-century British poet.
Tenney, Tenneyson, Tennie, Tennis, Tennison, Tenny, Tenson

Teo (Vietnamese) a form of Tom.

Teobaldo (Italian, Spanish) a form of Theobald.

Teócrito (Greek) God's chosen one.

Teodoro (Italian, Spanish) a form of Theodore.
Teodore, Teodorico

Teodosio (Greek) he who gives to God.

Teófano (Greek) friend of God; loved by God.

Teófilo (Greek) loved by God.

Teppo (French) a familiar form of Stephen.

Tequan (American) a combination of the prefix Te + Quan.
Tequinn, Tequon

Terance (Latin) a form of Terrence.
Terriance

Tercio, Tertulio (Greek) third child of the family.

Terell (German) a form of Terrell.
Tarell, Tereall, Terel, Terelle, Tyrel

Teremun (Tiv) father's acceptance.

Terence 🅱🅶 (Latin) a form of Terrence.
Teren, Teryn

Terencio (Spanish) a form of Terrence.

Teri 🅶🅱 (Greek) reaper. A familiar form of Theresa.

Terra 🅶🅱 (Latin) earth. (Japanese) swift arrow. (American) forms of Tara.

Terran (Latin) a short form of Terrance.
Teran, Teren, Terran, Terren

Terrance 🅱🅶 (Latin) a form of Terrence.
Tarrance, Terran

Terrell 🅱🅶 (German) thunder ruler.
Terell, Terrail, Terral, Terrale, Terrall, Terreal, Terrel, Terrelle, Terrill, Terryal, Terryel, Tirel, Tirrel, Tirrell, Turrell, Tyrel, Tyrell

Terrence (Latin) smooth.
Tarrance, Tearence, Terance, Terence, Terencio, Terrance, Terren, Terrin, Terry, Torrence, Tyreese

Terri 🅶🅱 (English) a form of Terry.

Terrick (American) a combination of the prefix Te + Derrick.
Teric, Terick, Terik, Teriq, Terric, Terrik, Tirek, Tirik

Terrill (German) a form of Terrell.
Teriel, Teriell, Terril, Terryl, Terryll, Teryll, Teryl, Tyrill

Terrin (Latin) a short form of Terrence.
Terin, Terrien, Terryn, Teryn, Tiren

Terris (Latin) son of Terry.

Terron (American) a form of Tyrone.
Tereon, Terion, Terione, Teron, Terone, Terrion, Terrione, Terriyon, Terrone, Terronn, Terryon, Tiron

Terry **BG** (English) a familiar form of Terrence. See also Keli.
Tarry, Terrey, Terri, Terrie, Tery

Tertius (Latin) third.

Teseo (Greek) founder.

Teshawn (American) a combination of the prefix Te + Shawn.
Tesean, Teshaun, Teshon

Tess **GB** (Greek) a short form of Theresa.

Tessa **GB** (Greek) reaper.

Teva (Hebrew) nature.

Tevan (American) a form of Tevin.
Tevaughan, Tevaughn, Teven, Tevvan

Tevel (Yiddish) a form of David.

Tevin **BG** (American) a combination of the prefix Te + Kevin.
Teavin, Teivon, Tevan, Tevien, Tevinn, Tevon, Tevvin, Tevyn

Tevis (Scottish) a form of Thomas.
Tevish

Tevon (American) a form of Tevin.
Tevion, Tevohn, Tevone, Tevonne, Tevoun, Teyvon

Tewdor (German) a form of Theodore.

Tex (American) from Texas.
Tejas

Thabit (Arabic) firm, strong.

Thad (Greek, Latin) a short form of Thaddeus.
Thadd, Thade, Thadee, Thady

Thaddeus (Greek) courageous. (Latin) praiser. Bible: one of the Twelve Apostles. See also Fadey.
Tad, Taddeo, Taddeus, Thaddis, Thadeaus, Tadzio, Thad, Thaddaeus, Thaddaus, Thaddeau, Thaddeaus, Thaddeo, Thaddeous, Thaddiaus, Thaddius, Thadeaou, Thadeous, Thadeus, Thadieus, Thadious, Thadius, Thadus

Thady (Irish) praise.
Thaddy

Thai (Vietnamese) many, multiple.

Thaman (Hindi) god; godlike.

Than (Burma) million.
Tan, Thanh

Thane (English) attendant warrior.
Thain, Thaine, Thayne

Thang (Vietnamese) victorious.

Thanh (Vietnamese) finished.

Thaniel (Hebrew) a short form of Nathaniel.

Thanos (Greek) nobleman; bearman.
Athanasios, Thanasis

Thatcher (English) roof thatcher, repairer of roofs.
Thacher, Thatch, Thaxter

Thaw (English) melting ice.

Thayer (French) nation's army.
Thay

Thel (English) upper story.

Thenga (Yao) bring him.

Theo (English) a short form of Theodore.

Theobald (German) people's prince; bold people. See also Dietbald.
Teobaldo, Thebault, Theòbault, Thibault, Tibalt, Tibold, Tiebold, Tiebout, Toiboid, Tybald, Tybalt, Tybault

Theodore 🅱🅶 (Greek) gift of God. See also Feodor, Fyodor.
Téadóir, Teador, Ted, Teddy, Tedor, Tedorek, Tedorik, Telly, Teodomiro, Teodoro, Teodus, Teos, Tewdor, Theo, Theodor, Theódor, Theodors, Theodorus, Theodosios, Theodrekr, Tivadar, Todor, Tolek, Tudor

Theodoric (German) ruler of the people. See also Dedrick, Derek, Dirk.
Teodorico, Thedric, Thedrick, Thierry, Till

Theophilus (Greek) loved by God.
Teofil, Théophile, Theophlous, Theopolis

Theresa 🅶🅱 (Greek) reaper.

Theron (Greek) hunter.
Theran, Theren, Thereon, Therin, Therion, Therrin, Therron, Theryn, Theryon

Thian (Vietnamese) smooth.
Thien

Thibault (French) a form of Theobald.
Thibaud, Thibaut

Thierry (French) a form of Theodoric.
Theirry, Theory

Thom (English) a short form of Thomas.
Thomy

Thoma (German) a form of Thomas.

Thomas ☀ 🅱🅶 (Greek, Aramaic) twin. Bible: one of the Twelve Apostles. See also Chuma, Foma, Maslin.
Tam, Tammy, Tavish, Tevis, Thom, Thoma, Thomason, Thomaz, Thomeson, Thomison, Thommas, Thompson, Thomson, Tom, Toma, Tomas, Tomás, Tomasso, Tomcy, Tomey, Tomey, Tomi, Tommy, Toomas

Thompson (English) son of Thomas.
Thomason, Thomison, Thomsen, Thomson

Thor (Scandinavian) thunder. Mythology: the Norse god of thunder.
Thorin, Tor, Tyrus

Thorald (Scandinavian) Thor's follower.
Terrell, Terrill, Thorold, Torald

Thorbert (Scandinavian) Thor's brightness.
Torbert

Thorbjorn (Scandinavian) Thor's bear.
Thorburn, Thurborn, Thurburn

Thorgood (English) Thor is good.

Thorleif (Scandinavian) Thor's beloved.
Thorlief

Thorley (English) Thor's meadow.
Thorlea, Thorlee, Thorleigh, Thorly, Torley

Thorndike (English) thorny embankment.
Thorn, Thorndyck, Thorndyke, Thorne

Thorne (English) a short form of names beginning with "Thorn."
Thorn, Thornie, Thorny

Thornley (English) thorny meadow.
Thorley, Thorne, Thornlea, Thornleigh, Thornly

Thornton (English) thorny town.
Thorne

Thorpe (English) village.
Thorp

Thorwald (Scandinavian) Thor's forest.
Thorvald

Thuc (Vietnamese) aware.

Thurlow (English) Thor's hill.
Thurlo

Thurmond (English) defended by Thor.
Thormond, Thurmund

Thurston (Scandinavian) Thor's stone.
Thorstan, Thorstein, Thorsten, Thurstain, Thurstan, Thursten, Torsten, Torston

Tiago (Spanish) a form of Jacob.

Tiarra GB (Latin) a form of Tiara (see Girls' Names).

Tiberio (Italian) from the Tiber River region.
Tiberias, Tiberious, Tiberiu, Tiberius, Tibius, Tyberious, Tyberius, Tyberrius

Tibor (Hungarian) holy place.
Tiburcio

Tiburón (Spanish) shark.

Tichawanna (Shona) we shall see.

Ticho (Spanish) a short form of Patrick.

Ticiano (Spanish) a form of Tito.

Tico (Greek) adventurous one; happy, fortunate.

Tieler (English) a form of Tyler.
Tielar, Tielor, Tielyr

Tiennot (French) a form of Stephen.
Tien

Tiernan (Irish) lord.

Tierney GB (Irish) lordly.
Tiarnach, Tiernan

Tiffany GB (Latin) trinity. (Greek) a short form of Theophania (see Girls' Names).

Tige (English) a short form of Tiger.
Ti, Tig, Tighe, Ty, Tyg, Tyge, Tygh, Tyghe

Tiger (American) tiger; powerful and energetic.
Tige, Tigger, Tyger

Tiimu (Moquelumnan) caterpillar coming out of the ground.

Tiktu (Moquelumnan) bird digging up potatoes.

Tilden (English) tilled valley.
Tildon

Tilford (English) prosperous ford.

Till (German) a short form of Theodoric.
Thilo, Til, Tillman, Tilman, Tillmann, Tilson

Tilo (Teutonic) skillful and praises God.

Tilton (English) prosperous town.

Tim (Greek) a short form of Timothy.
Timmie, Timmy

Timin (Arabic) born near the sea.

Timmothy (Greek) a form of Timothy.
Timmathy, Timmithy, Timmoty, Timmthy

Timmy (Greek) a familiar form of Timothy.
Timmie

Timo (Finnish) a form of Timothy.
Timio

Timofey (Russian) a form of Timothy.
Timofei, Timofej, Timofeo

Timon (Greek) honorable.

Timoteo (Portuguese, Spanish) a form of Timothy.

Timothy ☆ BG (Greek) honoring God. See also Kimokeo.
Tadhg, Taidgh, Tiege, Tim, Tima, Timithy, Timka, Timkin, Timmothy, Timmy, Timo, Timofey, Timok, Timon, Timontheo, Timonthy, Timót, Timote, Timotei, Timoteo, Timoteus, Timothé, Timothée, Timotheo, Timotheos, Timotheus, Timothey, Timothie, Timthie, Tiomóid, Tisha, Tomothy, Tymon, Tymothy

Timur (Hebrew) a form of Tamar. (Russian) conqueror.
Timour

Tin (Vietnamese) thinker.

Tina GB (Spanish, American) a short form of Augustine.

Tincupuma, Tinquipoma (Quechua) he who creates much music and dance.

Tino (Spanish) venerable, majestic. (Italian) small. A familiar form of Antonio. (Greek) a short form of Augustine.
Tion

Tinsley (English) fortified field.

Tiquan (American) a combination of the prefix Ti + Quan.
Tiquawn, Tiquine, Tiquon, Tiquwan, Tiqwan

Tíquico (Greek) very fortunate person.

Tirso (Greek) crowned with fig leaves.

Tisha GB (Russian) a form of Timothy.
Tishka

Tishawn (American) a combination of the prefix Ti + Shawn.
Tishaan, Tishaun, Tishean, Tishon, Tishun

Tito (Italian) a form of Titus.
Titas, Titis, Titos

Titoatauchi, Tituatauchi (Quechua) he who brings luck in trying times.

Titu (Quechua) difficult, complicated.

Titus (Greek) giant. (Latin) hero. A form of Tatius. History: a Roman emperor.
Tite, Titek, Tito, Tytus

Tivon (Hebrew) nature lover.

TJ (American) a combination of the initials T. + J.
Teejay, Tj, T.J., T Jae, Tjayda

Tobal (Spanish) a short form of Christopher.
Tabalito

Tobar (Gypsy) road.

Tobi GB (Yoruba) great.

Tobias (Hebrew) God is good.
Tobia, Tobiah, Tobiás, Tobiath, Tobin, Tobit, Toby, Tobyas, Tuvya

Tobías (Hebrew) a form of Tobias.

Tobin (Hebrew) a form of Tobias.
Toben, Tobian, Tobyn, Tovin

Toby BG (Hebrew) a familiar form of Tobias.
Tobbie, Tobby, Tobe, Tobee, Tobey, Tobie

Todd BG (English) fox.
Tod, Toddie, Toddy

Todor (Basque, Russian) a form of Theodore.
Teodor, Todar, Todas, Todos

Toft (English) small farm.

Tohon (Native American) cougar.

Tokala (Dakota) fox.

Toland (English) owner of taxed land.
Tolan

Tolbert (English) bright tax collector.

Toller (English) tax collector.

Tolomeo (Greek) powerful in battle.

Tom (English) a short form of Tomas, Thomas.
Teo, Thom, Tommey, Tommie, Tommy

Toma (Romanian) a form of Thomas.
Tomah

Tomas (German) a form of Thomas.
Tom, Tomaisin, Tomaz, Tomcio, Tome, Tomek, Tomelis, Tomico, Tomik, Tomislaw, Tommas, Tomo, Tomson

Tomás (Irish, Spanish) a form of Thomas.
Tomas, Tómas, Tomasz

Tomasso (Italian) a form of Thomas.
Tomaso, Tommaso

Tombe (Kakwa) northerners.

Tomé (Hebrew) identical twin brother.

Tomey (Irish) a familiar form of Thomas.
Tome, Tomi, Tomie, Tomy

Tomi 🄶🄱 (Japanese) rich.
(Hungarian) a form of Thomas.

Tomlin (English) little Tom.
Tomkin, Tomlinson

Tommie 🄱🄶 (Hebrew) a form of Tommy.
Tommi

Tommy 🄱🄶 (Hebrew) a familiar form of Thomas.
Tommie, Tomy

Tonda (Czech) a form of Tony.
Tonek

Tong (Vietnamese) fragrant.

Toni 🄶🄱 (Greek, German, Slavic) a form of Tony.
Tonee, Tonie, Tonio, Tonis, Tonnie

Tonio (Portuguese) a form of Tony. (Italian) a short form of Antonio.
Tono, Tonyo

Tony 🄱🄶 (Greek) flourishing. (Latin) praiseworthy. (English) a short form of Anthony. A familiar form of Remington.
Tonda, Tonek, Toney, Toni, Tonik, Tonio, Tonny

Tooantuh (Cherokee) spring frog.

Toomas (Estonian) a form of Thomas.
Toomis, Tuomas, Tuomo

Topa, Tupa (Quechua) honorific title; royal, majestic, glorious, noble, honorable.

Topher (Greek) a short form of Christopher, Kristopher.
Tofer, Tophor

Topo (Spanish) gopher.

Topper (English) hill.

Tor (Norwegian) thunder. (Tiv) royalty, king.
Thor

Torcuato (Latin) adorned with a collar or garland.

Tori **GB** (English) a form of Tory.

Torian (Irish) a form of Torin.
Toran, Torean, Toriano, Toriaun, Torien, Torrian, Torrien, Torryan

Toribio (Greek) he who makes bows.

Torin (Irish) chief.
Thorfin, Thorstein, Torian, Torion, Torrin, Toryn

Torkel (Swedish) Thor's cauldron.

Tormey (Irish) thunder spirit.
Tormé, Tormee

Tormod (Scottish) north.

Torn (Irish) a short form of Torrence.
Toran

Toro (Spanish) bull.

Torquil (Danish) Thor's kettle.
Torkel

Torr (English) tower.
Tory

Torrance (Irish) a form of Torrence.
Torance

Torren (Irish) a short form of Torrence.
Torehn, Toren

Torrence (Irish) knolls. (Latin) a form of Terrence.
Tawrence, Toreence, Torence, Torenze, Torey, Torin, Torn, Torr, Torrance, Torren, Torreon, Torrin, Torry, Tory, Torynce, Tuarence, Turance

Torrey (English) a form of Tory.
Toreey, Torie, Torre, Torri, Torrie, Torry

Toru (Japanese) sea.

Tory **GB** (English) familiar form of Torr, Torrence.
Torey, Tori, Torrey

Toshi-Shita (Japanese) junior.

Tovi (Hebrew) good.
Tov

Townley (English) town meadow.
Townlea, Townlee, Townleigh, Townlie, Townly

Townsend (English) town's end.
Town, Townes, Towney, Townie, Townsen, Townshend, Towny

Trabunco (Mapuche) meeting at the marsh.

Trace (Irish) a form of Tracy.
Trayce

Tracey 🅶🅱 (Irish) a form of Tracy.

Traci 🅶🅱 (Irish) a form of Tracy.

Tracy 🅶🅱 (Greek) harvester. (Latin) courageous. (Irish) battler.
Trace, Tracey, Tracie, Treacy

Trader (English) well-trodden path; skilled worker.

Trae (English) a form of Trey.
Trai, Traie, Tre, Trea

Traful (Araucanian) union.

Trahern (Welsh) strong as iron.
Traherne, Tray

Tramaine (Scottish) a form of Tremaine, Tremayne.
Tramain, Traman, Tramane, Tramayne, Traymain, Traymon

Tranamil (Mapuche) low, scattered light.

Traquan (American) a combination of Travis + Quan.
Traequan, Traqon, Traquon, Traqwan, Traqwaun, Trayquan, Trayquane, Trayqwon

Trashawn 🅱🅶 (American) a combination of Travis + Shawn.
Trasen, Trashaun, Trasean, Trashon, Trashone, Trashun, Trayshaun, Trayshawn

Traugott (German) God's truth.

Travaris (French) a form of Travers.
Travares, Travaress, Travarious, Travarius, Travarous, Travarus, Travauris, Traveress, Traverez, Traverus, Travoris, Travorus

Travell (English) traveler.
Travail, Travale, Travel, Travelis, Travelle, Trevel, Trevell, Trevelle

Traven (American) a form of Trevon.
Travin, Travine, Trayven

Travers (French) crossroads.
Travaris, Traver, Travis

Travion (American) a form of Trevon.
Traveon, Travian, Travien, Travione, Travioun

Travis 🅱🅶 (English) a form of Travers.
Travais, Travees, Traves, Traveus, Travious, Traviss, Travius, Travous, Travus, Travys, Trayvis, Trevais, Trevis

Travon 🅱🅶 (American) a form of Trevon.
Traevon, Traivon, Travone, Travonn, Travonne

Tray (English) a form of Trey.
Traye

Trayton (English) town full of trees.
Trayten

Trayvon (American) a combination of Tray + Von.
Trayveon, Trayvin, Trayvion, Trayvond, Trayvone, Trayvonne, Trayvyon

Treavon (American) a form of
Trevon.
Treavan, Treavin, Treavion

Trecaman (Mapuche) majestic
steps of the condor.

Tredway (English) well-worn
road.
Treadway

Tremaine, Tremayne BG
(Scottish) house of stone.
*Tramaine, Tremain, Tremane,
Treymaine, Trimaine*

Trent BG (Latin) torrent, rapid
stream. (French) thirty.
Geography: a city in northern
Italy.
Trente, Trentino, Trento, Trentonio

Trenton (Latin) town by the rapid
stream. Geography: the capital of
New Jersey.
*Trendon, Trendun, Trenten,
Trentin, Trenttton, Trentyn, Trinten,
Trintin, Trinton*

Trequan (American) a
combination of Trey + Quan.
*Trequanne, Trequaun, Trequian,
Trequon, Treqwon, Treyquane*

Treshawn (American) a
combination of Trey + Shawn.
*Treshaun, Treshon, Treshun,
Treysean, Treyshawn, Treyshon*

Treston (Welsh) a form of Tristan.
Trestan, Trestin, Trestton, Trestyn

Trev (Irish, Welsh) a short form of
Trevor.

Trevaughn (American) a combi-
nation of Trey + Vaughn.
*Trevaughan, Trevaugn, Trevaun,
Trevaune, Trevaunn, Treyvaughn*

Trevelyan (English) Elian's
homestead.

Trevin (American) a form of
Trevon.
*Trevian, Trevien, Trevine,
Trevinne, Trevyn, Treyvin*

Trevion (American) a form of
Trevon.
*Trevione, Trevionne, Trevyon,
Treyveon, Treyvion*

Trevis (English) a form of Travis.
Treves, Trevez, Treveze, Trevius

Trevon BG (American) a combi-
nation of Trey + Von.
*Traven, Travion, Travon, Tre,
Treavon, Trévan, Treveyon, Trevin,
Trevion, Trevohn, Trevoine,
Trévon, Trevone, Trevonn,
Trevonne, Treyvon*

Trevor BG (Irish) prudent.
(Welsh) homestead.
*Travor, Treavor, Trebor, Trefor,
Trev, Trevar, Trevares, Trevarious,
Trevaris, Trevarius, Trevaros,
Trevarus, Trever, Trevore,
Trevores, Trevoris, Trevorus,
Trevour, Trevyr, Treyvor*

Trey (English) three; third.
Trae, Trai, Tray, Treye, Tri, Trie

Treyvon (American) a form of Trevon.
Treyvan, Treyven, Treyvenn, Treyvone, Treyvonn, Treyvun

Trigg (Scandinavian) trusty.

Trina GB (Greek) pure.

Trini (Latin) a short form of Trinity.

Trinity GB (Latin) holy trinity.
Trenedy, Trini, Trinidy

Trip, Tripp (English) traveler.

Tristan BG (Welsh) bold. Literature: a knight in the Arthurian legends who fell in love with his uncle's wife.
Treston, Tris, Trisan, Tristain, Tristán, Tristano, Tristen, Tristian, Tristin, Triston, Tristyn, Trystan

Tristano (Italian) a form of Tristan.

Tristen BG (Welsh) a form of Tristan.
Trisden, Trissten

Tristin BG (Welsh) a form of Tristan.
Tristian, Tristinn

Triston BG (Welsh) a form of Tristan.

Tristram (Welsh) sorrowful. Literature: the title character in Laurence Sterne's eighteenth-century novel *Tristram Shandy*.
Tristam

Tristyn (Welsh) a form of Tristan.
Tristynne

Troilo (Egyptian) he who was born in Troy.

Trot (English) trickling stream.

Trowbridge (English) bridge by the tree.

Troy BG (Irish) foot soldier. (French) curly haired. (English) water. See also Koi.
Troi, Troye, Troyton

True (English) faithful, loyal.
Tru

Truesdale (English) faithful one's homestead.

Truitt (English) little and honest.
Truett

Truman (English) honest. History: Harry S. Truman was the thirty-third U.S. president.
Trueman, Trumain, Trumaine, Trumann

Trumble (English) strong; bold.
Trumball, Trumbell, Trumbull

Trustin (English) trustworthy.
Trustan, Trusten, Truston

Trygve (Norwegian) brave victor.

Trystan (Welsh) a form of Tristan.
Tryistan, Trysten, Trystian, Trystin, Trystn, Tryston, Trystyn

Tsalani (Nguni) good-bye.

Tse (Ewe) younger of twins.

Tu BG (Vietnamese) tree.

Tuaco (Ghanaian) eleventh-born.

Tuan (Vietnamese) goes smoothly.

Tubal (Hebrew) he who tills the soil.

Tucker BG (English) fuller, tucker of cloth.
Tuck, Tuckie, Tucky, Tuckyr

Tudor (Welsh) a form of Theodore. History: an English ruling dynasty.
Todor

Tug (Scandinavian) draw, pull.
Tugg

Tuketu (Moquelumnan) bear making dust as it runs.

Tukuli (Moquelumnan) caterpillar crawling down a tree.

Tulio (Italian, Spanish) lively.
Tullio

Tullis (Latin) title, rank.
Tullius, Tullos, Tully

Tully (Irish) at peace with God. (Latin) a familiar form of Tullis.
Tull, Tulley, Tullie, Tullio

Tumaini (Mwera) hope.

Tumu (Moquelumnan) deer thinking about eating wild onions.

Tung (Vietnamese) stately, dignified. (Chinese) everyone.

Tungar (Sanskrit) high; lofty.

Tupac (Quechua) Lord.

Tupacamaru (Quechua) glorious Amaru, an Incan lord.

Tupacapac (Quechua) glorious and kind-hearted lord.

Tupacusi (Quechua) happy and majestic.

Tupaquiupanqui, Tupayupanqui (Quechua) memorable and glorious lord.

Tupi (Moquelumnan) pulled up.

Tupper (English) ram raiser.

Turi (Spanish) a short form of Arthur.
Ture

Turk (English) from Turkey.

Turner BG (Latin) lathe worker; wood worker.

Turpin (Scandinavian) Finn named after Thor.

Tut (Arabic) strong and courageous. History: a short form of Tutankhamen, an Egyptian king.
Tutt

Tutu (Spanish) a familiar form of Justin.

Tuvya (Hebrew) a form of Tobias.
Tevya, Tuvia, Tuviah

Tuwile (Mwera) death is inevitable.

Tuyen (Vietnamese) angel.

Twain (English) divided in two. Literature: Mark Twain (whose real name was Samuel Langhorne Clemens) was one of the most prominent nineteenth-century American writers.
Tawine, Twaine, Twan, Twane, Tway, Twayn, Twayne

Twia (Fante) born after twins.

Twitchell (English) narrow passage.
Twytchell

Twyford (English) double river crossing.

Txomin (Basque) like the Lord.

Ty 🅱🅶 (English) a short form of Tyler, Tyrone, Tyrus.
Tye

Tyee (Native American) chief.

Tyger (English) a form of Tiger.
Tige, Tyg, Tygar

Tylar (English) a form of Tyler.
Tyelar, Tylarr

Tyler ☀ 🅱🅶 (English) tile maker.
Tieler, Tiler, Ty, Tyel, Tyeler, Tyelor, Tyhler, Tylar, Tyle, Tylee, Tylere, Tyller, Tylor, Tylyr

Tylor 🅱🅶 (English) a form of Tyler.
Tylour

Tymon (Polish) a form of Timothy. (Greek) a form of Timon.
Tymain, Tymaine, Tymane, Tymeik, Tymek, Tymen

Tymothy (English) a form of Timothy.
Tymithy, Tymmothy, Tymoteusz, Tymothee, Timothi

Tynan (Irish) dark.
Ty

Tynek (Czech) a form of Martin.
Tynko

Tyquan (American) a combination of Ty + Quan.
Tykwan, Tykwane, Tykwon, Tyquaan, Tyquane, Tyquann, Tyquine, Tyquinn, Tyquon, Tyquone, Tyquwon, Tyqwan

Tyra 🅶🅱 (Scottish) a form of Tyree.

Tyran (American) a form of Tyrone.
Tyraine, Tyrane

Tyree 🅱🅶 (Scottish) island dweller. Geography: Tiree is an island off the west coast of Scotland.
Tyra, Tyrae, Tyrai, Tyray, Tyre, Tyrea, Tyrée

Tyreese (American) a form of Terrence.
Tyreas, Tyrease, Tyrece, Tyreece, Tyreice, Tyres, Tyrese, Tyresse, Tyrez, Tyreze, Tyrice, Tyriece, Tyriese

Tyrel, Tyrell 🅱🅶 (American) forms of Terrell.
Tyrelle, Tyrrel, Tyrrell

Tyrick (American) a combination
of Ty + Rick.
*Tyreck, Tyreek, Tyreik, Tyrek,
Tyreke, Tyric, Tyriek, Tyrik, Tyriq,
Tyrique*

Tyrin (American) a form of
Tyrone.
Tyrinn, Tyrion, Tyrrin, Tyryn

Tyron (American) a form of
Tyrone.
Tyrohn, Tyronn, Tyronna, Tyronne

Tyrone (Greek) sovereign. (Irish)
land of Owen.
*Tayron, Tayrone, Teirone, Terron,
Ty, Tyerone, Tyhrone, Tyran, Tyrin,
Tyron, Tyroney, Tyronne, Tyroon,
Tyroun*

Tyrus (English) a form of Thor.
Ty, Tyruss, Tyryss

Tyshawn (American) a
combination of Ty + Shawn.
*Tyshan, Tyshaun, Tyshauwn,
Tyshian, Tyshinn, Tyshion, Tyshon,
Tyshone, Tyshonne, Tyshun,
Tyshunn, Tyshyn*

Tyson BG (French) son of Ty.
*Tison, Tiszon, Tyce, Tycen Tyesn,
Tyeson, Tysen, Tysie, Tysin Tysne,
Tysone*

Tytus (Polish) a form of Titus.
Tyus

Tyvon (American) a combination
of Ty + Von.
*Tyvan, Tyvin, Tyvinn, Tyvone,
Tyvonne*

Tywan (Chinese) a form of
Taiwan.
*Tywain, Tywaine, Tywane,
Tywann, Tywaun, Tywen, Tywon,
Tywone, Tywonne*

Tzadok (Hebrew) righteous.
Tzadik, Zadok

Tzion (Hebrew) sign from God.
Zion

Tzuriel (Hebrew) God is my rock.
Tzuriya

Tzvi (Hebrew) deer.
Tzevi, Zevi

U

Uaine (Irish) a form of Owen.

Ubadah (Arabic) serves God.

Ubaid (Arabic) faithful.

Ubaldo (Germanic) he of daring
thoughts.

Uberto (Italian) a form of Hubert.

Uche (Ibo) thought.

Uchu (Quechua) hot like pepper.

Ucumari (Quechua) he who has
the strength of a bear.

Uday (Sanskrit) to rise.

Udell (English) yew-tree valley.
Dell, Eudel, Udale, Udall, Yudell

Udit (Sanskrit) grown; shining.

Udo (Japanese) ginseng plant.
(German) a short form of Udolf.

Udolf (English) prosperous wolf.
Udo, Udolfo, Udolph

Ugo (Italian) a form of Hugh,
Hugo.

Ugutz (Basque) a form of John.

Uilliam (Irish) a form of William.
Uileog, Uilleam, Ulick

Uinseann (Irish) a form of
Vincent.

Uistean (Irish) intelligent.
Uisdean

Uja (Sanskrit) growing.

Uku (Hawaiian) flea, insect;
skilled ukulele player.

Ulan (African) first-born twin.

Ulbrecht (German) a form of
Albert.

Ulf (German) wolf.

Ulfred (German) peaceful wolf.

Ulfrido (Teutonic) he imposes
peace through force.

Ulger (German) warring wolf.

Ulises (Latin) a form of Ulysses.
Ulishes, Ulisse, Ulisses

Ullanta (Aymara) warrior who
sees everything from his
watchtower.

Ullantay (Quechua) lord Ollanta.

Ullock (German) sporting wolf.

Ulmer (English) famous wolf.
Ullmar, Ulmar

Ulmo (German) from Ulm,
Germany.

Ulpiano, Ulpio (Latin) sly as a
fox.

Ulric (German) a form of Ulrich.
Ullric

Ulrich (German) wolf ruler; ruler
of all. See also Alaric.
*Uli, Ull, Ulric, Ulrick, Ulrik, Ulrike,
Ulu, Ulz, Uwe*

Ulrico (Germanic) noble as a
king.

Ultman (Hindi) god; godlike.

Ulyses (Latin) a form of Ulysses.
Ulysee, Ulysees

Ulysses (Latin) wrathful. A form
of Odysseus.
*Eulises, Ulick, Ulises, Ulyses,
Ulysse, Ulyssees, Ulysses,
Ulyssius*

Umang (Sanskrit) enthusiastic.
Umanga

Umar (Arabic) a form of Omar.
Umair, Umarr, Umayr, Umer

Umberto (Italian) a form of
Humbert.
Uberto

Umi (Yao) life.

Umit (Turkish) hope.

Unai (Basque) shepherd.
Una

Unay (Quechua) previous; remote, underlying.

Uner (Turkish) famous.

Unika GB (Lomwe) brighten.

Unique GB (Latin) only, unique.
Uneek, Unek, Unikque, Uniqué, Unyque

Unwin (English) nonfriend.
Unwinn, Unwyn

Upshaw (English) upper wooded area.

Upton (English) upper town.

Upwood (English) upper forest.

Urban (Latin) city dweller; courteous.
Urbain, Urbaine, Urbane, Urbano, Urbanus, Urvan, Urvane

Urbane (English) a form of Urban.

Urbano (Italian) a form of Urban.

Urcucolla (Quechua) hill; the god Colla.

Uri (Hebrew) a short form of Uriah.
Urie

Uriah (Hebrew) my light. Bible: a soldier and the husband of Bathsheba. See also Yuri.
Uri, Uria, Urias, Urijah

Urian (Greek) heaven.
Urihaan

Urías (Greek) light of the lord.

Uriel BG (Hebrew) God is my light.
Urie

Urso (Latin) bear.

Urson (French) a form of Orson.
Ursan, Ursus

Urtzi (Basque) sky.

Usamah (Arabic) like a lion.
Usama

Usco, Uscu (Quechua) wild cat.

Uscouiyca, Uscuiyca (Quechua) sacred; wild cat.

Useni (Yao) tell me.
Usene, Usenet

Usi (Yao) smoke.

Ustin (Russian) a form of Justin.

Usuy (Quechua) he who brings abundances.

Utatci (Moquelumnan) bear scratching itself.

Uthman (Arabic) companion of the Prophet.
Usman, Uthmaan

Uttam (Sanskrit) best.

Uturuncu (Quechua) jaguar; tiger; the bravest.

Uturuncu Achachi (Quechua) he who has brave ancestors, jaguar ancestors.

Uwe (German) a familiar form of Ulrich.

Uzi (Hebrew) my strength.
Uzzia

Uziel (Hebrew) God is my strength; mighty force.
Uzie, Uzziah, Uzziel

Uzoma (Nigerian) born during a journey.

Uzumati (Moquelumnan) grizzly bear.

V GB (American) an initial used as a first name.

Vachel (French) small cow.
Vache, Vachell

Vaclav (Czech) wreath of glory.
Vasek

Vadin (Hindi) speaker.
Vaden

Vail BG (English) valley.
Vaile, Vaill, Vale, Valle

Val BG (Latin) a short form of Valentin.

Valborg (Swedish) mighty mountain.

Valdemar (Swedish) famous ruler.

Valdo (Teutonic) he who governs, the monarch.

Valentin (Latin) strong; healthy.
Val, Valencio, Valenté, Valentijn, Valentine, Valentino, Valenton, Valentyn, Velentino

Valentín (Latin) a form of Valentin.

Valentino (Italian) a form of Valentin.

Valerian (Latin) strong; healthy.
Valeriano, Valerii, Valerio, Valeryn

Valerie GB (Russian) a form of Valerii.

Valerii (Russian) a form of Valerian.
Valera, Valerie, Valerij, Valerik, Valeriy, Valery

Valfredo (Germanic) peaceful king.

Valfrid (Swedish) strong peace.

Valin (Hindi) a form of Balin. Mythology: a tyrannical monkey king.

Vallis (French) from Wales.
Valis

Valter (Lithuanian, Swedish) a form of Walter.
Valters, Valther, Valtr, Vanda

Van (Dutch) a short form of Vandyke.
Vander, Vane, Vann, Vanno

Vance BG (English) thresher.

Vanda GB (Lithuanian) a form of Walter.
Vander

Vandyke (Dutch) dyke.
Van

Vanessa GB (Greek) butterfly.

Vanya (Russian) a familiar form of Ivan.
Vanechka, Vanek, Vanja, Vanka, Vanusha, Wanya

Vardon (French) green knoll.
Vardaan, Varden, Verdan, Verdon, Verdun

Varian (Latin) variable.

Varick (German) protecting ruler.
Varak, Varek, Warrick

Vartan (Armenian) rose producer; rose giver.

Varun (Hindi) rain god.
Varron

Vasant (Sanskrit) spring.
Vasanth

Vashawn (American) a combination of the prefix Va + Shawn.
Vashae, Vashan, Vashann, Vashaun, Vashawnn, Vashon, Vashun, Vishon

Vasilis (Greek) a form of Basil.
Vas, Vasaya, Vaselios, Vashon, Vasil, Vasile, Vasileior, Vasileios, Vasilios, Vasilius, Vasilos, Vasilus, Vasily, Vassilios, Vasylko, Vasyltso, Vazul

Vasily (Russian) a form of Vasilis.
Vasilek, Vasili, Vasilii, Vasilije, Vasilik, Vasiliy, Vassili, Vassilij, Vasya, Vasyenka

Vasin (Hindi) ruler, lord.

Vasu (Sanskrit) wealth.

Vasyl (German, Slavic) a form of William.
Vasos, Vassily, Vassos, Vasya, Vasyuta, VaVaska, Wassily

Vaughn BG (Welsh) small.
Vaughan, Vaughen, Vaun, Vaune, Von, Voughn

Veasna (Cambodian) lucky.

Ved (Sanskrit) sacred knowledge.

Vedie (Latin) sight.

Veer (Sanskrit) brave.

Vegard (Norwegian) sanctuary; protection.

Velvel (Yiddish) wolf.

Venancio (Latin) a fan of hunting.

Vencel (Hungarian) a short form of Wenceslaus.
Venci, Vencie

Venceslao (Slavic) crowned with glory.

Venedictos (Greek) a form of Benedict.
Venedict, Venediktos, Venka, Venya

Veniamin (Bulgarian) a form of Benjamin.
Venyamin, Verniamin

Venkat (Hindi) god; godlike. Religion: another name for the Hindu god Vishnu.

Ventura (Latin) he who will be happy.

Venturo (Spanish) food fortune.

Venya (Russian) a familiar form of Benedict.
Venedict, Venka

Vere (Latin, French) true.

Vered (Hebrew) rose.

Vergil (Latin) a form of Virgil. Literature: a Roman poet best known for his epic poem *Aenid*.
Verge

Vern (Latin) a short form of Vernon.
Verna, Vernal, Verne, Verneal, Vernel, Vernell, Vernelle, Vernial, Vernine, Vernis, Vernol

Vernados (German) courage of the bear.

Verner (German) defending army.
Varner

Verney (French) alder grove.
Vernie

Vernon (Latin) springlike; youthful.
Vern, Varnan, Vernen, Verney, Vernin

Vero (Latin) truthful, sincere, credible.

Verrill (German) masculine. (French) loyal.
Verill, Verrall, Verrell, Verroll, Veryl

Vespasiano (Latin) name of the Roman emperor from the first century.

Vian (English) full of life.

Vic (Latin) a short form of Victor.
Vick, Vicken, Vickenson

Vicente 🅱🇬 (Spanish) a form of Vincent.
Vicent, Visente

Vicenzo (Italian) a form of Vincent.

Vicky 🇬🇧 (Latin) a familiar form of Victoria.

Victoir (French) a form of Victor.

Victor (Latin) victor, conqueror.
Vic, Victa, Victer, Victoir, Victoriano, Victorien, Victorin, Victorio, Viktor, Vitin, Vittorio, Vitya, Wikoli, Wiktor, Witek

Víctor (Spanish) a form of Victor.

Victoria 🇬🇧 (Latin) a form of Victor.

Victorio (Spanish) a form of Victor.
Victorino

Victoro (Latin) victor.

Vidal (Spanish) a form of Vitas.
Vida, Vidale, Vidall, Videll

Vidar (Norwegian) tree warrior.

Videl (Spanish) life.

Vidor (Hungarian) cheerful.

Vidur (Hindi) wise.

Viho (Cheyenne) chief.

Vijay (Hindi) victorious.

Vikas (Hindi) growing.
Vikash, Vikesh

Vikram (Hindi) valorous.
Vikrum

Vikrant (Hindi) powerful.
Vikran

Viktor (German, Hungarian, Russian) a form of Victor.
Viktoras, Viktors

Vilfredo (Germanic) peaceful king.

Vilhelm (German) a form of William.
Vilhelms, Vilho, Vilis, Viljo, Villem

Vili (Hungarian) a short form of William.
Villy, Vilmos

Viliam (Czech) a form of William.
Vila, Vilek, Vilém, Viliami, Viliamu, Vilko, Vilous

Viljo (Finnish) a form of William.

Ville (Swedish) a short form of William.

Vimal (Hindi) pure.

Vin (Latin) a short form of Vincent.
Vinn

Vinay (Hindi) polite.

Vince (English) a short form of Vincent.
Vence, Vint

Vincent BG (Latin) victor, conqueror. See also Binkentios, Binky.
Uinseann, Vencent, Vicente, Vicenzo, Vikent, Vikenti, Vikesha, Vin, Vince, Vincence, Vincens, Vincente, Vincentius, Vincents, Vincenty, Vincenzo, Vinci, Vincien, Vincient, Vinciente, Vincint, Vinny, Vinsent, Vinsint, Wincent

Vincente (Spanish) a form of Vincent.
Vencente

Vincenzo (Italian) a form of Vincent.
Vincenz, Vincenza, Vincenzio, Vinchenzo, Vinzenz

Vinci (Hungarian, Italian) a familiar form of Vincent.
Vinci, Vinco, Vincze

Vinny (English) a familiar form of Calvin, Melvin, Vincent.
Vinnee, Vinney, Vinni, Vinnie

Vinod (Hindi) happy, joyful.
Vinodh, Vinood

Vinson (English) son of Vincent.
Vinnis

Vipul (Hindi) plentiful.

Viraj (Hindi) resplendent.

Virat (Hindi) very big.

Virgil (Latin) rod bearer, staff bearer.
Vergil, Virge, Virgial, Virgie, Virgilio

Virgilio (Spanish) a form of Virgil.
Virjilio

Virginio (Latin) he is pure and simple.

Virote (Tai) strong, powerful.

Vishal (Hindi) huge; great.
Vishaal

Vishnu (Hindi) protector.

Vitaliano, Vitalicio (Latin) young and strong.

Vitas (Latin) alive, vital.
Vidal, Vitus

Vito (Latin) a short form of Vittorio.
Veit, Vidal, Vital, Vitale, Vitalis, Vitas, Vitin, Vitis, Vitus, Vitya, Vytas

Vítor (Latin) victor.

Vittorio (Italian) a form of Victor.
Vito, Vitor, Vitorio, Vittore, Vittorios

Vitya (Russian) a form of Victor.
Vitenka, Vitka

Vivek (Hindi) wisdom.
Vivekinan

Vivian GB (Latin) full of life.

Viviano (Spanish) small man.

Vladimir (Russian) famous prince. See also Dima, Waldemar, Walter.
Bladimir, Vimka, Vlad, Vladamir, Vladik, Vladimar, Vladimeer, Vladimer, Vladimere, Vladimire, Vladimyr, Vladjimir, Vladka, Vladko, Vladlen, Vladmir, Volodimir, Volodya, Volya, Vova, Wladimir

Vladimiro (Spanish) a form of Vladimir.

Vladislav (Slavic) glorious ruler. See also Slava.
Vladik, Vladya, Vlas, Vlasislava, Vyacheslav, Wladislav

Vlas (Russian) a short form of Vladislav.

Volker (German) people's guard.
Folke

Volney (German) national spirit.

Von (German) a short form of many German names.

Vova (Russian) a form of Walter.
Vovka

Vuai (Swahili) savior.

Vulpiano (Latin) sly as a fox.

Vyacheslav (Russian) a form of Vladislav. See also Slava.

W

W BG (American) an initial used as a first name.

Waban (Ojibwa) white.
Wabon

Wade (English) ford; river crossing.
Wad, Wadesworth, Wadi, Wadie, Waed, Waid, Waide, Wayde, Waydell, Whaid

Wadley (English) ford meadow.
Wadleigh, Wadly

Wadsworth (English) village near the ford.
Waddsworth

Wagner (German) wagoner, wagon maker. Music: Richard Wagner was a famous nineteenth-century German composer.
Waggoner

Wahid (Arabic) single; exclusively unequaled.
Waheed

Wahkan (Lakota) sacred.

Wahkoowah (Lakota) charging.

Wain (English) a short form of Wainwright. A form of Wayne.

Wainwright (English) wagon maker.
Wain, Wainright, Wayne,
Wayneright, Waynewright,
Waynright, Wright

Waite (English) watchman.
Waitman, Waiton, Waits, Wayte

Wakefield (English) wet field.
Field, Wake

Wakely (English) wet meadow.

Wakeman (English) watchman.
Wake

Wakiza (Native American) determined warrior.

Walcott (English) cottage by the wall.
Wallcot, Wallcott, Wolcott

Waldemar (German) powerful; famous. See also Vladimir.
Valdemar, Waldermar, Waldo

Walden (English) wooded valley. Literature: Henry David Thoreau made Walden Pond famous with his book *Walden*.
Waldi, Waldo, Waldon, Welti

Waldino (Teutonic) having an open and bold spirit.

Waldo (German) a familiar form of Oswald, Waldemar, Walden.
Wald, Waldy

Waldron (English) ruler.

Waleed (Arabic) newborn.
Waled, Walid

Walerian (Polish) strong; brave.

Wales (English) from Wales.
Wael, Wail, Wali, Walie, Waly

Walford (English) Welshman's
ford.

Walfred (German) peaceful ruler.
Walfredo, Walfried

Wali (Arabic) all-governing.

Walker 🅱🅶 (English) cloth
walker; cloth cleaner.
Wallie, Wally

Wallace (English) from Wales.
*Wallach, Wallas, Wallie, Wallis,
Wally, Walsh, Welsh*

Wallach (German) a form of
Wallace.
Wallache

Waller (German) powerful.
(English) wall maker.

Wally (English) a familiar form of
Walter.
Walli, Wallie

Walmond (German) mighty ruler.

Walsh (English) a form of
Wallace.
Welch, Welsh

Walt (English) a short form of
Walter, Walton.
Waltey, Waltli, Walty

Walter (German) army ruler,
general. (English) woodsman.
See also Gautier, Gualberto,
Gualtiero, Gutierre, Ladislav,
Vladimir.
Valter, Vanda, Vova, Walder,

*Wally, Walt, Waltli, Walther,
Waltr, Wat, Waterio, Watkins,
Watson, Wualter*

Walther (German) a form of
Walter.

Walton (English) walled town.
Walt

Waltr (Czech) a form of Walter.

Walworth (English) fenced-in
farm.

Walwyn (English) Welsh friend.
*Walwin, Walwinn, Walwynn,
Walwynne, Welwyn*

Wamblee (Lakota) eagle.

Wang (Chinese) hope; wish.

Wanikiya (Lakota) savior.

Wanya 🅱🅶 (Russian) a form of
Vanya.
Wanyai

Wapi (Native American) lucky.

Warburton (English) fortified
town.

Ward (English) watchman,
guardian.
Warde, Warden, Worden

Wardell (English) watchman's
hill.

Wardley (English) watchman's
meadow.
Wardlea, Wardleigh

Ware (English) wary, cautious.

Warfield (English) field near the weir or fish trap.

Warford (English) ford near the weir or fish trap.

Warley (English) meadow near the weir or fish trap.

Warner (German) armed defender. (French) park keeper.
Werner

Warren (German) general; warden; rabbit hutch.
Ware, Waring, Warrenson, Warrin, Warriner, Worrin

Warton (English) town near the weir or fish trap.

Warwick (English) buildings near the weir or fish trap.
Warick, Warrick

Washburn (English) overflowing river.

Washington (English) town near water. History: George Washington was the first U.S. president.
Wash

Wasili (Russian) a form of Basil.
Wasyl

Wasim (Arabic) graceful; good-looking.
Waseem, Wasseem, Wassim

Watende (Nyakyusa) there will be revenge.

Waterio (Spanish) a form of Walter.
Gualtiero

Watford (English) wattle ford; dam made of twigs and sticks.

Watkins (English) son of Walter.
Watkin

Watson (English) son of Walter.
Wathson, Whatson

Waverly GB (English) quaking aspen-tree meadow.
Waverlee, Waverley

Wayland (English) a form of Waylon.
Weiland, Weyland

Waylon (English) land by the road.
Wallen, Walon, Way, Waylan, Wayland, Waylen, Waylin, Weylin

Wayman (English) road man; traveler.
Waymon

Wayne (English) wagon maker. A short form of Wainwright.
Wain, Wanye, Wayn, Waynell, Waynne, Wene, Whayne

Wazir (Arabic) minister.

Webb (English) weaver.
Web, Weeb

Weber (German) weaver.
Webber, Webner

Webley (English) weaver's meadow.
Webbley, Webbly, Webly

Webster (English) weaver.

Weddel (English) valley near the ford.

Wei-Quo (Chinese) ruler of the country.
Wei

Welborne (English) spring-fed stream.
Welborn, Welbourne, Welburn, Wellborn, Wellborne, Wellbourn, Wellburn

Welby (German) farm near the well.
Welbey, Welbie, Wellbey, Wellby

Weldon (English) hill near the well.
Weldan

Welfel (Yiddish) a form of William.
Welvel

Welford (English) ford near the well.

Wells (English) springs.
Welles

Welsh (English) a form of Wallace, Walsh.
Welch

Welton (English) town near the well.

Wemilat (Native American) all give to him.

Wemilo (Native American) all speak to him.

Wen (Gypsy) born in winter.

Wenceslaus (Slavic) wreath of honor.
Vencel, Wenceslao, Wenceslas, Wenzel, Wenzell, Wiencyslaw

Wendell (German) wanderer. (English) good dale, good valley.
Wandale, Wendall, Wendel, Wendle, Wendy

Wene (Hawaiian) a form of Wayne.

Wenford (English) white ford.
Wynford

Wentworth (English) pale man's settlement.

Wenutu (Native American) clear sky.

Werner (English) a form of Warner.
Wernhar, Wernher

Wes (English) a short form of Wesley.
Wess

Wesh (Gypsy) woods.

Wesley ⒷⒼ (English) western meadow.
Wes, Weseley, Wesle, Weslee, Wesleyan, Weslie, Wesly, Wessley, Westleigh, Westley, Wezley

West (English) west.

Westbrook (English) western brook.
Brook, West, Westbrooke

Westby (English) western farmstead.

Westcott (English) western cottage.
Wescot, Wescott, Westcot

Westley (English) a form of Wesley.
Westlee, Westly

Weston BG (English) western town.
West, Westen, Westin

Wetherby (English) wether-sheep farm.
Weatherbey, Weatherbie, Weatherby, Wetherbey, Wetherbie

Wetherell (English) wether-sheep corner.

Wetherly (English) wether-sheep meadow.

Weylin (English) a form of Waylon.
Weylan, Weylyn

Whalley (English) woods near a hill.
Whaley

Wharton (English) town on the bank of a lake.
Warton

Wheatley (English) wheat field.
Whatley, Wheatlea, Wheatleigh, Wheatly

Wheaton (English) wheat town.

Wheeler (English) wheel maker; wagon driver.

Whistler (English) whistler, piper.

Whit (English) a short form of Whitman, Whitney.
Whitt, Whyt, Whyte, Wit, Witt

Whitby (English) white house.

Whitcomb (English) white valley.
Whitcombe, Whitcumb

Whitelaw (English) small hill.
Whitlaw

Whitey (English) white skinned; white haired.

Whitfield (English) white field.

Whitford (English) white ford.

Whitley GB (English) white meadow.
Whitlea, Whitlee, Whitleigh

Whitman (English) white-haired man.
Whit

Whitmore (English) white moor.
Whitmoor, Whittemore, Witmore, Wittemore

Whitney GB (English) white island; white water.
Whit, Whittney, Widney, Widny

Whittaker (English) white field.
Whitacker, Whitaker, Whitmaker

Wicasa (Dakota) man.

Wicent (Polish) a form of
Vincent.
Wicek, Wicus

Wichado (Native American)
willing.

Wickham (English) village
enclosure.
Wick

Wickley (English) village
meadow.
Wilcley

Wid (English) wide.

Wies (German) renowned
warrior.

Wikoli (Hawaiian) a form of
Victor.

Wiktor (Polish) a form of Victor.

Wilanu (Moquelumnan) pouring
water on flour.

Wilbert (German) brilliant;
resolute.
Wilberto, Wilburt

Wilbur (English) wall
fortification; bright willows.
*Wilber, Wilburn, Wilburt, Willbur,
Wilver*

Wilder (English) wilderness, wild.
Wylder

Wildon (English) wooded hill.
Wilden, Willdon

Wile (Hawaiian) a form of Willie.

Wiley (English) willow meadow;
Will's meadow.
Whiley, Wildy, Willey, Wylie

Wilford (English) willow-tree
ford.
Wilferd

Wilfred (German) determined
peacemaker.
*Wilferd, Wilfredo, Wilfrid,
Wilfride, Wilfried, Wilfryd, Will,
Willfred, Willfried, Willie, Willy*

Wilfredo (Spanish) a form of
Wilfred.
*Fredo, Wifredo, Wilfrido,
Willfredo*

Wilhelm (German) determined
guardian.
Wilhelmus, Willem

Wiliama (Hawaiian) a form of
William.
Pila, Wile

Wilkie (English) a familiar form
of Wilkins.
Wikie, Wilke

Wilkins (English) William's kin.
*Wilkens, Wilkes, Wilkie, Wilkin,
Wilks, Willkes, Willkins*

Wilkinson (English) son of little
William.
Wilkenson, Willkinson

Will (English) a short form of
William.
Wil, Wilm, Wim

Willard (German) determined and brave.
Williard

Willem (German) a form of William.
Willim

William ★ BG (English) a form of Wilhelm. See also Gilamu, Guglielmo, Guilherme, Guillaume, Guillermo, Gwilym, Liam, Uilliam, Wilhelm.
Bill, Billy, Vasyl, Vilhelm, Vili, Viliam, Viljo, Ville, Villiam, Welfel, Wilek, Wiliam, Wiliama, Wiliame, Will, Willaim, Willam, Willeam, Willem, Williams, Willie, Willil, Willis, Willium, Williw, Willyam, Wim

Williams (German) son of William.
Wilams, Willaims, Williamson, Wuliams

Willie BG (German) a familiar form of William.
Wile, Wille, Willi, Willia, Willy

Willis (German) son of Willie.
Willice, Wills, Willus, Wyllis

Willoughby (English) willow farm.
Willoughbey, Willoughbie

Wills (English) son of Will.

Willy (German) a form of Willie.
Willey, Wily

Wilmer (German) determined and famous.
Willimar, Willmer, Wilm, Wilmar, Wylmar, Wylmer

Wilmot (Teutonic) resolute spirit.
Willmont, Willmot, Wilm, Wilmont

Wilny (Native American) eagle singing while flying.

Wilson BG (English) son of Will.
Wilkinson, Willson, Wilsen, Wolson

Wilt (English) a short form of Wilton.

Wilton (English) farm by the spring.
Will, Wilt

Wilu (Moquelumnan) chicken hawk squawking.

Win BG (Cambodian) bright. (English) a short form of Winston and names ending in "win."
Winn, Winnie, Winny

Wincent (Polish) a form of Vincent.
Wicek, Wicenty, Wicus, Wince, Wincenty

Winchell (English) bend in the road; bend in the land.

Windsor (English) riverbank with a winch. History: the surname of the British royal family.
Wincer, Winsor, Wyndsor

Winfield (English) friendly field.
Field, Winfred, Winfrey, Winifield, Winnfield, Wynfield, Wynnfield

Winfried (German) friend of peace.

Wing (Chinese) glory.
Wing-Chiu, Wing-Kit

Wingate (English) winding gate.

Wingi (Native American) willing.

Winslow (English) friend's hill.

Winston (English) friendly town; victory town.
Win, Winsten, Winstin, Winstonn, Winton, Wynstan, Wynston

Winter GB (English) born in winter.
Winterford, Wynter

Winthrop (English) victory at the crossroads.

Winton (English) a form of Winston.
Wynten, Wynton

Winward (English) friend's guardian; friend's forest.

Wit (Polish) life. (English) a form of Whit. (Flemish) a short form of DeWitt.
Witt, Wittie, Witty

Witek (Polish) a form of Victor.

Witha (Arabic) handsome.

Witter (English) wise warrior.

Witton (English) wise man's estate.

Wladislav (Polish) a form of Vladislav.
Wladislaw

Wolcott (English) cottage in the woods.

Wolf (German, English) a short form of Wolfe, Wolfgang.
Wolff, Wolfie, Wolfy

Wolfe (English) wolf.
Wolf, Woolf

Wolfgang (German) wolf quarrel. Music: Wolfgang Amadeus Mozart was a famous eighteenth-century Austrian composer.
Wolf, Wolfegang, Wolfgans

Wood (English) a short form of Elwood, Garwood, Woodrow.
Woody

Woodfield (English) forest meadow.

Woodford (English) ford through the forest.

Woodrow (English) passage in the woods. History: Thomas Woodrow Wilson was the twenty-eighth U.S. president.
Wood, Woodman, Woodroe, Woody

Woodruff (English) forest ranger.

Woodson (English) son of Wood.
Woods, Woodsen

Woodville (English) town at the edge of the woods.

Woodward (English) forest warden.
Woodard

Woody (American) a familiar form of Elwood, Garwood, Woodrow.
Wooddy, Woodie

Woolsey (English) victorious wolf.

Worcester (English) forest army camp.

Wordsworth (English) wolf-guardian's farm. Literature: William Wordsworth was a famous British poet.
Worth

Worie (Ibo) born on market day.

Worth (English) a short form of Wordsworth.
Worthey, Worthington, Worthy

Worton (English) farm town.

Wouter (German) powerful warrior.

Wrangle (American) a form of Rangle.
Wrangler

Wray (Scandinavian) corner property. (English) crooked.
Wreh

Wren (Welsh) chief, ruler. (English) wren.

Wright (English) a short form of Wainwright

Wrisley (English) a form of Risley.
Wrisee, Wrislie, Wrisly

Wriston (English) a form of Riston.
Wryston

Wuliton (Native American) will do well.

Wunand (Native American) God is good.

Wuyi (Moquelumnan) turkey vulture flying.

Wyatt ☆ BG (French) little warrior.
Wiatt, Wyat, Wyatte, Wye, Wyeth, Wyett, Wyitt, Wytt

Wybert (English) battle bright.

Wyborn (Scandinavian) war bear.

Wyck (Scandinavian) village.

Wycliff (English) white cliff; village near the cliff.
Wyckliffe, Wycliffe

Wylie (English) charming.
Wiley, Wye, Wyley, Wyllie, Wyly

Wyman (English) fighter, warrior.

Wymer (English) famous in battle.

Wyn (Welsh) light skinned; white. (English) friend. A short form of Selwyn.
Win, Wyne, Wynn, Wynne

Wyndham (Scottish) village near the winding road.
Windham, Wynndham

Wynono (Native American) first-born son.

Wythe (English) willow tree.

Xabat (Basque) savior.

Xaiver (Basque) a form of Xavier.
Xajavier, Xzaiver

Xan (Greek) a short form of Alexander.
Xane

Xander (Greek) a short form of Alexander.
Xande, Xzander

Xanthus (Latin) golden haired.
Xanthos

Xarles (Basque) a form of Charles.

Xavier ☀ BG (Arabic) bright. (Basque) owner of the new house. See also Exavier, Javier, Salvatore, Saverio.
Xabier, Xaiver, Xavaeir, Xaver, Xavian, Xaviar, Xavior, Xavon, Xavyer, Xever, Xizavier, Xxavier, Xzavier, Zavier

Xenophon (Greek) strange voice.
Xeno, Zennie

Xenos (Greek) stranger; guest.
Zenos

Xerxes (Persian) ruler. History: a king of Persia.
Zerk

Ximenes (Spanish) a form of Simon.
Ximenez, Ximon, Ximun, Xymenes

Xochiel, Xochtiel (Nahuatl) flower.

Xylon (Greek) forest.

Xzavier (Basque) a form of Xavier.
Xzavaier, Xzaver, Xzavion, Xzavior, Xzvaier

Yacu (Quechua) water.

Yadid (Hebrew) friend; beloved.
Yedid

Yadira GB (Hebrew) friend.

Yadon (Hebrew) he will judge.
Yadean, Yadin, Yadun

Yael GB (Hebrew) a form of Jael.

Yafeu (Ibo) bold.

Yagil (Hebrew) he will rejoice.

Yago (Spanish) a form of James.

Yaguatí (Guarani) leopard.

Yahto (Lakota) blue.

Yahya (Arabic) living.
Yahye

Yair (Hebrew) he will enlighten.
Yahir

Yakecen (Dene) sky song.

Yakez (Carrier) heaven.

Yakov (Russian) a form of Jacob.
*Yaacob, Yaacov, Yaakov, Yachov,
Yacoub, Yacov, Yakob, Yashko*

Yale (German) productive.
(English) old.

Yamqui (Aymara) title of nobility,
master.

Yan, Yann **BG** (Russian) forms of
John.
Yanichek, Yanick, Yanka, Yannick

Yana (Native American) bear.

Yanamayu (Quechua) black
river.

Yancy (Native American)
Englishman, Yankee.
*Yan, Yance, Yancey, Yanci,
Yansey, Yansy, Yantsey, Yauncey,
Yauncy, Yency*

Yanick, Yannick (Russian)
familiar forms of Yan.
*Yanic, Yanik, Yannic, Yannik,
Yonic, Yonnik*

Yanka (Russian) a familiar form
of John.
Yanikm

Yanni (Greek) a form of John.
*Ioannis, Yani, Yannakis, Yannis,
Yanny, Yiannis, Yoni*

Yanton (Hebrew) a form of
Johnathon, Jonathon.

Yao (Ewe) born on Thursday.

Yaphet (Hebrew) a form of
Japheth.
Yapheth, Yefat, Yephat

Yarb (Gypsy) herb.

Yardan (Arabic) king.

Yarden (Hebrew) a form of
Jordan.

Yardley (English) enclosed
meadow.
*Lee, Yard, Yardlea, Yardlee,
Yardleigh, Yardly*

Yarom (Hebrew) he will raise up.
Yarum

Yaron (Hebrew) he will sing; he
will cry out.
Jaron, Yairon

Yasashiku (Japanese) gentle;
polite.

Yash (Hindi) victorious; glory.

Yasha (Russian) a form of Jacob,
James.
Yascha, Yashka, Yashko

Yashwant (Hindi) glorious.

Yasin (Arabic) prophet.
*Yasine, Yasseen, Yassin, Yassine,
Yazen*

Yasir (Afghan) humble; takes it easy. (Arabic) wealthy.
Yasar, Yaser, Yashar, Yasser

Yasuo (Japanese) restful.

Yates (English) gates.
Yeats

Yatin (Hindi) ascetic.

Yauar (Quechua) blood.

Yauarguacac (Quechua) he sheds tears of blood.

Yauarpuma (Quechua) puma blood.

Yauri (Quechua) lance, needle; copper.

Yavin (Hebrew) he will understand.
Jabin

Yawo (Akan) born on Thursday.

Yazid (Arabic) his power will increase.
Yazeed, Yazide

Yechiel (Hebrew) God lives.

Yedidya (Hebrew) a form of Jedidiah. See also Didi.
Yadai, Yedidia, Yedidiah, Yido

Yegor (Russian) a form of George. See also Egor, Igor.
Ygor

Yehoshua (Hebrew) a form of Joshua.
Yeshua, Yeshuah, Yoshua, Y'shua, Yushua

Yehoyakem (Hebrew) a form of Joachim, Joaquín.
Yakim, Yehayakim, Yokim, Yoyakim

Yehudi (Hebrew) a form of Judah.
Yechudi, Yechudit, Yehuda, Yehudah, Yehudit

Yelutci (Moquelumnan) bear walking silently.

Yeoman (English) attendant; retainer.
Yoeman, Youman

Yeremey (Russian) a form of Jeremiah.
Yarema, Yaremka, Yeremy, Yerik

Yervant (Armenian) king, ruler. History: an Armenian king.

Yeshaya (Hebrew) gift. See also Shai.

Yeshurun (Hebrew) right way.

Yeska (Russian) a form of Joseph.
Yesya

Yestin (Welsh) just.

Yevgenyi (Russian) a form of Eugene.
Gena, Yevgeni, Yevgenij, Yevgeniy

Yigal (Hebrew) he will redeem.
Yagel, Yigael

Yirmaya (Hebrew) a form of Jeremiah.
Yirmayahu

Yishai (Hebrew) a form of Jesse.

Yisrael (Hebrew) a form of Israel.
Yesarel, Yisroel

Yitro (Hebrew) a form of Jethro.

Yitzchak (Hebrew) a form of
Isaac. See also Itzak.
Yitzak, Yitzchok, Yitzhak

Yngve (Swedish) ancestor; lord,
master.

Yo (Cambodian) honest.

Yoakim (Slavic) a form of Jacob.
Yoackim

Yoan (German) a form of Johan,
Johann.
Yoann

Yoav (Hebrew) a form of Joab.

Yochanan (Hebrew) a form of
John.
Yohanan

Yoel (Hebrew) a form of Joel.

Yogesh (Hindi) ascetic. Religion:
another name for the Hindu god
Shiva.

Yohan, Yohann (German) forms
of Johan, Johann.
*Yohane, Yohanes, Yohanne,
Yohannes, Yohans, Yohn*

Yohance (Hausa) a form of John.

Yonah (Hebrew) a form of Jonah.
Yona, Yonas

Yonatan (Hebrew) a form of
Jonathan.
*Yonathan, Yonathon, Yonaton,
Yonattan*

Yong (Chinese) courageous.
Yonge

Yong-Sun (Korean) dragon in the
first position; courageous.

Yoni (Greek) a form of Yanni.
Yonis, Yonnas, Yonny, Yony

Yoofi (Akan) born on Friday.

Yooku (Fante) born on
Wednesday.

Yoram (Hebrew) God is high.
Joram

Yorgos (Greek) a form of George.
Yiorgos, Yorgo

York (English) boar estate; yew-
tree estate.
*Yorick, Yorke, Yorker, Yorkie,
Yorrick*

Yorkoo (Fante) born on Thursday.

Yosef (Hebrew) a form of Joseph
See also Osip.
*Yoceph, Yoosuf, Yoseff, Yoseph,
Yosief, Yosif, Yosuf, Yosyf,
Yousef, Yusif*

Yoselin **GB** (Latin) a form of
Jocelyn.

Yóshi (Japanese) adopted son.
Yoshiki, Yoshiuki

Yoshiyahu (Hebrew) a form of
Josiah.
*Yoshia, Yoshiah, Yoshiya,
Yoshiyah, Yosiah*

Yoskolo (Moquelumnan)
breaking off pine cones.

Yosu (Hebrew) a form of Jesus.

Yotimo (Moquelumnan) yellow jacket carrying food to its hive.

Yottoko (Native American) mud at the water's edge.

Young (English) young.
Yung

Young-Jae (Korean) pile of prosperity.

Young-Soo (Korean) keeping the prosperity.

Youri (Russian) a form of Yuri.

Yousef (Yiddish) a form of Joseph.
Yousaf, Youseef, Yousef, Youseph, Yousif, Youssef, Yousseff, Yousuf

Youssel (Yiddish) a familiar form of Joseph.
Yussel

Yov (Russian) a short form of Yoakim.

Yovani (Slavic) a form of Jovan.
Yovan, Yovanni, Yovanny, Yovany, Yovni

Yoyi (Hebrew) a form of George.

Yrjo (Finnish) a form of George.

Ysidro (Greek) a short form of Isidore.

Yu (Chinese) universe.
Yue

Yudell (English) a form of Udell.
Yudale, Yudel

Yuki BG (Japanese) snow.
Yukiko, Yukio, Yuuki

Yul (Mongolian) beyond the horizon.

Yule (English) born at Christmas.

Yuli (Basque) youthful.

Yuma (Native American) son of a chief.

Yunus (Turkish) a form of Jonah.

Yupanqui (Quechua) he who honors his ancestors.

Yurac (Quechua) white.

Yurcel (Turkish) sublime.

Yuri GB (Russian, Ukrainian) a form of George. (Hebrew) a familiar form of Uriah.
Yehor, Youri, Yura, Yure, Yuric, Yurii, Yurij, Yurik, Yurko, Yurri, Yury, Yusha

Yusif (Russian) a form of Joseph.
Yuseph, Yusof, Yussof, Yusup, Yuzef, Yuzep

Yustyn (Russian) a form of Justin.
Yusts

Yusuf (Arabic, Swahili) a form of Joseph.
Yusef, Yusuff

Yutu (Moquelumnan) coyote out hunting.

Yuval (Hebrew) rejoicing.

Yves (French) a form of Ivar, Ives.
Yvens, Yvon, Yyves

Yvon (French) a form of Ivar, Yves.
Ivon, Yuvon, Yvan, Yvonne

Yvonne GB (French) a form of Yvon.

Z

Z BG (American) an initial used as a first name.

Zac (Hebrew) a short form of Zachariah, Zachary.
Zacc

Zacarias (Portuguese, Spanish) a form of Zachariah.
Zacaria, Zacariah

Zacary (Hebrew) a form of Zachary.
Zac, Zacaras, Zacari, Zacariah, Zacarias, Zacarie, Zacarious, Zacery, Zacory, Zacrye

Zaccary (Hebrew) a form of Zachary.
Zac, Zaccaeus, Zaccari, Zaccaria, Zaccariah, Zaccary, Zaccea, Zaccharie, Zacchary, Zacchery, Zaccury

Zaccheus (Hebrew) innocent, pure.
Zacceus, Zacchaeus, Zacchious

Zach (Hebrew) a short form of Zachariah, Zachary.

Zachari (Hebrew) a form of Zachary.
Zacheri

Zacharia (Hebrew) a form of Zachary.
Zacharya

Zachariah BG (Hebrew) God remembered.
Zac, Zacarias, Zacarius, Zacary, Zaccary, Zach, Zacharias, Zachary, Zacharyah, Zachory, Zachury, Zack, Zakaria, Zako, Zaquero, Zecharia, Zechariah, Zecharya, Zeggery, Zeke, Zhachory

Zacharias (German) a form of Zachariah.
Zacarías, Zacharais, Zachariaus, Zacharius, Zackarias, Zakarias, Zecharias, Zekarias

Zacharie BG (Hebrew) a form of Zachary.
Zachare, Zacharee, Zachurie, Zecharie

Zachary ✨ BG (Hebrew) a familiar form of Zachariah. History: Zachary Taylor was the twelfth U.S. president. See also Sachar, Sakeri.
Xachary, Zac, Zacary, Zaccary, Zach, Zacha, Zachaery, Zachaios, Zacharay, Zacharey, Zachari, Zacharia, Zacharias, Zacharie, Zacharry, Zachaury, Zachery, Zachory, Zachrey, Zachry, Zachuery, Zachury, Zack, Zackary, Zackery, Zackory, Zakaria, Zakary, Zakery, Zakkary, Zechary, Zechery, Zeke

Zachery (Hebrew) a form of Zachary.
Zacheray, Zacherey, Zacheria, Zacherias, Zacheriah, Zacherie, Zacherius, Zackery

Zachory (Hebrew) a form of Zachary.

Zachry (Hebrew) a form of Zachary.
Zachre, Zachrey, Zachri

Zack (Hebrew) a short form of Zachariah, Zachary.
Zach, Zak, Zaks

Zackary (Hebrew) a form of Zachary.
Zack, Zackari, Zacharia, Zackare, Zackaree, Zackariah, Zackarie, Zackery, Zackhary, Zackie, Zackree, Zackrey, Zackry

Zackery (Hebrew) a form of Zachery.
Zackere, Zackeree, Zackerey, Zackeri, Zackeria, Zackeriah, Zackerie, Zackerry

Zackory (Hebrew) a form of Zachary.
Zackoriah, Zackorie, Zacorey, Zacori, Zacory, Zacry, Zakory

Zadok (Hebrew) a short form of Tzadok.
Zaddik, Zadik, Zadoc, Zaydok

Zadornin (Basque) Saturn.

Zafir (Arabic) victorious.
Zafar, Zafeer, Zafer, Zaffar

Zahid (Arabic) self-denying, ascetic.
Zaheed

Zahir (Arabic) shining, bright.
Zahair, Zahar, Zaheer, Zahi, Zair, Zaire, Zayyir

Zahur (Swahili) flower.

Zaid (Arabic) increase, growth.
Zaied, Zaiid, Zayd

Zaide (Hebrew) older.

Zaim (Arabic) brigadier general.

Zain (English) a form of Zane.
Zaine

Zakaria (Hebrew) a form of Zachariah.
Zakaraiya, Zakareeya, Zakareeyah, Zakariah, Zakariya, Zakeria, Zakeriah

Zakariyya (Arabic) prophet. Religion: an Islamic prophet.

Zakary (Hebrew) a form of Zachery.
Zak, Zakarai, Zakare, Zakaree, Zakari, Zakarias, Zakarie, Zakarius, Zakariye, Zake, Zakhar, Zaki, Zakir, Zakkai, Zako, Zakqary, Zakree, Zakri, Zakris, Zakry

Zakery (Hebrew) a form of Zachery.
Zakeri, Zakerie, Zakiry

Zaki (Arabic) bright; pure. (Hausa) lion.
Zakee, Zakia, Zakie, Zakiy, Zakki

Zakia BG (Swahili) intelligent.

Zakkary (Hebrew) a form of Zachary.
Zakk, Zakkari, Zakkery, Zakkyre

Zako (Hungarian) a form of Zachariah.

Zale (Greek) sea strength.
Zayle

Zalmai (Afghan) young.

Zalman (Yiddish) a form of Solomon.
Zaloman

Zamiel (German) a form of Samuel.
Zamal, Zamuel

Zamir (Hebrew) song; bird.
Zameer

Zan (Italian) clown.
Zann, Zanni, Zannie, Zanny, Zhan

Zana **GB** (Spanish) a form of Zanna (see Girls' Names).

Zander (Greek) a short form of Alexander.
Zandore, Zandra, Zandrae, Zandy

Zane **BG** (English) a form of John.
Zain, Zayne, Zhane

Zanis (Latvian) a form of Janis.
Zannis

Zanvil (Hebrew) a form of Samuel.
Zanwill

Zaquan (American) a combination of the prefix Za + Quan.
Zaquain, Zaquon, Zaqwan

Zaqueo (Hebrew) pure, innocent.

Zareb (African) protector.

Zared (Hebrew) ambush.
Zaryd

Zarek (Polish) may God protect the king.
Zarik, Zarrick, Zerek, Zerick, Zerric, Zerrick

Zavier (Arabic) a form of Xavier.
Zavair, Zaverie, Zavery, Zavierre, Zavior, Zavyr, Zayvius, Zxavian

Zayit **BG** (Hebrew) olive.

Zayne (English) a form of Zane.
Zayan, Zayin, Zayn

Zdenek (Czech) follower of Saint Denis.

Zeb (Hebrew) a short form of Zebediah, Zebulon.
Zev

Zebedee (Hebrew) a familiar form of Zebediah.
Zebadee

Zebediah (Hebrew) God's gift.
Zeb, Zebadia, Zebadiah, Zebedee, Zebedia, Zebidiah, Zedidiah

Zebulon (Hebrew) exalted, honored; lofty house.
Zabulan, Zeb, Zebulan, Zebulen, Zebulin, Zebulun, Zebulyn, Zev, Zevulon, Zevulun, Zhebulen, Zubin

Zechariah **BG** (Hebrew) a form of Zachariah.
Zecharia, Zecharian, Zecheriah, Zechuriah, Zekariah, Zekarias, Zeke, Zekeria, Zekeriah, Zekerya

Zed (Hebrew) a short form of Zedekiah.

Zedekiah (Hebrew) God is mighty and just.
Zed, Zedechiah, Zedekias, Zedikiah

Zedidiah (Hebrew) a form of Zebediah.

Zeeman (Dutch) seaman.

Zeév (Hebrew) wolf.
Zeévi, Zeff, Zif

Zeheb (Turkish) gold.

Zeke (Hebrew) a short form of Ezekiel, Zachariah, Zachary, Zechariah.

Zeki (Turkish) clever, intelligent.
Zeky

Zelgai (Afghan) heart.

Zelig (Yiddish) a form of Selig.
Zeligman, Zelik

Zelimir (Slavic) wishes for peace.

Zemar (Afghan) lion.

Zen (Japanese) religious. Religion: a form of Buddhism.

Zenda GB (Czech) a form of Eugene.
Zhek

Zeno (Greek) cart; harness. History: a Greek philosopher.
Zenan, Zenas, Zenon, Zino, Zinon

Zenón (Greek) he who lives.

Zenzo (Italian) a form of Lorenzo.

Zephaniah (Hebrew) treasured by God.
Zaph, Zaphania, Zeph, Zephan

Zephyr BG (Greek) west wind.
Zeferino, Zeffrey, Zephery, Zephire, Zephram, Zephran, Zephrin

Zero (Arabic) empty, void.

Zeroun (Armenian) wise and respected.

Zeshawn (American) a combination of the prefix Ze + Shawn.
Zeshan, Zeshaun, Zeshon, Zishaan, Zishan, Zshawn

Zesiro (Luganda) older of twins.

Zeus (Greek) living. Mythology: chief god of the Greek pantheon.

Zeusef (Portuguese) a form of Joseph.

Zev (Hebrew) a short form of Zebulon.

Zevi (Hebrew) a form of Tzvi.
Zhvie, Zhvy, Zvi

Zhane GB (English) a form of Zane.

Zhek (Russian) a short form of Evgeny.
Zhenechka, Zhenka, Zhenya

Zhìxin (Chinese) ambitious.
Zhi, Zhìhuán, Zhipeng, Zhi-yang, Zhìyuan

Zhora (Russian) a form of
George.
Zhorik, Zhorka, Zhorz, Zhurka

Zhuàng (Chinese) strong.

Zia 𝗚𝗕 (Hebrew) trembling;
moving. (Arabic) light.
Ziah

Zigfrid (Latvian, Russian) a form
of Siegfried.
*Zegfrido, Zigfrids, Ziggy, Zygfryd,
Zygi*

Ziggy (American) a familiar form
of Siegfried, Sigmund.
Ziggie

Zigor (Basque) punishment.

Zikomo (Nguni) thank-you.

Zilaba (Luganda) born while sick.
Zilabamuzale

Zimra (Hebrew) song of praise.
*Zemora, Zimrat, Zimri, Zimria,
Zimriah, Zimriya*

Zimraan (Arabic) praise.

Zinan (Japanese) second son.

Zindel (Yiddish) a form of
Alexander.
Zindil, Zunde

Zion (Hebrew) sign, omen;
excellent. Bible: the name used to
refer to Israel and to the Jewish
people.
Tzion, Zyon

Ziskind (Yiddish) sweet child.

Ziv (Hebrew) shining brightly.
(Slavic) a short form of Ziven.

Ziven (Slavic) vigorous, lively.
Zev, Ziv, Zivka, Zivon

Ziyad (Arabic) increase.
Zayd, Ziyaad

Zlatan (Czech) gold.
Zlatek, Zlatko

Zoe 𝗚𝗕 (Greek) life.

Zoé (Hindu) life.

Zoey 𝗚𝗕 (Greek) a form of Zoe.

Zohar 𝗕𝗚 (Hebrew) bright light.
Zohair

Zollie, Zolly (Hebrew) forms of
Solly.
Zoilo

Zoltán (Hungarian) life.

Zorba (Greek) live each day.

Zorion (Basque) a form of Orion.
*Zoran, Zoren, Zorian, Zoron,
Zorrine, Zorrion*

Zorya (Slavic) star; dawn.

Zósimo (Greek) he who fights.

Zotikos (Greek) saintly, holy.
Religion: a saint in the Eastern
Orthodox Church.

Zotom (Kiowa) a biter.

Zsigmond (Hungarian) a form of
Sigmund.
Ziggy, Zigmund, Zsiga

Zuberi (Swahili) strong.

Zubin (Hebrew) a short form of
  Zebulon.
  Zubeen

Zuhayr (Arabic) brilliant, shining.
  Zyhair, Zuheer

Zuka (Shona) sixpence.

Zuriel (Hebrew) God is my rock.

Zygmunt (Polish) a form of
  Sigmund.

Also from Meadowbrook Press

✦ *The Official Lamaze Guide*
The first official guide to pregnancy and childbirth presenting the Lamaze method of natural childbirth, this book gives expectant mothers confidence in their ability to give birth free of unnecessary medical intervention, and provides detailed information for couples to deal with whatever issues arise.

✦ *Pregnancy, Childbirth, and the Newborn*
More complete and up-to-date than any other pregnancy guide, this remarkable book is the "bible" for childbirth educators. Now revised with a greatly expanded treatment of pregnancy tests, complications, and infections; an expanded list of drugs and medications (plus advice for uses); and a brand-new chapter on creating a detailed birth plan.

✦ *The Simple Guide to Having a Baby*
All the basic knowledge first-time parents need for a successful pregnancy and childbirth. This is a simple, just-the-facts guide for expectant parents who want only the most important, down-to-earth how-to information covering health during pregnancy, labor and delivery, and care for a new baby.

✦ *First-Year Baby Care*
This is one of the leading baby-care books to guide you through your baby's first year. Newly revised, it contains the latest, greatest information on the basics of baby care, including bathing, diapering, medical facts, and feeding your baby.

**We offer many more titles written to delight, inform, and entertain.
To order books with a credit card or browse our full
selection of titles, visit our website at:**

www.meadowbrookpress.com

or call toll-free to place an order, request a free catalog, or ask a question:

1-800-338-2232

Meadowbrook Press • 5451 Smetana Drive • Minnetonka, MN • 55343